Arrhythmia Recognition

The Art of Interpretation

Lead I

Lead II   Lead III

Tomas B. Garcia, MD, FACEP

Geoffrey T. Miller, NREMT-P

JONES AND BARTLETT PUBLISHERS

Sudbury, Massachusetts

BOSTON   TORONTO   LONDON   SINGAPORE

Jones and Bartlett Publishers

World Headquarters
Jones and Bartlett Publishers
40 Tall Pine Drive
Sudbury, MA 01776
978-443-5000
info@jbpub.com
www.jbpub.com

Jones and Bartlett Publishers Canada

6339 Ormindale Way
Mississauga, ON L5V 1J2
CANADA

Jones and Bartlett Publishers International

Barb House, Barb Mews
London W6 7PA
UK

Cover and Illustration Credits: pg. i. Proportions of the human figure, c. 1492 (Vitruvian Man) (pen & ink on paper) by Leonardo da Vinci (1452-1519) Galleria dell' Accademia, Venice, Italy/Bridgeman Art Library.

Production Credits
Chief Executive Officer: Clayton Jones
Chief Operating Officer: Don W. Jones, Jr.
Executive V.P. & Publisher: Robert W. Holland, Jr.
V.P., Design and Production: Anne Spencer
V.P., Sales and Marketing: William Kane
V.P., Manufacturing and Inventory Control: Therese Bräuer
Publisher: Kimberly Brophy
Associate Managing Editor: Carol E. Brewer
Associate Editor: Elizabeth Petersen
Production Editor: Scarlett L. Stoppa
Production Assistant: Carolyn Rogers
Director of Marketing: Alisha Weisman
Director, Interactive Technology: Adam Alboyadjian
Interactive Technology Manager: Dawn Mahon Priest
Design and Composition: Nesbitt Graphics, Inc.
Cover Design: Kristin Ohlin
Printing and Binding: Imago
Cover Printer: Imago

ISBN-13: 978-0-7637-2246-3
ISBN-10: 0-7637-2246-4

Library of Congress Cataloging-in-Publication Data
Garcia, Tomas B., 1952-
    Arrhythmia recognition : the art of interpretation / Tomas
B. Garcia,
Geoffrey T. Miller.-- 1st ed.
        p. ; cm.
Includes bibliographical references and index.
    ISBN 0-7637-2246-4 (pbk. : alk. paper)
  1. Arrhythmia--Diagnosis. 2. Electrocardiography--Interpretation.
    [DNLM: 1. Arrhythmia--diagnosis. 2. Electrocardiography.
WG 330
G216t 2004] I. Miller, Geoffrey T. II. Title.
    RC685.A65G335 2004
    616.1'28075--dc22
6048   2003016920

Printed in Malaysia
12 11 10 09 08   10 9 8 7 6 5 4

Brief Table of Contents

Table of Contents

Features

This text contains an astounding assortment of full color illustrations, rhythm strips, and self-tests to facilitate comprehension of critical concepts and help students synthesize the information learned.

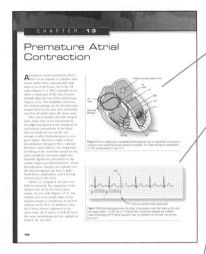

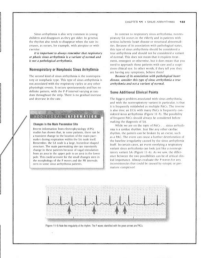

Full-color illustrations aid comprehension of difficult concepts.

Rhythm strips appear within chapters to illustrate and explain important points.

Additional Information boxes provide a more in-depth discussion of chapter topics.

Clinical Pearls highlight points that are important in treatment.

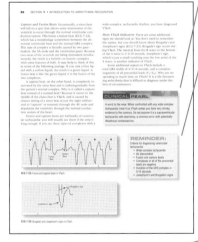

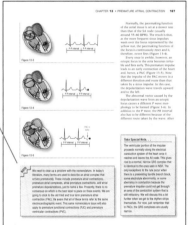

Reminder boxes highlight points that the student should keep in mind while reading.

Note boxes highlight specific points of controversy or difficulty.

Arrhythmia Recognition boxes summarize distinguishing factors of the rhythms discussed in the chapter.

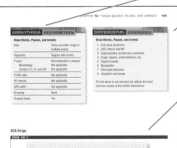

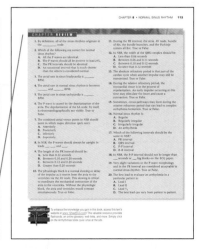

Differential Diagnosis boxes give a list of potential causes for the rhythms discussed in the chapter.

End-of-chapter rhythm strips allow students to synthesize the information learned in the chapter. Every strip is accompanied by an explanation.

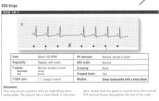

End-of-chapter multiple-choice quizzes allow students to review the knowledge they have just learned.

Features

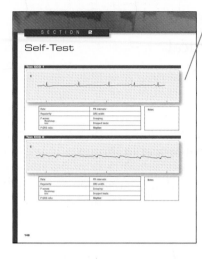

End-of-section tests allow students to synthesize the information learned in the section.

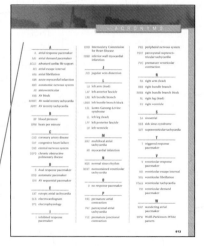

Every end-of-section test is explained.

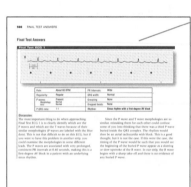

The text concludes with a final self-test of 75 rhythm strips, complete with interpretations.

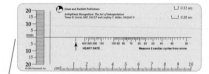

A heart rate calculator ruler is included on the inside front cover—use this to measure and read ECG strips.

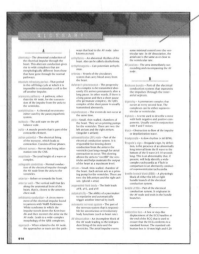

A comprehensive glossary provides definitions of terminology used in the text.

An acronym list provides easy quick-reference of the acronyms used in the field of electrocardiography and in this text.

Student Resources

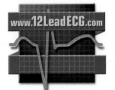

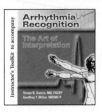

www.12LeadECG.com/Arrhythmias contains the following student resources to enhance learning and help arrhythmia recognition skills:

- Practice rhythm strips
- Rhythm quizzes
- Terminology flashcards
- Online glossary
- Web links

Also in the Series...

Once you've finished reading *Arrhythmia Recognition*, you'll want to read the following texts in the series to familiarize yourself with the subject of 12-lead electro-cardiography. These texts present 12-lead ECG interpretation in the same clear, graphics-intensive, ECG-intensive style seen in this text.

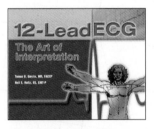

12-Lead ECG: The Art of Interpretation
ISBN: 0-7637-1284-1
This all-encompassing text is designed to make you a fully advanced interpreter of ECGs.

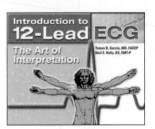

Introduction to 12-Lead ECG: The Art of Interpretation
ISBN: 0-7637-1961-7
This introductory-level text is designed to give beginners a basic knowledge of ECG interpretation.

Instructor Resources

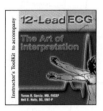

Instructor's ToolKit to accompany Arrhythmia Recognition: The Art of Interpretation
ISBN: 0-7637-3135-8
This CD contains PowerPoint presentations, lecture outlines, and an image bank including all of the images that appear in this text.

Instructor's ToolKit to accompany 12-Lead ECG: The Art of Interpretation
ISBN: 0-7637-1962-5
This CD contains the 232 real-life, full-size ECGs that appear in *12-Lead ECG: The Art of Interpretation*, to enhance your classroom presentations.

Ordering Information

For a complete listing of our EMS products, or to place your order online, please visit www.EMSzone.com. To order Jones and Bartlett products by phone, fax, or e-mail, please contact us at:

Jones and Bartlett Publishers
40 Tall Pine Drive
Sudbury, MA 01776
Phone: (978) 443-5000
Fax: (978) 443-8000
info@jbpub.com

Dedications and Biographies

To all of the courageous men and women of the armed forces, EMS, fire, and law enforcement departments around our country. You put your lives on the line every day to protect us and our freedom. I thank you. God bless you and keep you all safe from harm.

Tomas B. Garcia, MD, FACEP

Dr. Tomas B. Garcia received his undergraduate degree from Florida International University. While applying to medical school, Dr. Garcia was licensed and practiced as an EMT in the state of Florida. Dr. Garcia received his medical degree from the University of Miami. He completed his internship and residency at Jackson Memorial Hospital in Miami, Florida and subsequently received board certification in both Internal Medicine and Emergency Medicine.

Dr. Garcia taught and practiced in the Emergency Department of the Brigham and Women's Hospital/Harvard Medical School in Boston, Massachusetts and Grady Memorial Hospital/Emory Medical School in Atlanta, Georgia.

His main area of interest is emergency cardiac care, and he lectures nationally on topics related to these issues. He is creating an Internet site devoted to medical education and emergency cardiac care issues at www.heartstuff.com.

To all of the students, clinicians, researchers, and instructors who selflessly devote themselves to learning, understanding, sharing, and providing care to those in need. I thank you for your dedication and effort.

Geoffrey Tobias Miller, NREMT-P

Geoffrey T. Miller, a nationally registered paramedic, is the assistant director of emergency medical skills training at the University of Miami School of Medicine Center for Research in Medical Education, where he develops innovative EMS curricula and assessment systems that are used by prehospital providers and medical schools throughout the United States.

Previously, he worked as a Paramedic Firefighter with Alachua County Fire Rescue before moving into EMS education where he served as associate professor of emergency medical services programs at Santa Fe Community College in Gainesville, Florida. Miller is actively involved in academic research and publication in EMS education. He has coauthored several books and articles. He is a frequent speaker at state and national conferences.

A member of numerous professional organizations and committees, Miller is currently serving as president of the Florida Association of Emergency Medical Services Educators. In 2000, Miller was recognized as the Paramedic Instructor of the Year by the Florida Association of Emergency Medical Services Educators. In 2003, he was recognized as the EMS Educator of the Year by the State of Florida Department of Health Bureau of Emergency Medical Services.

You can contact Mr. Miller via e-mail at gmiller@med.miami.edu.

Acknowledgments

The decision to write a comprehensive text is easy in most cases. You see a need, you have a concept, and the decision to write the book is made. It is in implementing the idea that the enormity of the decision becomes apparent. Thankfully, many people along the way help in achieving our goals.

First and foremost is God. Throughout my life you have opened and closed doors for me in very strange ways. However, the path that you have helped me see has always led me to exactly where I needed to be at that moment. I trust you, and in you, with all my heart and soul.

I would like to give a special hug to my Martica, who took care of me, rubbed my neck, soothed my mind, beat me at Chinese checkers (occasionally. . .), and overall helped me keep my sanity.

I would like to thank Don Corn for his insight and expertise in graphics management and the printing process. You started me on the L-O-N-G process of learning to manipulate art with a computer, and I will always be in your debt for your encouragement and your support. I would also like to thank his wife, Janice, who was always just a phone call away and was always ready to spend the time to hear my rantings.

I would like to thank Jones and Bartlett Publishers for their support of my projects. I would especially like to thank Carol Brewer, my editor and friend, for her tireless work on all of my projects. You have been supportive and kind to a fault. J&B does not know how lucky they are to have you! I would also like to give special thanks to Scarlett Stoppa, whose expertise and hard work in polishing the appearance of this book have transformed it into a beautiful work of "art." I also thank Kimberly Brophy and Larry Newell for their unwavering support and commitment. Finally, I would like to thank all of the copy editors and production folk who spent countless hours putting this "art" piece together.

Finally, I would like to remind my son Daniel that he always has been, and always will be, the most important part my life. To my mom, my sister, and the rest of the "Garcia" crew: I love you all deeply. You are the glue that keeps me together in this life.

Tomas B. Garcia, MD, FACEP

Lao-Tze is quoted as saying:
"If you tell me, I will listen.
If you show me, I will see.
But if you let me experience,
I will learn."

There have been many who have provided me these experiences. They have shaped and driven me over the years. I am thankful for every one of them:

My mother, father, brother, and family for your understanding and support throughout my life.

Jena, for being there during my less-than-best moments and most importantly for sharing the truly great ones.

Andy Carlisle, for opening my eyes to the excitement of EMS. Dr. Pete Gianas and Cliff Chapman for keeping them open.

Steve Everett, friend and mentor, for showing me how much more there is to teaching, for sharing your wisdom with me, and for generally listening to me ramble on over the years.

Dr. Michael S. Gordon, all my friends and colleagues at the CRME (Center for Research in Medical Education), and the M.I.A.M.I. (Miami International Alliance for Medical-Education Innovation) Group, your knowledge and talent for teaching has been a tremendous inspiration.

My work family at the EMST (CRME, Emergency Medical Skills Training Division), Al, David Lee, Eva, Jill, Joe, Maria, and Obie. Thanks for putting up with me and my occasional wild ideas.

My students, for asking all the questions (I'm still not sure how you fit some of them into our discussions) that allow me to learn with you.

Jones and Bartlett Publishers, for their commitment to this project and the hard work from all involved.

Geoffrey Tobias Miller, NREMT-P

Jones & Bartlett Publishers and the authors would like to thank the following people for reviewing this text.

Toni J. Galvan, RN, MSN, CCRN, CEN
Texas Tech University Health Sciences Center
School of Nursing
Lubbock, Texas

Guy H. Haskell, PhD, NREMT-P
Emergency Medical and Safety Services Consultants
Bloomington, Indiana

Leo C. Kelly, PA
Providence Hospital
Washington, DC
Loudoun County Fire-Rescue
Loudoun County, Virginia

Jennifer McCarthy, BS, MICP
Union County College
Plainfield, New Jersey

Eric C. Nager, MD, FAAEM
Franklin Square Hospital
Baltimore County Fire Department
Baltimore, Maryland

Stephen J. Rahm, NREMT-P
Kendall County EMS Training Institute
Boerne, Texas

Joyce B. Vazzano, RN, MSN
Johns Hopkins University
School of Nursing
Baltimore, Maryland

Foreword

Arrhythmia Recognition: The Art of Interpretation

One of the most important skills for any clinician to master is the ability to recognize and evaluate a rhythm strip. This information is as basic as knowing how to use a stethoscope. However, as our reliance on newer and more advanced technology has increased, our basic clinical and diagnostic skills have begun to deteriorate.

Arrhythmia recognition is, by its very nature, cloaked in objective criteria. We need these criteria to differentiate between the various rhythm abnormalities and to allow us some objectivity when assigning the various treatment strategies. However, if objective criteria were the only variables involved in evaluating a rhythm, computers would have taken over the job of interpreting ECGs and rhythm strips long ago. But, as we all know, computer assisted interpretation has pretty much been a failure to date. Why? Because arrhythmia recognition is primarily an *art*. Computers don't do well with art.

An appreciation of art requires deep, thoughtful study and mastery of a subject and that requires time. However, in our busy, hectic lives, most of us cannot dedicate that much time and effort to just this one aspect of clinical practice. We barely have enough time to keep up with all of the new information, let alone going over the basic information. In addition, our clinical instructors and educators have to spend more and more time on paperwork and securing reimbursement, and they, therefore, have less and less time to devote to teaching.

So, we rely on specialists to give us a final interpretation for our patient's strips and ECGs. However, here is an interesting fact: More cardiologists fail the boards because of an inability to interpret ECGs than for any other reason. Training difficulties apply to them as well.

Furthermore, the American Heart Association 2000 guidelines requires *all* clinicians taking care of patients to be able to differentiate between supraventricular and ventricular tachycardias. This can be a tough assignment when the supraventricular tachycardia presents with wide QRS complexes. In addition, we need to be able to differentiate between the various tachyarrhythmias and administer the appropriate drug to each one. You see, our ability to treat arrhythmias has expanded to allow treatment for the individual pathways and mechanisms involved. In other words, you better know what the arrhythmia is and the pathways and mechanisms that cause it.

Our old ideas about arrhythmias as well have changed with the onset of electrophysiology as a medical subspecialty. Newer techniques bring newer insights and treatment. We need to come face-to-face with this new mindset and come up with new and creative approaches to medical education and training. Hopefully, this book is just one of those small steps.

We can no longer rely on books that present just a few isolated facts and give you a bunch of strips. We need to understand the why's and how's and be able to distinguish between the various possibilities. We cannot afford to fall back on traditional systems of learning arrhythmia recognition for the patient's sake and because of our ever-increasing problem—medical malpractice.

In order to understand and interpret rhythm strips and ECGs thoroughly, we need to approach the material with three main objectives in mind: 1) We need to understand the objective criteria for each arrhythmia; 2) We need to fully understand the mechanisms involved and the subtleties that can develop within that one rhythm category and in any one patient; 3) We need to be able to put our electrocardiographic findings together with the history, physical exam, and laboratory data to arrive at the correct diagnosis for our patient. ECGs and rhythm strips do not live in a vacuum. In this book, we will meet these objectives head on.

We will provide you with the objective criteria that are particular to that one rhythm and then we will discuss the mechanisms and subtleties of each rhythm abnormality. In addition, we will give you various examples of each of the arrhythmias so that you can see these subtleties in action. We will try to provide you with examples that cover the full spectrum of how the arrhythmia presents, including strips in which the QRS complexes are tall, short, wide, narrow, positive, negative, and isoelectric.

At the end of each chapter, we will provide you with a synopsis of the rhythm, which basically organizes everything in a nutshell for you. This will be very helpful when you just want a quick review or when you just need to look up some quick facts about the rhythm.

Being able to interpret the arrhythmia without knowing the potential clinical causes is not a very healthy way to approach arrhythmia recognition. As such, we are providing a differential diagnosis block at the end of each of the chapters to point you in the right clinical direction. Please note that these differential diagnosis boxes are not all-inclusive but contain the major culprits in which the rhythm abnormality is found.

The chapters conclude with a review containing fill-in-the-blank, multiple-choice, and true and false questions. The purpose of these questions is not to provide you with unanswerable challenges but to re-emphasize the important take-home messages of the chapter.

Each section ends with a review test in which we provide you with some unknowns. You should spend the time to solve each of the rhythm strips and to understand them. Once you have completed your evaluation, you can turn to the answers for confirmation and further discussion. This is a feature that we feel will strengthen your understanding by providing you with some "individualized" instruction about each of the strips.

The book ends with two of my favorite features—a chapter on putting it all together and the final test. I like to think of these two features as working together to put the finishing touches on your study of the topic. The chapter on putting it all together is geared towards strengthening the art of interpretation to the maximum. In this chapter, we try to reinforce the need to evaluate all of the information at your disposal to interpret the rhythm. These sources of information include the history, physical exam, and laboratory data, as well as the ECG and the rhythm strip.

Many of you will be very upset that we did not include treatment strategies in this book. The reason that we did not present this information is that it typically takes about 2 to 3 years to bring a book from conception to print. Most of the information that you find in medical textbooks, including the references, is obsolete by the time the book hits the shelves. If not, it will be obsolete very shortly afterwards. The only thing more dangerous than a lack of information is wrong information. We encourage you to go on the Internet and review the latest treatment strategies for the vari-

ous rhythms as you finish each chapter. This way, you will have the most current and up-to-date information available.

A Little More About the Art

When I teach medical students physical diagnosis, they spend the first couple of weeks merely observing patients from afar. They are not to talk to or examine the patient. Their only duty is to answer one simple question: Is the patient sick or not sick? They only have about 10 to 15 seconds to make up their minds, so that they cannot rationalize too much. Their decision has to be made from the gut, based on information that they gain through observation either consciously or unconsciously. It sounds complicated and yet students amaze me with how quickly they learn this task and how effectively they put these lessons to use. This internal decision maker is an innate part of us all and will never steer you wrong. All you have to do is develop it.

So what does this have to do with rhythm strips? Simple—we are going to use the same approach to learn arrhythmia recognition. *The only way to learn arrhythmias is to look at thousands of them and answer the question, "sick or not sick."* Most findings are not as unique from person to person, but instead they vary from person to person and even within the same person at various times (kind of like fingerprints). If you only see one sample strip for each pathology but never see that picture-perfect example again in your life, you will never be able to diagnose it in your patient.

The complex language that is used in electrocardiography can be confusing and overwhelming. Most people buy an advanced textbook on arrhythmias, begin to read it, and then quickly give up. Sound familiar? You have to be very competent at electrocardiography and arrhythmia recognition to be able to understand the written word describing the possible variations. Most of us are visual learners. The simple way to learn about the rhythms, and the one that has been largely underutilized, is to use extensive graphics and to show various examples of each abnormality in order to develop a feel for what you are looking at. After a while, you will begin to feel your gut telling you whether the patient is "sick or not sick."

The process of learning to interpret rhythm strips is not unlike learning to throw a ball. You can read about the throw, the trajectories, the spin, and the accuracy, but unless you see a few balls thrown and throw hundreds or thousands yourself, you will never really learn know how to throw a ball. In the same way, you need to see hundreds of strips before you become comfortable. By the time you finish this book, you will be comfortable with the terminology and the concepts.

I have been asked by a few hundred students to teach them what they *really* need to know. I can sum up the answer in one short, concise statement: you need to know the changes that your specific patient presented you on their strip! You never know what will be important at any one point in your career; any one fact can cost the patient his or her life and will cost you countless hours of guilt, and possibly millions of dollars! Arrhythmia interpretation is the same whether you are an EMT, paramedic, nurse, resident, attending physician, or a cardiologist. You cannot learn just enough to get by. Does a resident need to know the changes of hyperkalemia that can lead to a lethal arrhythmia? Does a paramedic or nurse need to know that paroxysmal atrial tachycardia with block is associated with digoxin toxicity? To whom is it more important to know that a patient with a prolonged QT interval can develop torsade de pointes? It is important to you if you are the only one around at the time. Passing the buck to a higher level doesn't work with arrhythmias because you may not have enough time to pass it!

In closing, I would like to state that you need to look at everything at your disposal and trust yourself when you are interpreting a rhythm strip. *Don't let anyone talk you out of something that you know is true.* Just smile at them and do what is best for the patient. You will not go wrong. Remember that an expert is someone who knows one more fact than you do. However, that one fact may not be relevant to your case so you may be the true expert!

Tomas B. Garcia, MD, FACEP

Learning How to Interpret Arrhythmias

Dip, squiggle, pause, bump, blip, repeat, another case of the infamous "funk-a-cardia." During my formative student years, when presented with a complicated-looking rhythm that challenged my ability to interpret, I fell back to this trusty (however inadequate) choice, much to my instructor's chagrin. Fortunately, the frustration of not understanding prompted me to seek out those individuals and resources that led me to realize what I was seeing. It also reinforced in me a great trait, a "habit for learning."

To paraphrase Aristotle, excellence is not an act, but a habit. To put it another way, Michael Jordan did not become one of the greatest basketball players of all time just because he woke up one morning and decided to.

He spent many thousands of hours practicing and sharpening his knowledge and skill for the game. As you begin to learn and understand the arrhythmias covered in this text, be patient and develop a strong practice "habit" that will lead you to an understanding of the material.

The text you are about to read is meant as a guide and "pointer-outer" to get you familiar with the recognition of cardiac arrhythmias. As you begin your study, we encourage you to seek out as many opportunities as possible to develop your "habit" of arrhythmia recognition. Look to your instructors, clinical experts and peer groups, as they are a tremendous wealth of knowledge and experience. Remember, none of us picked up a book and became experts in one reading; rather, we have honed our skills in the art of arrhythmia interpretation through deliberate and repetitive practice.

This text has essentially two purposes. First, it is a teaching text designed for all levels of healthcare providers who are learning arrhythmias for the first time. Second, it is a reference for those already familiar with cardiac arrhythmias and their presentation. We hope that it will prove a valuable aid to those who are learning and those who continue to learn.

One of your first goals is to understand the basics, the foundation upon which everything else depends. While building this foundation, you will answer the question, "What is normal?" It takes a clear understanding of what a good thing looks like to be able to comprehend the bad. While I agree that some of the absolute worst arrhythmias, like asystole or ventricular fibrillation, may be some of the easiest to spot, there are many more that are not so obvious. Many of these are every bit as problematic and potentially lethal for the patient. This book is designed to build your level of understanding of why and how these changes occur in the cardiac electrical conduction system and provide a background as to their significance in the context of patient care.

We have systematically ordered the book to guide you from the top to the bottom of the conduction system as it relates to the development and presentation of arrhythmias. This building process will aid your understanding in an objective-structured, stair-step approach. At the conclusion of each chapter you will be presented with a brief quiz and practice strips to give you an opportunity to evaluate your own progress. We have included detailed explanations to assist you in your interpretation and understanding. Additionally, there are arrhythmia self-assessments at the end of each section that evaluate your ability to differentiate the various arrhythmias within. Finally at the end of the text, a comprehensive assessment is provided to test your ability to put it all together.

As you begin to learn and understand the objective criteria for the various arrhythmias it is important to understand how to use this information. The findings on a monitor attached to a patient are only a piece of a much greater puzzle. The patient's problem is the sum of all of its parts. Never forget that there is a tremendous amount of critical diagnostic information acquired through one of the most cost-effective evaluations that can be performed: the history and physical. Along the way we have included differential diagnosis information related to specific arrhythmias. This information may be critical in determining your interpretation and will certainly direct your course of therapy.

As our understanding of cardiac care advances, we must become more precise at recognizing cardiac arrhythmias, even (if not especially) the difficult ones. Therapies are more often focused at specific, unique problems rather than a broad-based, one-shot cure all. The setting in which you practice arrhythmia interpretation is not the most important part. It is equally vital for the recovery room personnel to recognize problematic arrhythmias as it is for the paramedic responding in the field or the cardiologist during an angioplasty in the cath lab. Each level of healthcare provider plays an essential role in the health and well-being of the patients we care for. Essential to this is the ability to recognize and manage patients with arrhythmias. With greater emphasis on creating patient safety systems within healthcare organizations, we are again challenged with the responsibility of accuracy.

Undoubtedly things will change. Even as this text goes to press, there will be that "one-more" paper published that provides new evidence to our understanding of cardiovascular disease, electrophysiology, emergency cardiac care, etc. The challenge to all of us is to embrace change and continue to seek and acquire better understandings of these changes. Learning will always be a piece of what you practice in any medical profession.

If you study just to remember, you will forget. But, if you study to understand, you will remember. We hope that through the many examples and variety of methods that explain these sometimes complex ideas, you will find it easier to understand and master the art of arrhythmia interpretation. Remember, this is the first step in your learning adventure. Now go out and experience the art of arrhythmia interpretation and practice, practice, practice your learning habit.

Geoffrey Tobias Miller, NREMT-P

Introduction to Arrhythmia Recognition

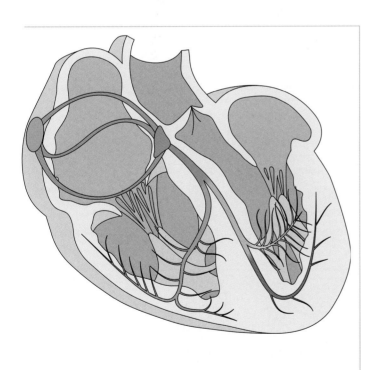

CHAPTER 1

Anatomy

Gross Anatomy

Since you are reading a book on electrocardiography, we assume that you have some basic knowledge of anatomy. However, a review is never a bad thing, so we are going to cover the basic anatomy of the heart and then concentrate on the electrical conduction system.

The heart sits in the middle of the chest at a slight angle pointing downward, to the left, and slightly anterior. Take a look at Figure 1-1.

Now, let's look at the heart itself. First, from an anterior view, and then in cross-section.

Anterior View

The right ventricle (RV) dominates the anterior view (Figure 1-2). Most of the anterior surface of the ventricles consists of the RV surface. A key point to remember is that, though the RV dominates this visual view, the left ventricle (LV) dominates the electrical view. We will review this in more detail in Chapter 3 when we discuss vectors.

The Heart in Cross Section

Figure 1-3 shows a cross-sectional view of the heart. In the following sections, we will cover the function of the heart as a pump and review the electrical conduction system in greater detail.

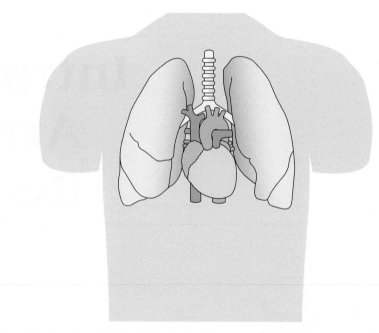

Figure 1-1: Location of the heart in the chest cavity.

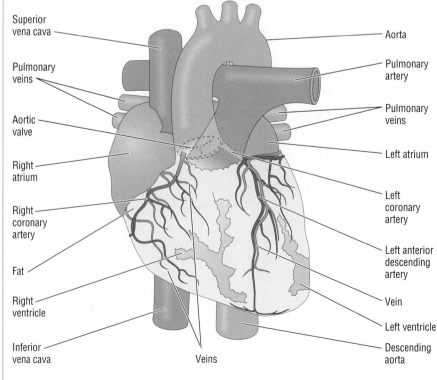

Superior vena cava

Pulmonary veins

Aortic valve

Right atrium

Right coronary artery

Fat

Right ventricle

Inferior vena cava

Veins

Aorta

Pulmonary artery

Pulmonary veins

Left atrium

Left coronary artery

Left anterior descending artery

Vein

Left ventricle

Descending aorta

Figure 1-2: Anterior view of the heart.

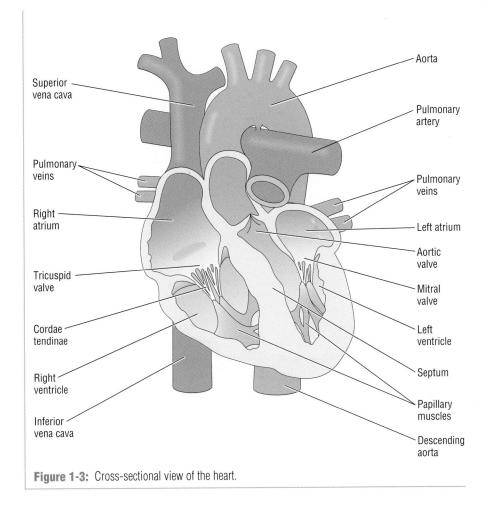

Figure 1-3: Cross-sectional view of the heart.

The Heart as a Pump

The heart consists of four main chambers: the two atria and the two ventricles. The atria empty into their corresponding ventricles. The left ventricle empties into the peripheral circulatory system, and the right ventricle empties into the pulmonary system. Veins bring blood to the heart, while arteries take blood away from the heart. As Figure 1-4 shows, this is a closed system. Blood circulates inside this closed system over and over, taking up oxygen in the lungs and giving it up to the peripheral tissues. This is a simplistic explanation of a very complicated system, but it will suffice for our purposes at this time.

Pump Function Simplified

It is simplest to think of the circulatory system as an engineer would: as a system of interconnected pumps and pipes.

Take a look at Figure 1-5 on the next page. We see that there are four pumps in sequence. The two small primer pumps are the atria, whose sole purpose is to push a small amount of blood into the two larger ones, the ventricles. The ventricles differ in size and in the amount of pressure that they can generate. Because of the one-way valves found in the venous system, blood can only flow forward.

Cardiac Output

Blood pressure is critical to life. We need blood pressure to act as the driving force to move blood through the circulatory system in order to deliver oxygen and nutrients to every cell. How does the body maintain blood pressure? It is maintained by both passive and active means. In this section, we will first go over the passive system and then we will discuss the active system.

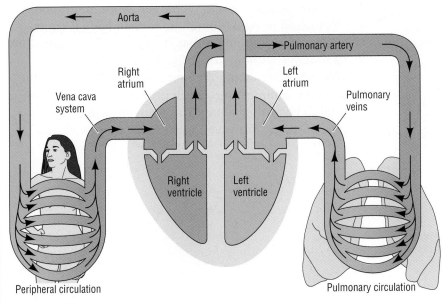

Figure 1-4: The heart as a pump.

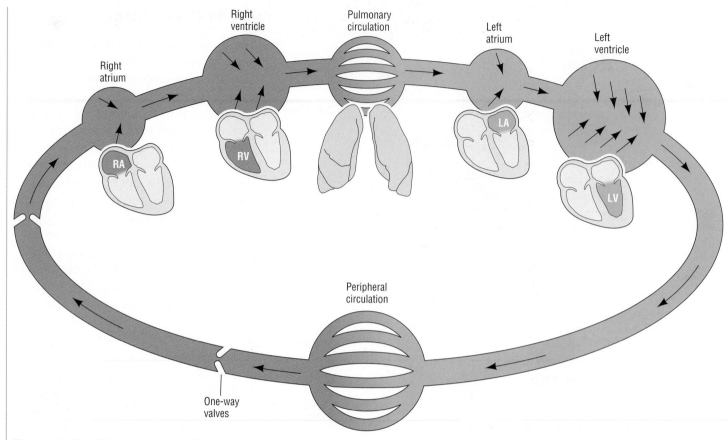

Figure 1-5: Simplified pump function of the circulatory system.

Passive Pumping

Suppose you put an extra 70 mL of fluid into a fluid-filled, solid-walled pipe such as a PVC or copper pipe (Figure 1-6). What changes would the extra fluid create in the tube? The pressure in the tube would build up dramatically with every cc of fluid you put into it (Figure 1-7). The pressure would force fluid to run out the open end of the pipe in order to relieve the pressure. That system works well when you have a short amount of pipe and a strong pump. The longer the pipe, the stronger the pump needed.

In one pound of fat tissue in the human body there is one-quarter mile of tubing (Figure 1-8). We can assume that this is true for other types of tissue as well.

How many miles of tubing are in your entire vascular system? A lot! The pump needed to push blood through such a tubing system, if it were rigid, would need to be very strong indeed. What do you suppose such strong forces would do to your red cells, white cells, and platelets? They would destroy them. Therefore, this type of system would not work in our bodies.

Instead of rigid tubing, the human body is composed of *elastic* tubing. Elastic tubing can bend and allow us to move without any difficulty. It is compressible, allowing external muscle movement to help pump the blood by compressing or milking the tube, causing the fluid to be pushed along. The main advantage to this type of tubing, however, is its elastic properties. Its

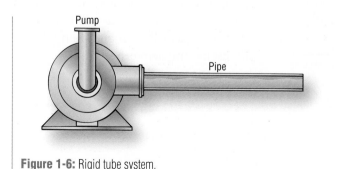

Figure 1-6: Rigid tube system.

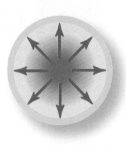

Figure 1-7: Pressure inside the pipe.

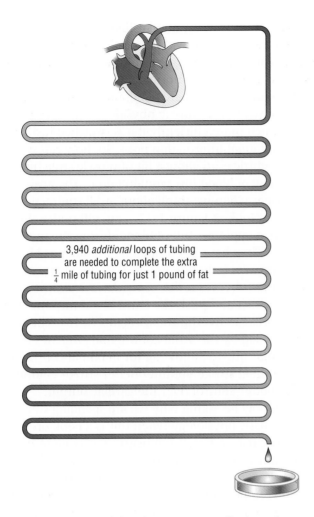

3,940 *additional* loops of tubing are needed to complete the extra $\frac{1}{4}$ mile of tubing for just 1 pound of fat

Figure 1-8: Every pound of fat has about one-quarter mile of vascular tubing in it to allow perfusion of every cell.

elasticity allows the blood vessel to simply distend in order to accommodate for the extra fluid whenever the heart pumps (Figure 1-9).

What would happen to the pressure inside the tube now? It would build up inside the tube but the distension would distribute the pressure a bit more smoothly. What happens to an elastic band when you stretch it? It wants to go back to its original shape. This built-up energy places constant, smooth pressure on the blood, causing it to flow out in a smooth fashion, avoiding high shearing pressures and turbulence (Figure 1-9). The distended arterial walls are, in essence, acting like an additional pump helping to push the blood forward through the circulatory system.

The slow, constant pressure of a distended elastic arterial system wanting to return to normal is the passive way in which the circulatory system functions. Now let's go over the active system that causes the arterial distension in the first place.

Active Pumping

The blood pressure is maintained actively by the amount of blood that the heart pumps out into the vascular system every minute—in other words, the **cardiac output**. Cardiac output is, in turn, composed of two variables: the *stroke volume* and the *heart rate*. The stroke volume is the amount of blood that the heart ejects during any one contraction. This amount is usually around 70 cc of blood per contraction. Heart rate, as you can imagine, refers to the number of times the heart beats in one minute.

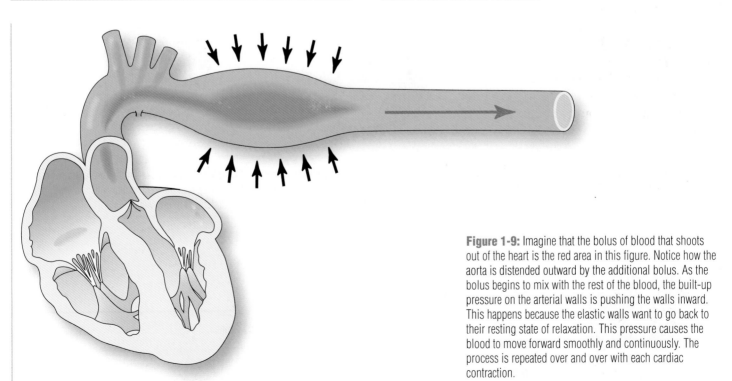

Figure 1-9: Imagine that the bolus of blood that shoots out of the heart is the red area in this figure. Notice how the aorta is distended outward by the additional bolus. As the bolus begins to mix with the rest of the blood, the built-up pressure on the arterial walls is pushing the walls inward. This happens because the elastic walls want to go back to their resting state of relaxation. This pressure causes the blood to move forward smoothly and continuously. The process is repeated over and over with each cardiac contraction.

Cardiac output is mathematically calculated by taking the amount of blood that the heart can eject in one contraction and then multiplying this by the number of contractions per minute. In other words:

Cardiac Output = Stroke Volume × Heart Rate

In order to maintain a good hemodynamic balance, the cardiac output has to be within the normal range. Notice however, that you can maintain an adequate cardiac output by altering the two variables. For example, suppose that the stroke volume was 40 cc/min (instead of the normal 70 cc/min). Can you figure out a way that the cardiac output for the heart can be maintained within the normal range? One way would be by increasing the heart rate. That is the reason why, when someone has lost a significant amount of blood (resulting in decreased stroke volume because there is less blood to pump), a tachycardia develops as a compensatory mechanism. The body tries to overcome the deficiency in blood and stroke volume by increasing heart rate.

Now let's take a closer look at the concept of stroke volume. At the end of systole, the ventricles have just emptied their contents into the arterial system (Figure 1-10). How does the heart fill up the ventricles again? If you remember from basic physiology, the largest amount of ventricular filling occurs during early diastole, when the atrioventricular valves open up and a rush of blood floods the ventricular chamber (Figure 1-11). This is known as the *rapid filling phase of diastole.*

After the rapid ventricular filling phase of diastole, the ventricles are full with blood. If the ventricles were to beat at this point, the stroke volume of the heart would be at the lower end of normal for most people. Why? Because the ventricles are filled, but not overfilled. It is a well-known fact in muscle physiology that a muscle contracts much more efficiently if it is stretched just a bit (see Additional Information box). So, how can we overfill the ventricles to allow a bit of muscle stretching? Passive inflow of blood just wouldn't do it. The answer is made clear when we think about atrial contraction.

If you look at Figure 1-12, you will notice that the atria are completely full of blood during the middle of diastole. They have been filled by the venous blood which is constantly flowing back to the heart. At the end of diastole, when the ventricles are almost full, the atria contract and push the extra blood into the ventricles in order to overfill them (Figure 1-13). The overfilling provided by the atrial contraction stretches the ventricular muscle, allowing for maximal contractility and maximal stroke volume. Better stroke volume means better control over the cardiac output.

You may be asking why we are spending so much time on basic physiology when this is a book on arrhythmias. The reason is that the heart rate is one of the most important variables in the maintenance of cardiac output. As we saw earlier, the other main variable is the stroke volume. In many cases, arrhythmias will affect either one or both of these variables profoundly. In order to understand the clinical implications of arrhythmias,

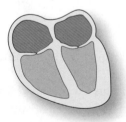

Figure 1-10: This figure shows the heart in late systole. The atria are full but the ventricles are empty.

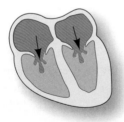

Figure 1-11: In early diastole, the AV valves open, allowing a large amount of blood to rush into the ventricles. This is the rapid filling phase of diastole.

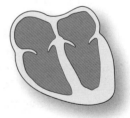

Figure 1-12: In mid-diastole, the ventricles are full. Notice that the ventricular walls, however, are not distended in any way.

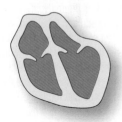

Figure 1-13: The atrial contraction allows an extra amount of blood to enter the ventricles, causing them to stretch and overfill. The slight stretch in the ventricular muscle caused by the atrial kick will maximize stroke volume and cardiac output.

Muscle Tension

When a muscle is at its normal length (Figure 1-14), the amount of tension that it can produce is a set amount. In other words, a muscle can only produce just so much tension. On the other hand, if the muscle were stretched, the amount of tension that it could produce would be increased (Figure 1-15).

The heart muscle is no exception to this rule. If the heart were only allowed to fill by passive means such as the inflow of blood, the heart muscle would not be stretched. The amount of force that the heart could use to contract would be less than if the muscle were stretched somewhat. (Textbooks on physiology refer to this finding as the Frank-Starling mechanism or law.) The atrial kick allows the heart to "overfill" a bit and stretch the muscle, maximizing myocardial contraction.

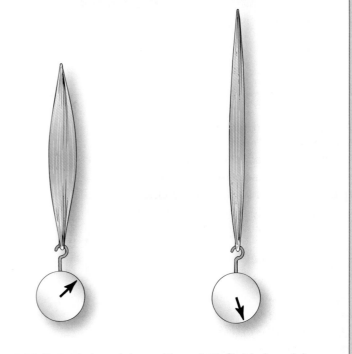

Figure 1-14: Unstretched muscle has less tension than stretched muscle.

Figure 1-15: Stretched muscle has better functionality.

you need to understand the concept of cardiac filling and cardiac output very clearly. We will constantly refer back to this section throughout the book.

Now let's take a closer look at how heart rate affects stroke volume. What do you think happens to the stroke volume of the heart at very fast heart rates? Remember from our previous discussion on the rapid filling phase that most of the blood volume entering the ventricle occurs during very early diastole right after the AV valves open up (Figure 1-16). At very fast ventricular rates, the ventricles do not have time to fill adequately because the rapid filling phase is shortened (Figure 1-17). The net result is that the ventricles are not filled to capacity or overfilled at the end of diastole. Now when they contract, the amount of blood that is expelled is less than optimal. Less than optimal ejection means a decrease in cardiac output. In other words, the cardiac output will diminish because the stroke volume will be greatly decreased. Decreased cardiac output could very easily cause or lead to hemodynamic instability. That is how and why a tachycardia or rapid heart rate can kill.

The Electrical Conduction System

The cardiac impulse is essentially bioelectrical energy. From our own experience in life, we know that electric-

ity travels everywhere it can, as fast as it can. In the heart, one way that bioelectrical energy can travel is by direct cell-to-cell transmission of the impulse (Figure 1-18). This form of impulse transmission is slow and would lead to unsynchronized mechanical contraction of the heart. In this section, we are going to begin to look at a group of specialized cells in the heart that make up a specialized system known as the electrical conduction system.

In the last few pages, we discussed the need for controlled contraction of the atria in order to superfill the ventricles. So, let's begin our look at the electrical conduction system by asking a simple question: If transmission occurred throughout the atria by any means available (cell-to-cell transmission, specialized conduction system, etc.), how can you trigger the atria and not trigger the ventricles at the same time (Figure 1-18)?

If the electrical impulse traveled freely from the atria to the ventricles, then both the atria and the ventricles would contract almost simultaneously. This simultaneous stimulation would not allow the main priming function of the ventricles to occur. In order to prime the ventricles, the atria must contract just before the ventricles begin to contract. Sequential contraction has to happen because once the ventricles contract, the increased force of the ventricular contraction shuts the

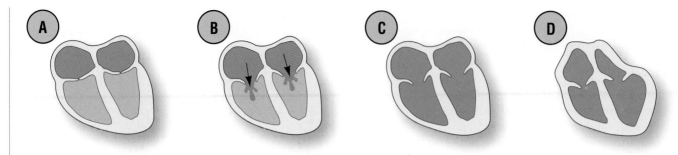

Figure 1-16: Normal rapid filling phase and the overfilling caused by atrial contraction during normal heart rates.

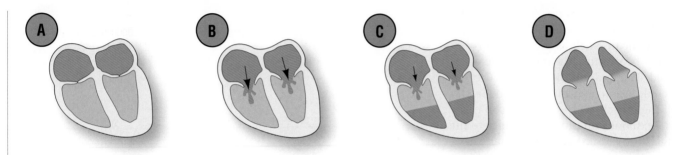

Figure 1-17: Impaired rapid filling phase is shown on Examples A to C. The small amount of blood added by the atrial kick is not enough to overcome the decreased blood volume in the ventricles. The net result is that the stroke volume, and hence the cardiac output, will be greatly decreased.

atrioventricular (AV) valves. If the valves are closed, no blood can go through them. The blood pumped by the atria would not overfill the ventricles, but would instead be forced back into the circulatory system.

Nature, in its infinite wisdom, overcame this problem with some elegant solutions. First, it made the atrioventricular septum a wall of nonconductive tissue between the atria and the ventricles (Figure 1-19). This created a firewall between the atria and the ventricles, completely stopping the conduction of the impulse before it reached the ventricles. This alone was not a great solution. Now, how does the impulse reach the ventricles? It can't. Enter elegant solution #2, the AV node.

The only electrical communication between the atria and the ventricles is a small amount of gatekeeping tissue known as the *atrioventricular (AV) node* (Figure 1-20). The AV node slows the conduction of the impulse from the atria to the ventricles just enough to allow the atria to finish their mechanical contraction.

Think of the AV node as a guarded gate at an apartment complex. When you first drive up to the guard gate, the gate is down and you need to pull your car to a stop. The guard asks you a bunch of questions, calls the person in the apartment and asks if they are ready to receive you, and then opens the gate. Only after the gate opens can you drive through without causing your car some serious damage. The guard, the gatekeeper,

has effectively slowed your arrival to maximize the effectiveness of the owner of the apartment. This is exactly what the AV node does in the heart. The atrial impulse reaches the AV node and wants to pass. The AV node slows down the conduction until the ventricles are ready. When the ventricles are ready, the gate is opened completely and the impulse travels through to stimulate the ventricles. This slowing-down function of the AV node is known as the *physiologic block* (Figure 1-21).

As we all know, arrhythmias can be quite deadly. Oftentimes hemodynamic compromise occurs because arrhythmias can cause asynchronous, ineffective contraction of the heart. The asynchronous contraction decreases cardiac output, which, in turn, decreases blood pressure and tissue perfusion. No circulation plus no delivery of oxygen or nutrients to the cells equals no life. The sequential, orderly, and controlled means of transmitting the electrical impulse through the AV node and its physiologic block are critical to life.

The electrical conduction system of the heart is made up of specialized cells (Figure 1-22). Some of these are specialized for pacemaking functions and some for the transmission of the impulses that travel through them. We will break down the system in the following paragraphs and describe the functions of each of the parts in greater detail.

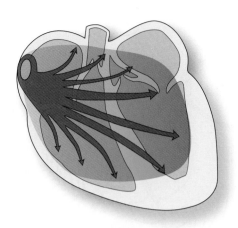

Figure 1-18: If the heart were composed of just muscle tissue, the electrical impulse would travel unimpeded from the atria to the ventricles, causing simultaneous contraction of the atria and ventricles.

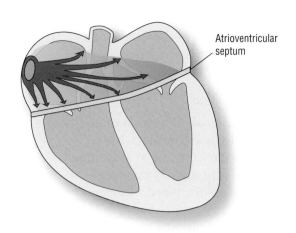

Figure 1-19: The AV septum represents a nonconductive wall between the atria and the ventricles. If the AV septum did not have any communication between the atria and the ventricles, the impulse would never reach the ventricles.

The main function of the system is to create an electrical impulse and transmit it in an organized manner to the rest of the myocardium. This is an electrochemical process that creates electrical energy that is picked up by the electrodes when we perform an electrocardiogram (ECG). (More on this in Chapter 3.)

The specialized conduction system is interwoven with the myocardial tissue itself, and is only distin-

guishable with certain stains under a microscope. So in looking at Figure 1-23, keep in mind that the system is actually in the heart walls. The atrial myocytes are innervated by direct contact from one cell to another; the first cell innervates the second, the second innervates the third, and so on. The internodal pathways transmit the impulse from the sino atrial (SA) node to the AV node. The Purkinje system encircles the entire ventri-

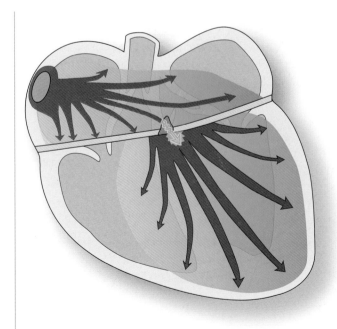

Figure 1-20: The AV node represents the only communication between the atria and the ventricles. It functions as the gatekeeper for the electrical impulse.

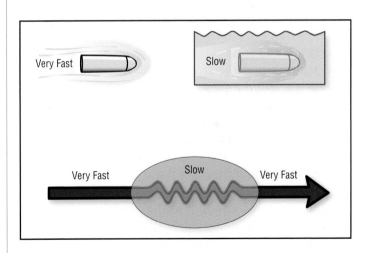

Figure 1-21: Just as a bullet travels faster through the air than through water, so the electrical impulse travels faster through the specialized conduction system and the myocardium than through the AV node. The AV node slows down the conduction of the impulse, causing the physiologic block.

cles, just under the endocardium, and is the final component of the conduction system. The Purkinje cells innervate the myocardial cells themselves.

Pacemaker Function

What is the pacemaker function of the heart, and why do we need it? The pacemaker dictates the rate at which the heart will cycle through its pumping action to circulate the blood. The pacemaker creates an organized beating of all of the cardiac cells, in a specialized sequence, to produce effective pumping action. It sets the pace that all of the other cells will follow. Let's look at an analogy.

Imagine that each cell of the heart represents a single musician. When we have a few dozen of these musicians, we have an orchestra—the heart. Now, if each musician decides to play whenever he or she wants to, they would make an unrecognizable jumble of sound. The musicians need a beat or signal to cue them when to start to play, direct them when to come into the piece and when to leave, and coordinate their actions to create a beautiful melody. In music, that pacemaker is the underlying beat kept by the drummer or the conductor. In sections that are swift, the beat increases. In sections that are slow and soft, the beat decreases. The same thing happens in the heart; during exercise the pace speeds up, and during rest it slows.

As we have mentioned, there are specialized cells whose function is to create an electrical impulse and act as the heart's pacemaker. The main area that fills this important function is the SA node, found in the muscle of the right atrium. This area responds to the needs of the body, controlling the beat based on information it receives from the nervous, circulatory, and endocrine systems. The main pacemaker paces at a rate of 60 to 100 beats per minute (BPM), with an average of 70.

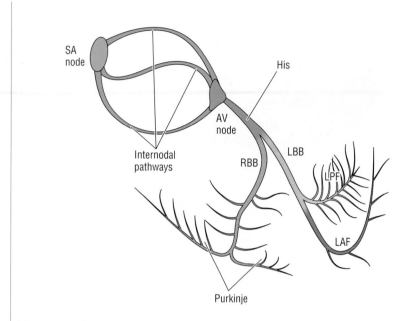

Figure 1-22: The electrical conduction system.

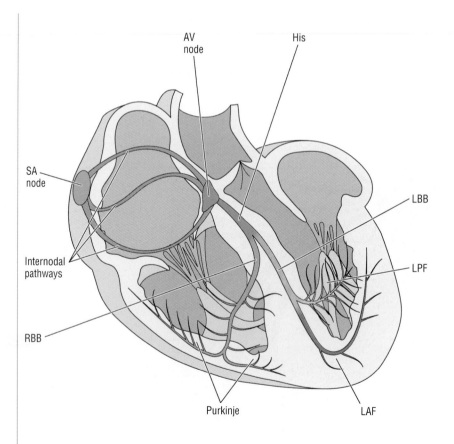

Figure 1-23: The electrical conduction system of the heart.

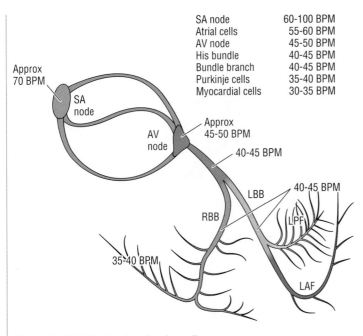

SA node	60-100 BPM
Atrial cells	55-60 BPM
AV node	45-50 BPM
His bundle	40-45 BPM
Bundle branch	40-45 BPM
Purkinje cells	35-40 BPM
Myocardial cells	30-35 BPM

Figure 1-24: Intrinsic rates of pacing cells.

Pacemaker Settings

One thing we know about the body is that everything has a backup. Every cell in the conduction system is capable of setting the pace (Figure 1-24). However, the intrinsic rate of each type of cell is slower than the cells that precede it. This means that the fastest pacer is the SA node, the next fastest is the AV node, and so on. The fastest pacer sets the pace because it causes all the ones that come after it to reset after each beat. In this way, the slower pacers will never fire. If the faster pacer doesn't fire for some reason, the next fastest will be there as a backup to ensure function that is as close to normal as possible.

The Sinoatrial (SA) Node

The SA node, the heart's main pacemaker, is found in the wall of the right atrium at its junction with the superior vena cava (Figure 1-25). Its blood supply comes from the right coronary artery in 59% of cases. In 38%, the blood supply originates from the left coronary artery, and in the last 3%, it arises from both.

Figure 1-25: SA node.

The Internodal Pathways

There are three internodal pathways: anterior, middle, and posterior. Their main purpose is to transmit the pacing impulse from the SA node to the AV node. In addition, there is a small tract of specialized cells known as the Bachman Bundle that transmits the impulses through the inter-atrial septum. All of these pathways are found in the walls of the right atrium and the inter-atrial septum.

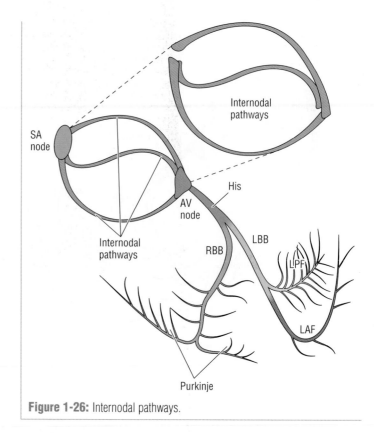

Figure 1-26: Internodal pathways.

The Atrioventricular (AV) Node

The AV node is located in the wall of the right atrium just next to the opening of the coronary sinus, the largest vein of the heart, and the septal leaflet of the tricuspid valve. It is responsible for slowing down conduction from the atria to the ventricles just long enough for atrial contraction to occur. This slowing allows the atria to "overfill" the ventricles and helps maintain the output of the heart at a maximum level. The AV node is always supplied by the right coronary artery.

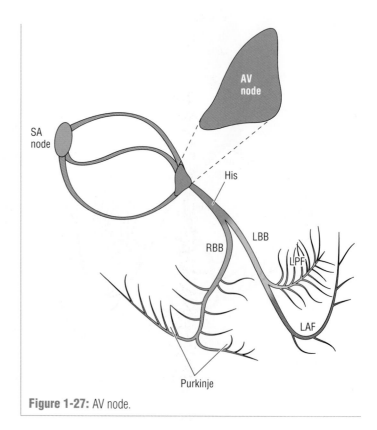

Figure 1-27: AV node.

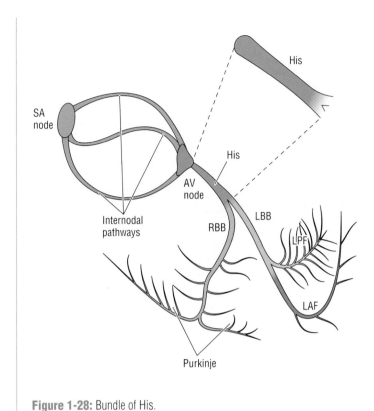

Figure 1-28: Bundle of His.

The Bundle of His

The Bundle of His starts at the AV node and eventually gives rise to both the right and left bundle branches. It is found partially in the walls of the right atrium, and in the interventricular septum. The His bundle is the only route of communication between the atria and the ventricles.

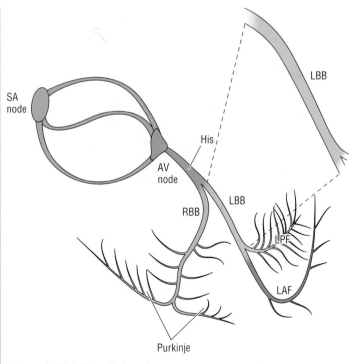

Figure 1-29: Left bundle branch.

The Left Bundle Branch (LBB)

The left bundle begins at the end of the His bundle and travels through the interventricular septum. The left bundle gives rise to the fibers that will innervate the LV and the left face of the interventricular septum. It first connects to a small set of fibers that innervate the upper segment of the interventricular septum. This will be the first area to depolarize, meaning that the heart's cells fire. The left bundle ends at the beginning of the left anterior (LAF) and left posterior fascicles (LPF).

The Right Bundle Branch (RBB)

The right bundle, which starts at the His bundle, gives rise to the fibers that will innervate the RV and the right face of the interventricular septum. It terminates in the Purkinje fibers associated with it.

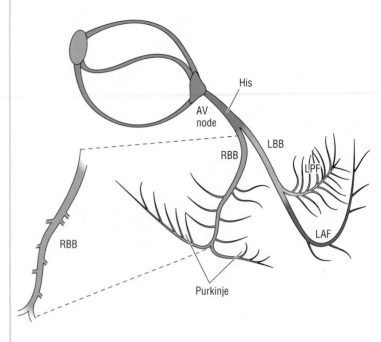

Figure 1-30: Right bundle branch.

The Left Anterior Fascicle (LAF)

The LAF, also known as the left anterior superior fascicle, travels through the left ventricle to the Purkinje cells that innervate the anterior and superior aspects of the left ventricle. It is a single-stranded fascicle, in comparison to the LPF.

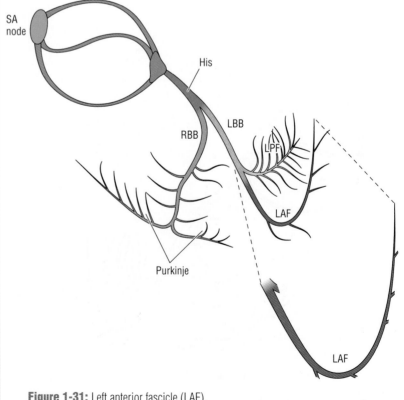

Figure 1-31: Left anterior fascicle (LAF).

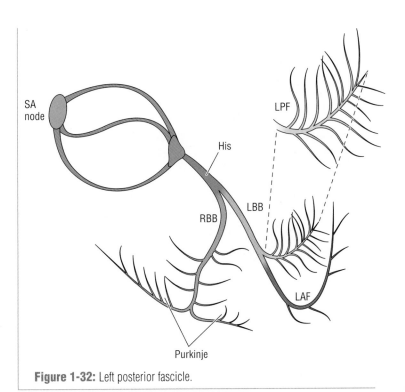

Figure 1-32: Left posterior fascicle.

The Left Posterior Fascicle (LPF)

The LPF is a fan-like structure leading to the Purkinje cells that will innervate the posterior and inferior aspects of the left ventricle. It is very difficult to block this fascicle because it is so widely distributed, rather than being just one strand.

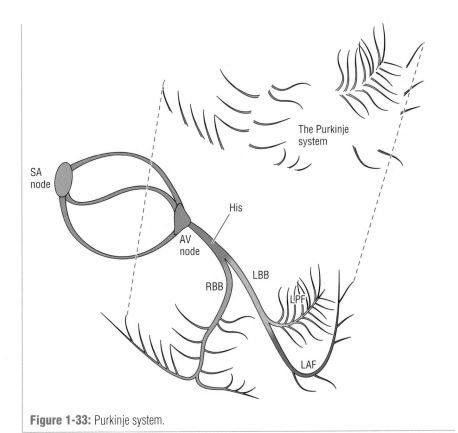

Figure 1-33: Purkinje system.

The Purkinje System

The Purkinje system is made up of individual cells just beneath the endocardium. They are the cells that directly innervate the myocardial cells and initiate the ventricular depolarization cycle.

When it comes to arrhythmias, the anatomy of the heart is easy. You need to know and understand the electrical conduction thoroughly and you need to know that there are four arrhythmogenic zones in the heart (Figure 1-34). The four zones are:

1. SA node (sinus)
2. Atrial
3. AV node (nodal)
4. Ventricular

The first three zones, the SA node, atria, and the AV node can be classified together as *supraventricular* because they encompass everything above the ventricles.

Basically, all of the arrhythmias that we will review in this book have their source of origin in one of these four zones (Figure 1-35). We will review each of these rhythms in great detail in their individual chapters. For now, it is just important to understand the concept of the four zones. In Chapter 37, we will review this chart again with a focus on diagnosing the individual arrhythmias.

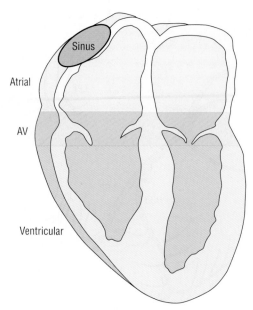

Figure 1-34: Four arrhythmogenic zones.

Sinus	Atria	Nodal/Bundles	Ventricles
Sinus Bradycardia	Ectopic Atrial	Junctional Junctional Escape First-degree AV Block	Ventricular Escape Idioventricular Accelerated Idioventricular
Normal Sinus Rhythm	Ectopic Atrial	Accelerated Junctional First-degree AV Block	Accelerated Idioventricular
Sinus Tachycardia	Atrial Tachycardia Atrial Flutter	First-degree AV Block Junctional Tachycardia AV Nodal Reentry Tach AV Reentry Tach	AV Reentry Tach Ventricular Tachycardia Torsade de Pointes Polymorphic VTach Ventricular Fibrillation
Sinus Arrhythmia PAC	Atrial Flutter	PJC Second-degree AV Block Third-degree AV Block	PVC
	Atrial Fibrillation Wandering Atrial Pacemaker Multifocal Atrial Tachycardia Variable Atrial Flutter		
	PAT with block Atrial Flutter	Second-degree AV Block Third-degree AV Block	
SA block SA Pause/arrest	Atrial Fibrillation	Junctional Junctional Escape Accelerated Junctional Junctional Tachycardia AVNodal Reentry Tach AV Reentry Tach	Asystole Ventricular Escape Idioventricular Accelerated Idioventricular Ventricular Tachycardia Torsade de Pointes Polymorphic VTach Ventricular Fibrillation

Figure 1-35: The cardiac rhythms based on the four arrhythmogenic zones.

CHAPTER **REVIEW**

1. Visually, the right ventricle dominates the anterior view of the heart. True or False.

2. The right ventricle pumps the blood through the peripheral circulation. True or False.

3. Which of the statements below is **incorrect:**
   A. The electrical conduction system of the heart is made up of specialized cells.
   B. The conduction system is interwoven into the myocardial tissue.
   C. The conduction system is visible under the microscope without special stains.
   D. The internodal pathways transmit the impulse between the SA node and the AV node.

Match the following correctly:

4. ____ SA node   A. 40–45 BPM
5. ____ Atrial cells   B. 30–35 BPM
6. ____ AV node   C. 60–100 BPM
7. ____ His bundle   D. 35–40 BPM
8. ____ Purkinje cells   E. 55–60 BPM
9. ____ Myocardial cells F. 45–50 BPM

10. The AV node is always supplied by:
    A. The left anterior descending artery
    B. The posterior descending artery
    C. The right coronary artery
    D. The left circumflex artery
    E. The first diagonal artery

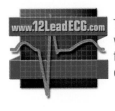

To enhance the knowledge you gain in this book, access this text's website at www.12leadECG.com! This valuable resource provides flashcards, an online glossary, web links, and more. Simply click on the Arrhythmias book cover once at the site.

CHAPTER 2

Electrophysiology

Why do you need to know about the generation of electrical activity in a cell and the effect of electrolytes on the electrocardiogram (ECG) or rhythm strip? Because, before you can understand what a rhythm strip does, you need to know how it gets its information. Electrolytes are the means by which the cell develops "electricity." You also need to know about electrolytes because imbalances can cause life-threatening problems. For example, if you knew that peaked, sharp T waves were a sign of hyperkalemia (elevated potassium), or that a prolonged QT interval could be a sign of hypocalcemia or hypomagnesemia, you might avert a serious arrhythmia. It takes only minutes in some cases to go from peaked T waves to asystole. (By the way, pacers do not work in hyperkalemia!) A little knowledge about electrolytes and their effects on the ECG patterns can save the patient—and you.

To understand why the ECG is altered by an electrolyte abnormality, we will review the way in which the myocardial cell becomes polarized and depolarized, and the biochemical mechanisms that allow the cell to contract. We will try to make the concepts as painless as possible, so bear with us. This is intended to be only a very basic discussion of the topic, which you can supplement with a good physiology textbook as needed.

Mechanics of Contraction

Imagine that the heart is made up of a series of small barrels or cells (Figure 2-1). Each of these barrels is made up of two halves that slide over each other and are held together by interlocking pieces (actin and myosin proteins). The actin molecules are attached to the outside edges of the barrel wall, and the myosin molecules are interspersed between the actin molecules.

The outsides of the barrels (cells) are fused together to form long bands, or myofibrils (Figure 2-2). These bands, in turn, are held together side-to-side by wire (connective tissue) to form sheets, which are covered with fluid (extracellular fluid). The main function of the bands is to contract and expand. When one of the barrels contracts, the whole sheet shortens by a small amount. When all of the barrels contract, the whole

sheet shortens significantly. The sheet returns to its starting size as all of the barrels relax. The sheets are arranged to form the four sacs that constitute the heart: two small, thin ones on top (the atria) and two large, thick ones on bottom (the ventricles).

Ion Movement and Polarity

The fluid inside and outside of the barrel contains water, salts, and proteins. The fluids are not the same, however; the concentrations of salt molecules and proteins are different in each one. In liquids, salts break

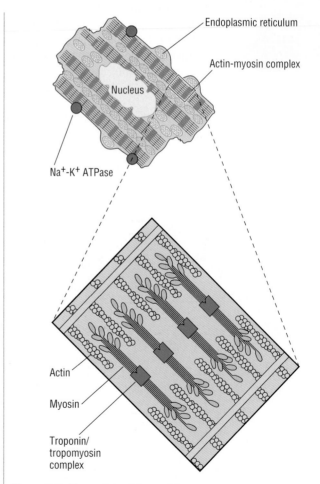

Figure 2-1: Myocardial cell (myocyte).

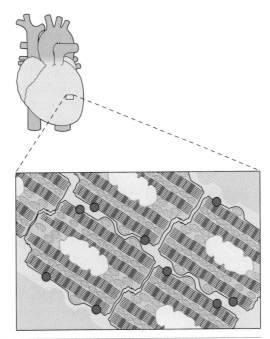

Figure 2-2: Barrels are held together, forming myofibrils and sheets.

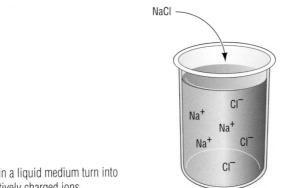

Figure 2-3: Salts in a liquid medium turn into positively and negatively charged ions.

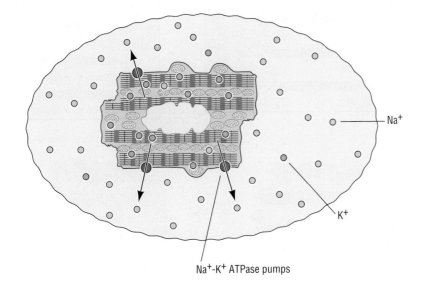

Na$^+$-K$^+$ ATPase pumps

Figure 2-4: Solutions inside and outside the barrel are different. The pump (dark blue dots) maintains the right number of ions on both sides of the wall.

down into positively and negatively charged particles known as ions (Figure 2-3). In other words, an ion is a positively or negatively charged particle in a solution. In the body, the main positively charged ions are sodium (Na+), potassium (K+), and calcium (Ca++). Chloride (Cl−) is the main negatively charged ion.

If the cell were not alive, the concentrations of all of the ions and charges would be the same on both sides of the barrel wall (the cell membrane). However, a live cell maintains differences in these concentrations across the cell membrane (Figure 2-4). The inside of the cell has a higher potassium concentration, whereas the outside has a higher concentration of sodium. The higher positive charge outside the cell thus causes relatively more negative charge inside the cell. The outside of the cell wall also has more calcium, which adds to the greater positive charge outside the cell. This difference between the charges outside and inside of the cell wall is known as its electrical potential.

Charges and ions naturally want to cancel themselves out and maintain neutrality. The cell wall is not a completely impermeable membrane. It is semi-permeable, because it contains small leaks that let some of the ions into and out of the cell. The natural tendency is for sodium to enter and potassium to exit. To maintain an electrical potential, the cell must have some way of pushing the ions around against their wishes. Enter the sodium-potassium ATPase pumps (dark blue dots in figures). The pumps actively move ions around to maintain the resting concentration and charge of the cell. How does the pump do that? The pump uses ATP, the body's fuel pellet, to push out two sodium ions (two positive charges) and bring in one potassium ion (one positive charge). The result is a greater number of positive charges outside the barrel than inside. In other words, the outside solution has a positive charge, while the inner solution has a more negative charge. Because of this pumping action, the electrical potential of the resting myocyte is approximately −70 to −90 mV.

As time passes, the number of ions entering into the cell starts to offset the effect of the pump, and the inside of the cell becomes less negative (increasing numbers of positively charged sodium ions are leaking in). This pattern of slowly increasing the cell's electrical potential is referred to as phase 4 of the action potential (Figure 2-5).

Membrane Channels and Action Potential Phases

Eventually, the cell becomes so positive that a new set of channels opens. The point at which the channels open is called the threshold potential, and the channels are the fast sodium channels. Think of this as a one-way valve at the end of a tube. When the positive charges inside the cell reach a certain point, the valve opens. Because it is a one-way valve, ions can only enter the cell, and what is the most common ion outside the cell? Sodium! This influx of sodium makes the cell even more positive, and the cycle continues. The rapid increase in sodium ions causes the cell to "spike," or fire. This is called phase 0 (Figure 2-5). The impulse is transmitted down the cell, which begins to influence the cell next to it, and so on, until they are all stimu-

lated. At this point, the cell is no longer polarized, or negatively charged; it is now depolarized, and just as positive as the outside solution.

The next phase, when the cell is at its peak positive charge, is phase 1. At this point, some negatively charged chloride ions enter the cell and cause the influx of sodium to slow down. This initial slowdown slams shut the one-way valve on the rapid sodium channels. Two more types of channels now open: the slow sodium channels and the calcium channels, and a slow "plateau" phase begins—phase 2. The slow sodium channels are responsible for a slow influx of sodium ions, but not to the degree of the fast sodium channels. The calcium channels open and begin to allow calcium to enter the cell. Calcium is a double positive ion; it has two positive charges instead of one. The influx of calcium and the slow influx of sodium help maintain the cell in the depolarized state.

This is where the fun starts: calcium is needed for the cell to contract. Calcium acts like a key, activating a clamp composed of the proteins troponin and tropomyosin. The clamp brings together the two ratcheting proteins, actin and myosin, and allows them to move along each other and cause the cell to contract (Figure 2-6). Without calcium, the right key configuration is not present to unlock and free the clamping pro-

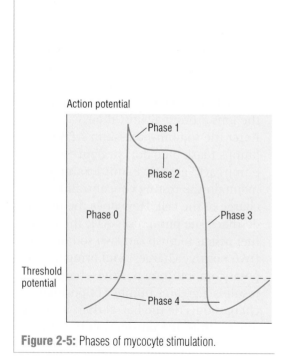

Figure 2-5: Phases of myocyte stimulation.

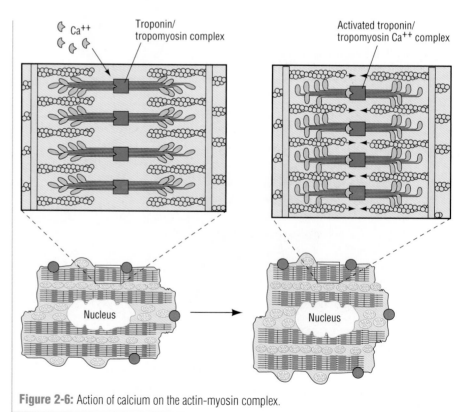

Figure 2-6: Action of calcium on the actin-myosin complex.

teins, and the actin and myosin do not come close enough together to engage their "teeth" with each other. The more calcium, the faster the clamping action, and the longer the contraction is maintained.

Next is phase 3. In this phase, some potassium channels open and allow potassium to escape the inside of the cell. During this phase of rapid repolarization, the exit of positive ions imparts a relatively negative charge to the inside of the cell (repolarizes it).

After the cell reaches resting potential, the whole process begins again. The Na-K ATPase pump begins to move sodium out and potassium in, the cell leaks, and it slowly creeps back up to the threshold potential to fire again. One critical point to understand about phase 4 is that different myocytes reach the threshold potential at different rates. Which ones reach it first? The ones that maintain the pacemaking function of the heart, the sinoatrial (SA) nodal cells. In sequence, the next ones are the atrial cells, the atrioventricular (AV) nodal cells, the bundle cells, the Purkinje cells, and finally the ventricular myocytes. Isn't it interesting that the independent rate for each of these systems is slower than the ones before? This is the body's protective mechanism, rather than having just one set of cells responsible for the pacing function. If all of the cells in the SA node die, then the next fastest phase 4 belongs to the atrial myocytes; they will fire before the other cells, and will set the pace. This continues down the line, as needed.

Introduction to the Nervous System and Cardiac Function

Now that we have an idea of how the bioelectrical energy is created in the heart and how the muscle contracts, let's turn our attention to how the brain and the heart communicate to control the hemodynamic status of the body. This communication uses chemical messengers and receptors to transport the information back and forth between the various organs. Understanding how these chemical messengers and receptors work, and how we can manipulate them in treatment, is critical to our study of arrhythmias.

Anatomically, the nervous system is made up of the *central nervous system* (CNS; brain and spinal cord) and various types of *peripheral nerves*. The two major types of peripheral nerves we will be discussing are the *afferent* nerves (Latin: *ad*, to + *ferre*, to bear), which carry sensory impulses from all parts of the body to the brain and *efferent* nerves (Latin: *efferens*, to bring out), which

Moving On

As a closing thought, imagine that there are millions of action potentials occurring throughout the heart. Each individual cell is polarizing and depolarizing about 70 to 100 times each minute, and there are quite a few million myocytes in the heart. This translates to millions or billions of action potentials occurring each minute. Miraculously, they will all act in unison, thanks to the electrical conduction system we reviewed in Chapter 1. The sum of these collective electrical discharges will create one large electrical current—the electric axis of the heart. In the next few chapters, we will see how the ECG machine measures these electrical potentials and changes them into the patterns that we will learn to recognize on an ECG tracing. We will see how the normal heart gives off some characteristic waves and complexes and how these complexes are altered in pathologic states.

Laying down the foundation for electrocardiography may appear tedious. It is important, however, if we really want to understand and interpret the ECG or rhythm strip correctly. Remember, it isn't enough just to read the rhythm strip; you must understand what causes the tracings, and the pathology it represents, in order to translate that information into a diagnosis. In turn, that diagnosis will be used to guide therapy—therapy that could save your patient's life.

carry messages from the brain to the muscles and all other organs of the body.

Functionally, the nervous system is divided into two primary components: the central nervous system (CNS) and the peripheral nervous system (PNS). The PNS is further subdivided into several subdivisions, which we will discuss further later on in this chapter (Figure 2-7).

Central Nervous System (CNS)

The CNS consists of the brain and spinal cord and functions as the control center for all other nervous system function. One could easily think of the CNS like a CPU (central processing unit) in a home computer. The CPU in a computer carries out all calculations coordinating

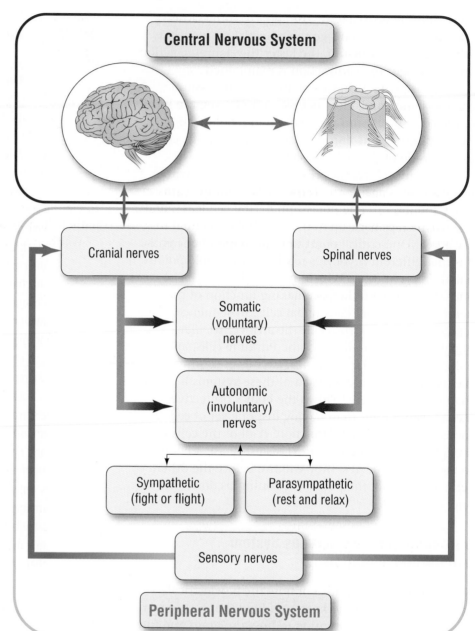

Figure 2-7: The human nervous system is composed of the central nervous system and the peripheral nervous system. The CNS receives its information about the outside world, and responds to that information, via the peripheral nervous system. The sensory nerves are responsible for sensing the environment. They transmit their data to the CNS (see green arrows) via the afferent portion of the PNS (cranial nerves and spinal nerves). The CNS then sends information back to the body via the efferent portion of the PNS (see blue arrows) to respond to the environment. That response could either effect muscle movement or it can invoke the autonomic nervous system (ANS). The ANS controls the "fight or flight" response and all of our internal organs.

all incoming and outgoing information through various cables and connections. The CNS receives input from various receptors throughout the body, interprets the stimulus received via these sensory neurons, makes decisions, and directs actions to be carried out. These messages are then sent back out to the body via motor neurons or effectors, which carry out the desired action in various muscles and glands throughout the body. Computers work in a very similar manner—the CPU interprets data from the keyboard, mouse, disk drives, and so forth, and makes decisions and produces output actions such as printing. The whole system is connected

by cables that function like the efferent and afferent nerves, sending and receiving information back and forth between the various components.

Peripheral Nervous System (PNS)

The peripheral nervous system (PNS) consists of all nervous tissue outside of the brain and spinal cord and is subdivided into two divisions, the *somatic* and *autonomic* nervous system. Of these two, we will spend the majority of our discussion on the autonomic nervous system, because this area has the greatest direct effect on cardiac function.

Autonomic Nervous System The autonomic nervous system (ANS) sends sensory impulses from internal structures (such as the blood vessels, the heart, and organs of the chest, abdomen, and pelvis) through afferent autonomic nerves to the brain. The responses to these stimuli are carried back to the organ systems by efferent autonomic nerves, which cause appropriate responses from the heart, vascular system, and other organs of the body to change the way they are functioning or behaving. We are rarely aware that this exchange of information is occurring, as these messages do not reach our consciousness, but cause a reflexive or automatic response.

The ANS is considered to be "automatic" or involuntary because we cannot control or dictate functions under its control to happen. The ANS is divided into two further subdivisions: the *sympathetic nervous system* and the *parasympathetic nervous system*. These two systems have opposing effects and are constantly in a tug-of-war over control of the body (Figure 2-8). The sympathetic system causes a "speeding up" of the system while the parasympathetic "slows down" the system.

The heart, like most of our major organs and glands, receives both sympathetic and parasympathetic stimuli. The sympathetic stimulus increases the heart rate and contractility of the muscle, while the parasympathetic impulses decrease the rate. The constant tug-of-war between these two different sets of stimuli determines the final heart rate and contractility status.

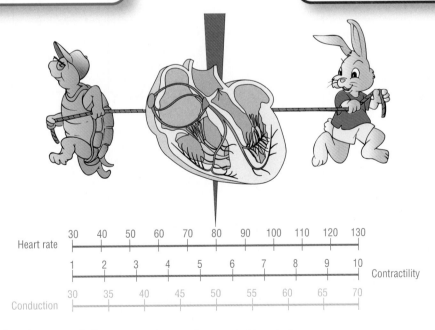

Parasympathetic:

1. Slows rate
2. Decreases contractility
3. Slows conduction through the AV node.

Main chemical messenger:
Acetylcholine

Sympathetic:

1. Speeds up rate
2. Increases contractility
3. Speeds conduction through the AV node.

Main chemical messenger:
Epinephrine

Figure 2-8: The sympathetic and parasympathetic nervous systems are in a constant tug-of-war, competing for final control over the body's response to stimuli.

Sympathetic Nervous System and the Heart

Also known as the "fight or flight" response, the sympathetic nervous system is dominant during periods of stress or activity. Control of the heart rate and force of contraction in response to stress is primarily under the control of the sympathetic nervous system. Sympathetic nerve fibers stimulate all parts of the atria and ventricles. Stimulation of the sympathetic nervous system causes the release of various chemical messengers including *epinephrine* and *norepinephrine* (Figure 2-9).

Epinephrine is the sympathetic nervous system's primary chemical messenger that activates a specific type of receptor in the heart known as the beta-1 ($ß_1$) adrenergic receptors. The results of epinephrine's effect on the heart are an increased heart rate (positive chronotropic effect), increased conduction velocity (positive dromotropic effect), and finally an increased force of contraction in the ventricular muscle itself (positive inotropic effect). Epinephrine causes a shortening of phase 4 of the action potential, essentially

---

ADDITIONAL INFORMATION

Sympathetic Nervous System

Adrenergic: Relating to nerve fibers that release norepinephrine or epinephrine.

Sympathomimetic: Effects resembling those caused by stimulation of the sympathetic nervous system, such as the effects seen following the injection of epinephrine into a patient.

Sympatholytic: Interfering with or inhibiting the effect of the impulses from the sympathetic nervous system.

An easy way to remember these two terms:

> When you ***mimic*** something, you imitate it (sympatho***mimetic***).
> When you ***lyse*** it, you dissolve it (sympatho***lytic***).

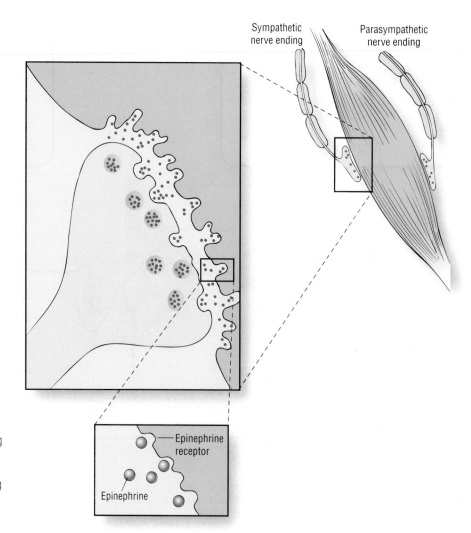

Figure 2-9: Two nerve endings are ending in their neuromuscular junctions (area where the nerve ending and the muscles meet). The close up shows some vesicles filled with chemical messengers or neurotransmitters, which are released from the nerve ending to the gap between the cells. The neurotransmitters cross the gap and attach to the receptors on the surface of the myocardial cell in order to affect it.

speeding up the pacemaking action of the SA node and all of the other pacemaker cells as well.

Parasympathetic Nervous System and the Heart
Parasympathetic nerve fibers also stimulate the atria, ventricles and, especially, the sinoatrial (SA) and atrioventricular (AV) nodes. The main efferent pathway from the CNS to the heart occurs via the *vagus* nerve (cranial nerve 10). The primary neurotransmitter, or chemical messenger, of the parasympathetic nervous system is *acetylcholine*. Acetylcholine influences the system by slowing the rate of depolarization, essentially making cardiac cells less excitable.

In the SA node, the slowing qualities of acetylcholine decrease the rate of firing for the pacemaking cells, which in turn reduces the heart rate. Another effect of acetylcholine is to decrease the conduction velocity through the AV node—this can create a temporal separation between the contraction of the atria and ventricles. Sometimes the effect on the AV node can actually cause a complete block, essentially shutting down all communication between the atria and the ventricles.

In closing, this discussion was intended as a brief introduction into the autonomic nervous system and its control over the heart. As you can see, the effect of the ANS on arrhythmia generation and management strategies is extensive. However, for our purposes, this brief discussion should suffice. Further discussion of the various chemical messengers and receptors is more appropriate for a textbook on pharmacology or an advanced text on arrhythmias.

ADDITIONAL **INFORMATION**

Parasympathetic Nervous System

Parasympathomimetic: Effects resembling those caused by stimulation of the parasympathetic nervous system.

Parasympatholytic: Interfering with or inhibiting impulses from the parasympathetic nervous system.

Cholinergic: Liberating acetylcholine or an agent that produces the effects of acetylcholine.

CHAPTER REVIEW

1. Which of the following is **incorrect:**
   A. Na^+
   B. K^-
   C. Ca^{++}
   D. Cl^-
   E. K^+

2. There is a high concentration of sodium inside of the cell. True or False.

3. There is a high concentration of potassium outside the cell. True or False.

4. The electrical potential of the resting myocytes is:
   A. +70 to +90 mV
   B. +100 to +120 mV
   C. Approximately zero
   D. −70 to −90 mV
   E. −100 to −120 mV

5. The sodium-potassium ATPase pumps use ATP to push two sodium ions out and bring one potassium ion into the cell. This creates a net negative charge inside the cell. True or False.

6. Actin and myosin are the protein chains that shorten the myocytes. Which *ion* acts like a key that allows the troponin/ tropomyosin complex to clamp these two together so they can interact?
   A. Sodium
   B. Potassium
   C. Calcium
   D. Magnesium
   E. Chloride

7. The cell is polarized in the normal resting state prior to firing. True or False.

8. The cell fires when the action potential is reached. The cell is polarized during this process. True or False.

9. Which one of the following has the fastest pacemaking function:
   A. SA node
   B. Atrial myocytes
   C. AV node
   D. Bundle branches
   E. Ventricular myocytes

10. The electrochemical activity of polarization-depolarization is measurable by the ECG. True or False.

11. The central nervous system primarily controls the heart and other organs through the _____ _____ _____.

12. The autonomic nervous system is further subdivided into the _____ nervous system and the _____ nervous system.

13. The two subsystems are constantly in a tug-of-war over which one will control the effects of the body. In the heart, the sympathetic nervous system _____ the rate and _____ contractility, while the parasympathetic nervous system _____ the rate and _____ contractility.

14. The primary chemical messenger for the sympathetic nervous system is _____.

15. The primary chemical messenger for the parasympathetic nervous system is _____.

16. _____ is a chemical messenger that speeds conduction through the AV node.

17. _____ is a chemical messenger that slows down conduction through the AV node.

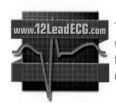
To enhance the knowledge you gain in this book, access this text's website at www.12leadECG.com! This valuable resource provides flashcards, an online glossary, web links, and more. Simply click on the Arrhythmias book cover once at the site.

CHAPTER 3

Vectors and the Basic Beat

Imagine each cell giving rise to its own electrical impulse. These impulses vary in intensity and direction. We use the term vector to describe these electrical impulses. A vector is a diagrammatic way to show the strength and the direction of the electrical impulse. For example, suppose the amount of electrical activity generated by a cell is worth $1.00 and is directed to the top of the page. We'll call that line Vector A (Figure 3-1). Now, another cell has an electrical discharge that is worth $2.00 and faces the upper right corner. The latter, Vector B, will be twice as big as Vector A. Well, as you can imagine, the heart has a few million of these individual vectors (Figure 3-2).

Adding and Subtracting Vectors

Vectors represent amounts of energy and direction. They add up when they are going in the same direction, and cancel each other out if they point in opposite directions. If they are at an angle to each other, they add or subtract energy and change directions when they meet (Figure 3-3). This is a brief introduction to vector mathematics. A good physics book will give you additional information.

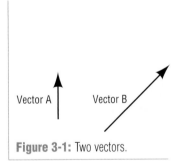

Figure 3-1: Two vectors.

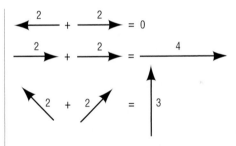

Figure 3-3: Examples of adding vectors.

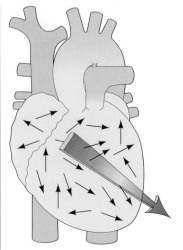

Figure 3-2: The heart contains millions of vectors.

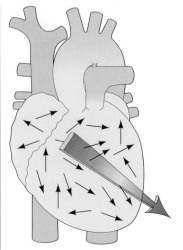

Figure 3-4: Sum of all ventricular vectors = electrical axis.

The Electrical Axis of the Heart

Now, take the sum of all of the millions of vectors found in the ventricles of the heart. We'll wait a few minutes while you add them up. That final vector, after all of the addition, subtraction, and direction changes, is known as the electrical axis of the ventricle (Figure 3-4). In the same way, each wave and segment has its own respective vector. There is a P-wave vector, a T-wave vector, an ST segment vector, and a QRS vector. The ECG is a measurement of these vectors as they pass under an electrode. That's it! It is an electronic representation of the electrical movement of the main vectors passing under an electrode, or a lead. In the next pages, we are only going to discuss the QRS vector.

Electrodes and Waves

The electrodes are sensing devices that pick up the electrical activity occurring beneath them. When a positive electrical impulse is moving away from the electrode (Figure 3-5, A), the ECG machine converts it into a negative (downward) wave. When a positive wave moves toward an electrode, the ECG records a positive (upward) wave (Figure 3-5, C). When the electrode is somewhere in the middle (Figure 3-5, B), the ECG shows a positive deflection for the amount of energy that is coming toward it and a negative wave for the amount going away from it. This is similar to the Doppler effect. We are all familiar with this effect when an ambulance approaches us with its siren on. As it moves closer, it gets louder; as it gets further away, the noise diminishes.

Leads Are Like Pictures of the Heart

So, the electrodes (leads) pick up the electrical activity of the vectors, and the ECG machine converts them to waves. Think of each set of waves as a picture. Now, imagine that we place various elec-

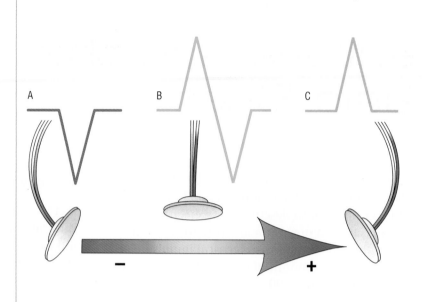

Figure 3-5: Three different ECGs resulting from the same vector, due to different lead placements.

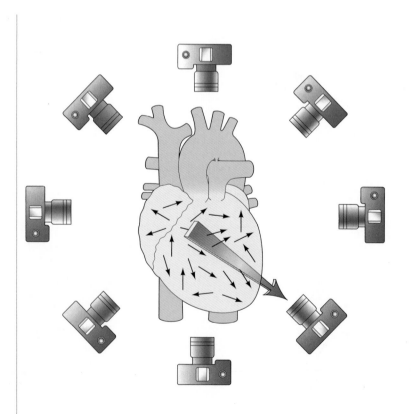

Figure 3-6: Leads view the heart from different angles.

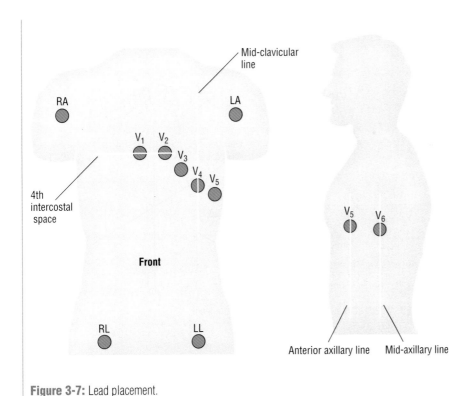

Figure 3-7: Lead placement.

Figure 3-8: Leads I, II, and III.

trodes—or cameras, for this analogy—at certain angles to the main axis (Figure 3-6). We would get multiple pictures of the heart from a three-dimensional perspective. Think of an ECG as a picture album, and it will be easy. To make matters more interesting, suppose we gave you multiple photographs of a toy elephant, including some reference for scale. Would you be able to put them together three-dimensionally in your mind's eye? Of course you would! This is all an ECG is meant to give us: a three-dimensional picture of the heart's electrical axes. From this picture, we can get all sorts of information about where pathologic processes—such as infarcts, hypertrophy, and blocks—are occurring.

Lead Placement (Where to Put the "Cameras")

All right, so where do you place the cameras, or electrodes? You place them over the areas shown in Figure 3-7. The limb leads (extremity leads)—the right arm (RA), left arm (LA), right leg (RL), and left leg (LL)—are placed at least 10 cm from the heart. It doesn't matter if you place the arm leads on the shoulders or the arms, as long as they're 10 cm from the heart. The precordial leads (chest leads), however, have to be placed exactly. Position V_1 and V_2 on each side of the sternum at the fourth intercostal space. To find the space, first isolate the Angle of Louis. This is a hump located near the top third of the sternum. Start feeling down your sternum from the top, and you'll feel it. It is located next to the second rib. The space directly beneath it is the second intercostal space. Count down two more spaces and you're there. V_4 is at the fifth intercostal space in the mid-clavicular line. Follow the diagram for the remaining positions.

How the Machine Manipulates the Leads

The ECG machine reads the positive and negative poles of the limb electrodes to produce leads I, II, and III on the ECG

(Figure 3-8). In other words, the camera is placed at the positive pole and aimed down the lead in question. In physics, two vectors (or in this case leads) are equal as long as they are parallel and of the same intensity and polarity. Therefore, we can move the leads from the locations shown in Figure 3-8 to a point passing through the center of the heart, and they will be the same (Figure 3-9, A). By doing some complicated vector manipulation, the machine comes up with three additional leads (Figure 3-9, B).

The Two Lead Systems

The Hexaxial System

Now, let's combine A and B from Figure 3-9. Using the same principle as before—that leads can be moved as long as the resultant lead is parallel and of the same polarity—we can produce the hexaxial system (Figure 3-10). Think of this as a system of analyzing vectors that cuts the center of the heart along a plane, creating a front half and a back half. It would be as if there were a glass sheet dividing the body from ear to ear. In anatomical terminology, this is called a coronal cut. Keep in mind as you proceed that what you are evaluating is how the vector would project on the two-dimensional glass sheet and not on the three-dimensional anterior or posterior parts of the heart.

The hexaxial system gives rise to the six limb leads: I, II, III, aVR, aVL, and aVF. Traditionally, the side of the lead that has the positive electrode, or pole, is the one that has the lead name at its end (Figure 3-9). Hence, the positive pole of lead I is at the right side of the circle, the positive pole of aVF is down, and so on. Also, note that the leads are 30 degrees apart. This will be very useful when we talk about axis.

The Precordial System

Remember the precordial leads—the ones on the chest itself? Think of these leads as sitting on a plane that is perpen-

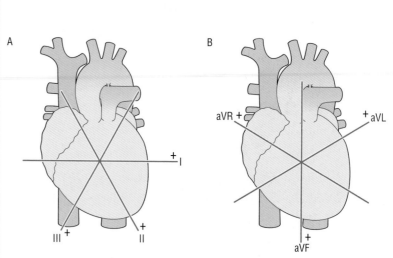

Figure 3-9: Vector manipulation results in three more leads.

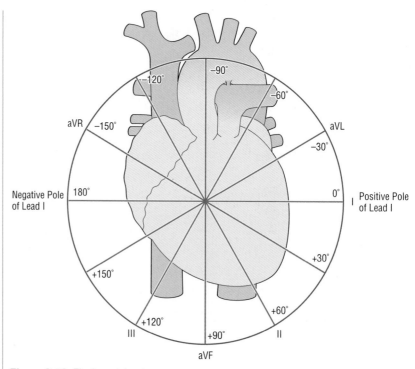

Figure 3-10: The hexaxial system.

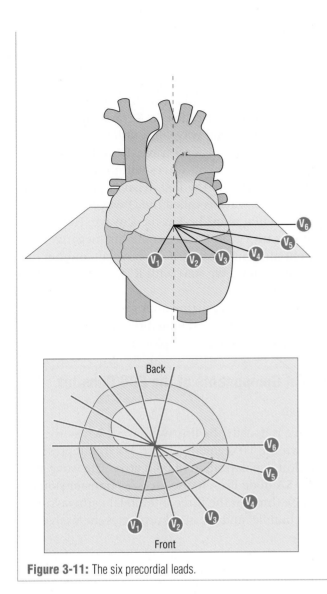

Figure 3-11: The six precordial leads.

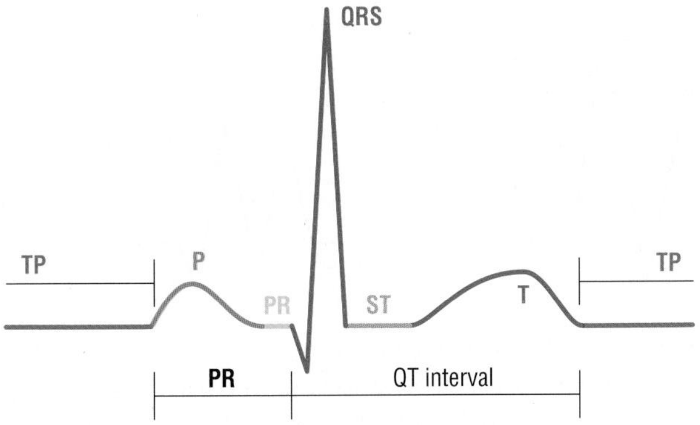

dicular to the limb leads. Again imagine a glass sheet, this time splitting the body through the center of the heart, into top and bottom halves. This is called a transverse plane. The result is a cross section, with six leads produced by the six chest electrodes (Figure 3-11).

The Basic Beat

Well, if you've gotten this far, you're ready for some true ECG interpretation! This is where we start looking at what all of those lines mean. We'll begin with the basic beat, or complex. This is one cycle of the heart represented electrocardiographically. We are going to break down the complex into its component parts. In this section of the book, we will just introduce you to the concepts involved with each of the components. In Part 2 we'll show you actual examples and their variations as they appear clinically. Let's get started.

Introduction to Basic Components

Figure 3-12 shows the basic components of the ECG complex. Here are some basic definitions. A wave is a deflection from the baseline that represents some cardiac event. For instance, the P wave represents atrial depolarization. A segment is a specific portion of the complex as it is represented on the ECG. For example, the segment between the end of the P wave and the beginning of the Q wave is known as the PR segment. An interval is the distance, measured as time, occurring between two cardiac events. The time interval between the beginning of the P wave and the beginning of the QRS complex is known as the PR interval. Note that there is a PR interval, as well as a PR segment. In addition to the waves shown in Figure 3-12, there are a few others not mentioned below, such as the R' (R prime) wave and the U wave, which we will talk about individually. There are also other intervals that we are going to cover, such as the R-R interval

Figure 3-12: Basic components of the ECG complex.

and the P-P interval. Making sure that you understand the definitions of the basic terms will help prevent confusion. In Figure 3-12, we have labeled the waves and segments with colored letters and the intervals with black letters for easier identification.

Wave Nomenclature

A wave represents an electrical event in the heart, such as atrial depolarization, atrial repolarization, ventricular depolarization, ventricular repolarization, or transmission through the His bundles, and so on. Waves can be single, isolated, positive, or negative deflections; biphasic deflections with both positive and negative components; or combinations that have multiple positive and negative components. Waves are deflections from the baseline. What is the baseline? It is a line from one TP segment to the next.

Let's look at what that means in Figure 3-13. Note that the QRS complex is a combination of two or more waves. To be completely correct, these waves should be named according to size, location, and direction of deflection. Tall or deep waves in the QRS complex are given capital letters: Q, R, S, R'. Small waves are given small letters: q, r, s, r'. This is why the example in Figure 3-13 is called a qRs wave. This standard is unfortunately not followed as rigorously as you might expect. Many authors simply use all capital letters. In this book, we will follow the standard nomenclature with capital and small letters.

R' and S' Waves Just to make matters more interesting, let's look at some problems with the QRS waves. Changes occurring in the QRS complex can lead to bizarre complexes, and their waves are named differently if they change directions and cross the baseline. Such a wave is called an X' (X prime) wave, in which X is not an actual wave, but rather a term that can stand for either an R or S wave. R' and S' (R prime and S prime) refer to extra waves within the QRS complex. By definition, the first negative wave that we reach after the P wave is called the Q wave. The first positive deflection after the P is the R wave. Here is where it gets tricky: an S wave is the first negative component after an R wave. If we now get another upward component, we start with R'. The next negative component is S'.

A positive wave occurring after the S' would then be an R" wave (read as R double prime), and so on. Figure 3-14 shows some examples.

Individual Components of the ECG Complex

The P Wave

The P wave is usually the first wave we reach as we travel down the TP segment (Figure 3-15). It represents the electrical depolarization of both atria. The wave starts when the SA node fires. It also includes transmission of the impulse through the three internodal pathways, the Bachman bundle, and the atrial myocytes themselves.

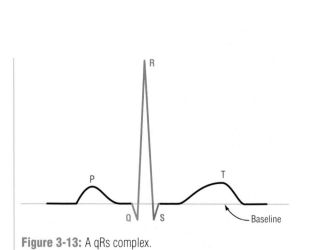

Figure 3-13: A qRs complex.

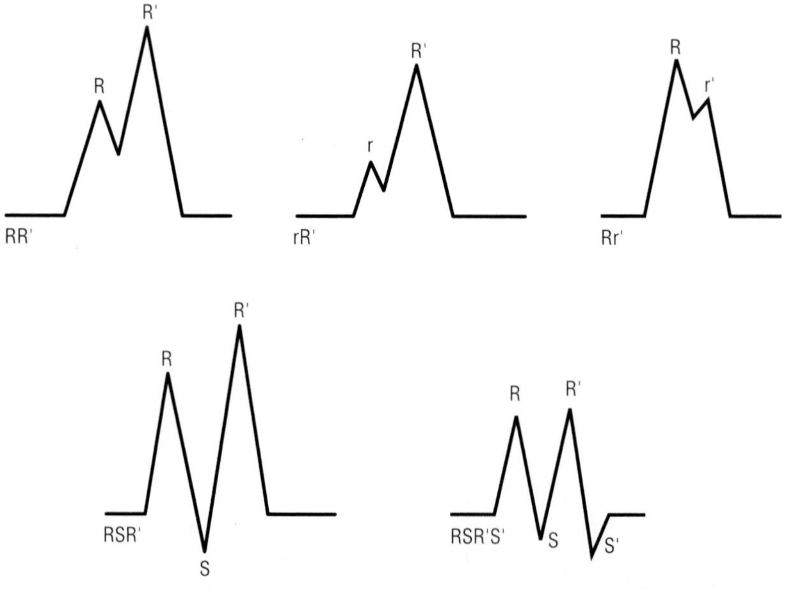

Figure 3-14: R' and S' complexes (NOTE: The top row does not technically contain S waves. The term S wave only applies to negative components, or components that fall below the baseline. However, it is common for people to refer to any dip in a notched R wave as an S wave, regardless of whether or not it falls below the baseline. By following this logic further, most authors and clinicians refer to the second peak as the R' wave. Although this nomenclature is technically incorrect, it is so common that people accept this as the norm.)

The duration of the wave itself can vary between 0.08 and 0.11 seconds in normal adults. The axis of the P wave is usually directed downward and to the left, the direction the electrical impulse travels on its journey to the atrioventricular node and the atrial appendages.

The Tp Wave

The Tp wave, which represents repolarization of the atria, deflects in the opposite direction of the P wave (Figure 3-16). It is usually not seen because it occurs at the same time as the QRS wave and is obscured (buried) by that more powerful complex. However, you can sometimes see it when there is no QRS after the P wave. This occurs in AV dissociation or nonconducted beats. You may also see it in PR depression, or in the ST segment depression present in very fast sinus tachycardias. It appears as ST depression because the QRS comes sooner in the cycle, and the Tp wave—if it is negative—draws the ST segment downward.

The PR Segment

The PR segment occupies the time frame between the end of the P wave and the beginning of the QRS complex (Figure 3-17). It is usually found along the baseline. It can, however, be depressed by less than 0.8 mm under normal circumstances; anything greater than that is pathological. It is pathologically depressed in pericarditis, and when there is an atrial infarct (a rare occurrence).

The PR Interval

The PR interval represents the time period from the beginning of the P wave to the beginning of the QRS complex (Figure 3-18). It includes the P wave and the PR segment, both discussed previously. The PR interval

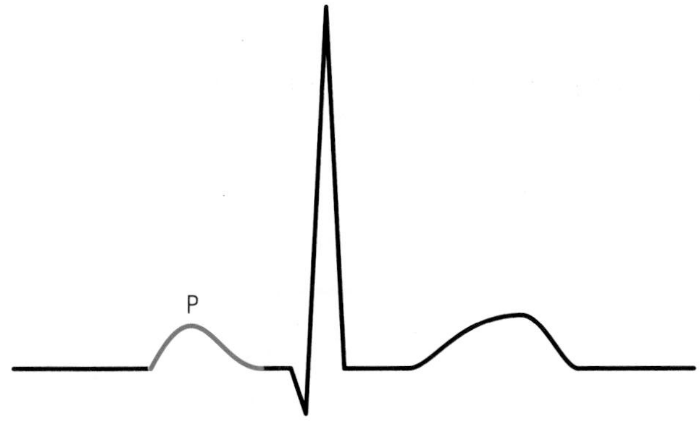

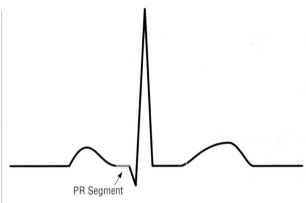

Figure 3-15: The P wave.
Cardiac event represented by the P wave: Atrial depolarization
Normal duration: 0.08 to 0.11 seconds
Axis: 0 to +75°, downward and to the left

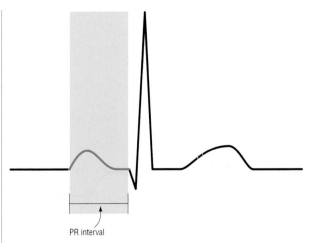

Figure 3-17: The PR segment.
Cardiac event represented by the PR segment:
Transmission of the electrical depolarization wave through the AV node, His bundles, bundle branches, and Purkinje system

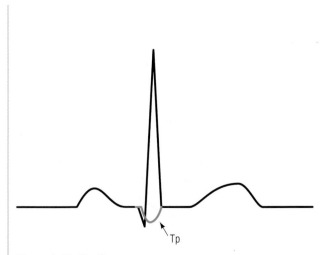

Figure 3-16: The Tp wave.
Cardiac event represented by the Tp wave: Atrial repolarization
Normal duration: Usually not seen
Wave orientation: Opposite to the P wave

Figure 3-18: The PR interval.
Cardiac events represented by the PR interval: Impulse initiation, atrial depolarization, atrial repolarization, AV node stimulation, His bundle stimulation, bundle branch, and Purkinje system stimulation
Normal duration: 0.11 to 0.20 seconds

covers all of the events from the initiation of the electrical impulse in the sinoatrial (SA) node up to the moment of ventricular depolarization. The normal duration is from 0.12 seconds to 0.20 seconds. If the PR interval is shorter than 0.11 seconds, it is considered shortened. A PR interval longer than 0.20 seconds is a first-degree AV block, which we will talk about in a later section. The PR interval can be quite long, sometimes 0.40 seconds or greater. The term PQ interval is sometimes used interchangeably if there is a Q wave as the initial component of the QRS complex.

The QRS Complex

The QRS complex represents ventricular depolarization. It is composed of two or more waves (Figure 3-19). Each wave has its own name or label. These can become quite complex. The main components are the Q, R, and S waves. By convention, the Q wave is the first negative deflection after the P wave. The Q wave can be present or absent. The R wave is the first positive deflection after the P. This will be the initial wave of the QRS complex if there is no Q present. The first negative deflection after the R wave is the S wave. If there are additional components in the QRS complex, they will be named as prime waves (see Figure 3-14).

Q Wave Significance The Q wave can be benign, or it can be a sign of dead myocardial tissue. A Q wave is considered significant if it is 0.03 seconds or wider, or its height is equal to or greater than one-third the height of the R wave (Figure 3-20). If it meets either of these criteria, it indicates a myocardial infarction (MI) over the region involved. If it doesn't, it is not a significant Q wave (Figure 3-21). Insignificant Q waves are

commonly found in I, aVL, and V$_6$, where they are due to septal innervation. These are therefore called septal Qs.

The Intrinsicoid Deflection The intrinsicoid deflection is measured from the beginning of the QRS complex to the beginning of the negative downslope of the R wave in leads that begin with an R wave and do not contain a Q wave (Figure 3-22). It represents the amount of time it takes the electrical impulse to travel from the Purkinje system in the endocardium to the surface of the epicardium immediately under an electrode. It is shorter (up to 0.035 seconds) in the right precordial

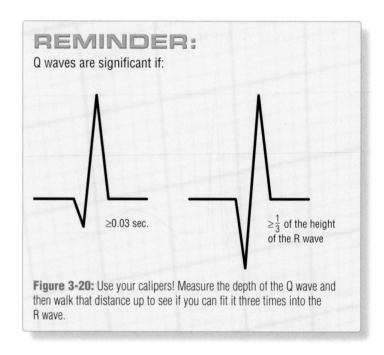

REMINDER:
Q waves are significant if:

≥0.03 sec.

≥$\frac{1}{3}$ of the height of the R wave

Figure 3-20: Use your calipers! Measure the depth of the Q wave and then walk that distance up to see if you can fit it three times into the R wave.

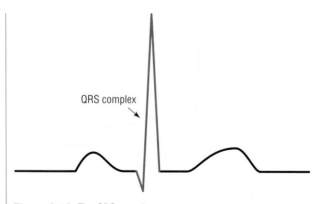

QRS complex

Figure 3-19: The QRS complex.
Cardiac event represented by the QRS complex: Ventricular depolarization
Normal duration: 0.06 to 0.11 seconds
Axis: −30 to + 105°, downward and to the left

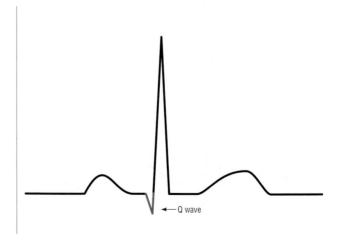

Q wave

Figure 3-21: Insignificant Q wave.

leads, V_1 through V_2, because the right ventricle is thin in comparison with the left. It is longer (up to 0.045 seconds) in the left precordial leads, V_5 to V_6, because of the left ventricle's greater thickness. Now, can you imagine what would cause the intrinsicoid deflection to be prolonged? You will see a longer intrinsicoid deflection if there is a thicker myocardium, as in ventricular hypertrophy, or when it takes longer for the electrical system to conduct that area, because of an intraventricular conduction delay such as, for instance, a left bundle branch block.

The ST Segment

The ST segment is the section of the ECG cycle from the end of the QRS complex to the beginning of the T wave. The point where the QRS complex ends and the ST segment begins is called the J point (Figure 3-23). Many times, a clear J point cannot be identified because of ST segment elevation. The ST segment is usually found along the baseline. However, it can vary up to 1 mm from baseline in the limb leads of normal patients, and up to 3 mm in the right precordials of some patients. This is caused either by left ventricular hypertrophy or by what is referred to as the early repolarization pattern.

Now, having made the statements about ST elevation and normal variants above, we need to make a clarification that you will hear many more times. Any ST elevation in a symptomatic patient should be consid-ered significant and representative of myocardial injury or infarction until proven otherwise. Don't make the mistake of calling an acute MI a normal variant! Just because an ST segment is not elevated enough to meet the guidelines for the administration of thrombolytics (presently 1 mm in two contiguous leads) does not mean that it is benign. You must have a high index of suspicion in these cases and try to obtain an old ECG to compare.

The ST segment represents an electrically neutral time for the heart. The ventricles are between depolarization (QRS complex) and repolarization (T wave). Mechanically, this represents the time that the myocardium is maintaining contraction in order to push the blood out of the ventricles. As you can imagine, very little blood would be expelled if the ventricles only contracted for 0.12 seconds.

The T Wave

The T wave represents ventricular repolarization (Figure 3-24). It is the next deflection—either positive or negative—that occurs after the ST segment and should begin in the same direction as the QRS complex.

Why should the T wave be in the same direction as the QRS? If it represents repolarization, shouldn't it be opposite the QRS? For the answer, we need to go back to the concept of ventricular excitation. The Purkinje system is near the endocardium; therefore, electrical depolarization should begin in the endocardium and move

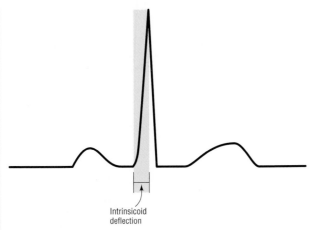

Figure 3-22: The intrinsicoid deflection.
Upper limit of normal for the intrinsicoid deflection:
In right precordials = 0.035 seconds
In left precordials = 0.045 seconds

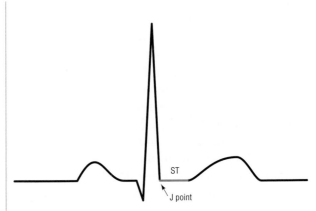

Figure 3-23: The J point.
Cardiac event represented by the ST segment: Electrically neutral period between ventricular depolarization and repolarization.
Normal location: At the level of the baseline
Axis: Inferior and to the left

out toward the epicardium (Figure 3-25, top arrow).

You would expect repolarization to occur in the same direction because the cell that was first depolarized should be the first to repolarize, but this is not the case. Because of increased pressure on the endocardium during contraction, the repolarization wave travels in the opposite direction, from the epicardium back to the endocardium (Figure 3-25, bottom arrow). Remember, a negative wave—and repolarization is a negative wave—traveling away from the electrode is perceived the same as a positive wave moving toward it. Hence, the normal T wave should be in the same direction as the QRS. There are exceptions in some pathological states.

The T wave should be asymmetrical, with the first part rising or dropping slowly and the latter part moving much faster (Figure 3-26). The way to check for symmetry of the T wave, if the ST segment is elevated, is to draw a perpendicular line from the peak of that wave to the baseline and then compare the symmetry of the two sides, ignoring the ST segment (Figure 3-27). Symmetric Ts can be normal, but are usually a sign of pathology.

The QT interval

The QT interval is the section of the ECG complex encompassing the QRS complex, the ST segment, and the T wave—from the beginning of the Q to the end of the T (Figure 3-28). It represents all of the events of ventricular systole, from the beginning of ventricular depolarization to the end of the repolarization cycle. The interval varies with heart rate, electrolyte abnormalities, age, and sex. A prolonged QT is a harbinger of possible arrhythmias, especially torsade de pointes. This is not a common occurrence, but it is life threatening. The QT interval should be shorter than one half

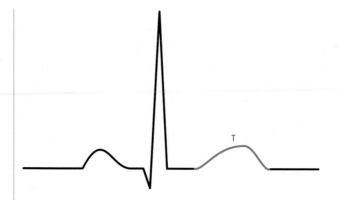

Figure 3-24: The T wave.
Cardiac event represented by the T wave: Ventricular repolarization
Axis: Downward and to the left, similar to the QRS axis

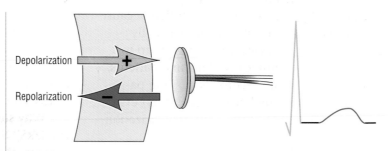

Figure 3-25: Depolarization and repolarization.

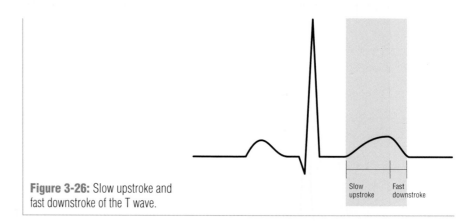

Figure 3-26: Slow upstroke and fast downstroke of the T wave.

Slow upstroke   Fast downstroke

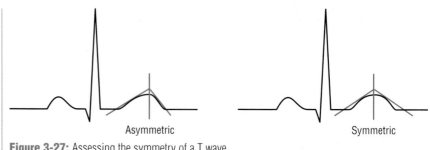

Asymmetric   Symmetric

Figure 3-27: Assessing the symmetry of a T wave.

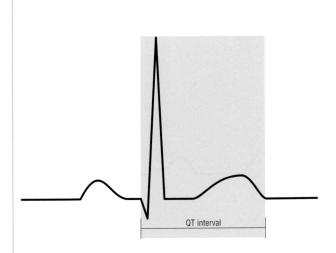

Figure 3-28: The QT interval.
Cardiac events represented by the QT interval: All the events of ventricular systole
Normal duration: Variable, especially with heart rate. Usually less than half of the R-R inteveral

REMINDER:

QTc = QT + 1.75 (ventricular rate − 60)
Cardiac events represented by the QTc interval: All the events of ventricular systole
Normal duration: 0.410 seconds
Prolonged QTc interval: >0.419 seconds

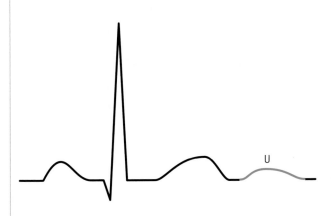

Figure 3-29: The U wave.
Cardiac event represented by the U wave: Unknown
Important points: Low voltage; deflects in the same direction as the T wave
Clinical importance: Usually benign. The most important clinical significance of a U wave is that it could potentially be a sign of hypokalemia.

of the preceding R-R interval (the interval between the peaks of the two preceding R waves). There are various formulas to evaluate the significance of a QT interval, but the most useful one is to evaluate the QTc (discussed next).

The QTc Interval The QTc interval stands for the QT corrected interval. What is it corrected for? Heart rate. As the heart rate decreases, the QT interval lengthens; conversely, as the heart rate increases, the QT interval shortens. This makes it hard to calculate the interval at which the QT is normal. By calculating the QTc interval, we can state that normal is around 0.410 seconds or 410 milliseconds. Giving a little leeway, we will say that anything above 0.419 seconds is lengthened. The formula for calculating the QTc appears in the box that follows. Most ECG machines will automatically calculate the interval for you.

The U Wave

The U wave is a small, flat wave sometimes seen after the T wave and before the next P wave (Figure 3-29). Various theories have arisen about what it represents, including ventricular depolarization and endocardial repolarization. Nobody knows for sure. It can be seen in normal patients, especially in the presence of bradycardia. It can also be seen in hypokalemia (low potassium). One valuable point is that there can be no possibility of hyperkalemia in the presence of a U wave (more about this later). The only other clinical significance of the U is that it can sometimes cause an inaccuracy in measuring the QT interval. This can lead to a longer-than-accurate value because some machines may include this interval in their measurements. ECG computers are notorious for this miscalculation.

Additional Intervals

There are a few additional intervals that we will cover as the text continues. However, let's talk about two of the most common ones now. First, there is the R-R interval, the distance between identical points (usually the peaks) of two consecutive QRS complexes (Figure 3-30). You will be measuring this often to evaluate the rhythm. Regular rhythms are those that have consistent R-R intervals.

Another is the P-P interval, the distance between two identical points on one P wave and the next (Figure 3-30). This interval will be very useful in evaluating the patient for rhythm abnormalities. Examples include Wenckebach second-degree heart block, atrial flutter, and third-degree heart block. We will discuss these rhythm abnormalities later in the book.

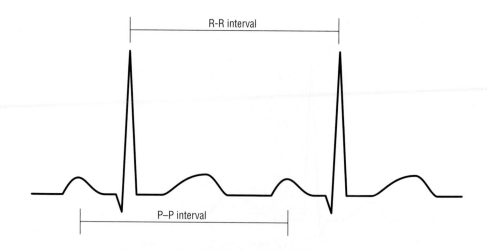

Figure 3-30: The P-P interval and the R-R interval.

CLINICAL PEARL

The true baseline of the ECG is a line drawn from the TP of one complex to the TP of another. The PR segment should fall on this line, but many times it does not. Fluctuations from the baseline may signify pathology.

CHAPTER **REVIEW**

1. Which of the following is **correct:**
   A. A vector is a diagrammatic way to show the *strength* of an electrical impulse.
   B. A vector is a diagrammatic way to show the *direction* of an electrical impulse.
   C. Both A and B are correct.
   D. Both A and B are incorrect.

2. The electrical axis of the heart is a vector representing the summation of all of the individual vectors that make ventricular depolarization. True or False.

3. Which of the following statements is **incorrect:**
   A. Electrodes are sensing devices that pick up electrical activity taking place beneath them.
   B. A positive electrical wave moving toward an electrode is represented on the ECG as a positive wave.
   C. A positive electrical wave moving away from an electrode is represented on the ECG as a negative wave.
   D. A positive electrical wave moving toward an electrode is represented on the ECG as an isoelectric segment.

4. An electrical lead is like a camera taking a picture of the electrical axis from its particular vantage point. A 12-lead ECG is like a picture album representing the "shots" taken by the 12 individual leads in a systematic format. True or False.

5. The baseline is a straight line drawn between the ____ of one complex to the ____ of the succeeding complex.
   A. PR segment–PR segment
   B. Beginning of one P–beginning of the next P
   C. TP segment–TP segment
   D. QT interval–QT interval
   E. None of the above

6. The P wave represents atrial repolarization and innervation of the atrial myocytes. True or False.

7. The PR segment and the PR interval both represent the same time frame. True or False.

8. The normal duration for the PR interval is _____ seconds.
   A. 0.08–0.10
   B. 0.11–0.15
   C. 0.11–0.20
   D. 0.20–0.24
   E. None of the above

9. The normal duration for the QRS interval is _____ seconds.
   A. 0.06–0.08
   B. 0.06–0.11
   C. 0.08–0.14
   D. 0.12–0.20
   E. None of the above

10. Q waves are significant if:
    A. They are $\geq$ 0.03 seconds (one little block) wide
    B. They are deeper than $1/3$ the height of the R wave
    C. Both A and B are correct
    D. Both A and B are incorrect
    E. None of the above

11. The T wave represents ventricular repolarization. True or False.

12. The T waves are usually asymmetrical. True or False.

13. The QT should always be more than $1/2$ the preceding R-R interval. True or False.

14. The U wave is a small, flat wave seen after the T wave and before the next P wave. True or False.

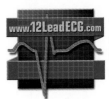

To enhance the knowledge you gain in this book, access this text's website at www.12leadECG.com! This valuable resource provides flashcards, an online glossary, web links, and more. Simply click on the Arrhythmias book cover once at the site.

CHAPTER 4

The Rhythm Strip, Tools, and Calculating Rates

Boxes and Sizes

The pen will record the ECG waves and segments onto the paper. To keep things simple, we have drawn straight horizontal lines to represent the complexes in Figure 4-1.

The ECG paper passes under the pen at a rate of 25 mm/sec. Each little box is, therefore, $1/25$th of a second, or 0.04 seconds. Because a big box is made up of five little boxes, it represents 5×0.04 sec $= 0.20$ sec, so five big boxes make 1 second.

There are usually some small marks along the bottom of the strip every 3 seconds so that you can keep tabs on the time more easily. The lead should be appropriately labeled by the machine or the person obtaining the strip for easy identification. In addition, the patient's name and hospital number (when appropriate) should be labeled at the beginning or end of the strip.

When we talk about the vertical height of a wave or segment, we use millimeters; for instance, a wave that is five little boxes high would, in reality, be five millimeters high. Likewise, a darker big box is five millimeters high.

It will be very useful to keep these measurements in mind, especially when we discuss rates and widths of waves and segments. Everything on the rhythm strip is measured in millimeters or milliseconds, and you will use these measurements to describe your findings when examining the strip.

As an example, a wave can be described as being 15 mm high and 0.06 seconds wide. This would tell us that the height of the wave is 15 little boxes or three big boxes, and the width is 1.5 little boxes. With a bit of practice, you'll have this mastered.

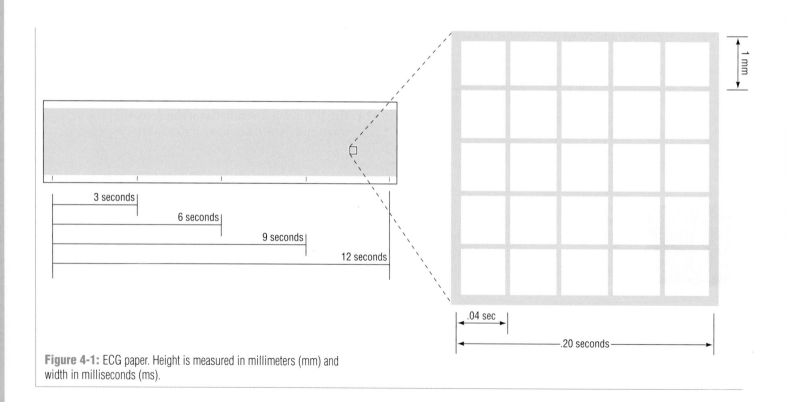

Figure 4-1: ECG paper. Height is measured in millimeters (mm) and width in milliseconds (ms).

Calibration

Sometimes, at the beginning or end of each ECG strip, you will find a steplike structure called a calibration box. The standard box is 10 mm high and 0.20 seconds wide (Figure 4-2, A). The calibration box is there to confirm that the ECG recording conforms to the standard format.

Occasionally, you will find that an ECG has been formatted in half-standard calibration (Figure 4-2, B). This is usually done when the complexes are so tall that they run into each other. You will know that it is half-standard because there will be an additional step halfway up the box that lasts for half the width of the standard box. When you see this stairlike configuration, you are at half-standard.

The only other calibration you will run across is one in which the paper speed is set to 50 mm/sec, instead of the traditional 25 mm/sec. In this case, the calibration box will be 0.40 seconds wide (Figure 4-2, C).

Temporal Relationship of Multiple-Lead Strips

Quite frequently, you may obtain an ECG that has three or more leads occurring simultaneously in real time. The leads that are to be viewed will be programmed by the person obtaining the strip directly on the machine. The resulting strip will present the leads, one on top of the other.

When you have a multiple-lead strip, it is critical to remember that the events shown on the paper are occurring at the same exact time across all the visible leads when viewed vertically. For example, imagine that we have a transparent ruler with a red line running through it, placed on top of the ECG (Figure 4-3). As we move the ruler across the paper, each event that is touching that perpendicular red line occurred at the same moment. The ECG machine's computer is capable of measuring three or more leads at once and representing them on the ECG simultaneously. Please note that only those events touching the red line occurred simultaneously. Always check that the tips of the complexes are found along the same vertical line on the ECG paper. This protects you against making a mistake in interpreting the complexes.

Why Is Temporal Spacing Important?

Why are we making such a big deal about this temporal spacing thing? Consider a situation such as the one shown in Figure 4-4. To simplify matters, we have represented the complexes as stars, both five- and six-pointed. As you are interpreting the rhythm strip,

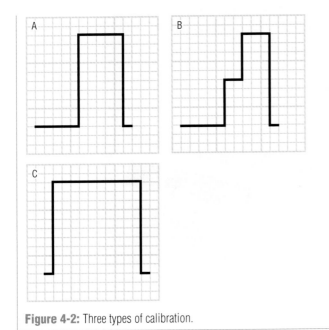

Figure 4-2: Three types of calibration.

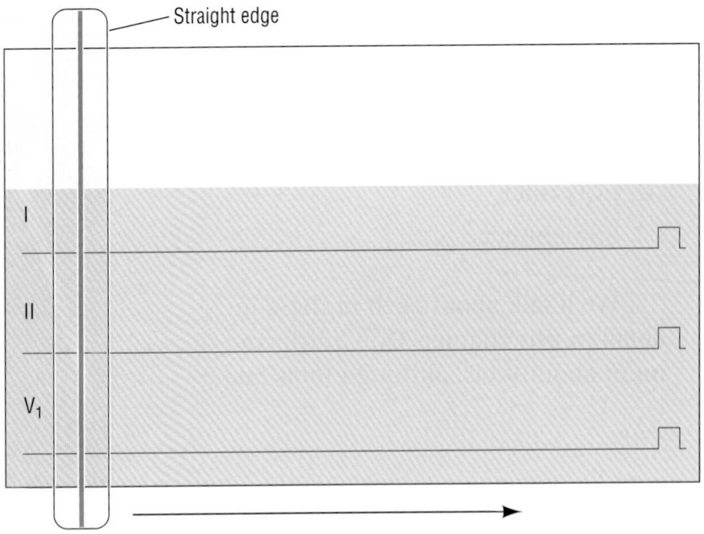

Figure 4-3: The red line represents time; events that touch the red line occurred simultaneously.

you notice on the lead V₁ rhythm strip that the fifth and sixth complexes are different—they are six-pointed stars instead of the baseline five-pointed ones. You can use this information to alter your interpretation appropriately in the other leads where the sixth point may not be as clearly visible. If you did not have a multiple-lead rhythm strip to show you that these two aberrant complexes were different, you could easily misinterpret the strip. Thanks to the multiple-lead rhythm strip, when you interpret the complexes appearing in leads I and II, you will take into account that the morphology of these QRS complexes is different from the others, and you can make the right interpretation and diagnosis.

Let's make the point crystal clear: this knowledge could dramatically alter your final diagnosis. It can—and we are trying not to be too dramatic here—save the patient's life. For a great example, have a look at the example at the end of Chapter 33. Among other things, temporal spacing is very important in determining rhythms, intervals, ST segment changes, premature complexes, and aberrantly conducted beats.

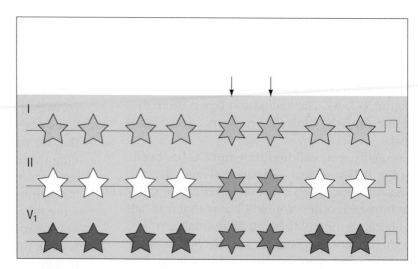

Figure 4-4: Different types of stars represent different morphologies.

> ## REMINDER:
>
> When interpreting an ECG, always check the format! Make sure that the rhythm strip is temporally related to the complexes above. (In some cases, it isn't.)

ECG Tools

There are various tools that make reading and interpreting the ECG much easier (Figure 4-5). These include:

1. Calipers
2. ECG ruler
3. Straight edge

We'll talk about each of these in detail in this chapter. One quick comment about tools: although tools make

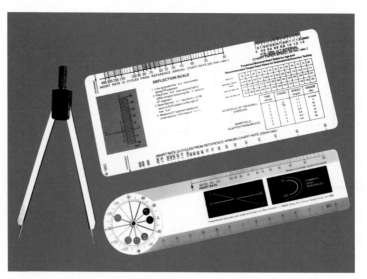

Figure 4-5: Calipers and an ECG ruler with an axis wheel and straight edge.

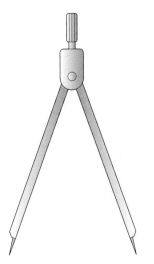

Figure 4-6: Measuring distances on the ECG with calipers.

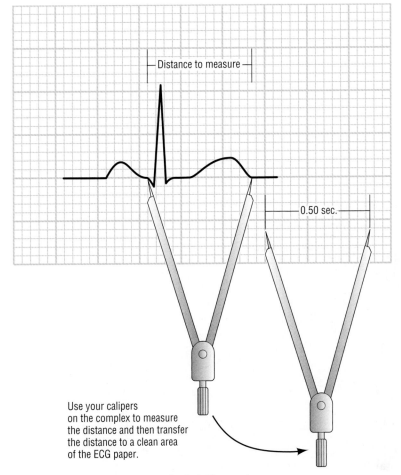

Distance to measure

0.50 sec.

Use your calipers on the complex to measure the distance and then transfer the distance to a clean area of the ECG paper.

Figure 4-7: Total width of the complex is 0.50 seconds.

your job easier, it is important not to completely depend upon them. If you do, you will feel helpless when they are not available.

Calipers: The Clinician's Best Friend

In our opinion, it is almost impossible to interpret arrhythmias with any degree of accuracy if you do not use calipers (Figure 4-6). This is a strong statement, but it is true. It is possible to measure intervals and waves without calipers. It is even possible to evaluate consistency when you are evaluating the rhythm. We have seen people do all kinds of creative markings on pieces of paper to transfer the heights and widths of complexes. However, for accuracy and dependability, nothing beats the ECG calipers. If you don't own a set, go to your nearest medical bookstore or drafting supply house to get one. Always have them with you when you work clinically. It will simplify your life.

How do you use the calipers? Place one of the pins at the beginning of the object you are measuring, and move the other pin to the end. Then you can transfer that distance to an uncluttered part of the ECG paper to evaluate the height or the time of the measured object. The following are some simple ways to use calipers.

How to Use Your Calipers

Once you have measured the distance, it is easier to calculate the actual time frame on a cleaner, less cluttered area of the ECG paper (Figure 4-7). Remember, the big boxes are 0.20 seconds; there are two of these in Figure 4-7, for a total of 0.40 seconds. The small boxes are 0.04 seconds, and there are two and a half of these for a total of 0.10 seconds.

Now, suppose you want to see if the distance between three complexes is the same. First, measure the distance between complex A and complex B. Then, without lifting the right pin, swing the left pin to see if the distance from B to C is equal (Figure 4-8). By not moving the right pin, you are ensuring that the distances are the same. Swinging one pin over the other like this is called "walking."

You can walk the calipers back and forth across a strip to check the regularity of the complexes. You can also take that distance and move it anywhere you want on the paper. This technique is useful in determining third-degree heart blocks and many other ECG or rhythm abnormalities. Take your calipers and practice on some of the rhythm strips in the back of this book. Make sure you do some measurements as well.

Comparing Widths

Explaining this one is a bit of overkill, but we really want you to understand the usefulness of the calipers. Suppose you wanted to see if distance A is the same as or longer than distance B (Figure 4-9). Position the calipers to measure distance A, then move them—transferring the distance accurately—to see if B is the same.

You will be using this technique for a great many comparisons in looking for atrioventricular blocks, aberrant beats, premature atrial contractions (PACs), premature ventricular contractions (PVCs), and so on. If you don't know what those things mean, don't worry about it; you will after you have looked over Chapter 7.

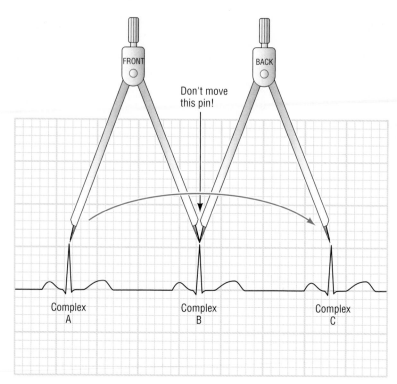

Figure 4-8: Walking the calipers. The distances are equal.

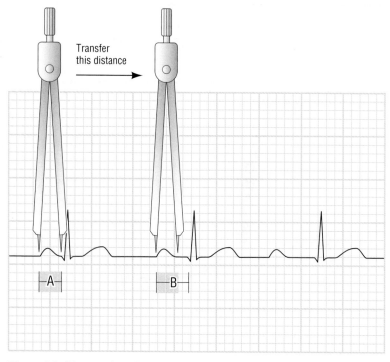

Figure 4-9: Distances A and B are not the same.

ECG Rulers

ECG rulers (Figure 4-10) are not needed if you have a pair of calipers. Most rulers have one side that measures the rate, and a metric ruler on the other. If you have a set of calipers and the ECG paper, you already have the same thing. ECG rulers also have some ECG criteria that are standard knowledge.

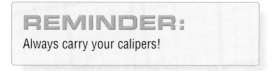

REMINDER:
Always carry your calipers!

Straight Edge

Straight edges are useful in evaluating the baseline and determining whether there is any elevation or depression present. You can use the ruler provided in this book or a piece of paper, even the ECG paper folded in on itself (without creasing the paper—messy ECGs are tough to read). The best straight edges are clear with a line in the middle so you can see the whole area in question without obstructing any of the complex. You can then use the straight line to evaluate the baseline. If you wish to create additional rulers, make a copy of the one in Figure 4-11 on overhead transparency film. Your neighborhood copy store should be able to accommodate you, preferably in color.

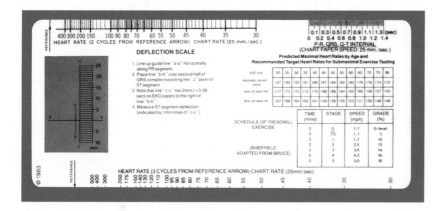

Figure 4-10: Straight edge ruler.

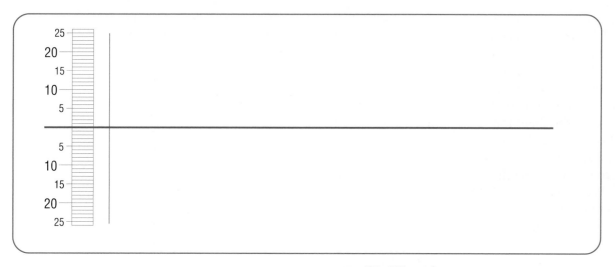

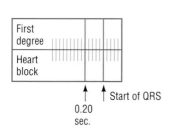

First degree

Heart block

↑ Start of QRS

0.20 sec.

If the QRS complex fits inside this box it is normal width. If it fits outside this box it is a bundle branch block.

0.12 seconds i.d.

Figure 4-11: ECG straight edge.

The Rate

When evaluating the rate of the complexes, first keep in mind that the P wave rate may be different from the QRS rate. For the purposes of this discussion, we consider QRS rates only. The same principles can be applied to obtain the P wave rate, if needed.

The rate can be obtained in various ways. If you have a computerized interpretation at the top of the ECG, you can usually use the rate that is given. Keep in mind, however, that this rate may be wrong. If it appears to be the wrong rate, calculate it yourself. One way of calculating the rate is to use a ruler, such as the one mentioned earlier in this chapter. There are also ways of calculating rate using the rhythm strip itself and your basic knowledge of the time intervals involved. Using your calipers with these techniques will be very helpful. Let's look at some of those ways now.

Establishing the Rate

Normal and Fast Rates

The easiest way to calculate the rate is to use the method illustrated in Figure 4-12. Find a QRS complex that starts on a thick line; this will be your starting point. Next, go to the exact spot on the next QRS complex—your end point. By tradition, we try to use the tip of the tallest wave on the QRS complex. However, you can use any spot as long as it is consistent. Then just count the thick lines in between the two spots, using the numbers shown in Figure 4-12. You will have to memorize this sequence, but it is more than worth your trouble.

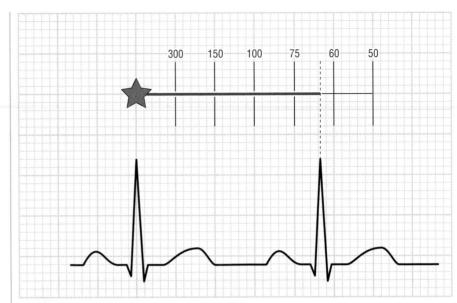

Figure 4-12: The rate is approximately 65–70 BPM.

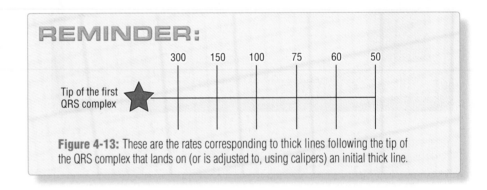

Figure 4-13: These are the rates corresponding to thick lines following the tip of the QRS complex that lands on (or is adjusted to, using calipers) an initial thick line.

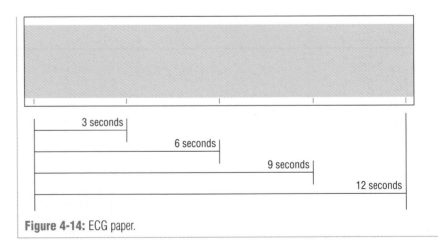

Figure 4-14: ECG paper.

Let's practice calculating some rates. . .

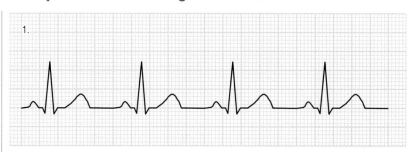

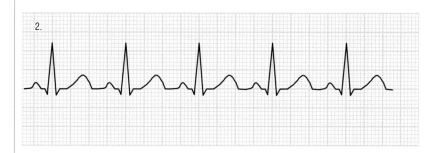

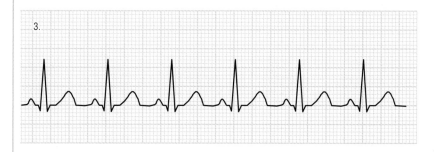

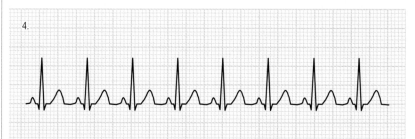

Figure 4-15: Answers: 1. 60 BPM, 2. 75 BPM, 3. About 80-85 BPM, 4. Approximately 130 BPM

Another way to calculate the rate is to use your calipers to measure from the top of one complex to the top of the next. Then move the calipers—maintaining the measured distance—so that the left tip rests on a thick line, and calculate the rate as above for the distance between the two tips. The advantage here is that you don't have to hunt down a QRS that lands on a thick line to use as a starting point.

Bradycardic Rates

Do you remember the concept in Figure 4-14? Knowing these time intervals will be very useful when you are calculating bradycardic rhythms. Can you think of how to use these intervals to calculate the rate generally, but especially in irregular and slow rhythms?

It's simple. Just count the number of cycles present in a 6-second strip, and multiply that number by 10. This will give you the number of beats in 60 seconds. You could also count the number of cycles in a 12-second strip and multiply by 5. Remember to use the fractional parts of cycles in your calculations, for example, 3.5 cycles in 6 seconds gives a rate of 35 beats per minute (3.5 cycles × 10 = 35 BPM).

> **REMINDER:**
> (cycles in 6 sec.) × 10 = BPM

Calculate the rates...

1.

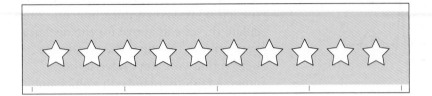

2.

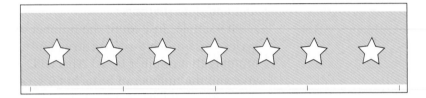

3.

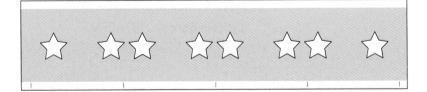

4.

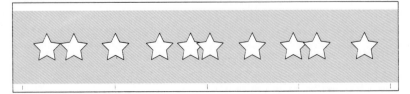

Figure 4-16: Answers: 1. Because the rhythm is regular, we can use either the 6-second or 12-second strip to figure out that there is a rate of: 5 (the # of beats in 6 seconds) × 10 = 50 BPM. 2. This set has approximately 3.5 beats × 10 = 35 BPM. 3. When the beats are irregular, it is more accurate to use the 12-second strip and multiply that number by 5. This gives us a rate of: 8 beats × 5 = 40 BPM 4. The rate is: 10 beats × 5 = 50 BPM

CHAPTER **REVIEW**

1. The paper on an ECG normally moves at:
   A. 50 mm/sec
   B. 75 mm/sec
   C. 25 cm/sec
   D. 25 mm/sec
   E. None of the above

2. The width of each small box represents:
   A. 0.04 seconds
   B. 0.02 seconds
   C. 0.40 seconds
   D. 0.20 seconds
   E. None of the above

3. The small boxes on ECG paper measure:
   A. 1 cm by 0.20 seconds
   B. 1 mm by 0.20 seconds
   C. 1 cm by 0.04 seconds
   D. 1 mm by 0.04 seconds
   E. None of the above

4. The big boxes on the ECG paper measure:
   A. 5 mm by 0.20 seconds
   B. 1 mm by 0.20 seconds
   C. 5 mm by 0.04 seconds
   D. 1 mm by 0.04 seconds
   E. None of the above

5. A wave that is 10 small boxes high and three small boxes wide is described as being:
   A. 1.0 mm by 0.3 seconds
   B. 10 mm by 0.12 seconds
   C. 12 mm by 0.3 seconds
   D. 12 mm by 0.10 seconds
   E. None of the above

6. A distance of 2 big boxes and 2 little boxes wide is described as being:
   A. 22 mm wide
   B. 0.22 seconds wide
   C. 0.48 seconds wide
   D. 4.8 seconds wide
   E. None of the above

7. When calculating rates, the numbers to remember are:
   A. 300–160–90–75–60–50
   B. 300–150–100–75–60–50
   C. 300–150–80–70–60–50
   D. 400–160–100–75–60–50
   E. None of the above

8. When calculating bradycardic rhythms, we take the number of complexes found during a 6-second interval on the ECG and multiply that number by 10. The product is the heart rate as beats per minute. True or False.

9. What is the rate if there are 3.5 beats in a 6-second strip?
   A. 3.5 BPM
   B. 35 BPM
   C. 350 BPM
   D. 3500 BPM
   E. None of the above

10. What is the rate if there are 3.5 beats in a 12-second strip?
    A. 3.5 BPM
    B. 35 BPM
    C. 17.5 BPM
    D. 175 BPM
    E. None of the above

11. What is the rate if there are five beats in a 6-second strip?
    A. 5 BPM
    B. 15 BPM
    C. 50 BPM
    D. 150 BPM
    E. None of the above

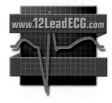

To enhance the knowledge you gain in this book, access this text's website at www.12leadECG.com! This valuable resource provides flashcards, an online glossary, web links, and more. Simply click on the Arrhythmias book cover once at the site.

CHAPTER 5

Basic Concepts in Arrhythmia Recognition

Introduction

Before we start looking at some actual patient strips and learning about each of the arrhythmias in depth, let's take a look at some concepts that will come up over and over again. We are going to address these issues using common terms and simplifying the evaluation of the strips as much as possible.

Many books address these topics as they arise in a particular rhythm strip. This book covers topics that are seen daily in rhythm strip analysis and then begins to cover the rarer topics. While some commonly seen rhythms may not be simple to understand, it is necessary to be able to recognize them.

The topics in this chapter include artifact, prematurity, the various types of pauses, ectopic foci, reentry, and aberrancy. Please be aware that this chapter merely introduces the material. These topics will be covered in much greater detail in the clinical sections of this book.

Artifact

Artifacts are false abnormalities of the baseline present on an ECG or rhythm strip that are due to sources other than the patient's bioelectrical impulses (Figure 5-1).

The sources of these abnormalities can be anything from movement on the part of the patient, movement of the electrical leads (wires), muscle tremors, and interference from external electrical equipment.

Many times the artifact can be easily identified and discounted. Other times, the artifact can be mistaken for the patient's rhythm or an arrhythmic event. In those cases, the artifact may lead to a misdiagnosis of the rhythm and result in inappropriate, sometimes dangerous, or unnecessary treatment.

In some circumstances, as in Figure 5-2, the entire rhythm strip can be altered by the artifact. In this example, the clinicians could easily have misdiagnosed the rhythm for a very dangerous rhythm known as ventricular tachycardia. Sometimes the artifact presents for only a short time, as in Figure 5-3. A quick way to verify your rhythm abnormality is to change the lead that your monitor is viewing, since many times the artifact will present in only one lead. If any questions remain, remember to view the "company that the arrhythmia keeps" (Figure 5-4). What we mean by this statement is that the arrhythmia does not occur in a void. Take a look at your patient and their clinical scenario before deciding on a course of action.

There is no easy way to tell what is artifact and what is the normal morphological appearance of a

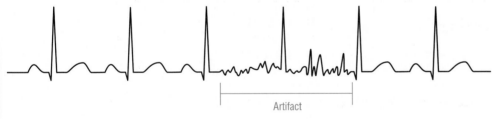

Figure 5-1: Artifact caused by a moving lead wire can result in a misdiagnosis of the rhythm.

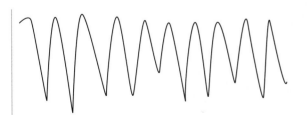

Figure 5-2: This patient was wrestling with her child. The movement of the leads caused the clinician to believe that the patient was in ventricular tachycardia. The rhythm returned to normal when the patient stopped moving.

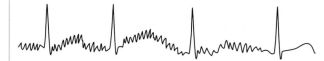

Figure 5-3: Interference by an electrical appliance in the room was the cause of this artifact. Turning off the machine caused the baseline to return to normal.

Figure 5-4: *No, this patient was not in an asystolic cardiac arrest!* The lead fell off his chest. When in doubt, take a look at your patient. A person cannot be sitting up eating dinner and be in asystole (lack of any electrical activity in the heart) at the same time. Remember to always look at "the company that the arrhythmia keeps."

rhythm. Unfortunately, it takes a lot of time and experience in strip interpretation before you get the hang of it. A word of wisdom is to always look at what is abnormal and concentrate on that spot. Usually, that is where the answer lies, even if it is just artifact.

Premature Complexes

A *premature complex* is basically one that arrives ahead of schedule. The complex occurs early or prematurely compared to where it should have occurred along the strip. In musical terms, the premature complex breaks the cadence of the rhythm. Take a look at Figure 5-5. Can you find the premature complex? Of course—it is represented by the sixth gold rectangle on the strip.

Premature complexes can be sinus, atrial, junctional, or ventricular in origin. The morphology of the complex will reflect their site of origin.

While we are on the topic of prematurity, there are some terms that you will frequently see related to premature complexes that recur at a regular interval. If the premature complex arrives every second beat, we refer to this presentation as *bigeminy* (Figure 5-6). If the premature complex arrives every third beat, we refer to this as *trigeminy*. As you can well imagine, every fourth beat is *quadrigeminy*, and so forth. The common thread among all these rhythms is the sequential repetitive occurrence of the premature complex.

Escape Complexes and Rhythms

An *escape complex* is almost the opposite of a premature complex. Instead of occurring early in the cadence of the rhythm, it occurs late in the cadence (Figure 5-8). In order to understand how an escape complex occurs, remember that all cardiac tissue has the ability to func-

Figure 5-5: Can you spot the premature complex in the strip?

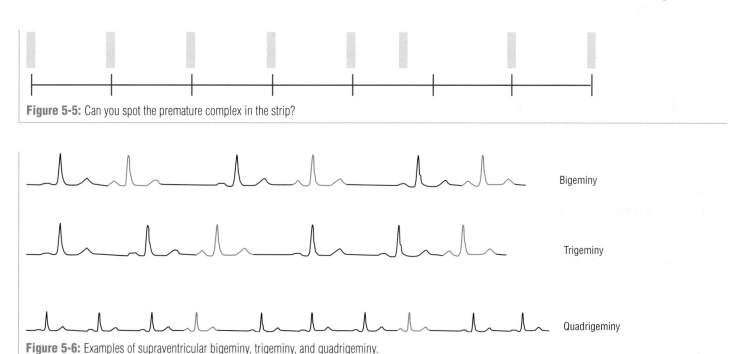

Bigeminy

Trigeminy

Quadrigeminy

Figure 5-6: Examples of supraventricular bigeminy, trigeminy, and quadrigeminy.

An Arrhythmia Versus an Event

At this point, we need to review some terminology. *A cardiac rhythm refers to the cadence or sequence of how the cardiac complexes occur.* Cardiac rhythms can be normal or abnormal and do not necessarily refer to a pathological process. Normally, the sinus node acts as the pacemaker and the impulse proceeds down the normal electrical conduction system to innervate both the atria and the ventricles sequentially.

An arrhythmia refers to a cardiac rhythm that is pathological in nature, and is one that is created or transmitted differently than the normal process. It can begin somewhere outside the sinus node. It can travel through different pathways other than the normal electrical conduction system. It can occur at rates outside of the normal range. It can be hemodynamically stable or it can cause hemodynamic instability. It can be fast or slow, wide or narrow.

We also should understand the difference between a rhythm and a rhythm with an overlying cardiac event that momentarily alters the cadence of the underlying rhythm. Suppose you had a strip with a clearly visible, regular cadence on it. Suddenly another pacemaker in

the heart became irritable and fired early. The cadence of the rhythm is altered by the event (Figure 5-7), but this is not a new arrhythmia. It is a normal rhythm with a premature complex. Always remember, *an event is not a rhythm.*

Why the distinction? Usually novice clinicians will focus on the event and not the rhythm itself. It is usually the underlying arrhythmia that will cause the hemodynamic compromise, not the single event. Let's use an analogy to think about this another way. In Emergency Medicine, we are involved in the care of trauma patients. For a trauma patient, one of the most impressive wounds, *visually,* is a scalp laceration. They normally cause small rivers of blood to drip down the face and can be quite dramatic. However, how many people actually die from a laceration to the scalp? Very, very few. On the other hand, a blunt liver laceration does not have a impressive visual presentation, but is often a killer. The clinician needs to look past the dramatic presentation of the scalp laceration and concentrate on the blunt injury that can kill the patient. That same mentality is how you need to approach an arrhythmia; concentrate on the rhythm and just be aware of the single event.

Figure 5-7   Event

tion as a potential pacemaker for the heart. The sinus node has the fastest pacing cycle; the ventricular muscle has the slowest (Figure 5-9). When the primary pacemaker fails for whatever reason, the next one in succession will take over the main role.

The reason this fail-safe pacemaking system exists is so that if one pacemaker fails, there are other pacemakers to keep the heart going and the person does not die. In an escape complex, the pacemaker that is setting the main rhythm fails and the next one takes over. This can occur either for one complex, or for however long it is needed.

An *escape rhythm* occurs when the primary pacemaker fails for a prolonged period of time. Once again,

the next pacemaker in succession will usually take over pacemaking function for the heart.

Ectopic Foci and Their Morphologies

The basic beat was discussed in depth in Chapter 3. This section deals with variations in the morphology of the complex based on where the complex originated in the heart. The exact location or focus that acts as the main pacemaker for a complex dictates the appearance of the complex. This is due to many factors and we will address them individually in the pages to come. For now, take a look at Figure 5-10 to get an overall impression of the location of a particular focus and its associated morphology characteristics.

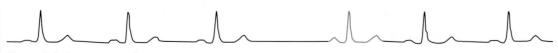

Figure 5-8: An escape complex.

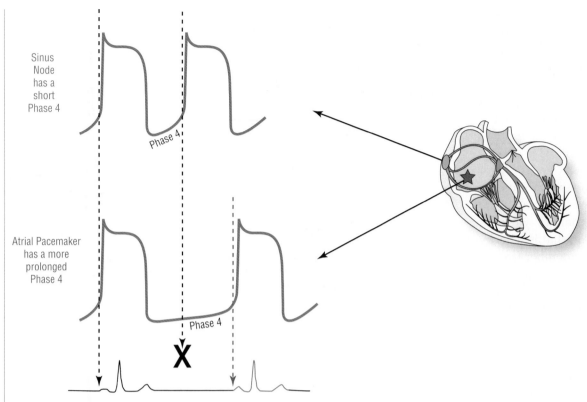

Figure 5-9: When the atrial pacemaker fails to pace at the expected time, the next pacemaker will fire according to its schedule. This creates an escape complex (see blue arrow).

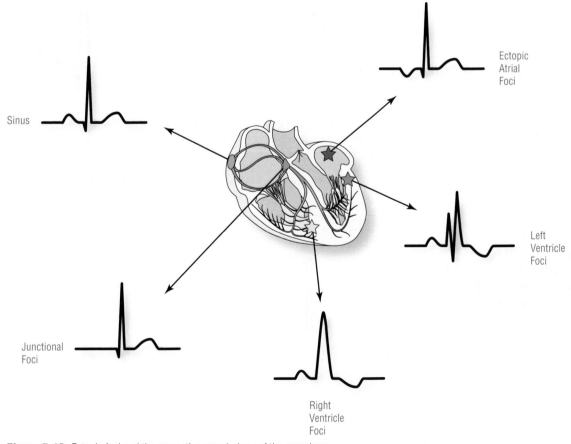

Figure 5-10: Ectopic foci and the respective morphology of the complexes.

There are many factors that affect the morphology of the complexes on an ECG. The main ones include the actual pacemaker site and the route that the impulse has to take to cause depolarization of the entire heart. These topics will be discussed in much greater detail as needed in subsequent sections of the book, but for now we will have an introductory discussion.

Let's start off by looking at the ectopic atrial sites. Since we are talking about atrial sites, the changes will be seen in the P waves and that is where we will begin. If you remember from Chapter 3, a positive vector heading toward an electrode will be interpreted on the ECG as a positive wave (Figure 5-11). A positive vector headed away from an electrode will be interpreted as a negative wave on the ECG (Figure 5-12). Vectors dictate morphology; directions of the depolarization waves on the heart dictate vector direction and vector size.

When you have an ectopic focus acting as the pacemaker for a complex, the angle and direction of the main atrial vector (also known as the *P wave axis*) will be different from one that originated in the sinus node. For simplicity, Figure 5-12 shows a vector that originated in the inferior aspect of the left atria and travels superiorly, backward, and to the right. This vector is seen by the electrodes for leads II, III, and aVF as heading away from them, and so will give rise to a completely negative or inverted P wave. As you can imagine, there are quite a large number of possible ectopic pacemakers, and therefore, quite a large number of possible P wave morphologies. ***The important thing clinically, is that ectopic P waves are all different morphologically from the sinus P waves.*** Picking up on these differences is key to making the correct diagnosis.

Now, let's turn our attention to the AV node. When the AV node functions as the primary pacemaker for a complex, one of two things will happen: (1) There will be no P waves; or (2) The P wave will always be inverted in leads II, III, and aVF.

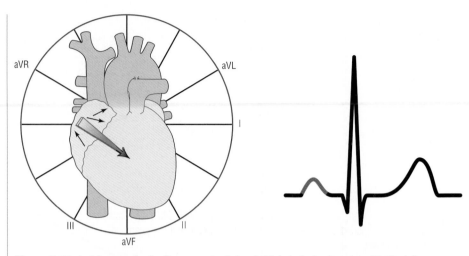

Figure 5-11: In this example, the P wave vector is headed inferiorly, backward, and to the left. Leads I and II see a positive vector headed toward them, and this is represented electrocardiographically as a positive P wave in those leads.

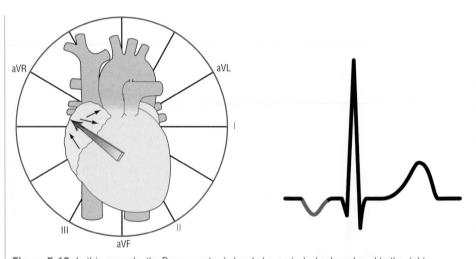

Figure 5-12: In this example, the P wave vector is headed superiorly, backward, and to the right. Leads I and II see a positive vector headed away from them, and this is represented electrocardiographically as a negative P wave in those leads.

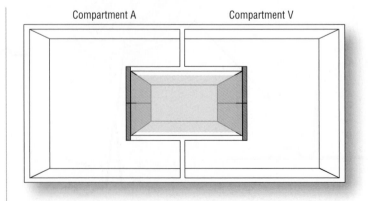

Figure 5-13: A large container with a central lock and two gates in the middle. The gates and the lock allow controlled communication between the two sides of the containers.

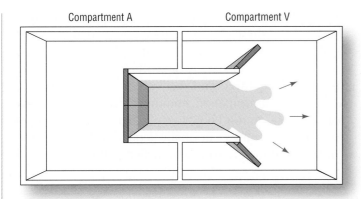

Figure 5-14: If the lock in the middle of the container were filled with water and the right gate opened, the water would flow into compartment V and spread evenly throughout that side of the container.

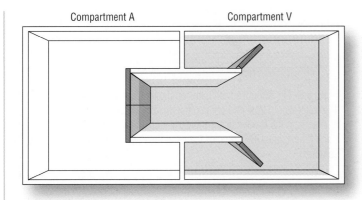

Figure 5-15: The right side of the gate was opened, releasing the contents and filling compartment V.

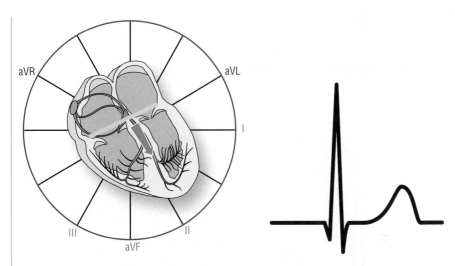

Figure 5-16: The impulse that originated in a junctional focus caused normal conduction down the electrical conduction system. The ventricles depolarized normally, forming a QRS complex with a normal morphology.

Earlier, in Chapter 1, we saw that the AV node is the only connection between the atria and the ventricles under normal circumstances. If it were not for the AV node, the atria and ventricles would actually function completely oblivious to each other. The AV node is, essentially, the gatekeeper for the heart, allowing communication to proceed back and forth. We saw that the gate can either be opened, allowing impulses to travel back and forth between the atria and the ventricles, or it can be closed, blocking impulse transmission between the two.

Now, suppose you had a large empty container meant to hold water with two sides, compartments A and V (Figure 5-13). There is a wall in the middle acting as a dam to prevent water from traveling back and forth between the two sides. The dam has a lock in the middle with two gates that could be opened to allow movement of water back and forth between the compartments. Suppose you filled the lock, right between two gates, with water (Figure 5-14). What would happen if you opened the gate on the right? The water would flow into compartment V. Compartment A would be dry and unaware of the flooding occurring in compartment V.

The same thing can happen when the AV node acts as the primary pacemaker. The junctional focus fires, causing an impulse to start to develop. This is equivalent to filling the lock with water. In our analogy, the next step would be to open the right side of the gate and allow the water to fill compartment V (Figure 5-15). In the heart, the impulse that originated in the junctional focus travels down the electrical conduction pathway, causing a normal depolarization of the ventricles (Figure 5-16). This is represented on the ECG as a normal-looking QRS complex with no P waves. There are no P waves because the AV node did not allow the impulse to travel retrogradely into the atria. To put it another way, the left side of the gate was not opened.

This is what occurs if the AV node does not allow the impulse generated in a junctional focus from traveling retrogradely or backward into the atria. This is one possibility. Now let's turn our attention to the other possibility.

Suppose that both gates on the lock were opened up simultaneously. What would happen to the water in the lock? It would flow into both compartments at the same time (Figure 5-17). This is exactly what happens when a junctional focus fires as the pacemaker of the complex. In this case, the P wave and the QRS complex would both be formed at exactly the same time, leading to a buried P wave (Figure 5-18). The morphology of the QRS complex may be slightly altered or it may appear normal.

If the junctional focus were closer to the atrial side of the AV node, the retrograde conduction to the atria would occur faster than ventricular depolarization and the P wave would come sooner in the cycle. This morphologically causes a shortened PR interval.

Ectopic Foci in the Ventricles

We have seen how the morphological changes of the complexes are caused when an ectopic focus in the atria and AV node act as the primary pacemaker. Now, we turn our attention to what happens when the ventricles act as the ectopic focus.

The first thing to notice about any ventricular ectopic focus is that it will lead to very broad, bizarre-looking QRS complexes (Figure 5-19). In addition, the site of the ventricular focus will alter the morphology in its own way. Both of these changes can be understood more easily if you keep in mind that ECG morphology is dictated by vectors. So, you already have the knowledge base to figure out why this occurs. Let's see how it happens.

Use your imagination, and the information you have learned so far in this book, to try to figure out the process. How do the ventricles normally depolarize? The impulse comes down the electrical conduction pathway and

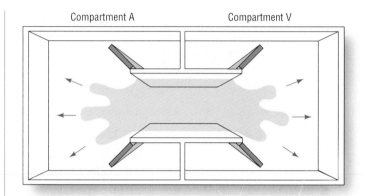

Figure 5-17: Suppose both gates on the lock opened up at the same time. The water would flow into both compartments simultaneously. In the AV node, this leads to the P wave occurring early (causing a short PR interval) or at the same time as the QRS complex (causing the P wave to be buried in the QRS complex).

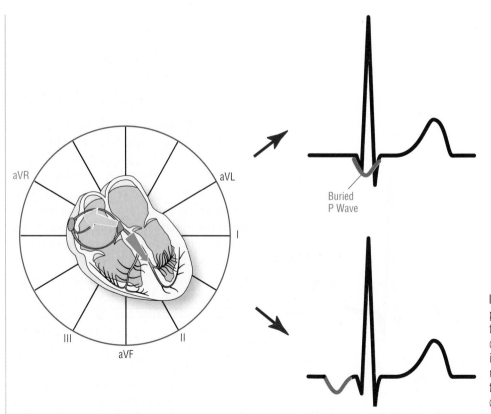

Figure 5-18: If a junctional focus acts as a primary pacemaker for a complex, the PR interval is shorter than expected or the P wave is buried in the QRS complex. The P-wave morphology would always be inverted in leads II, III, and aVF because of the direction of the vector (see yellow vector) caused by the retrograde atrial conduction of the junctional complex.

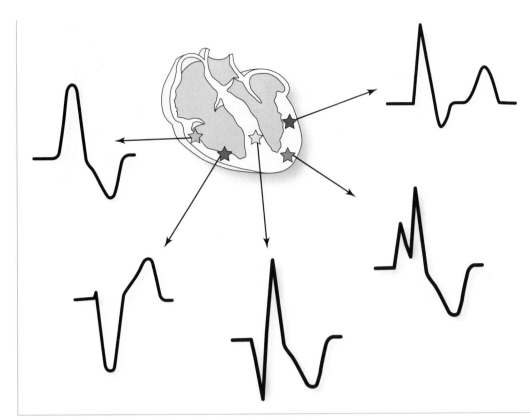

Figure 5-19: The firing of a ventricular ectopic focus leads to the formation of wide, bizarre-looking QRS complexes. The figure shows various types of possible QRS morphologies, but the actual appearance of a QRS cannot be predicted completely based on the location of the ectopic focus. In addition, the morphology will change based on the lead used to view the complexes.

spreads through the His bundles, the left and right bundle branches, and finally reaches the Purkinje system. The Purkinje system, in turn, stimulates the nearest myofibrils. From that point on, one myofibril stimulates an adjoining myofibril and the rest of the process of ventricular depolarization occurs via direct cell-to-cell stimulation. The organized sequential stimulation of the first set of myofibrils at the same time throughout both the left and right ventricles greatly shortens the process of ventricular depolarization, leading to a nice, normal-looking QRS complex.

Now, what happens when an ectopic focus acts as a primary pacemaker? Is the electrical conduction system stimulated simultaneously, providing a synchronized depolarization wave to occur in both ventricles? The answer is no. When an ectopic ventricular focus fires, the only cells that become stimulated by the depolarization are the ones in direct contact with the ectopic focus. When they, in turn, fire, they only stimulate their surrounding myofibrils, and so forth. This is a process of direct cell-to-cell stimulation that is very time consuming and does not lead to synchronized mechanical contraction. In Figure 5-20, the cell-to-cell depolarization wave is represented by the concentric waves moving outward from the ectopic focus.

How would this direct cell-to-cell transmission of the ventricular depolarization wave look morphologically on an ECG? It depends on the vector that it forms, but it would definitely be wide because of the slow nature of the conduction. Remember, what leads to a nice,

tight QRS complex is the *synchronized* conduction of the depolarization wave. An ectopic focus leads to *asynchronous* depolarization, which is very slow. Time on an ECG is demonstrated in the horizontal direction, hence the wide presentation on the complexes.

Now on to why the complexes are bizarre in appearance. Under normal circumstances, the synchronous depolarization of both ventricles leads to the formation of three almost simultaneous vectors (Figure 5-21). These vectors give rise to distinct morphological ECG representations that form the QRS complex: the Q wave, the R wave, and the S wave. With the firing of a ventricular pacemaker, do you have the formation of the same three distinct vectors, or do you have the formation of a haphazard series of vectors? The answer is a haphazard series of vectors. How these vectors align temporally will decide the final morphology of the QRS complex.

Aberrancy

In electrocardiography, *aberrancy* relates to electrical impulses that travel along nonestablished pathways in order to depolarize the heart. For example, the atrial and ventricular ectopic focus that we covered above are aberrantly conducted. Another aspect of the term that you will very frequently hear, and the main reason for this section, is when a complex is partially transmitted along the normal electrical pathway and then becomes aberrantly conducted because of some obstruction. Let's start off this discussion by going into this process in more detail.

Suppose you had a dry riverbed. Suddenly there was a big storm leading to a buildup of water that caused a flash flood. The rising waters would take the path of least resistance which, in this case, would be the dry riverbed (Figure 5-22). Now, suppose a beaver had built a dam across that riverbed at some time in the past. What would happen to the water flow when it hit the beaver dam? The water flow would smash into it and have to flow around the obstruction, taking any route it could. Would the flow around the obstruction be smooth as it would have been in the normal riverbed? No, because the water would have to go over millions of tiny obstacles, constantly change directions depending on elevation, and so forth. That flow creates turbulence. Turbulence, even though it is full of energy, is actually much slower moving than smooth, laminar flow. Let's recap: The water flows smoothly and faster before the obstruction. Once it meets the obstruction, it needs to find a way around it. That causes a slow, turbulent flow of the water to develop.

The same process can sometimes occur in the heart (Figure 5-23). The most common scenario is as follows: A normal electrical impulse is traveling down the electrical conduction system. Suddenly it hits an area that is *refractory* (temporarily unable to transmit the impulse) and it continues on from that spot by direct cell-to-cell transmission. As we saw before when we discussed ectopic foci, direct cell-to-cell transmission of the electrical impulse is slow and leads to aberrant vectors. Slow transmission of the impulse leads to wide complexes. Aberrant vectors lead to morphological differences in the complexes. So, what we end up with many times is a complex that starts out looking normal and like its neighboring complexes but suddenly there is a shift, and it looks totally different at the end.

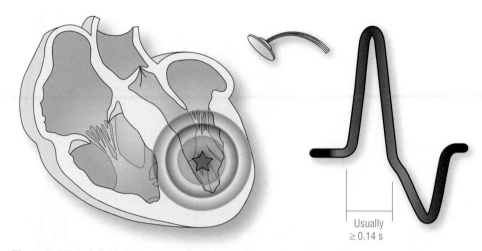

Figure 5-20: An irritable focus, represented by the red star, acts as a pacemaker and causes an impulse to occur. This gives rise to a depolarization wave that radiates outward by direct cell-to-cell transmission throughout **both** of the ventricles. Note the color-coded sections of the depolarization wave and the complex.

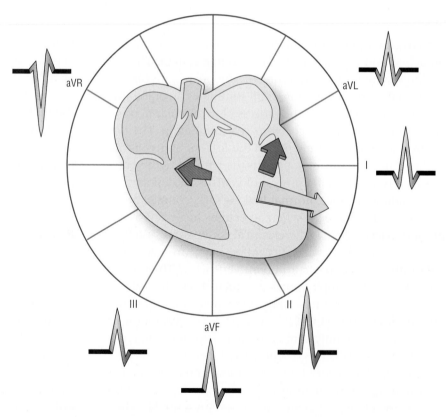

Figure 5-21: The synchronous depolarization of the ventricles by the electrical conduction system gives rise to three main vectors. The first one, represented by the red vector, will give rise to the Q wave. The second vector, represented by the yellow vector, will give rise to the R wave. The third vector, the blue vector, gives rise to the S wave. The three vectors are represented on the QRS complexes (as they appear in their particular leads) by their respective colors.

Fusion

Before we were born, our particular genetic material was created by taking some of the genetic material of our mothers and some of the genetic material of our fathers. We are, in essence, a fusion of the genetic material of both of our parents. We can resemble one parent more than another, but we will never be identical to either one. Keep this concept in mind as you read on.

In this section, we are going to be addressing an issue that will come up again and again throughout the book, the concept of *fusion*. Fusion refers to the merging together or melding of two or more waves and vectors that are occurring at the same, or nearly the same, moment in time. The final result is that the complexes that are formed have characteristics of both of the parent waves or vectors, but they are never morphologically identical to either. The *fusion complexes* thus formed are different in morphology from the rest of the strip as each of the parents adds their input into the final product.

The confusion in electrocardiography among beginners is that, in reality, fusion is actually two different electrocardiographic phenomena with one name. The first is an isolated electrocardiographic summation or fusion of waves occurring from two different complexes. An example of this type of fusion is when the T wave from one complex fuses with the P wave that causes the complex immediately after it. This leads to the buried P

phenomenon, which we will discuss at great length later on in the book. This type of fusion occurs mostly during premature or fast rhythms and is fairly evident on the ECG because of the events that are occurring around it.

The second type of fusion is an actual fusion of two entire complexes that are occurring simultaneously. An example of this type of fusion is one in which two ectopic foci in the atria, the ventricles, or both are firing at the same time. The result is that both depolarization

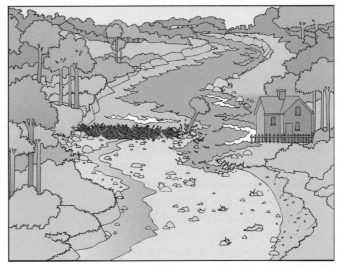

Figure 5-22: A flash flood on a river hits an obstruction. The water must find a way around the obstruction. causing turbulence and slower, abnormal flow.

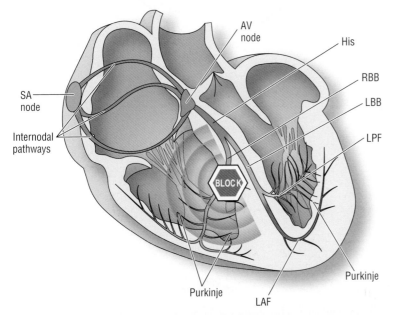

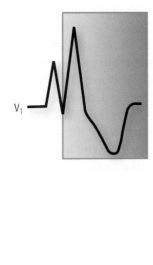

Figure 5-23: When the impulse hits an area of refractoriness in the right bundle branch, for example, the impulse is forced to continue by direct cell-to-cell transmission throughout the rest of the right ventricle. This leads to a complex that starts out normal and then ends up with a very bizarre appearance.

waves begin to form and eventually crash into one another. The complexes formed during this type of fusion are more difficult to differentiate and can be easily mistaken for completely ectopic beats.

Please be aware that nowhere else have we seen fusion broken down in this manner. However, these issues are constantly being questioned by students as they begin to learn electrocardiography and arrhythmia interpretation. To our knowledge the literature just has never separated the two concepts. We feel breaking it down simplifies learning the two individual concepts.

The Isolated Electrocardiographic Type of Fusion

We have touched on this type of fusion before, when we talked about the buried P waves and how they alter the appearance of either the QRS complex or the T wave (depending on the actual burial site of the P wave). We want you to notice, however, that this type of fusion is actually just an *electrocardiographic* phenomenon. This is not an actual physical fusion of two waves occurring during the same complex but rather the waves are actually part of two *different* complexes adding themselves up on the ECG (Figure 5-24).

To put it another way, the fusion of the two waves in this type of isolated fusion occurs only at the level of the strip because the two separate events are occurring at the same time. The result is that the two electrical vectors are interacting on the ECG only, but **the forces of one vector are not affecting the actual shape of the other vector; the forces are just adding up on the ECG.**

Actual Fusion

The other type of fusion is when the waves actually merge and fuse in the heart. In this case, the ECG lead then picks up that information and transfers it to the strip. This is a subtle difference from isolated electrocardiographic fusion. We call this type of fusion

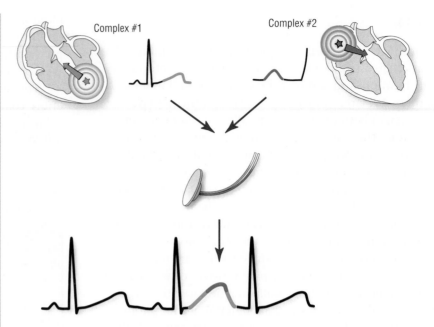

Figure 5-24: Buried P waves. Two different waves are both occurring simultaneously. One is the ventricular repolarization wave of complex #1 (blue vector) and the other is an atrial depolarization wave of complex #2 (green vector). The net result of the two vectors is an *electrocardiographic* fusion complex. The fusion of the two waves alters the morphology of the T wave in the rhythm strip.

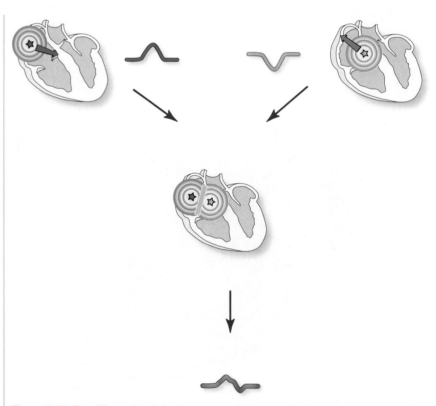

Figure 5-25: Two different depolarization waves are both occurring simultaneously, one arising from the SA node, the other from an ectopic atrial focus. The net result of the two waves is a fusion complex. The fusion complex has characteristics of both individual waves.

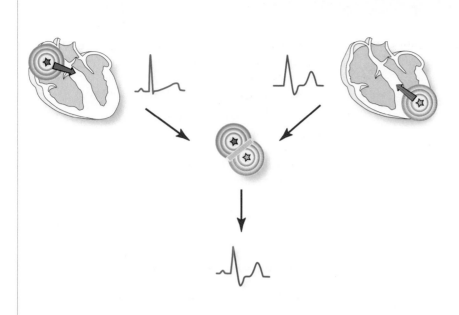

Figure 5-26: Two different depolarization waves are both occurring simultaneously, one arising from the SA node and then spreading to the ventricles via the AV node, the other originating from a ventricular ectopic focus. The net result of the two ventricular waves is a fusion complex. The fusion complex has characteristics of both individual waves. Note that the fusion did not occur with the P wave, just the QRS complexes.

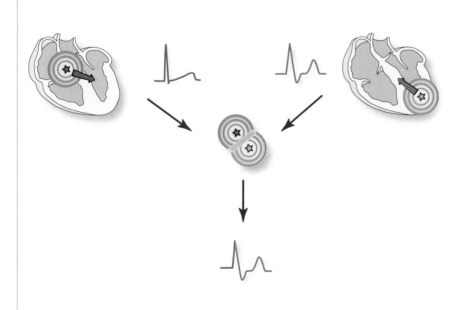

Figure 5-27: Two different depolarization waves are both occurring simultaneously, one arising from the AV node, the other from a ventricular ectopic focus. The net result of the two waves is a fusion complex of the QRS complexes, just like the one we saw in Figure 5-26. The fusion complex has characteristics of both individual waves. Note that there is no visible P wave in this figure when compared to Figure 5-26.

"actual fusion" to help distinguish it. Graphically, an example of this is represented by Figure 5-25, where two atrial foci are firing at the same time.

Suppose you had a complex that originated in the SA node (Figure 5-25, green vector). The depolarization wave would begin in the SA node and begin to spread normally throughout the atria. This depolarization wave would give rise to a normal P wave. Now, suppose that you had another depolarization wave start elsewhere in the atria or AV junctional area (Figure 5-25, blue vector). This wave would have no way of knowing that there already was a wave coming towards it from the SA node. This wave would start to give rise to an inverted P wave with an abnormal P wave axis and differing morphology from the sinus P wave.

Eventually, the two waves would crash into each other and cancel each other out. But, before they did that they would have had to create some sort of an electrocardiographic representation. The problem lies in that both of these waves are occurring at the exact same time. Electrocardiographically, the waves would fuse or mix with each other to create a complex that has some of the characteristics of the sinus wave and some of the characteristics of the ectopic wave. How much the fusion wave resembles either of the two parent waves depends on the timing of the two waves and their proximity to the leads. The depolarization wave that started the earliest would have the closest morphological appearance to the start of the final fusion wave. The middle and the end would be up for grabs.

The exact same concept of fusion is at work when a normally transmitted atrial complex fuses with an ectopic ventricular complex (Figure 5-26) or when a junctional complex fuses with an ectopic ventricular complex (Figure 5-27). Fusion complexes between an atrial P wave and a junctional ectopic pacemaker are quite common, and we shall see some examples when we start to examine actual patient strips.

CHAPTER **REVIEW**

1. Artifacts relate to complexes that arise at odd times or intervals from the underlying rhythm. True or False.

2. Things that commonly lead to artifact formation include (circle all that apply):
   A. Atrial premature contractions
   B. Moving lead wires
   C. Ventricular rhythms
   D. Muscle tremors
   E. Interference from an external electrical apparatus

3. Artifact can frequently lead to diagnostic errors in the proper identification of cardiac arrhythmias. True or False.

4. You walk in and find that your patient's monitor shows a straight line and they are sitting up talking with their friends. The most common cause is:
   A. Cardiac arrest.
   B. Fine ventricular fibrillation.
   C. The chest lead fell off the patient.
   D. The patient is an android.

5. A premature complex is a complex that arrives before the expected time according to the cadence of the underlying rhythm. True or False.

6. Premature complexes can originate in the:
   A. Sinus node
   B. Atrial muscle tissue
   C. AV node
   D. Ventricles
   E. All of the above

7. An escape complex occurs late in the cadence of the underlying rhythm momentarily. It occurs when the principal pacemaker fails and is replaced by the next available pacemaker in the pacemaker hierarchy of the heart and the electrical conduction system. True or False.

8. An escape rhythm occurs when the failure of the primary pacemaker lasts for an extended period of time, causing the next available pacemaker in the hierarchy to take over the entire pacing function for as long as needed. This is a protective mechanism to assure survival. True or False.

9. Two of the main factors that determine the morphology of complexes include the:
   A. Location of the initiating focus or pacemaker.
   B. Size of the initiating bioelectrical impulse.
   C. Route of conduction that the impulse travels through the heart.
   D. Patient's state of consciousness.
   E. A and C

10. Ectopic P waves are all morphologically different from sinus P waves. True or False.

11. An ectopic atrial pacemaker firing near the AV node will cause the P wave morphology to appear:
    A. Upright in lead II, III, and aVF
    B. Upright in lead V_1
    C. Inverted in lead II, III, and aVF
    D. Inverted in lead V_1

12. An ectopic complex originating in the AV node may be transmitted retrogradely to the atria or may actually never cause atrial depolarization by blocking retrograde conduction. True or False.

13. The morphology of ectopic ventricular complexes should always be narrow, and slightly different from the appearance of the normal sinus complex. True or False.

14. An electrical impulse can travel normally down the electrical conduction system and then hit an area that is refractory to impulse propagation. The subsequent impulse propagation would then continue aberrantly via direct cell-to-cell transmission from the point of obstruction (area that is refractory). The result can be an aberrantly conducted complex that has a normal morphological appearance at the onset but then changes abruptly. True or False.

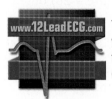

To enhance the knowledge you gain in this book, access this text's website at www.12leadECG.com! This valuable resource provides flashcards, an online glossary, web links, and more. Simply click on the Arrhythmias book cover once at the site.

Relevant Topics in Basic Electrocardiography

Introduction

Arrhythmia recognition is based on basic electrocardiography. It is impossible to really understand and work with arrhythmias without having at least some rudimentary information on basic ECG interpretation. This is a fact that eludes many authors and educators, and is probably one of the major reasons why people can understand the principles of arrhythmias but constantly miss the diagnoses on actual strips.

In this chapter, we will give you a basic tour of electrocardiography. We will primarily focus on relevant information that is going to affect your ability to recognize and interpret arrhythmias. These topics include the three-dimensional picture of the heart, the electrical axes of the heart (including the P-wave axis), and left and right bundle branch blocks.

We will cover the three-dimensional capabilities of electrocardiography because it will become increasingly important to you to isolate the pathologies involved in the various arrhythmias. We will cover the electrical axes because the waves we see on the ECG are graphical representations of the individual axes for those waves: the P-wave we see on the strip is a graphical representation of the P-wave axis; the QRS complex is a graphical representation of the main ventricular axis. Finally, why study the bundle branch block morphologies? Because they are representative of the way ectopic ventricular pacemakers cause aberrant morphology on the ECG and rhythm strip. If you understand how the bundle branch blocks are formed, it will be much easier for you to understand how ventricular complexes are formed and how aberrancy develops and affects morphology.

At the end of this chapter, you will not be able to interpret ECGs, but you will have a working knowledge of these points, and more importantly, you will know how to apply that knowledge clinically in your everyday practice. As you proceed through this book, you will notice that the information in this chapter will continually strengthen your ability to interpret arrhythmias and make their individual pathologic processes a little clearer.

Basic Information

We are going to begin our discussion by examining the typical layout of an ECG. Figure 6-1 shows the placement of the various leads in the standard format used by most ECG machines. There is, however, great variation in this system among the many manufacturers of ECG equipment. You should get used to the format that is used at your institution.

Some formats do not include a rhythm strip at the bottom. We believe this puts one at a great disadvantage in interpreting ECGs. Another disadvantage of some formats is that they provide a rhythm strip, but don't show it in temporal relationship to the complexes above the strip. In other words, the complexes on the rhythm strip do not coincide with the ones that are above it on the ECG paper. Usually, you look at the rhythm strip and see which are the aberrant beats. Then, you can look up and see which complexes in the top part of the ECG are the aberrant ones. If you don't have this temporal relationship between the rhythm strip and the leads themselves, it will be difficult to distinguish normal from aberrant beats on this type of ECG.

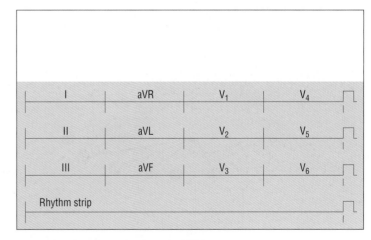

Figure 6-1: Locations of leads on the ECG paper.

If you remember, Chapter 3 discussed how leads are like cameras. All electrocardiography is based on the principle of taking multiple "pictures" of an electrical event from different camera angles or leads. There are 12 leads in a full 12-lead ECG. That means that we are looking at the heart from 12 different angles. Looking at the electrical events from this many angles allows us to formulate a three-dimensional picture of the heart and pinpoint pathology to the various regions.

In Figure 6-2, we are combining the limb leads (leads I, II, III, aVR, aVL, and aVF) and the precordial leads (leads V_1 through V_6) into one functional system. These two planes divide the heart in such a way that we can formulate that three-dimensional picture mentioned above. Let's look at some examples of how we can clinically use this information to isolate various myocardial infarction sites.

Suppose a patient had an inferior myocardial infarction (heart attack). Where would you see the changes on an ECG? Looking at Figure 6-2, what are the leads that face the bottom of the heart? They are leads II, III, and aVF! So, if you saw ECG changes consistent with an acute myocardial infarction (AMI) in leads II, III, and aVF, you would know that the patient was having an inferior wall MI (IWMI). See? You're getting good already. Now, suppose the ECG shows changes in leads V_1 and V_2. They run along the septum—hence a septal wall MI. V_3 and V_4 are the most anterior (anterior wall MI), and the lateral leads are I, aVL, V_5, and V_6. Get the picture? Let's look at these areas individually.

Localizing an Area: Inferior Wall

Suppose you look at an ECG and see changes in leads II, III, and aVF. Unless you have memorized the pattern,

you would not know what area of the heart those changes represented. Because memorization is not the optimal way to remember (we forget 90% of what we learn that way), we need to come up with a logical way to remember this pattern. If you know the hexaxial and precordial systems, you will be able to recognize that the leads in question represent the inferior wall of the heart (Figure 6-3). Changes of ischemia or infarction on that area of the ECG would tell you that the patient was having either inferior wall ischemia or an inferior wall MI. If you know the system, there will be very few things about electrocardiography that you will not be able to work out.

Localizing Other Areas

You can also use this approach to localize the anterior, septal, and lateral walls (Figure 6-4) and events that involve more than one region—the inferolateral wall, for instance. This involves both the inferior and lateral areas. Can you figure out which leads are involved? (See Figure 6-5 for the answer.)

It would be nice if the ECG machine gave us a logical three-dimensional picture of the heart like the ones we have just seen, but unfortunately, life is not that kind. We have to formulate our own three-dimensional picture by looking at a flat piece of ECG paper with the 12 leads on it (Figure 6-6). The good thing is that the ECG leads are set up by regions. We took the liberty of color coding those regions for you as they appear on the paper so that it would be easier to visualize where the regions are found (Figure 6-7). Take a few minutes now and compare the two figures.

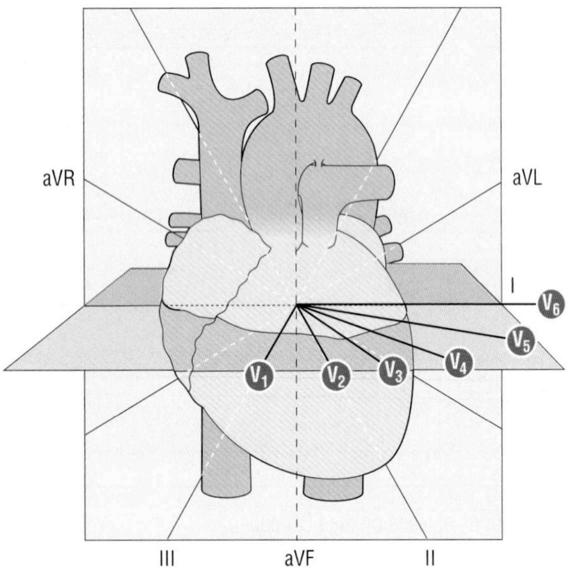

Figure 6-2: Leads in three dimensions.

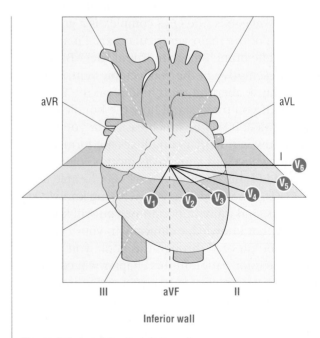

Figure 6-3: Localizing the inferior wall.

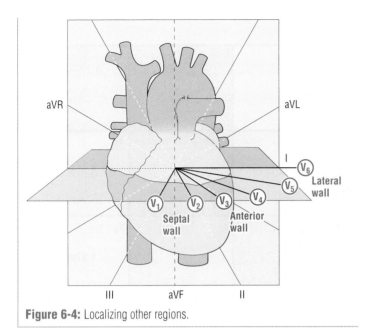

Figure 6-4: Localizing other regions.

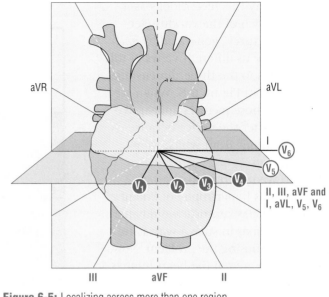

Figure 6-5: Localizing across more than one region.

As we mentioned earlier in this chapter, this is intended only as a very selective introduction to electrocardiography. The information above is needed in arrhythmia management because you need to understand what you are looking at when you get an ECG to evaluate the morphology of certain waves. Let's take, for example, P waves. In which lead, three-dimensionally, would you expect the P waves to be the most easily visualized? The first thing you should think about is where the P waves originate. They originate in the sinus node and travel outward throughout the atria. The lead that is the closest to the sinus node is V_1. It is also the lead where P waves are best viewed. If you ever have a question about a P wave, take a look at lead V_1.

As you can see, using full 12-lead ECGs as a tool to help your assessment when you are evaluating an arrhythmia opens up a whole new world. Waves and events are more clear in some leads than in others. Using all 12 leads greatly facilitates the chances of making a correct diagnosis. Now, let's move on to the axis.

The Electrical Axis

Up until now, we have touched on the concept of the electrical axis in various chapters. This tells you that just about everything in electrocardiography is related to the electrical axis and its graphic representation in the different leads. Before you begin this chapter, you should go back and review the information on vectors in Chapter 3.

The electrical axis, as we discussed there, is the sum total of all the vectors generated by the action potentials of the individual ventricular myocytes. We cannot evaluate the ventricular axis directly. Instead, we have to

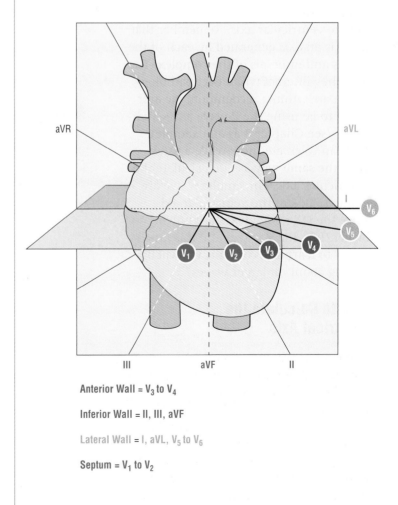

Anterior Wall = V_3 to V_4

Inferior Wall = II, III, aVF

Lateral Wall = I, aVL, V_5 to V_6

Septum = V_1 to V_2

Figure 6-6: ECG leads are set up by regions.

measure the way the vector looks as it travels under each of the various electrodes. The "pictures" generated by each of the leads give us different views of this axis as it relates to the three-dimensional state, as shown in Figure 6-8. When we examine how those pictures appear, we can piece together the vector because we know the locations from which they were taken.

How do we use the axis clinically? Suppose there is hypertrophy of one of the ventricles. That ventricle would alter the ventricular axis in such a way as to assist us in diagnosing the problem. Now, imagine that an area of the heart infarcts. The ventricular axis would definitely be altered by the lack of electrical activity generated in that dead zone. Suppose a section of the electrical conduction system is diseased or blocked. Do you think that would alter the electrical axis of the ventricle? It certainly would.

For now, we are going to be reviewing the ventricular axis. Remember that there is an axis generated by each of the waves and intervals of the complex. The way they interact will reflect pathology.

In arrhythmia recognition, we are going to be using the P wave axis extensively (see Chapter 8 as an example). You can calculate the P wave axis exactly the same way as you calculate the ventricular axis. For simplicity, we are going to look at the ventricular axis, since the QRS complexes are much bigger than the P waves and it is much easier to learn the concepts we will be talking about on larger waves.

How to Calculate the Electrical Axis

There are many ways to calculate the direction and intensity of the ventricular axis. We will show you a system that we feel is easy to understand and use. We will present a very simple system that breaks the hexaxial system down into four quadrants. Then we will show you how to determine the exact quadrant that holds the ventricular axis.

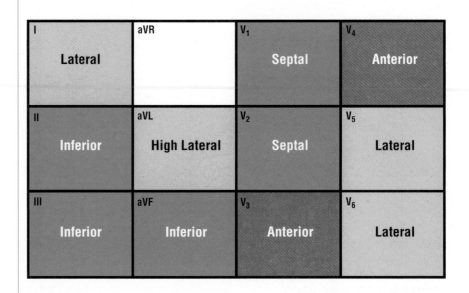

I	aVR	V₁	V₄
Lateral		Septal	Anterior
II	aVL	V₂	V₅
Inferior	High Lateral	Septal	Lateral
III	aVF	V₃	V₆
Inferior	Inferior	Anterior	Lateral

Figure 6-7: Color coding in this figure represents how the leads relate to various regions of the heart.

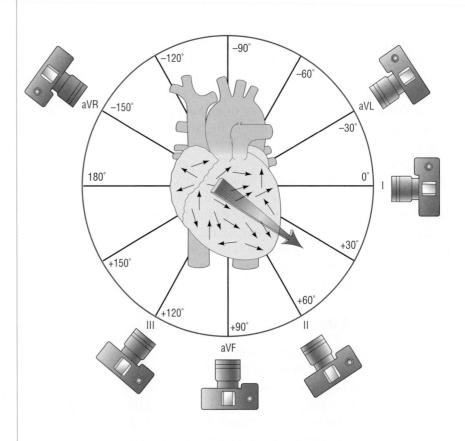

Figure 6-8: Locations of the leads determine the direction of the vector.

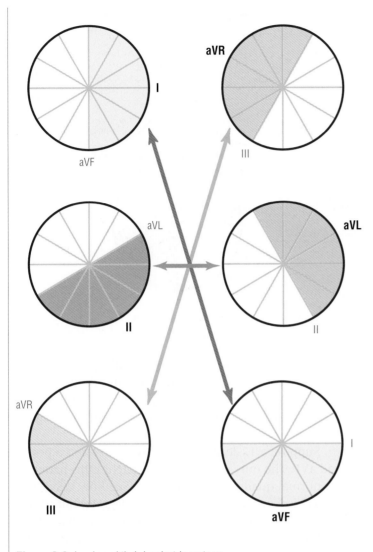

Figure 6-9: Leads and their isoelectric partners.

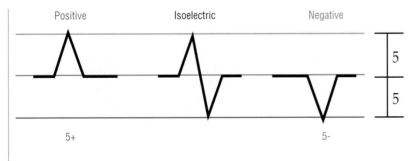

Figure 6-10: The QRS complex of positive, isoelectric, and negative leads.

The hexaxial system is represented by a circle with all of the leads enclosed. Remember that the entire circle is composed of six leads superimposed on each other? (Review this in Chapter 3 if you don't.) Each lead has a positive half and a negative half, as shown in Figure 6-9. For simplicity, we'll make the side with color and the lead label the positive half; the white and unlabeled side will always be the negative half.

Now, notice that the dividing line between each positive and negative half of a lead happens to fall on a lead that is at an exact 90° angle from it. This lead is referred to as the isoelectric lead, meaning that it is neither positive nor negative along that line (red labels in Figure 6-9). In other words, each lead has a corresponding isoelectric lead; I is isoelectric to aVF, II is isoelectric to aVL, III is isoelectric to aVR, and vice versa. This concept of the isoelectric lead will be very useful to us later on when we want to isolate the lead to within 10°.

On the ECG, any positive vector will be represented as taller or more positive. Any negative vector will appear as a deeper or more negative complex (Figure 6-10). A lead is considered positive if it is even a smidgen more positive than negative. (Webster's defines *smidgen* as a little teeny bit.) Likewise, it is considered negative if it is even a smidgen more negative than positive.

A lead is isoelectric when it is exactly the same distance positive as it is negative. There is only one isoelectric limb lead on the ECG because there is only one ventricular axis. All the other leads are either positive or negative.

When we plot the vector on the hexaxial system, a vector that is even slightly positive will be found on the positive half of the circle. By the same token, any negative complex has to be on the negative half of the circle. If it is exactly isoelectric, then it will fall directly along the isoelectric lead. If that occurs, you have a slight problem. The vector can point in one of two directions, either toward the negative or toward the positive pole. Note that both of these directions will be exactly isoelectric to the lead in question. How can we resolve this dilemma? At this point, you need to go back to the ECG and take a look at the complexes that are found in that isoelectric lead. If those complexes are positive, then the vector will point in the direction of the positive pole of the isoelectric lead. If the complexes are negative, then the vector will point toward the negative pole. This is your first introduction into how we will always use two leads to isolate the vector. This is an important, but difficult, point to understand. In Figure 6-11, for instance, vectors A, B, and C are all positive in lead I, and vectors D, E, and F are all negative in lead I.

Can you now see how the vector and the ECG are related? Because the vector cannot be seen, we use the complexes, and their relative positivity or negativity in each lead, to calculate the exact direction of the ventricular axis. Let's begin by seeing how to shorten the direction from 360° down to one of four 90° quadrants.

When we look at a 12-lead ECG, we do not know where the axis is pointing. To start isolating that direction, we want you to look at leads I and aVF (notice that these leads are isoelectric to each other). First, look at lead I and figure out whether it is positive or negative. Don't worry about how positive or negative right now; you only care about which half of the circle it falls into. If it is positive, it would have to be on the blue or positive side of the lead; if negative, it will fall in the white or negative half of the lead, as shown in Figure 6-12A. Next, look at lead aVF. Repeat the same thought process. Is it positive or negative in aVF? Place it in either the yellow or the white half, as referenced in Figure 6-12B. Because we know that yellow and blue make green, by overlapping these two circles, we create a new circle with four quadrants: one white, one blue, one yellow, and one green, as seen in Figure 6-12C.

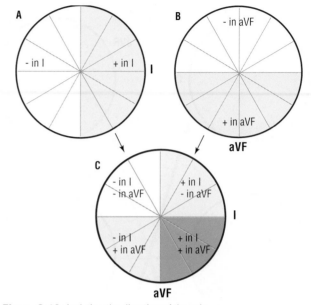

Figure 6-12: Isolating the direction of the axis.

Instead of saying positive or negative, we find it useful to say that a positive lead is taller than it is deep, hence ↑. A negative lead is deeper than it is tall, thus ↓. Using this system, you do not have to add the heights of the complex's components algebraically.

Suppose a 12-lead has a positive lead I and a positive lead aVF. The only quadrant that matches this pattern is the normal quadrant (Figure 6-13). See how easy? Next, we will isolate the axis to within 10 degrees, but for now let's just take baby steps in determining the quadrant.

We have seen that by looking at only leads I and aVF, we were able to break the hexaxial system down into four quadrants. We are going to name these four quadrants to make them easier to identify: Normal, left, right, and extreme right. These are shown in Figure 6-13.

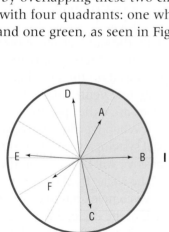

Figure 6-11: Positive and negative vectors in the hexaxial system.

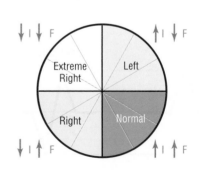

Figure 6-13: The four quadrants of the hexaxial system.

These are going to be very useful to us when we get ready to calculate the true axis as closely as possible. For now, we can just state that any axis that falls outside the normal quadrant should be considered abnormal. (In reality, the normal quadrant extends from −20° to +100°, not 0° to +90°, but the latter is close enough for now.) If the axis falls into the left quadrant, it is considered to have a *left axis deviation*. If it falls into either the right or extreme right, it has a *right axis deviation*.

Bundle Branch Blocks

In this section we will discuss the concept of the bundle branch block (BBB) to help you formulate a practical understanding of the electrocardiographic principles involved.

We need to start off our general discussion by revisiting the electrical conduction system (Figure 6-15). Notice that the bundle of His splits off into the left and right bundle branches (LBB and RBB). The LBB, in turn, divides into the left anterior and left posterior fascicles. Both the RBB and the two fascicles then split into smaller and smaller branches to form a network of terminal branches, which are collectively known as the Purkinje system (Figure 6-16). The Purkinje system allows the almost instantaneous firing of all of the ventricular cells at once.

Look at Figure 6-16. We want you to use your imagination to think about the ventricles of the heart as a flat sheet rather than a three-dimensional structure. Thinking about the system in this way will facilitate your understanding of the concepts.

Notice how the conduction system divides and innervates different areas of the heart. The left anterior fascicle innervates the superior and anterior aspects of the left ventricle (LV). The left posterior fascicle innervates the inferior and posterior aspects of the LV. The RBB

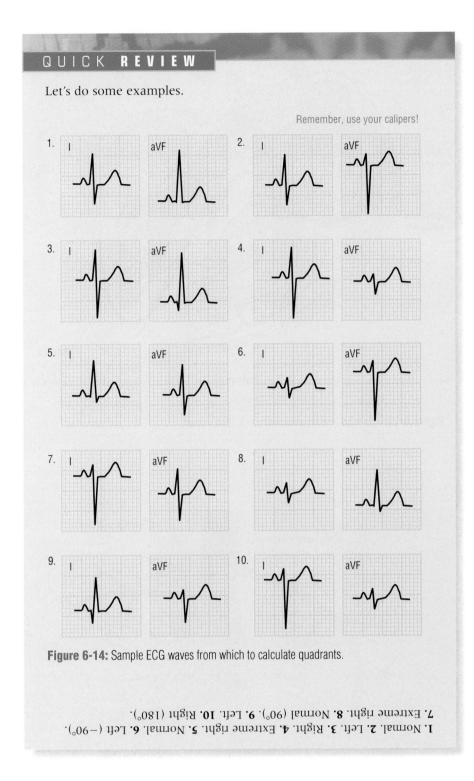

QUICK REVIEW

Let's do some examples.

Remember, use your calipers!

Figure 6-14: Sample ECG waves from which to calculate quadrants.

1. Normal. 2. Left. 3. Right. 4. Extreme right. 5. Normal. 6. Left (−90°). 7. Extreme right. 8. Normal (90°). 9. Left. 10. Right (180°).

innervates part of the septum and the right ventricle (RV).

Note that there is overlap of the different systems. This overlap is more prominent along the septum and along the border of the two fascicles.

What Happens If One Side Is Blocked?

OK, now suppose that the patient had an MI or something that blocks or destroys part of the conduction system (Figure 6-17)? Well, the normally functioning system would transmit the impulse down the section of normal pathway the same way it always does. The sections of the heart that are innervated by those fibers would then fire instantaneously and in a coordinated fashion. However, the section that is innervated by the blocked section would not receive a coordinated pulse. It would, instead, have to be depolarized by a slow transmission of the impulse that is spread directly from cell to cell (Figure 6-18), starting from somewhere along the septum and then spreading like a wave across the affected area of the heart.

Let's look at Figure 6-18 a little more closely. The impulse would travel down the left bundle normally. Hence, the LV and that section of the septum that is innervated by the LBB would fire normally. On the other hand, the rest of the septum, and the RV, would depolarize by the slower cell-to-cell route.

As you can imagine, this method of depolarizing the ventricles will give rise to abnormal-looking complexes on the ECG. Would the width of the QRS complex be increased? Yes. Why? *Because the slow cell-to-cell transmission requires a longer period of time to depolarize that section of the heart.* The net result is that the complexes are wider—greater than or equal to 0.12 seconds, to be exact.

Would the morphology be different? Yes, it would. Once again, the morphology of the complex is an electrocardiographic representation of the vectors occurring in the heart during depolarization and repolarization. By adding

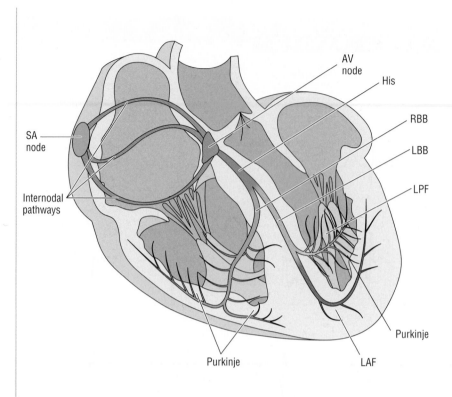

Figure 6-15: The heart and the electrical conduction system.

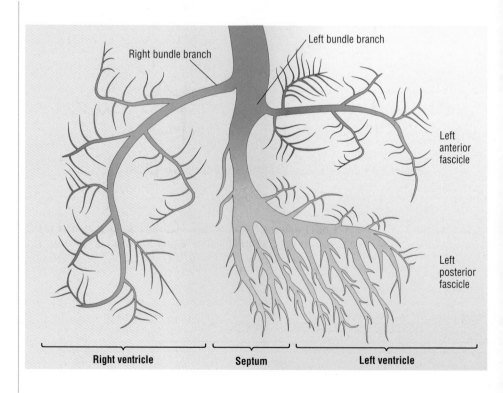

Figure 6-16: A closer look at the electrical conduction system.

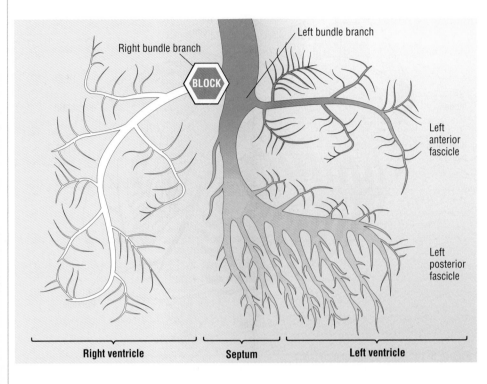

Figure 6-17: Bundle branch block.

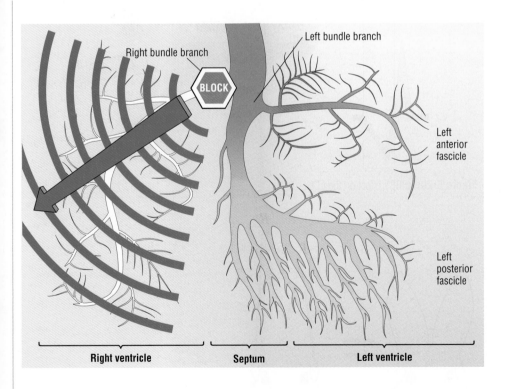

Figure 6-18: Slow depolarization caused by the bundle branch block.

the block, we have now created a slow-moving vector that was not there originally. In addition, since it occurs after the LBB has fired, the slow vector would be *unopposed*. This extra and unopposed vector will dramatically alter the appearance of the QRS complex.

Right Bundle Branch Block (RBBB)

The Major Morphologies Previously, we stated that the appearance of the QRS complex would be different from normal in both width and morphology. The good news is that there are only two major morphology patterns noted in bundle branch blocks: RBBB and LBBB. We will start with RBBB (Figure 6-19).

RBBB pattern is caused by a block of the right bundle branch somewhere near its inception. The fact that the left side of the heart depolarizes normally gives rise to a QRS complex that initially starts with a normal appearance. That is to say, the first 0.04 to 0.08 seconds of the QRS complex appear nice and tight, with the initial deflection headed in the exact direction we would ordinarily expect.

The end of the complex, however, is a different matter. This part appears wide and bizarre because of the vector labeled *4* in Figure 6-20. That slow, unopposed vector appears as a slow, slurring S wave in leads I and V_6. This occurs because vector 4 is heading toward the right, away from the electrodes placed at the lead I and V_6 sites.

In lead V_1, the pattern is a bit different. Here vector 1, which reflects septal depolarization, creates a small *r* wave. Next, the vectors marked 2 and 3 cause an S wave. The S wave does not get to complete, however, because vector 4 starts to oppose it. Shortly afterward, vector 4 comes into full, unopposed glory. Once again, the electrode at V_1 sees a large, unopposed vector coming at it, and represents this as a much taller R' wave. This is how the traditional rsR' or RSR' of RBBB in V_1 is formed. Many people refer to this complex as the "rabbit ears" for obvious reasons (see Figure 6-21).

We need to make one thing perfectly clear. We mentioned that a BBB gives rise to two major morphologies, but there are millions of minor morphologies depending on the location of the actual block, the direction of the slow depolarization wave, and so on. The net result is that the RSR' and the slurred S waves can have millions of minor differences, just as there are millions of different appearances to real rabbit ears (Figure 6-22).

This leads us to our next pearl of wisdom: *Never count on rabbit ears to make the diagnosis of RBBB!* Sometimes the complexes in lead V_1 will not look like rabbit ears at all but just like a big R wave, or an R wave with a slight hump. This lack of obvious rabbit ears is the main failure to diagnose RBBB. This can be a critical mistake in interpreting an ECG. Many patients have died and many unfortunate practitioners have been sued because of this failure to diagnose RBBB.

The most important thing to notice in lead V_1 is that you will always have positive complexes. You will never—we repeat, never—see negative complexes in lead V_1 in the presence of an RBBB. This is because of that unopposed vector, which causes a markedly positive complex in lead V_1.

So besides a positive complex in V_1, what should we look for to make the diagnosis of RBBB? The answer is the slurred S waves. Always look for the slurred S waves. They are much more consistent in appearance than the RSR' complex. This is the opposite of what is suggested by authors who encourage a dependence on observing rabbit ears. We hope this does not offend anyone, but this is a rookie mistake. If the QRS complex is greater than or equal to 0.12 seconds, look for the slurred S waves and a positive complex in lead V_1. If you see definite rabbit ears, then so much the better.

CLINICAL PEARL

Beware of rabbit ears! Look for the slurred S instead.

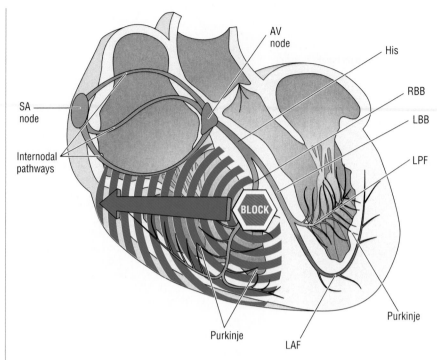

Figure 6-19: Right bundle branch block.

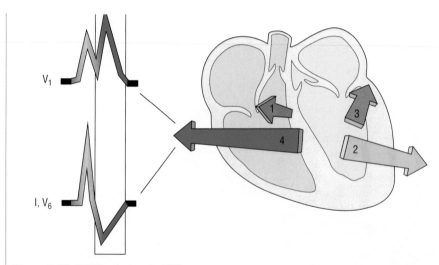

Figure 6-20: RBBB's effect on the ECG.

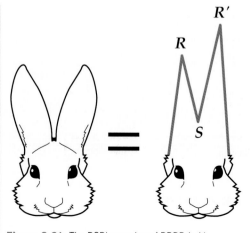

Figure 6-21: The RSR' complex of RBBB in V_1.

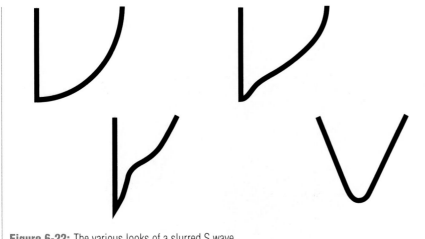

Figure 6-22: The various looks of a slurred S wave.

Complexes ≥ 0.12 seconds?
      ↘ *Yes*
   Slurred S waves in leads I and V₆?
         ↘ *Yes*
      Positive complexes in lead V₁?
            ↘ *Yes*
         Then it's RBBB!

Figure 6-23: Decision sequence for RBBB.

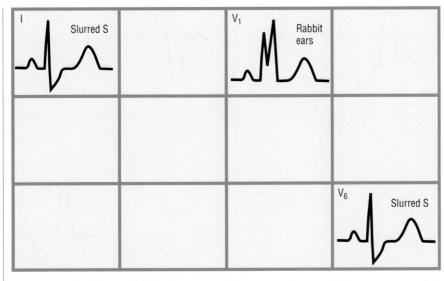

Figure 6-24: The ECG and RBBB.

Applying the Criteria for RBBB Get used to measuring intervals when you are calculating the rate on an ECG. Remember always to measure the widest lead. If you find wide complexes that are greater than or equal to 0.12 seconds wide, then you could be dealing with a bundle branch block.

You should next look for slurred S waves in leads I and V₆. If the S wave is fatter than the first part of the QRS complex and if the shape is slurred in any way, you can be quite confident that you are dealing with an RBBB.

Now look at V₁. If there are positive complexes in this lead, regardless of morphology, you have definitely identified an RBBB pattern. This is simple, fast, and very accurate! Figure 6-23 summarizes the sequence of observations to make in identifying RBBB. The following list, along with Figure 6-24, illustrates the three criteria:

1. QRS prolongation of ≥ 0.12 seconds
2. Slurred S wave in leads I and V₆
3. RSR' pattern in lead V₁

Left Bundle Branch Block (LBBB)

Remember these words of wisdom: whenever you look at an ECG that has a regular rhythm and say, "Gee whiz, that's an ugly gram!" you are probably looking at LBBB. The left bundle is always 0.12 seconds wide or more. So what makes these ECGs so ugly? They are usually composed of *monomorphic complexes* (either all positive or all negative) and have ST depression or elevation, and broad T waves. Note that the T waves should be *discordant*. This means that the last part of the QRS complex and the T wave should be electrically opposite each other. In other words, if the QRS complex is positive, then the T wave should be negative, or vice versa. If they both head in the same direction, it is called *concordant;* this is a sign of some pathologic process going on. The result of all of these findings is a "hunchback of Notre Dame" ECG.

The pathology involved in LBBB is caused by a block of the left bundle *or* of both fascicles of the left bundle. This block causes the electrical potential to travel down the right bundle first. Then ventricular depolarization proceeds from right to left by direct cell-to-cell transmission (Figure 6-25). The left ventricle is so big that the transmission is delayed, hence the 0.12 seconds or more criterion, and the complexes are not initially sharp as they were in the RBBB pattern. This slowed transmission with no sharp vectors gives rise to the broad, monomorphic complexes classically seen in LBBB. Furthermore, because the vector is proceeding from right to left, those complexes are negative in leads V_1 to V_2, and positive in I and V_5 to V_6. In other words: *If you look at V_1 and V_6, you will note that the complexes are all positive or all negative, respectively* (Figure 6-25). (Note: V_1 and V_2 may have a small *r* wave due to the initial vector produced by innervation through the right bundle.)

Because the vector arising from the right bundle is small and canceled by the large vector from the left ventricle, the complexes are generally similar in different people. This makes the recognition of the LBBB pattern easier than that of RBBB. Just remember to look in V_1 and V_6; if the complexes are broad, monomorphic, and all up or down, you've identified LBBB!

Criteria for Diagnosing LBBB As with RBBB, there are three main criteria for diagnosing LBBB (Figure 6-26):

1. Duration ≥ 0.12 seconds

2. Broad, monomorphic R waves in I and V_6, with no Q waves

3. Broad, monomorphic S waves in V_1; may have a small r wave

Just as there are never any certainties in life, let us say that there are no certainties in the appearance of the complexes. In general, as mentioned earlier, all LBBBs are similar to each other—

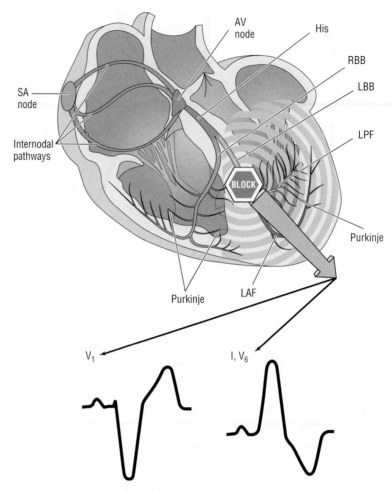

Figure 6-25: Left bundle branch block.

> **NOTE**
>
> The left bundle branch block pattern is like a rock thrown up in the air; it either goes all up or all down!

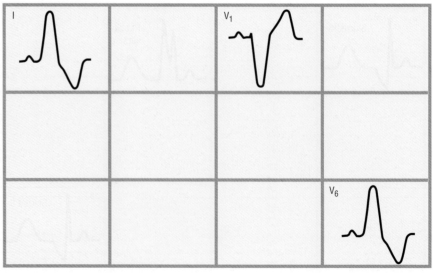

Figure 6-26: The ECG and LBBB.

much more so than just about any other type of ECGs when it comes to the appearance of the complexes. However, having said this, some of the complexes may have various small differences; the R waves can be notched in V_6, for instance (Figure 6-27). This notching can rarely be mistaken for an RSR' pattern, but it is not RSR'! Remember that rabbit ears are associated with RBBB and are found in V_1, not V_6.

There can also be some variations in the size of the R wave in V_1. Note, for instance, that the R wave can be narrow—less than 0.03 seconds (Figure 6-27). Wider R waves can be a sign of a previous posterior AMI; we will discuss more on this later.

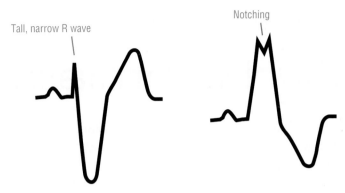

Figure 6-27: Here are some variations from the norm. Variations are not limited to the two examples shown in this illustration.

CHAPTER REVIEW

1. The entire ECG is:
   A. 3 seconds long
   B. 6 seconds long
   C. 9 seconds long
   D. 12 seconds long
   E. None of the above

2. The electrical axis is the sum total of all the vectors generated by the action potentials of all of the ventricular myocytes. True or False.

3. Which one is correct when we refer to the normal quadrant?
   A. Lead I is positive.
   B. Lead aVF is positive.
   C. Both A and B are correct.
   D. None of the above

4. Which one is correct when we refer to the left quadrant?
   A. Lead I is negative.
   B. Lead aVF is positive.
   C. Both A and B are correct.
   D. None of the above

5. Which one is correct when we refer to the right quadrant?
   A. Lead I is negative.
   B. Lead aVF is negative.
   C. Both A and B are correct.
   D. None of the above

6. Which one is correct when we refer to the extreme right quadrant?
   A. Lead I is negative.
   B. Lead aVF is negative.
   C. Both A and B are correct.
   D. None of the above

7. Because all RSR' complexes are close in appearance, all you need to diagnose RBBB is to identify their presence in V_1. True or False.

8. The three major criteria for diagnosing RBBB include:
   A. QRS ≥ 0.12 seconds
   B. Slurred S wave in leads I and V_6
   C. RSR' pattern in V_1
   D. All of the above
   E. None of the above

9. In RBBB, there can be a negative complex in V_1 or V_2. True or False.

10. The major criteria for diagnosing LBBB include:
    A. QRS ≥ 0.12 seconds
    B. Broad, monomorphic S wave in leads I and V_6
    C. Broad, monomorphic R wave in V_1
    D. All of the above
    E. None of the above

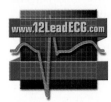

To enhance the knowledge you gain in this book, access this text's website at www.12leadECG.com! This valuable resource provides flashcards, an online glossary, web links, and more. Simply click on the Arrhythmias book cover once at the site.

CHAPTER 7

Arrhythmias: A Quick Review

This chapter is dedicated to the discussion of rhythms and arrhythmias. This will be a preliminary introduction to the subject. Individual arrhythmias are discussed in greater detail as they are encountered in the rest of the text. We recommend that you read the next section (Major Concepts) once, then proceed to the discussion of the individual rhythms, and finally return to reread Major Concepts. This will help to clarify the terminology.

Major Concepts

There are 10 points you should think about in an organized manner when approaching arrhythmias:

General:

1. Is the rhythm fast or slow?
2. Is the rhythm regular or irregular? If irregular, is it regularly irregular or irregularly irregular?

P waves:

3. Do you see any P waves?
4. Are all of the P waves the same?
5. Does each QRS complex have a P wave?
6. Is the PR interval constant?

QRS complexes:

7. Are the P waves and QRS complexes associated with one another?
8. Are the QRS complexes narrow or wide?
9. Are the QRS complexes grouped or not grouped?
10. Are there any dropped beats?

General

Is the rhythm fast or slow? Many rhythm abnormalities are associated with specific rate ranges. Therefore, it is very important to determine the rate of the rhythm in question. Decide if you are dealing with a tachycardia (> 100 BPM), a bradycardia (< 60 BPM), or a normal rate.

Is the rhythm regular or irregular? Do the P waves and QRS complexes follow a regular pattern with the same intervals separating them, or are the intervals different between some or all of the beats? This is a great tool to help you narrow down the rhythm, as you will see in the upcoming pages.

There is an additional question you must answer if the rhythm is irregular: Is it regularly irregular or irregularly irregular? At first glance, this statement can be confusing. A rhythm is regularly irregular if it has some form or regularity to the pattern of the irregular complex. An example would be a rhythm in which every third complex comes sooner than the preceding two. Therefore, the intervals would be long-long-short, long-long-short, in a repeating pattern that is predictable and recurring in its irregularity.

An irregularly irregular rhythm has no pattern at all. All of the intervals are haphazard and do not repeat, with an occasional, accidental exception. Luckily, there are only three irregularly irregular rhythms: atrial fibrillation, wandering atrial pacemaker, and multifocal atrial tachycardia. This is a differential diagnosis that you should commit to memory, as it will get you out of some tight spots.

P Waves

Do you see any P waves? The presence of P waves tells you that the rhythm in question has some atrial or supraventricular component. This is another major branch of the differential diagnosis of arrhythmias. The P waves, generated by the SA node or another atrial pacemaker, will usually reset any pacemaker down the chain.

Are all of the P waves the same? The presence of P waves that are identical means that they are being generated by the same pacemaker site. Identical P waves should have identical PR intervals unless an AV nodal block is present (more later). If the P waves are not identical, consider two possibilities: there is an additional pacemaker cell firing, or there is some other component of the complex superimposed on the P wave, such as a T wave occurring at the same moment as the P wave. The presence of three or more different P wave morphologies with different PR intervals defines either wandering atrial pacemaker or multifocal atrial tachycardia, both described later in this chapter.

Does each QRS complex have a P wave? An abnormal number of P waves in comparison to QRS complexes is an important point in determining whether you are dealing with some sort of AV nodal block.

Is the PR interval constant? Once again, this is extremely useful in identifying a wandering atrial pacemaker or multifocal atrial tachycardia. It is also helpful in evaluating premature atrial contractions (PACs) with and without aberrant conduction (slow conduction from cell to cell that produces abnormally wide QRS complexes).

QRS Complexes

Are the P waves and QRS complexes associated with one another? Is the P wave before a QRS complex responsible for the firing of that QRS (associated with it)? A positive answer to this question will help determine if the entire complex is a normal beat, a premature beat, or a low-grade AV nodal block. In the discussion of ventricular tachycardia, you may note that the presence of capture and fusion beats is critical to the diagnosis. In these cases, the P wave preceding the capture or fusion beat is responsible for the complex, in contrast to the other P waves that are dissociated from their respective QRSs.

Are the QRS complexes narrow or wide? Narrow complexes represent impulses that have traveled down the normal AV node/Purkinje network. These complexes are usually found in supraventricular rhythms, including junctional rhythms. Wide complexes indicate that the impulses did not follow the normal electrical conduction system, but instead were transmitted by direct cell-to-cell contact at some point in their travels through the heart. These wide complexes are found in premature ventricular contractions (PVCs), aberrantly conducted beats, ventricular tachycardia, and bundle branch blocks.

Are the QRS complexes grouped or not grouped? This is very useful in determining the presence of an AV nodal block or recurrent premature complexes, such as bigeminy (a repeating pattern of a normal complex followed by a premature complex) and trigeminy (a repeating pattern of two normal complexes followed by a premature complex).

Are there any dropped beats? Dropped beats occur in AV nodal blocks and sinus arrest.

Individual Rhythms

Supraventricular Rhythms

Normal Sinus Rhythm (NSR)

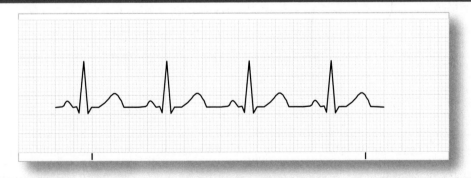

Rate:	60–100 BPM	PR interval:	Normal
Regularity:	Regular	QRS width:	Normal
P wave:	Present	Grouping:	None
P:QRS ratio:	1:1	Dropped beats:	None

Putting it all together:
This rhythm represents the normal state with the SA node functioning as the lead pacer. The intervals should all be consistent and within normal ranges. Note that this refers to the atrial rate; normal sinus rhythm (NSR) can occur with a ventricular escape rhythm or other ventricular abnormality if AV dissociation exists.

Sinus Arrhythmia

ECG 7-2

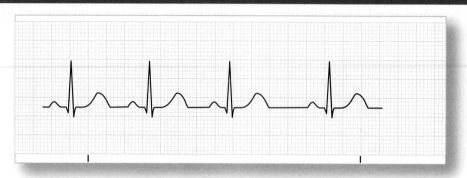

Rate:	60–100 BPM	PR interval:	Normal
Regularity:	Varies with respiration	QRS width:	Normal
P wave:	Normal	Grouping:	None
P:QRS ratio:	1:1	Dropped beats:	None

Putting it all together:

This rhythm represents the normal respiratory variation, becoming slower during exhalation and faster upon inhalation. This occurs because inhalation increases venous return by lowering intrathoracic pressure. Note that the PR intervals are the same; only the TP intervals (the interval from the end of the T wave of one complex to the beginning of the P wave of the next complex) vary with the respirations.

Sinus Bradycardia

ECG 7-3

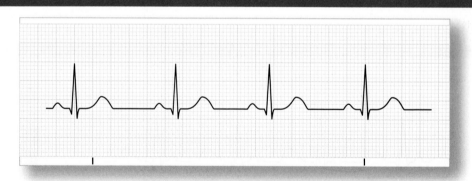

Rate:	Less than 60 BPM	PR interval:	Normal to slightly prolonged
Regularity:	Regular	QRS width:	Normal to slightly prolonged
P wave:	Present	Grouping:	None
P:QRS ratio:	1:1	Dropped beats:	None

Putting it all together:

The sinus beats are slower than 60 BPM. The origin may be in the SA node or in an atrial pacemaker. This rhythm can be caused by vagal stimulation leading to nodal slowing, or by medicines such as beta blockers, and is normally found in some well-conditioned athletes. The QRS complex, and the PR and QTc intervals, may slightly widen as the rhythm slows below 60 BPM. However, they will not widen past the upper threshold of the normal range for that interval. For example, the PR interval may widen, but it should not widen over the upper range of 0.20 seconds.

Sinus Tachycardia

ECG 7-4

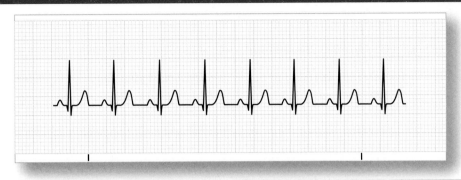

Rate:	Greater than 100 BPM	PR interval:	Normal to slightly shortened
Regularity:	Regular	QRS width:	Normal to slightly shortened
P wave:	Present	Grouping:	None
P:QRS ratio:	1:1	Dropped beats:	None

Putting it all together:

This can be caused by medications or by conditions that require increased cardiac output, such as exercise, hypoxemia, hypovolemia, hemorrhage, and acidosis.

Sinus Pause/Arrest

ECG 7-5

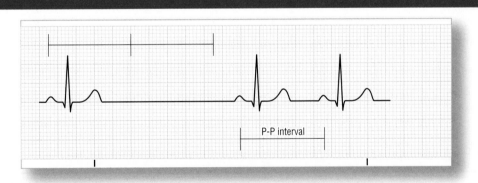

Rate:	Varies	PR interval:	Normal
Regularity:	Irregular	QRS width:	Normal
P wave:	Present except in areas of pause/arrest	Grouping:	None
P:QRS ratio:	1:1	Dropped beats:	Yes

Putting it all together:

A sinus pause is a variable time period during which there is no sinus pacemaker working. The time interval is not a multiple of the normal P-P interval. (A dropped complex that is a multiple of the P-P interval is known as an SA block, discussed next.) A sinus arrest is a longer pause, though there is no clear-cut criterion for how long a pause has to last before it is called an arrest.

Sinoatrial Block

ECG 7-6

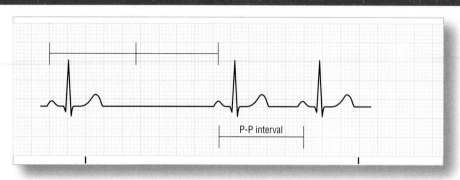

Rate:	Varies	PR interval:	Normal
Regularity:	Irregular	QRS width:	Normal
P wave:	Present except in areas of dropped beats	Grouping:	None
P:QRS ratio:	1:1	Dropped beats:	Yes

Putting it all together:

The block occurs in some multiple of the P-P interval. After the dropped beat, the cycles continue on time and as scheduled. The pathology involved is a nonconducted beat from the normal pacemaker.

Premature Atrial Contraction (PAC)

ECG 7-7

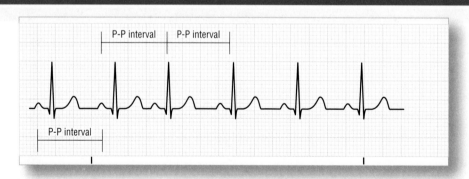

Rate:	Depends on the underlying rate	PR interval:	Varies in the PAC, otherwise normal
Regularity:	Irregular	QRS width:	Normal
P wave:	Present; in the PAC, may be a different shape	Grouping:	Sometimes
P:QRS ratio:	1:1	Dropped beats:	No

Putting it all together:

A premature atrial contraction (PAC) occurs when some other pacemaker cell in the atria fires at a rate faster than that of the SA node. The result is a complex that comes sooner than expected. Notice that the premature beat "resets" the SA node, and the pause after the PAC is not compensated; the underlying rhythm is disturbed and does not proceed at the same pace. This noncompensatory pause is less than twice the underlying normal P-P interval.

Ectopic Atrial Tachycardia

ECG 7-8

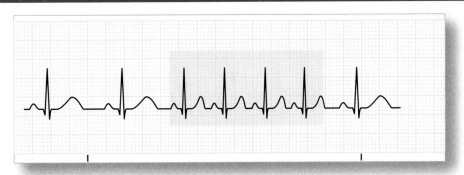

Rate:	100–180 BPM	PR interval:	Ectopic focus has a different interval
Regularity:	Regular	QRS width:	Normal, but can be aberrant at times
P wave:	Morphology of ectopic focus is different	Grouping:	None
P:QRS ratio:	1:1	Dropped beats:	None

Putting it all together:

Ectopic atrial tachycardia occurs when an ectopic atrial focus fires more quickly than the underlying sinus rate. The P waves and PR intervals are different because the rhythm is caused by an ectopic atrial pacemaker (a pacemaker outside of the normal SA node). The episodes are usually not sustained for an extended period. Because of the accelerated rate, some ST- and T-wave abnormalities may be present transiently.

Wandering Atrial Pacemaker (WAP)

ECG 7-9

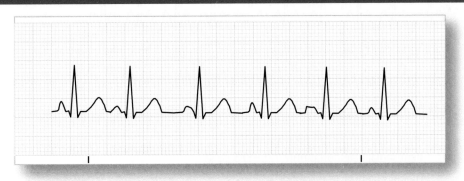

Rate:	100 BPM	PR interval:	Variable depending on the focus
Regularity:	Irregularly irregular	QRS width:	Normal
P wave:	At least three different morphologies	Grouping:	None
P:QRS ratio:	1:1	Dropped beats:	None

Putting it all together:

Wandering atrial pacemaker (WAP) is an irregularly irregular rhythm created by multiple atrial pacemakers each firing at its own pace. The result is an electrocardiogram (ECG) with at least three different P wave morphologies with their own intrinsic PR intervals. Think of each pacer firing from a different distance, and with a different P wave axis. The longer the distance, the longer the PR interval. The varying P wave axis causes differences in the morphology of the P waves.

Multifocal Atrial Tachycardia (MAT)

ECG 7-10

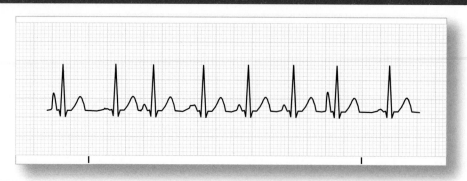

Rate:	Greater than 100 BPM	PR interval:	Variable
Regularity:	Irregularly irregular	QRS width:	Normal
P wave:	At least 3 different morphologies	Grouping:	None
P:QRS ratio:	1:1	Dropped beats:	None

Putting it all together:

Multifocal atrial tachycardia (MAT) is merely a tachycardic WAP. Both MAT and WAP are commonly found in patients with severe lung disease. The tachycardia can cause cardiovascular instability at times, so it should be treated. Treatment is difficult, and should be aimed at correcting the underlying problem.

Atrial Flutter

ECG 7-11

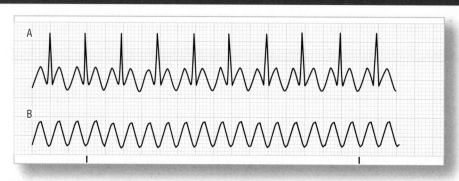

Rate:	Atrial rate commonly 250–350 BPM Ventricular rate commonly 125–175 BPM	PR interval:	Variable
Regularity:	Usually regular, but may be variable	QRS width:	Normal
P wave:	Saw toothed appearance, "F waves"	Grouping:	None
P:QRS ratio:	Variable, most commonly 2:1	Dropped beats:	None

Putting it all together:

The F waves appear in a saw toothed pattern such as those in this ECG. (QRSs have been removed from strip B to reveal F wave shape.) The QRS rate is usually regular and the complexes appear at some multiple of the P-P interval. The usual QRS response is 2:1 (this means that there are 2 F waves for each QRS complex). The ventricular response can also occur slower at rates of 3:1, 4:1, or higher. Sometimes the ventricular response will be irregular.

Rarely, you will have a truly variable ventricular response that does not fall on any multiple of the F-F interval. We call this an atrial flutter with a variable ventricular response.

In closing, keep in mind that the saw toothed appearance may not be obvious in all 12 leads. Whenever you see a ventricular rate of 150 BPM, look for the buried F waves of an atrial flutter with 2:1 block!

Atrial Fibrillation

ECG 7-12

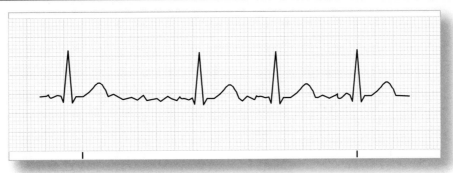

Rate:	Variable, ventricular response can be fast or slow	PR interval:	None
Regularity:	Irregularly irregular	QRS width:	Normal
P wave:	None; chaotic atrial activity	Grouping:	None
P:QRS ratio:	None	Dropped beats:	None

Putting it all together:

Atrial fibrillation is the chaotic firing of numerous atrial pacemaker cells in a totally haphazard fashion. The result is that there are no discernible P waves, and the QRS complexes are innervated haphazardly in an irregularly irregular pattern. The ventricular rate is guided by occasional activation from one of the pacemaking sources. Because the ventricles are not paced by any one site, the intervals are completely random.

Premature Junctional Contraction (PJC)

ECG 7-13

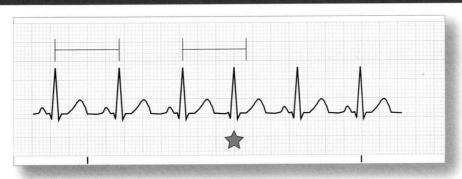

Rate:	Depends on underlying rhythm	PR interval:	None, short, or retrograde; if present, does not represent atrial stimulation of the ventricles
Regularity:	Irregular	QRS width:	Normal
P wave:	Variable (none, antegrade, or retrograde)	Grouping:	Usually none, but can occur
P:QRS ratio:	None; or 1:1 if antegrade or retrograde	Dropped beats:	None

Putting it all together:

A premature junctional contraction (PJC) is a beat that originates prematurely in the AV node. Because it travels down the normal electrical conduction system of the ventricles, the QRS complex is identical to the underlying QRSs. PJCs usually appear sporadically, but can occur in a regular, grouped pattern such as supraventricular bigeminy or trigeminy. There may be an ante-grade or retrograde P wave associated with the complex. An antegrade P wave is one that appears before the QRS complex. The PR interval is very short in these cases, and the P-wave axis will be abnormal (inverted in leads II, III, and aVF; more on these types of P waves in Chapter 21). A retrograde P is one that appears after the QRS complex.

Junctional Escape Beat

ECG 7·14

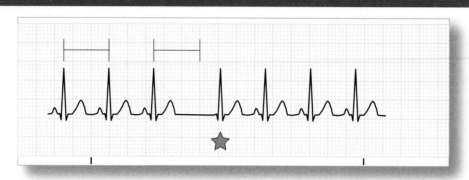

Rate:	Depends on underlying rhythm	PR interval:	None, short, or retrograde; if present, does not represent atrial stimulation of the ventricles
Regularity:	Irregular	QRS width:	Normal
P wave:	Variable (none, antegrade, or retrograde)	Grouping:	None
P:QRS ratio:	None, or 1:1 if antegrade or retrograde	Dropped beats:	Yes

Putting it all together:

An escape beat occurs when the normal pacemaker fails to fire and the next available pacemaker in the conduction system fires in its place. Remember that this was discussed in Chapter 1. The AV nodal pacer senses that the normal pacer did not fire. So, when its turn comes up and it reaches threshold potential, it fires. The distance of the escape beat from the preceding complex is always longer than the normal P-P interval.

Junctional Rhythm

ECG 7·15

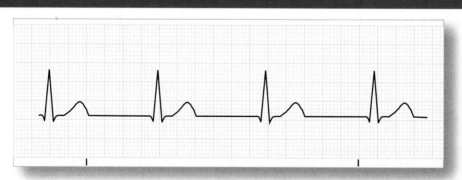

Rate:	40–60 BPM	PR interval:	None, short, or retrograde; if present, does not represent atrial stimulation of the ventricles
Regularity:	Regular	QRS width:	Normal
P wave:	Variable (none, antegrade, retrograde)	Grouping:	None
P:QRS ratio:	None, or 1:1 if antegrade or retrograde	Dropped beats:	None

Putting it all together:

A junctional rhythm arises as an escape rhythm when the normal pacemaking function of the atria and SA node is absent. It can also occur in the case of AV dissociation or third-degree AV block (more on this later).

Accelerated Junctional Rhythm

ECG 7-16

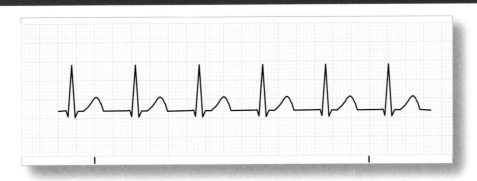

Rate:	60–100 BPM	PR interval:	None, short, or retrograde; if present, does not represent atrial stimulation of the ventricles
Regularity:	Regular	QRS width:	Normal
P wave:	Variable (none, antegrade, retrograde)	Grouping:	None
P:QRS ratio:	None, or 1:1 if antegrade or retrograde	Dropped beats:	None

Putting it all together:

This rhythm originates in a junctional pacemaker that, because it is firing faster than the normal pacemaker, takes over the pacing function. It is faster than expected for a normal junctional rhythm, pacing in the range of 60–100 BPM. If it exceeds 100 BPM, it is known as junctional tachycardia. As with other junctional pacers, the P waves can be absent or conducted in an antegrade or retrograde fashion.

Ventricular Rhythms

Premature Ventricular Contraction (PVC)

ECG 7-17

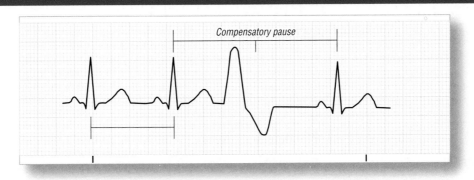

Rate:	Depends on the underlying rhythm	PR interval:	None
Regularity:	Irregular	QRS width:	Wide (≥ 0.12 seconds), bizarre appearance
P wave:	Not present on the PVC	Grouping:	Usually not present
P:QRS ratio:	No P waves on the PVC	Dropped beats:	None

Putting it all together:

A PVC is caused by the premature firing of a ventricular cell. The ventricular pacer fires before the normal SA node or supraventricular pacer, which causes the ventricles to be in a refractory state (not yet repolarized and unavailable to fire again) when the normal pacer fires. Hence, the ventricles do not contract at their normal time. However, the underlying pacing schedule is not altered, so the beat following the PVC will arrive on time. This is a *compensatory pause*.

Ventricular Escape Beat

ECG 7-18

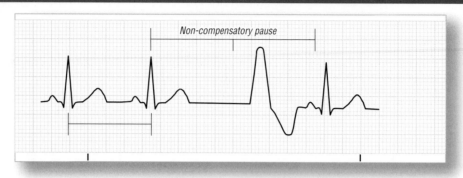

Non-compensatory pause

Rate:	Depends on the underlying rhythm	PR interval:	None
Regularity:	Irregular	QRS width:	Wide (≥ 0.12 seconds), bizarre appearance
P wave:	None in the PVC	Grouping:	None
P:QRS ratio:	None in the PVC	Dropped beats:	None

Putting it all together:

A ventricular escape beat is similar to a junctional escape beat, but the focus is in the ventricles. The pause is *non-compensatory* in this case because the normal pacer did not fire. (This is what led to the ventricular escape beat.) The pacer then resets itself on a new timing cycle, and may even have a different rate.

Idioventricular Rhythm

ECG 7-19

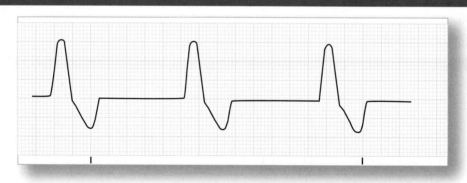

Rate:	20–40 BPM	PR interval:	None
Regularity:	Regular	QRS width:	Wide (≥0.12 seconds), bizarre appearance
P wave:	None	Grouping:	None
P:QRS ratio:	None	Dropped beats:	None

Putting it all together:

Idioventricular rhythm occurs when a ventricular focus acts as the primary pacemaker for the heart. The QRS complexes are wide and bizarre, reflecting their ventricular origin. This rhythm can be found by itself, or as a component of AV dissociation or third-degree heart block. (In these latter cases, there may be an underlying sinus rhythm with P waves present.)

CLINICAL PEARL

We usually try to stay away from treatment, but a word of caution: Do not treat this rhythm with antiarrhythmics! If you are successful in eliminating your last pacemaker, what do you have? Asystole.

Accelerated Idioventricular Rhythm

ECG 7·20

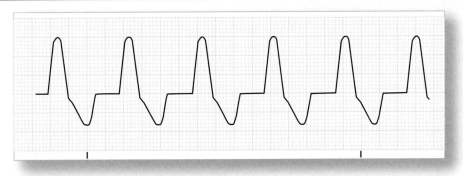

Rate:	40–100 BPM	PR interval:	None
Regularity:	Regular	QRS width:	Wide (≥ 0.12 seconds), bizarre appearance
P wave:	None	Grouping:	None
P:QRS ratio:	None	Dropped beats:	None

Putting it all together:

This is, basically, a faster version of an idioventricular rhythm. There are usually no P waves associated with it, in keeping with the ventricular source of the pacing. However, they can be present in AV dissociation or third-degree heart block.

Ventricular Tachycardia (VTach)

ECG 7·21

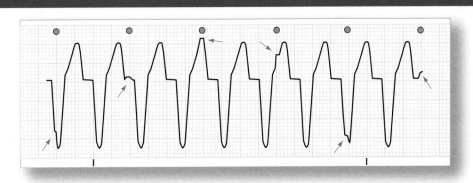

Rate:	100–200 BPM	PR interval:	None
Regularity:	Regular	QRS width:	Wide, bizarre
P wave:	Dissociated atrial rate	Grouping:	None
P:QRS ratio:	Variable	Dropped beats:	None

Putting it all together:

Ventricular tachycardia (VTach) is a very fast ventricular rate that is usually dissociated from an underlying atrial rate. In this ECG, you will notice irregularities of the QRS morphologies at regular intervals. These irregularities are the underlying sinus beats. (Blue dots indicate sinus beats, and arrows pinpoint the irregularities.) There are many criteria related to VTach, which we'll take a look at now.

Capture and Fusion Beats Occasionally, a sinus beat will fall on a spot that allows some innervation of the ventricle to occur through the normal ventricular conduction system. This forms a fusion beat (ECG 7-22), which has a morphology somewhere between the abnormal ventricular beat and the normal QRS complex. This type of complex is literally caused by two pacemakers, the SA node and the ventricular pacer. Because two areas of the ventricle are being stimulated simultaneously, the result is a hybrid—or fusion—complex with some features of both. It may help to think of this in terms of the following analogy. If you mix a blue liquid with a yellow liquid, the result is a green liquid. A fusion beat is like the green liquid; it is the fusion of the two complexes.

A capture beat, on the other hand, is completely innervated by the sinus beat and is indistinguishable from the patient's normal complex. Why is it called a capture beat instead of a normal beat? Because it occurs in the middle of the chaos that is VTach, and is caused by chance timing of a sinus beat at just the right millisecond to "capture" or transmit through the AV node and depolarize the ventricles through the normal conduction system of the heart.

Fusion and capture beats are hallmarks of ventricular tachycardia; you will usually see them if the strip is long enough. If you see these types of complexes with a wide-complex, tachycardic rhythm, you have diagnosed VTach.

More VTach Indicators There are some additional signs we should look at. You don't need to remember the names, but you should know about Brugada's and Josephson's signs (ECG 7-23). Brugada's sign occurs during VTach. The interval from the R wave to the bottom of the S wave is ≥ 0.10 seconds. Josephson's sign, which is just a small notching near the low point of the S wave, is another indicator of VTach.

Some additional aspects in VTach include a total QRS width of ≥ 0.16 seconds, and a complete negativity of all precordial leads (V_1–V_6). Why are we spending so much time on VTach? It is a life-threatening arrhythmia that is difficult to diagnose under the best of circumstances.

CLINICAL PEARL

A word to the wise: When confronted with any wide-complex tachycardia, treat it as VTach unless you have very strong evidence to the contrary. Do not assume it is a supraventricular tachycardia with aberrancy, a common error with potentially disastrous consequences.

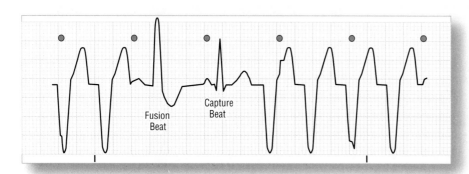

ECG 7-22: Fusion and capture beats in VTach.

REMINDER:

Criteria for diagnosing ventricular tachycardia:
- Wide-complex tachycardia
- AV dissociation
- Fusion and capture beats
- Complexes in all of the precordial leads are negative
- Duration of the QRS complex ≥ 0.16 seconds
- Josephson's and Brugada's signs

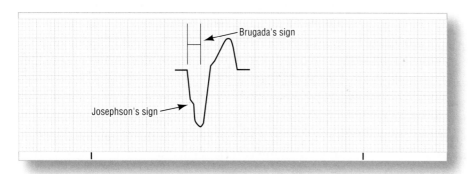

ECG 7-23: Brugada's and Josephson's signs in VTach.

Torsade de Pointes

ECG 7·24

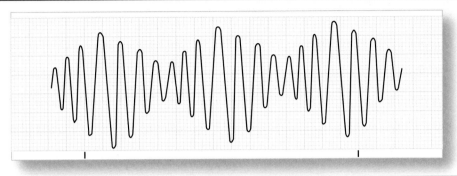

Rate:	200–250 BPM	PR interval:	None
Regularity:	Irregular	QRS width:	Variable
P wave:	None	Grouping:	Variable sinusoidal pattern
P:QRS ratio:	None	Dropped beats:	None

Putting it all together:

Torsade de pointes occurs with an underlying prolonged QT interval. It has an undulating, sinusoidal appearance in which the axis of the QRS complexes changes from positive to negative and back in a haphazard fashion. (The name, torsade de pointes, means twisting of points.) It can convert into either a normal rhythm or ventricular fibrillation. Be very careful with this rhythm, as it is a harbinger of death!

Ventricular Flutter

ECG 7·25

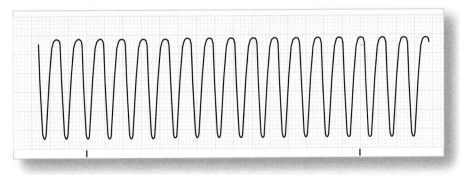

Rate:	200–300 BPM	PR interval:	None
Regularity:	Regular	QRS width:	Wide, bizarre
P wave:	None	Grouping:	None
P:QRS ratio:	None	Dropped beats:	None

Putting it all together:

Ventricular flutter is very fast VTach. When you can no longer tell if it is a QRS complex, a T wave, or an ST segment, you have VFlutter. The beats are coming so fast that they fuse into an almost straight sinusoidal pattern with no discernible components.

CLINICAL PEARL

When you see VFlutter at a rate of 300 BPM, you should think about the possibility of Wolf-Parkinson-White syndrome (WPW) with 1:1 conduction of an atrial flutter. (We know this may not mean much now, but it will later on.)

Ventricular Fibrillation (Vfib)

ECG 7-26

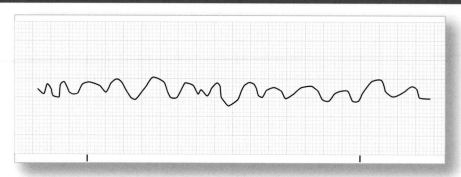

Rate:	Indeterminate	PR interval:	None
Regularity:	Chaotic rhythm	QRS width:	None
P wave:	None	Grouping:	None
P:QRS ratio:	None	Dropped beats:	No beats at all!

Putting it all together:

If you were going to draw a picture of cardiac chaos, this would be it. The ventricular pacers are all going haywire and firing at their own pace. The result is many small areas of the heart firing at once with no organized activity.

CLINICAL PEARL

If your patient looks fine and is wide awake and looking at you, a lead has fallen off and this is an artifact, not Vfib.

Heart Blocks

First-degree Heart Block

ECG 7-27

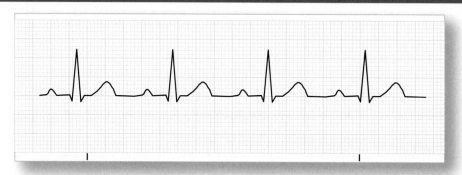

Rate:	Depends on underlying rhythm	PR interval:	Prolonged > 0.20 seconds
Regularity:	Regular	QRS width:	Normal
P wave:	Normal	Grouping:	None
P:QRS ratio:	1:1	Dropped beats:	None

Putting it all together:

First-degree heart block results from a prolonged physiologic block in the AV node. This can occur because of medication, vagal stimulation, and disease, among others. The PR interval will be greater than 0.20 seconds.

 NOTE A word of caution about the nomenclature of blocks: The rhythm disturbances we are looking at here are *AV nodal blocks.* There are also *bundle branch blocks,* a very different phenomenon.

Mobitz I Second-Degree Heart Block (Wenckebach)

ECG 7-28

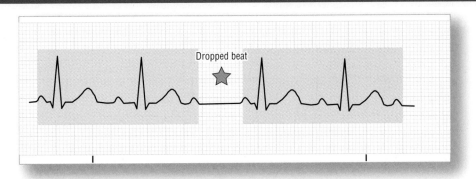

Rate:	Depends on underlying rhythm	PR interval:	Variable
Regularity:	Regularly irregular	QRS width:	Normal
P wave:	Present	Grouping:	Present and variable (see blue shading in ECG 7-28)
P:QRS ratio:	Variable: 2:1, 3:2, 4:3, 5:4, etc.	**Dropped beats:** Yes	

Putting it all together:

Mobitz I is also known as Wenckebach (pronounced WENN-key-bock). It is caused by a diseased AV node with a long refractory period. The result is that the PR interval lengthens between successive beats until a beat is dropped. At that point, the cycle starts again. The R-R interval, on the other hand, shortens with each beat.

Mobitz II Second-Degree Heart Block

ECG 7-29

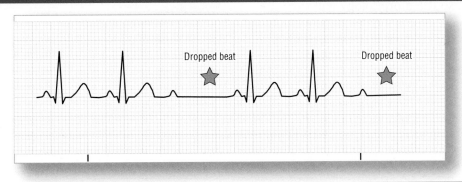

Rate:	Depends on underlying rhythm	PR interval:	Normal
Regularity:	Regularly irregular	QRS width:	Normal
P wave:	Normal	Grouping:	Present and variable
P:QRS ratio:	X:X–1; e.g., 3:2, 4:3, 5:4, etc. The ratio can also be variable on rare occasions.	**Dropped beats:** Yes	

Putting it all together:

In Mobitz II, there are grouped beats with one beat dropped between each group. The key point to remember is that the PR interval is the same in all of the conducted beats. This rhythm is caused by a diseased AV node, and it is a harbinger of bad things to come—namely, complete heart block.

CLINICAL PEARL

What if there is a 2:1 ratio of Ps to QRSs? Is this Mobitz I or Mobitz II? In reality, you can't tell. This example is named a 2:1 second-degree block (no type is specified). Because you can't tell, assume the worst—Mobitz II. You cannot go wrong by being overly cautious with a patient's life.

Third-Degree Heart Block

ECG 7-30

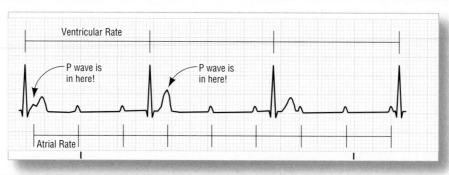

Rate:	Separate rates for the underlying (sinus) rhythm and the escape rhythm. They are dissociated from one another.	P:QRS ratio:	Variable
		PR interval:	Variable; no pattern
Regularity:	Regular, but P rate and QRS rate are different	QRS width:	Normal or wide
		Grouping:	None
P wave:	Present	Dropped beats:	None

Putting it all together:

This is a complete block of the AV node; the atria and ventricles are firing separately—each to its own drummer, so to speak. The sinus rhythm can be bradycardic, normal, or tachycardic. The escape beat can be junctional or ventricular, so the morphology will vary.

NOTE

Semantics alert: If there are just as many P waves as there are QRSs, but they are dissociated, it is known as AV dissociation rather than third-degree heart block.

CHAPTER **REVIEW**

1. Sinus arrhythmia is a normal respiratory variant. True or False.

2. A regular rhythm with a heart rate of 125 BPM with identical P waves occurring before each of the QRS complexes is:
   A. Sinus bradycardia
   B. Normal sinus rhythm
   C. Ectopic atrial tachycardia
   D. Atrial flutter
   E. Sinus tachycardia

3. If an entire complex is missing from a rhythm strip but the underlying rhythm is unchanged and maintains the same P-P or R-R interval (excluding the dropped beat), it is known as:
   A. Sinus bradycardia
   B. Atrial escape beat
   C. Sinus pause
   D. Sinoatrial block
   E. Junctional escape beat

4. An irregularly irregular rhythm of 65 BPM with at least three varying P-wave morphologies and PR intervals is known as:
   A. Atrial fibrillation
   B. Wandering atrial tachycardia
   C. Multifocal atrial tachycardia
   D. Atrial flutter
   E. Accelerated idioventricular rhythm

5. In atrial flutter, the flutter wave usually occurs at a rate of 250–350 BPM. True or False.

6. Atrial fibrillation is an irregularly irregular rhythm with no discernible P waves in any lead. True or False.

7. An irregularly irregular rhythm at 195 BPM with no discernible P waves is known as:
   A. Atrial fibrillation with a rapid ventricular response
   B. Multifocal atrial tachycardia
   C. Atrial flutter
   D. Ectopic atrial tachycardia
   E. Accelerated idioventricular rhythm

8. An accelerated junctional rhythm is a junctional rhythm over 100 BPM. True or False.

9. An idioventricular rhythm is caused by a ventricular focus acting as the primary pacemaker. The usual rate is in the range of 20–40 BPM. True or False.

10. Ventricular tachycardia is associated with:
    A. Capture beats
    B. Fusion beats
    C. Both A and B
    D. None of the above

11. A wide-complex tachycardia should always be considered and treated as ventricular tachycardia until proven otherwise. True or False.

12. Ventricular fibrillation has discernible complexes on close examination of the strip. True or False.

13. A grouped rhythm with PR intervals that prolong until a beat is dropped is known as:
    A. Wandering atrial pacemaker
    B. First-degree heart block
    C. Mobitz I second-degree heart block, or Wenckbach
    D. Mobitz II second-degree heart block
    E. Third-degree heart block

14. A grouped rhythm with dropped QRS complexes occurring either regularly or variably is known as:
    A. Wandering atrial pacemaker
    B. First-degree heart block
    C. Mobitz I second-degree heart block, or Wenckebach
    D. Mobitz II second-degree heart block
    E. Third-degree heart block

15. A rhythm with dissociated atrial and ventricular pacemakers, in which the atrial beat is faster than the ventricular rate, is known as:
    A. Wandering atrial pacemaker
    B. First-degree heart block
    C. Mobitz I second-degree heart block, or Wenckebach
    D. Mobitz II second-degree heart block
    E. Third-degree heart block

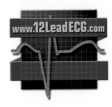

To enhance the knowledge you gain in this book, access this text's website at www.12leadECG.com! This valuable resource provides flashcards, an online glossary, web links, and more. Simply click on the Arrhythmias book cover once at the site.

Sinus Rhythms

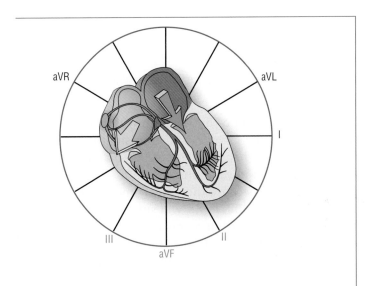

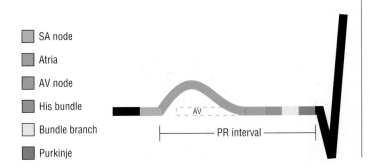

SA node
Atria
AV node
His bundle
Bundle branch
Purkinje

CHAPTER 8

Normal Sinus Rhythm

Introduction to Sinus Rhythms

The family of sinus rhythms have one thing in common: they all start at the SA node. The purpose of this introductory page is to lay down some basic foundation and terminology that we will continue to use throughout this book. For now, don't worry about understanding everything about each of the different sinus rhythms; we are going to review each of these in great detail in the coming pages.

Since, by definition, all of the complexes originate in the SA node, all the P waves for any one patient should be morphologically the same. In addition, since the impulses all travel down the normal electrical conduction system, the PR intervals should all be the same from complex to complex.

These are the two things common to all of the sinus rhythms (Figure 8-1):

1. *All the P waves are identical.*
2. *All the PR intervals are the same.*

Other things like the rate, regularity, and morphology will vary depending on the actual rhythm involved and the patient's individual anatomy, pathology, and variable neurohormonal state.

There are a couple of general terms we need to discuss at this point. The established normal rates for most people are from 60 to 100 beats per minute (BPM).

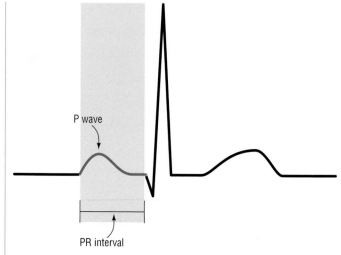

Figure 8-1: In all sinus rhythms, the P waves are identical.

When we encounter a rhythm strip with consistent morphology of the P waves and consistent PR intervals that has a regular heart rate between 60 and 100 BPM, we say that it is a normal sinus rhythm. This is a simplistic definition because there are some other criteria that we need to fulfill, but it will suffice for now. If the heart rate is irregular but meets the sinus rhythm criteria, we call it sinus arrhythmia (more on this later).

Bradycardia refers to slow rhythms, usually lower than 60 BPM. Therefore, a sinus bradycardia refers to a rhythm that meets the sinus rhythm criteria and is less than 60 BPM. Tachycardia refers to fast rhythms, faster than 100 BPM, to be exact. Once again, a sinus tachycar-

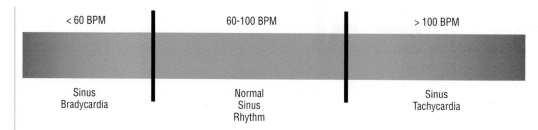

Figure 8-2: The regular sinus rhythms—sinus bradycardia, normal sinus rhythm, and sinus tachycardia—differ only in rate. Green is clinically insignificant and red signifies possible danger zones.

dia refers to a rhythm that matches the criteria we will outline for sinus rhythms but is faster than 100 BPM.

We want you to think of the regular sinus rhythms as a spectrum going from fast to slow (Figure 8-2). This is because, essentially, these three are exactly the same . . . just the rate is different. The clinical significance is highlighted by the color of the gradient. Green is clinically insignificant, whereas, red signifies possible danger zones. In general, when the rhythm is too slow or too fast, perfusion and cardiac function are compromised.

Characteristics of sinus rhythms are summarized in Table 8-1.

Normal Sinus Rhythm

Normal sinus rhythm (NSR) is the normal functioning rhythm of the heart. It is not an arrhythmia in the true sense of the word, because it is the normal state of functioning of the heart and not a pathological state. While the heart is in NSR, it cycles through automaticity, depolarization, and repolarization to produce the coordinated contraction and relaxation of the muscle needed to propel blood through the circulatory system.

Most textbooks spend just a few paragraphs, at most, to present this topic; however, we are going to present it more thoroughly because it is the foundation of arrhythmia recognition. Knowing how and why things occur will greatly facilitate your understanding of the more complex arrhythmias.

The Formation of the ECG

We begin to look at NSR by seeing how the traditional electrocardiographic pattern is created. In the figures, depolarization is depicted as a spreading red wave. The process of repolarization is represented as a spreading blue wave. While reviewing this section, keep in mind that this is a continuous process. There is no actual period of rest or inactivity and the cycle repeats over and over again because of the *automaticity* of the SA node. Figure 8-3 provides a review of the electrical conduction system.

The rate in NSR is between 60 and 100 beats per minute (BPM). Remember, by convention, any rhythms with rates below 60 BPM are considered bradycardias and any rhythms with rates above 100 BPM are considered tachycardias.

Rhythm	Characteristics
Normal sinus rhythm	• 60 to 100 BPM • All P waves are identical. • All PR intervals are identical. • Regular heart rate
Sinus bradycardia	• Slower than 60 BPM • All P waves are identical. • All PR intervals are identical.
Sinus tachycardia	• Faster than 100 BPM • All P waves are identical. • All PR intervals are identical.
Sinus arrhythmia	• Can have a normal rate, a bradycardic rate, or a tachycardic rate • All P waves are identical. • All PR intervals are identical. • Irregular heart rate

Table 8-1: Characteristics of Sinus Rhythms

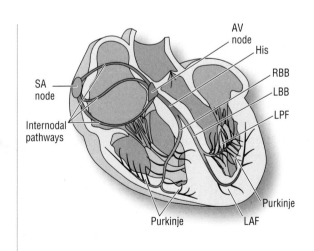

Figure 8-3: The electrical conduction system.

Cycle #1 (Figure 8-4A): The baseline is a period when the majority of the cardiac muscle is at rest. The SA node, however, is going through the process of automaticity and slowly depolarizing until the threshold potential is reached and the cells fire to start a new cardiac cycle.

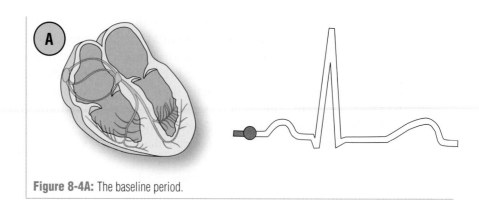

Figure 8-4A: The baseline period.

Cycle #2 (Figure 8-4B): At this point, the SA node is firing. The spread is being transmitted through the internodal pathways on its way to the AV node. This period is electrocardiographically neutral because there are not enough depolarized myocytes to create a measurable vector.

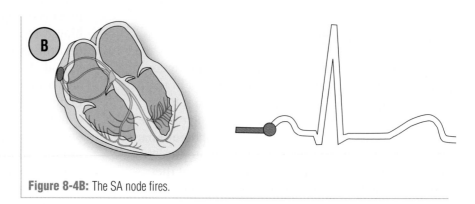

Figure 8-4B: The SA node fires.

Cycle #3 (Figure 8-4C): The right atria has now depolarized. This gives rise to a vector that heads to the right, slightly anteriorly, and down (yellow vector). In addition, many other things are occurring (see Additional Information box on the next page). The AV node is performing its main function by causing the physiologic block.

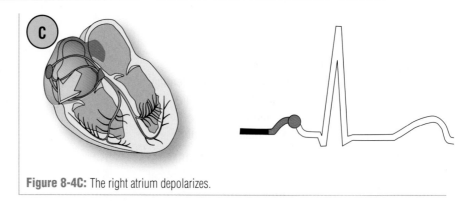

Figure 8-4C: The right atrium depolarizes.

Cycle #4 (Figure 8-4D): Both atria have depolarized completely. The SA node and the surrounding area have begun to repolarize. The left atrial vector is directed to the left, inferiorly, and slightly backwards (blue vector).

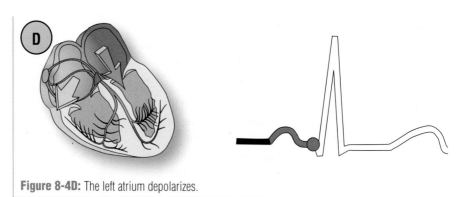

Figure 8-4D: The left atrium depolarizes.

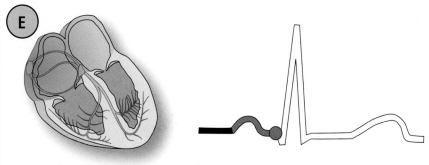

Cycle #5 (Figure 8-4E): At this point, depolarization of the left atria is almost complete and repolarization of the right atria is fairly well along.

Figure 8-4E: Depolarization is almost complete.

ADDITIONAL **INFORMATION**

Normal Sinus Rhythm

By definition, the SA node is always the primary pacemaker for the heart in NSR. Since there is only one pacemaker, *the P waves need to be identical*. In addition, since the distance and route taken to reach the AV node are the same, *the PR intervals have to be both normal and consistent.*

Since the impulse always starts at the SA node and spreads downward to depolarize the atria, the atrial vectors must always point inferiorly in NSR. In Figure 8-5, both the right atrial (yellow) vector and the left atrial (blue) vectors are heading inferiorly, directly toward leads II, III, and aVF of the hexaxial system. Positive vectors heading toward an electrode always gives rise to positive waves on an ECG. This means that, electrocardiographically, *the P wave must always be upright in leads II, III, and aVF during NSR.* If the P waves are negative in leads II, III, and aVF, the rhythm cannot be

NSR and there has to be an ectopic pacemaker (most commonly an ectopic atrial or a junctional pacemaker).

The PR interval represents a very busy time in the cardiac cycle. The atria, the AV node, bundle of His, both bundle branches, and the Purkinje system are all depolarizing and conducting the impulse (Figure 8-6). In addition, the AV node is performing its main function by causing a transient slowing of the impulse called the *physiologic block*. This slowing of the impulse is critical to coordinate the mechanical contraction of the atria in order to maximize ventricular filling. Without the block, the atria and ventricles would contract simultaneously.

The PR interval is considered normal if it is between 0.12 seconds to 0.20 seconds in length. It is shortened if it is less than or equal to 0.11 seconds and prolonged if it is greater than or equal to 0.21 seconds. Some authors consider 0.20 seconds to be borderline prolonged.

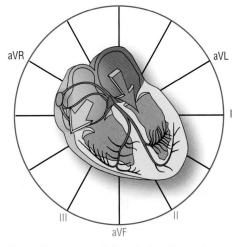

Figure 8-5: In normal sinus rhythm, the atrial vectors point inferiorly.

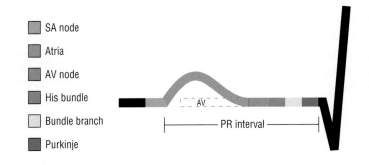

Figure 8-6: The PR interval.

Cycle #6 (Figure 8-4F): Repolarization has begun throughout most of the atria. The physiologic block is almost completed and the impulse is about to continue on to the ventricles.

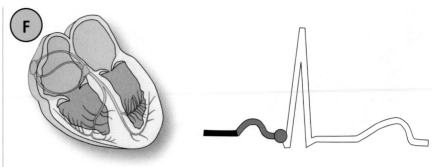

Figure 8-4F: Repolarization has begun throughout most of the atria.

Cycle #7 (Figure 8-4G): The physiologic block is completed and the impulse is proceeding through the bundle of His, the right and left bundles, the fascicles, and the Purkinje network. The impulse will be carried throughout most of the endocardium. Impulse spread will progress from endocardial surface to epicardial surface.

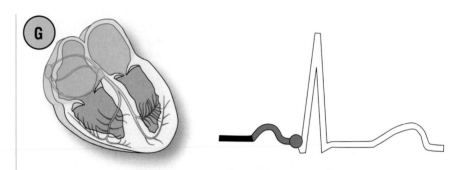

Figure 8-4G: The impulse is proceeding through the bundle of His, right and left bundles, and the Purkinje network.

Cycle #8 (Figure 8-4H): The very first area of the ventricles to depolarize is the upper septal area. It depolarizes from left to right giving rise to a small vector (pink vector) that is represented electrocardiographically as the septal Q waves.

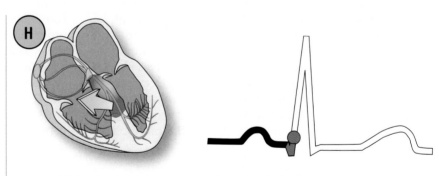

Figure 8-4H: The upper septal area of the ventricles starts to depolarize.

Cycle #9 (Figure 8-4I): The depolarization of the main portion of the left ventricle gives rise to a large vector (yellow vector) that is directed inferiorly, posteriorly, and backward. It gives rise to the large R wave depicted in this example.

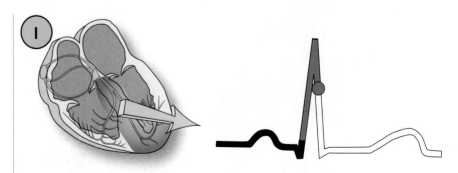

Figure 8-4I: Depolarization of the main portion of the left ventricle gives rise to a large R wave.

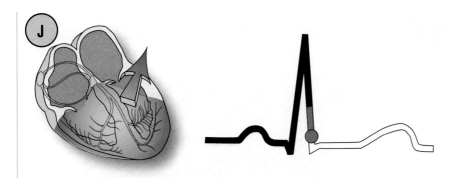

Figure 8-4J: The last portion of depolarization gives rise to an S wave.

Cycle #10 (Figure 8-4J): The last part of the left ventricle to depolarize is the upper, posterior part on the left. The positive depolarization wave going in that direction gives rise to a vector (blue vector) that is electrocardiographically represented as the S wave or terminal portion of the QRS complex.

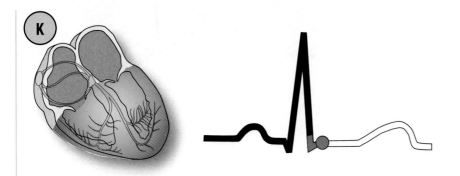

Figure 8-4K: Both ventricles have depolarized and the QRS complex is complete.

Cycle #11 (Figure 8-4K): At this point, both ventricles have depolarized. The QRS complex is complete. Since the depolarization of the ventricles occurred using the normal electrical conduction system, *the QRS complex should be normal in duration*. The normal QRS interval is within 0.06 and 0.11 seconds inclusive.

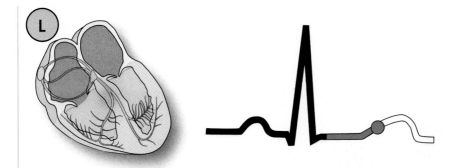

Figure 8-4L: The ventricles are completing depolarization and beginning to repolarize, giving rise to a T wave.

Cycle #12 (Figure 8-4L): This period represents a time when the ventricles are completing depolarization and are beginning to repolarize. The repolarization of the ventricles gives rise to the T wave. (See Additional Information box.)

Absolute Refractory Period

The early part of the T wave represents a period known as the *absolute refractory period*. If you notice on the graphic of the heart in cycle 12 and Figure 8-4L, most of the ventricle is still somewhat depolarized (represented by the pink areas). These areas would be *refractory* to any new impulses. In other words, since they are still depolarized (more positive), they would not be able to fire or conduct any new impulses. To use an analogy, let's think of a cannon. A loaded cannon can easily be fired by pulling the trigger. However, if you quickly pull the trigger again before the cannon has been adequately reloaded, it won't fire the second time even though the trigger was pulled.

Only some small isolated areas show complete repolarization (represented by the blue areas in the previous figures and blue cells in Figure 8-7) and would be available for another impulse. As more cells are repolarized, this can create a problem; as we shall see in the next Additional Information box.

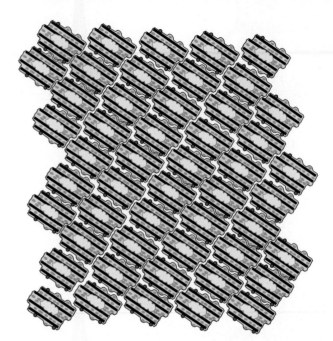

Figure 8-7: Only some cells are completely repolarized and ready for another impulse.

Cycle #13 (Figure 8-4M): The T wave is now well on its way electrocardiographically. This late part of the T wave, along the downward slope (see blue area), represents a period known as the *relative refractory period*. (See Additional Information box on the next page.)

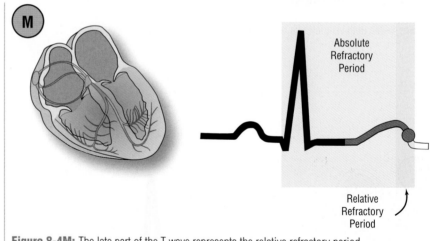

Figure 8-4M: The late part of the T wave represents the relative refractory period.

Cycle #14 (Figure 8-4N): This is the final phase. The heart is relaxing at this point. However, automaticity of all of the cells continues. Remember, in NSR the SA node will win the automaticity rate as it is the principal, and fastest, pacemaker for the heart. If the heart is functioning normally, this process will repeat over and over continuously.

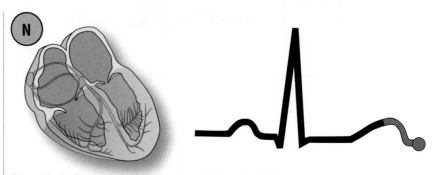

Figure 8-4N: The final phase. In this phase, the heart is relaxing.

Relative Refractory Period

During the relative refractory period many more cells are repolarized and ready to receive an impulse than during the absolute refractory period. As a result, transmission of impulses can occur, but often by very circuitous routes. Occasionally, a circular pathway is set up like the one in Figure 8-8. In this case, the impulse started out as a premature ventricular complex at the pacemaker cell labeled with the red star. Then, slowly, by direct cell-to-cell transmission, the impulse made its way around a segment of the heart. The transmission was so slow that by the time the impulse reached the original pacemaking area, that area was again repolarized. That means it was ready to receive a transmission again. This type of *circus movement* can cause serious *arrhythmogenic* consequences and is a set-up for ventricular tachycardia. We will spend a great deal more time on this later. This is just a small introduction to the topic of the absolute and relative refractory periods of the T wave.

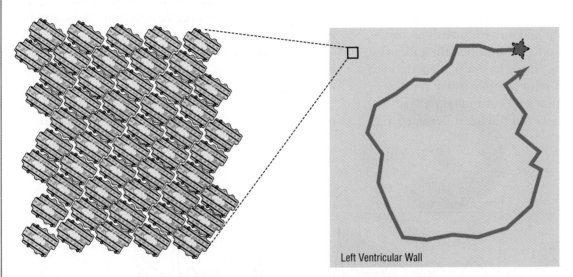

Left Ventricular Wall

Figure 8-8: When an impulse starts out as a premature ventricular complex at the pacemaker cell, the transmission can be so slow that by the time the impulse reaches the original pacemaking area, the area is again repolarized.

Regularity

Normal sinus rhythm is a regular rhythm. What we mean by this is that the complexes occur at a regular and consistent distance from each other. To use an analogy, think of how light posts are placed along the sides of the road. They are all placed at regular, recurring distances from each other along the roadside.

Why does this regularity occur? To understand why, we need to go back to the concept of automaticity and Phase 4 that we talked about in Chapter 2. Remember, Phase 4 is a very slow but continuous depolarization of the pacemaker cell from its most negative repolarization value until the threshold potential was reached and the cell fired. This slow, gradual Phase 4 is how the pacemaking function of the cardiac cells is created. The length of the Phase 4 cycle is very consistent and determines the pacemaking rate of the particular cell type involved.

Under normal circumstances, the SA node has the fastest Phase 4 of any of the cardiac cells and functions as the main pacemaker for the heart. By definition, NSR has the SA node as the main pacemaker to set the cardiac rate. This rate is very regular in most cases. Occasionally, slight variations in timing can occur. Variations of up to 0.16 seconds can occur occasionally and still be considered normal (Figure 8-9). In these cases, it is critical to remember that the P wave should have the same morphology as the sinus P wave and that the PR interval should be consistent with the regular complexes.

On a rhythm strip or ECG, the distance is measured from one spot on a complex to the same corresponding spot on the next complex. This distance is then transferred to the remaining beats. If the distance is the same, or close to it, we say that the rhythm is regular.

By tradition, the most common distance measured is called the *R-R interval* (R to R interval [Figure 8-10]).

This is the distance from the top of one QRS complex to the top of the next beat. The top of the QRS is used because it is usually very easily identifiable and easy to pinpoint with your calipers.

Another measurement that is constantly used is the *P-P interval* (Figure 8-11). You would calculate the distance the same way as the R-R interval, but you would use the top or the beginning of the P wave instead of the top of the R wave.

By definition, rhythms have to be either regular, regularly irregular, or irregularly irregular. We discussed the issues with regularity above. Now, let's turn our attention to the issues with irregularity.

Regularly Irregular Rhythms

To discuss irregularity, we need to understand the difference between a rhythm and a rhythm with an overlying cardiac *event* that momentarily alters the cadence of the underlying rhythm. Suppose you had a strip with an NSR clearly visible on it; for simplicity, we represented each complex with a gold bar in Figure 8-12. Suddenly another pacemaker in the heart became irri-

table and fired early. The morphology of either the P wave or the QRS complex generated by the secondary pacemaker would be different and early compared with the rest of the complexes around it. Let's use a blue circle in Figure 8-12 to represent this cardiac event. Would this new rhythm have a new name? The answer is no. What we say is that the patient has a normal sinus rhythm with a _____ (the blank will be filled in by the name of the event). For example, we would say that the patient had a normal sinus rhythm with a PVC.

This is an example of a *regularly irregular* rhythm. Let's break down this term a bit further in order to understand it more clearly. The first word "regularly" signifies that the underlying rhythm is regular. It could be any of the regular rhythms that we will discuss in this book, but it has to be a regular rhythm. The second word denotes the abnormal events that occur between or inside of the regular rhythm. That irregularity may occur once, twice, or be a recurring event at various intervals during the strip (Figure 8-13).

In some cases, the cardiac event may alter the rate of the original regular rhythm but the subsequent

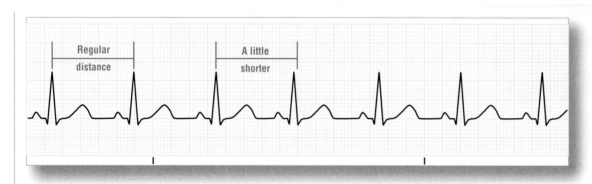

Figure 8-9: Notice the slight irregularity of the fourth complex. It is slightly early but has the same P wave morphology and PR intervals as the other beats. This is NSR.

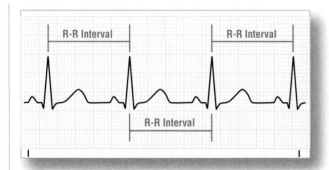

Figure 8-10: The R-R interval is the most common distance measured because it is easy to identify the top of the QRS complex.

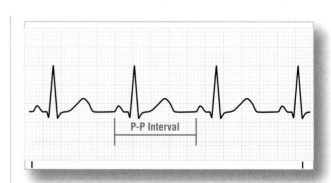

Figure 8-11: The P-P interval can also be used for measuring distance.

rhythm could still be regular. Look at Figure 8-14. At the start of the strip, we have a nice, slow, regular rhythm. Then a cardiac event occurs. After the event, the underlying rate or pacemaker has changed but the rhythm still remains regular. This is still considered a regularly irregular rhythm and is quite a common occurrence in many patients. We describe this rhythm by breaking down each component and mentioning them separately, for example, a normal sinus rhythm with a PVC followed by a sinus tachycardia.

Irregularly Irregular Rhythms

When a rhythm is completely chaotic and you cannot find any underlying regularity, we say that it is irregularly irregular. They are easy to spot because the ca-

dence of the complexes is completely haphazard. In addition, the P waves and PR intervals, if there are any, are almost always variable in morphology.

How does a rhythm become totally chaotic? Well, let's look at a case involving three different atrial pacemakers, each firing at its own intrinsic rate. In Figure 8-15 below, we have isolated the rhythm strip from the three different pacemakers: A, B, and C. For simplicity, we will use different colored bars to represent the complexes generated by each of the pacemakers.

Not a big deal, right? The rhythm for each of the three pacemakers is clearly delineated and easy to spot. Keep in mind that each one of those stars represents an entire complex, P wave, PR interval, QRS complex, and ST-T waves. Also keep in mind that each one of the P

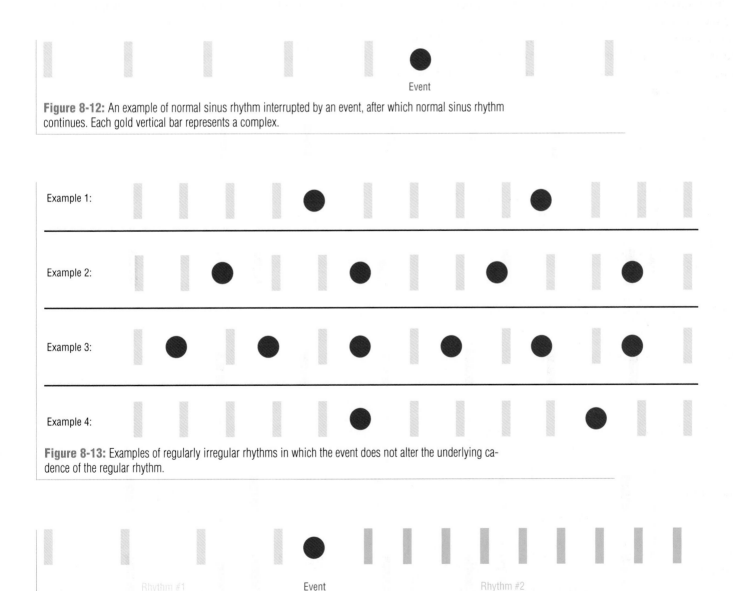

Figure 8-12: An example of normal sinus rhythm interrupted by an event, after which normal sinus rhythm continues. Each gold vertical bar represents a complex.

Example 1:

Example 2:

Example 3:

Example 4:

Figure 8-13: Examples of regularly irregular rhythms in which the event does not alter the underlying cadence of the regular rhythm.

Rhythm #1   Event   Rhythm #2

Figure 8-14: An example of normal sinus rhythm interrupted by an event, followed by sinus tachycardia.

waves and PR intervals may be different. Still not a problem—it is still easy to visualize.

Now, let's make all three pacemakers fire simultaneously in the same heart and have each one continue to fire at its own intrinsic rate. Can you visualize what the strip would look like?

Taking into account that some complexes would not be transmitted because they fall on the absolute refractory period, and the fact that some may not be transmitted for other unclear reasons, we can make a reasonable guess as to what the final strip would look like with these three pacemakers (Figure 8-16). As you can see, the final strip has very few repetitions of any R-R interval. This strip is typical of the chaotic and completely random pattern seen in an irregularly irregular rhythm.

To make matters a bit more complex, we need to remember that some complexes will fuse to form entirely new complex morphologies and completely different R-R intervals. To continue adding more complexity, suppose there were four pacemakers instead of three. What if there were five or six pacemakers? Now, you can begin to imagine the complexity found in irregularly irregular rhythms. Luckily for us, there are only three main irregularly irregular rhythms: wandering atrial pacemaker, multifocal atrial tachycardia, and atrial fibrillation. We will discuss each of these in great detail later on in the book. This is an initial introduction to the topic.

We have taken a serious look at how NSR is formed. We have reviewed the characteristics of NSR and some of the principles that are beautifully outlined by this rhythm, for example, regularity. Now, it is time to begin to actually look at some strips. In this book, we will try to show you various examples of each of the rhythms. We will show you some examples that are at the fast end of the spectrum, some that are at the slow end of the spectrum, some with positive complexes, and some with negative complexes. It is critical for you to apply the concepts we have learned to each strip. The concepts are what you will need to remember.

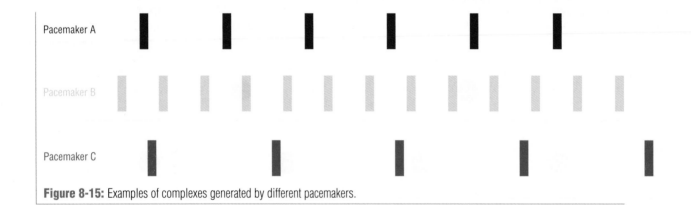

Figure 8-15: Examples of complexes generated by different pacemakers.

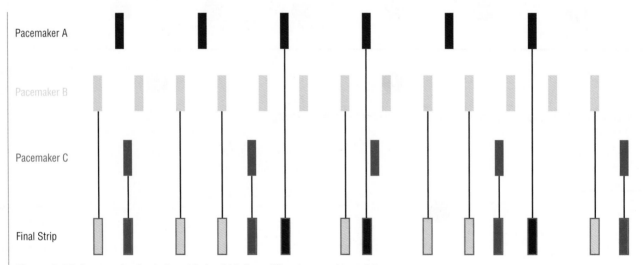

Figure 8-16: An example of a rhythm strip in which three different pacemakers exist.

ADDITIONAL **INFORMATION**

Nomenclature

A little problem with nomenclature . . .

Many authors state that in NSR the width of the QRS complex must be less than 0.12 seconds wide. They use the term *regular sinus rhythm* rather than *normal sinus rhythm* to describe rhythms with wide QRS complexes, but the methodology is not always spelled out. The majority of clinicians and authors use the terms interchangeably.

This text sticks with the strictest criteria and states that the QRS has to be normal width in order for the rhythm to be normal sinus rhythm. We will use the term *sinus rhythm* or *regular sinus rhythm* to describe strips with abnormally wide QRS complexes. Clinically, the important point to try to resolve is why the QRS complexes are wide in the first place.

ADDITIONAL **INFORMATION**

Slight Variations in P Waves and PR Intervals

We should clarify something about P morphology and PR morphology. Electrophysiology (EPS) studies have shown us that there can be some minimal differences in appearance between P waves and PR intervals that start in the same SA node (Figure 8-17). The reason for this is that the SA node is not just one single cell, or even one small area, but rather a fairly long spindle-shaped structure. The pacing cells can sometimes vary within the SA node, and these minor differences in location

can cause very minimal alterations in the morphology of the P and the length that the impulse has to travel to reach the AV node, hence the PR interval. When we say "identical" in this book, we mean that they are so similar as to almost guarantee the same site of origin. Pacemakers located outside the SA node would cause fairly obvious morphological differences that would be easy to identify.

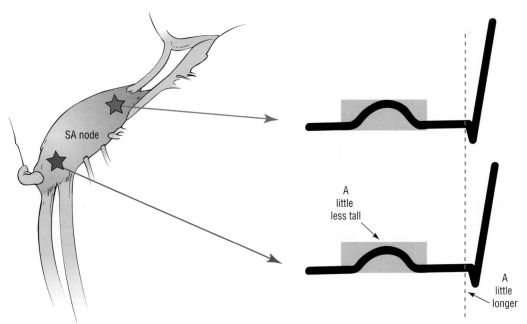

Figure 8-17: There can be slight differences in appearance between P waves and PR intervals that start in the same SA node.

ECG Strips

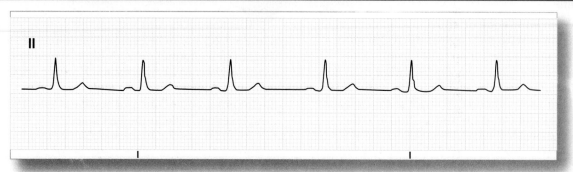

Discussion:

ECG 8-1 is a typical example of a normal sinus rhythm that is toward the slower end of the spectrum. It is just barely over 60 BPM, so it fits between the range of 60 and 100 BPM that is needed for NSR. The P waves are all the same morphology and the PR intervals are all identical. This is critical in determining the rhythm because it means that all of the complexes originated within the same pacemaker, in this case the sinus node. The P-P intervals are the same and the rhythm is very regular. The QRS complexes are all less than 0.12 seconds long and are similar in morphology. This rounds off all the necessary criteria for the diagnosis of NSR.

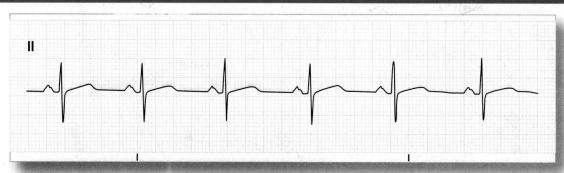

Rate:	Slightly over 60 BPM	PR intervals:	Normal, consistent
Regularity:	Regular	QRS width:	Normal
P waves:	Present	Rhythm:	**Normal sinus rhythm**

Discussion:

ECG 8-2 shows all of the characteristics of NSR. Notice that the QRS complexes are relatively isoelectric (the same distance in the positive and negative directions).

The orientation of the QRS complexes does not enter into the diagnosis of NSR in any way, and you should not worry too much about it for now.

ECG 8-3

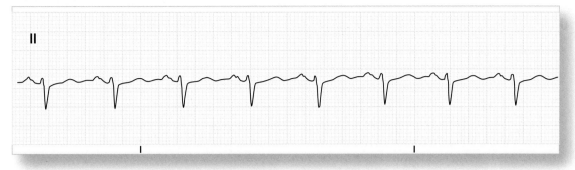

Rate:	Slightly over 80 BPM	PR intervals:	Normal, consistent
Regularity:	Regular	QRS width:	Normal
P waves:	Present	Rhythm:	**Normal sinus rhythm**

Discussion:

ECG 8-3 is also NSR. Notice that in this case, the complexes are all negative. Once again, the orientation of the complexes should not enter into the diagnosis. The P waves are notched but this is a normal finding.

ECG 8-4

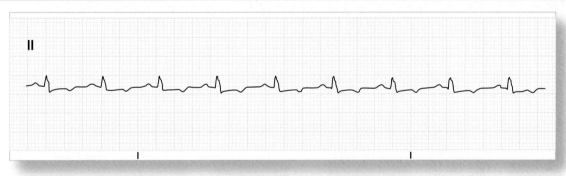

Rate:	Around 95 BPM	PR intervals:	Normal, consistent
Regularity:	Regular	QRS width:	Normal
P waves:	Present	Rhythm:	**Normal sinus rhythm**

Discussion:

This time we decided to show you an example of a rhythm strip with really small QRS complexes (ECG 8-4). Don't let the size of the QRS complexes or the flipped T waves fool you—it is still NSR. Remember, you cannot meet the criteria for small complexes on a rhythm strip; you need the whole ECG to make that determination.

ECG 8-5

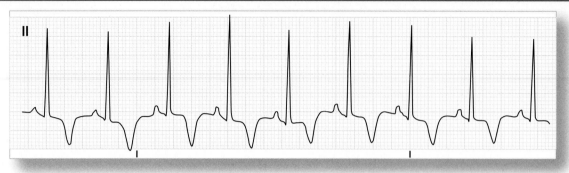

Rate:	Slightly under 100 BPM	PR intervals:	Normal, consistent
Regularity:	Regular	QRS width:	Normal
P waves:	Present	Rhythm:	**Normal sinus rhythm**

Discussion:

ECG 8-5 shows some pretty tall QRS complexes and some deep, inverted T waves. The rhythm, however, is NSR. Don't let the size of the complexes or any other pathology steer you from making the correct call on the rhythm. Remember, to really talk about cardiac pathology, you need a full 12-lead ECG and not just a rhythm strip.

ECG 8-6

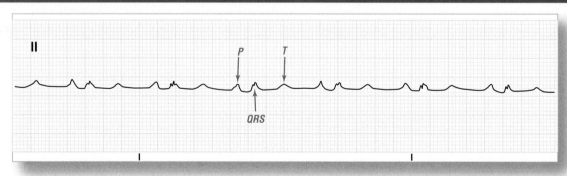

Rate:	Slightly over 65 BPM	PR intervals:	Normal, consistent
Regularity:	Regular	QRS width:	Normal
P waves:	Present	Rhythm:	**Normal sinus rhythm**

Discussion:

We decided it was time for the first curve ball. ECG 8-6 also shows some very small complexes. To simplify matters, we labeled the P wave, the QRS complex, and the T waves for easy identification. The morphology of some of the P waves shows some slight irregularities. Could this be multiple pacemakers at work? The answer is no. Notice that the PR intervals are the same and that the rhythm strip is very regular. Remember, different pacemakers would alter the regularity, the P wave morphology, and the PR interval. This is NSR.

This would be tough to figure out if it were a tachycardic rhythm, wouldn't it?

When Normal Sinus Rhythm Becomes More Tachycardic

ECG 8-7

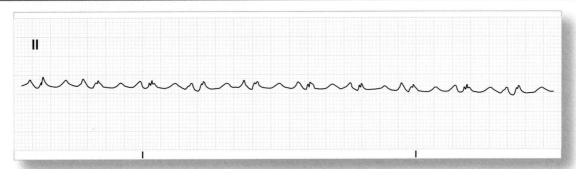

In ECG 8-7, the worst-case scenario comes true. This is the same patient as in ECG 8-6, but much more tachycardic. Now it is tougher to decide what is a P wave, what is a QRS complex, and what is a T wave. You can make some educated guesses, but that is a big risk to take when a life is at stake. Can you figure out a way to easily determine what is what?

The easiest thing to do is to change leads and see if you can get more distinctive complexes in that lead. Another method is to get a strip with simultaneous leads on it, or better yet an ECG, to identify the complexes better. Take a look at Figure 8-18. In this strip, two leads were obtained simultaneously. In lead III, the complexes are more distinctive and it is easy to identify the various parts of the complex. Now it is just a matter of following up an imaginary line from an obvious QRS complex on lead III and find the corresponding spot on lead II. That spot on lead II has to be the QRS complex. Do the same thing on the next obvious QRS complex and place your calipers between these two spots. Now, walk your calipers over and identify all of the other QRS complexes on the strip. The rhythm is easy to identify, even in lead II.

Here is a clinical pearl: Contrary to popular opinion, lead II is not always the best lead to identify rhythms. Which is the best lead? The answer is that it varies from patient to patient. In some patients, it will be lead II. In others, it may be lead V_1. In others, it may be aVL. You just never know. The take-home message is this: ***When you are dealing with a complex arrhythmia, obtain multiple leads or a full ECG.*** This makes identification easier and safer.

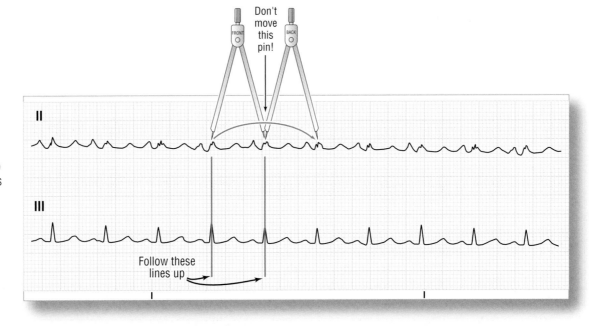

Figure 8-18: When attempting to measure complexes that are difficult to read, obtain a strip from another lead. This may help to clarify the ECG components and accurately measure the complexes.

A D D I T I O N A L **I N F O R M A T I O N**

Take-Home Points: Normal Sinus Rhythm

1. Atrial and ventricular rates are between 60 and 100 BPM.

2. Rhythm is regular.

3. All of the P waves are the same.

4. PR intervals have to be normal and should be the same throughout.

5. QRS width is normal.

(If the QRS complexes were wide but the other criteria were all met, we would say that the rhythm was sinus but not normal sinus.)

6. The P-P and R-R intervals should be the same throughout.

7. Very small irregularities in P wave morphology or in the PR are still within normal limits for NSR.

CHAPTER REVIEW

1. By definition, all of the sinus rhythms originate in the _____ node.

2. Which of the following are correct for normal sinus rhythm?
   A. All the P waves are identical.
   B. The P waves should all be positive in lead aVL.
   C. The PR intervals should be identical.
   D. An occasional interval that is much shorter than the others is considered normal.

3. The atrial rate in sinus bradycardia is _____ BPM.

4. The atrial rate in normal sinus rhythm is between _____ and _____ BPM.

5. The atrial rate in sinus tachycardia is _____ BPM.

6. The P wave is caused by the depolarization of the atria. The depolarization of the SA node, by itself, is electrocardiographically not visible. True or False.

7. The combined atrial vector points in NSR should point in which major direction (pick one):
   A. Anteriorly
   B. Posteriorly
   C. Inferiorly
   D. Superiorly

8. In NSR, the P waves should always be upright in leads ___, ___, and ____.

9. The length of the PR interval should be:
   A. Less than 0.12 seconds
   B. Between 0.10 and 0.20 seconds
   C. Between 0.12 and 0.20 seconds
   D. Greater than 0.20 seconds

10. The physiologic block is a normal slowing or delay of the impulse as it moves from the atria to the ventricles via the AV node. This slowing is critical to coordinate the mechanical contraction of the atria to the ventricles. Without the physiologic block, the atria and ventricles would contract simultaneously. True or False.

11. During the PR interval, the atria, AV node, bundle of His, the bundle branches, and the Purkinje system all fire. True or False.

12. In NSR, the width of the QRS complex should be:
    A. Less than 0.06 seconds
    B. Between 0.06 and 0.11 seconds
    C. Between 0.10 and 0.12 seconds
    D. Greater than 0.12 seconds

13. The absolute refractory period is that part of the cardiac cycle when another impulse may still be transmitted. True or False.

14. During the relative refractory period, the myocardial tissue is in the process of repolarization. An early impulse occurring at this time may stimulate the heart and cause a contraction. True or False.

15. Sometimes, circus pathways may form during the relative refractory period that can lead to complex arrhythmia formation. True or False.

16. Normal sinus rhythm is:
    A. Regular
    B. Regularly irregular
    C. Irregularly irregular
    D. An arrhythmia

17. Which of the following intervals should be the same in NSR?
    A. PR interval
    B. QRS interval
    C. P-P interval
    D. R-R interval

18. In NSR, the P-P interval should not be longer than ___ seconds or ___ big blocks on the ECG paper.

19. Very slight variations in the P wave morphology and in the PR interval are considered acceptable in normal sinus rhythm. True or False.

20. The best lead to evaluate an arrhythmia in a particular patient is:
    A. Lead I
    B. Lead II
    C. Lead V₁
    D. The best lead can vary from patient to patient.

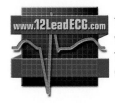

CHAPTER 9

Sinus Bradycardia

Sinus bradycardia (SB) refers to a rhythm that originates in the SA node and has a rate less than 60 BPM. If you look at Figure 9-1, you see that it lies on the left or slower end of the sinus spectrum. Sinus bradycardia has all of the characteristics of NSR except that the QRS complexes do not have to be less than 0.12 seconds. The P waves and PR intervals should all be the same morphology and duration.

So, where is the difference between NSR and SB? The answer lies in the Phase 4 interval of the cellular action potential (see Figure 9-2 and Chapter 2 for a review of the concepts). In sinus bradycardia, the SA node fires slower than in NSR. This means that the automaticity of the cells is prolonged temporally and you end up with a slower and longer Phase 4. Electrocardiographically, Phase 4 is represented by the TP segment (Figure 9-3). The slower the automaticity, the longer the TP segment, and vice versa.

Sinus bradycardia is easily identifiable because it has discrete complexes that are usually identical to the NSR complexes but separated by much longer TP segments (Figure 9-3). Once again, notice that the P waves, PR intervals, and QRS complexes are all identical. The QT interval and the duration of the T wave, on the other hand, may be a bit more prolonged in bradycardic rhythms due to their longer repolarization phases.

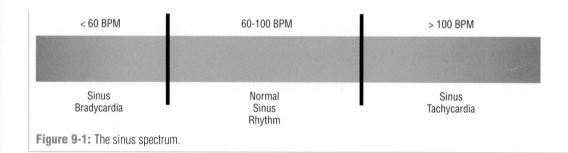

Figure 9-1: The sinus spectrum.

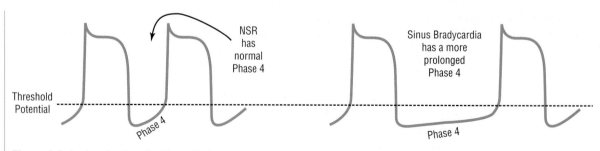

Figure 9-2: In sinus bradycardia, Phase 4 is longer.

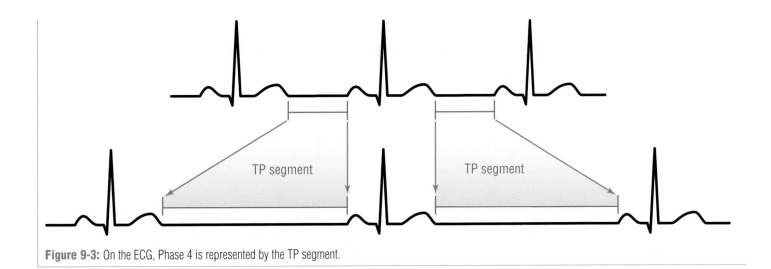

Figure 9-3: On the ECG, Phase 4 is represented by the TP segment.

When is Sinus Bradycardia Considered a Cardiac Emergency?

Sinus bradycardia is considered a cardiac emergency when there is significant hemodynamic compromise associated with it. If the patient is hypotensive or having chest pain, diaphoresis, and problems mentating, among other things, the heart rate must be increased either electrically (by using a pacemaker) or pharmaceutically (using atropine or a catecholamine-like agent like epinephrine, norepinephrine, or dopamine).

Most patients can tolerate heart rates between 50 and 60 BPM without too much difficulty. Sinus bradycardia typically becomes clinically significant when the heart rate drops below 50 BPM. This is because the slower the rate, the lower the cardiac output (remember: cardiac output = heart rate × stroke volume). Under normal circumstances, however, heart rates as slow as the low 40s may be normal for very well conditioned athletes and in some patients during sleep.

ARRHYTHMIA RECOGNITION

Sinus Bradycardia

Rate:	< 60 BPM
Regularity:	Regular
P wave:	Present
Morphology:	Same
Upright in II, III, and aVF:	Yes
P:QRS ratio:	1:1
PR interval:	Normal, consistent
QRS width:	Normal or wide
Grouping:	None
Dropped beats:	None

DIFFERENTIAL DIAGNOSIS

Sinus Bradycardia

1. Increased vagal tone
   a. Vomiting
   b. Carotid sinus massage
2. Myocardial infarction
3. Increased intracranial pressure
4. Hypoxemia or decreased ventilation
5. Hypothermia
6. Hypothyroidism
7. Drugs: beta blockers, calcium channel blockers, amiodarone, digitalis
8. Sick sinus syndrome
9. Electrolyte disorders
10. Athletes
11. Idiopathic

ECG Strips

ECG 9-1

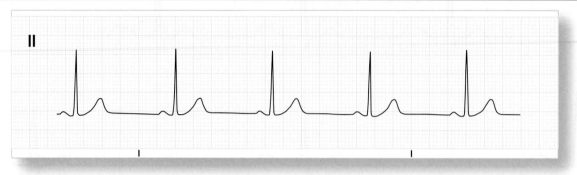

Rate:	Slightly under 60 BPM	PR intervals:	Normal, consistent
Regularity:	Regular	QRS width:	Normal
P waves:	Present	Rhythm:	**Sinus bradycardia**

Discussion:

ECG 9-1 is an excellent example of sinus bradycardia. Notice the long, flat TP segments between each of the complexes. The waves are all normal duration and morphology. Lead II shows upright P waves so that you know that the P wave axis is normal.

ECG 9-2

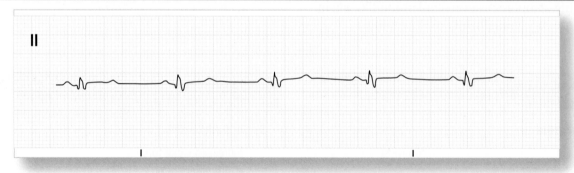

Rate:	About 55 BPM	PR intervals:	Normal, consistent
Regularity:	Regular	QRS width:	Normal
P waves:	Present	Rhythm:	**Sinus bradycardia**

Discussion:

The first thing to catch your eye in ECG 9-2 is the relatively small size of the QRS complexes. However, they are still easily identifiable. The intervals and waves are all normal. The only interval that may be slightly widened is the QRS interval. However, on close examination, we note that the complexes are about 0.11 seconds and within the normal limits. Once again, the P waves are upright in lead II. This is sinus bradycardia. If the QRS complexes were wider than 0.12 seconds, we would have two possibilities: (1) sinus bradycardia with aberrantly conducted ventricular complexes, and (2) sinus bradycardia with a bundle branch block. Comparison of this strip with others from the past would help answer the aberrancy question. An ECG would help distinguish the bundle branch block question easily. Comparison of this new ECG with an old one would help to distinguish if the bundle block is new.

ECG 9-3

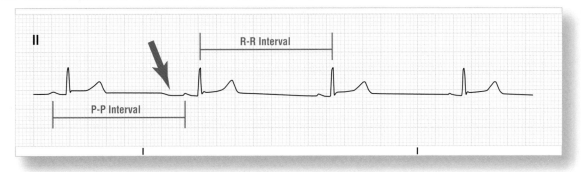

Rate:	Slightly under 45 BPM	PR intervals:	Normal, consistent
Regularity:	Regular	QRS width:	Normal
P waves:	Present	Rhythm:	**Sinus bradycardia**

Discussion:

ECG 9-3 shows a really slow rate with complexes that appear fairly normal. At first glance, it is obviously sinus bradycardia. Even though this diagnosis is correct, the criteria are a bit clouded. Take a look at the second P wave. Does the morphology look different? It is a bit different. Could it be a premature atrial contraction (PAC)? The answer is no, because the P-P and R-R intervals are the same throughout the entire strip. If the complex were a PAC, the abnormal P wave and its corresponding QRS complex should have occurred sooner than expected. This one came out exactly on time. So, what caused the morphology of that P wave to be dif-

ferent? Notice that right before the P wave, there is a dip in the baseline (see blue arrow). This dip almost breaks the P wave in two with the second half being normal. The dip is probably due to some movement of the patient or the leads. This dip, and not an ectopic P wave, is the cause of the alteration in the morphology of the P wave. The keys to making the diagnosis are the regularity and the overall similarities between all of the complexes. Remember to always look at the company the pathology keeps; if it is not there, think about the alternatives.

ECG 9-4

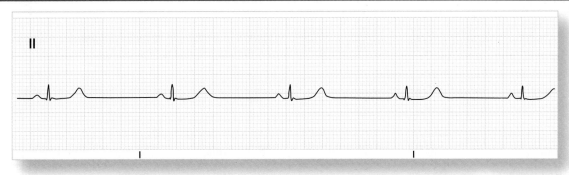

Rate:	About 45 BPM	PR intervals:	Normal, consistent
Regularity:	Regular	QRS width:	Normal
P waves:	Present	Rhythm:	**Sinus bradycardia**

Discussion:

ECG 9-4 also has some very small QRS complexes. The rate is very slow at 45 BPM. The P waves, PR intervals, and QRS complexes are all similar in morphology and duration. This is another example of sinus bradycardia.

You should clinically evaluate this patient, and anyone who is severely bradycardic, closely for any signs of hemodynamic insufficiency.

ECG 9-5

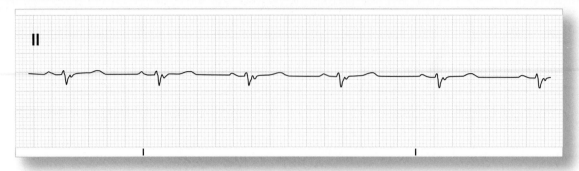

Rate:	Slightly under 60 BPM	PR intervals:	Normal, consistent
Regularity:	Regular	QRS width:	Normal
P waves:	Present	Rhythm:	**Sinus bradycardia**

Discussion:

ECG 9-5 meets all of the criteria for sinus bradycardia. The QRS complexes, if you measure them, are wider than 0.12 seconds. You will need to do some investigation to rule out aberrancy or another cause for the wide QRS complexes. When we performed an ECG and compared it to an old one, we found out that the patient had a long-standing bifascicular block with a right bundle branch block and a left anterior hemiblock. The P waves were identical to the ones found in prior ECGs and strips, so the rhythm is sinus bradycardia.

ECG 9-6

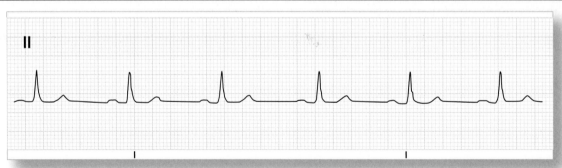

Rate:	Slightly under 60 BPM	PR intervals:	Prolonged, consistent
Regularity:	Regular	QRS width:	Normal
P waves:	Present	Rhythm:	**Sinus bradycardia**

Discussion:

Did you notice anything peculiar on ECG 9-6? If you did not, go back and examine it again, this time taking some extra time and measuring all of the intervals. The patient definitely has a rate less than 60 BPM and the P waves are upright in lead II. The QRS width is less than 0.12 seconds, which is normal. The problem lies in the PR interval. The PR interval is prolonged by being over 0.20 seconds (one big block). For now, just be aware of the problem and document it. Later on after we discuss AV blocks, you will call this sinus bradycardia with a first degree AV block.

C H A P T E R **R E V I E W**

1. The main pacemaker for a patient with sinus bradycardia is:
   A. SA node
   B. Ectopic atrial
   C. AV node
   D. Either A or B

2. In sinus bradycardia, the atrial rate must be _____ 60 BPM.

3. In sinus bradycardia, the main pacemaker is firing at a slow rate. For some patients, this slower rate can be normal. It is also seen normally in athletic individuals and in patients during sleep. True or False.

4. In sinus bradycardia, the entire complex is broader, leading to a slower rate. True or False.

5. What phase of the action potential is lengthened in sinus bradycardia?
   A. Phase 1
   B. Phase 2
   C. Phase 3
   D. Phase 4

6. A slightly prolonged QT interval and QTc are considered normal in sinus bradycardia. True or False.

7. The main electrocardiographic segment that is lengthened in sinus bradycardia is (pick the best one):
   A. PR interval
   B. QRS interval
   C. QT interval
   D. QTc

8. The P wave should be upright in leads ___, ___, and ___ in any sinus beat.

9. Myocardial infarctions can lead to sinus bradycardia. True or False.

10. Hemodynamically significant sinus bradycardia in a patient having an AMI should not be treated because they will get better as the patient's ischemia resolves. True or False.

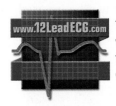

To enhance the knowledge you gain in this book, access this text's website at www.12leadECG.com! This valuable resource provides flashcards, an online glossary, web links, and more. Simply click on the Arrhythmias book cover once at the site.

Sinus Tachycardia

Sinus tachycardia (ST) refers to a rhythm that originates in the SA node and has a rate faster than 100 BPM. In Figure 10-1 we see that it lies on the right or faster end of the sinus spectrum. In most cases, sinus tachycardia has a rate between 100 and 160 BPM, but rates as high as 220 BPM can be seen. At higher rates, the diagnosis of sinus tachycardia becomes increasingly difficult and it can be confused with some of the other supraventricular tachycardias. We will discuss the differential diagnosis of narrow complex tachycardias in great detail in Chapter 27.

For any given patient, the heart rate is determined by a constant tug-of-war between the sympathetic and the parasympathetic divisions of the autonomic nervous system (Figure 10-2). If the parasympathetic dominates, the rhythm is slowed. If the sympathetic dominates, the rhythm is sped up. The effects of the sympathetic stimulation can go beyond the rate; it can sometimes cause minor morphological differences in the appearance of

the QRS complex. It can be difficult to distinguish pathological presentations from tachycardia-related changes.

Morphologically, sinus tachycardia has all of the characteristics of NSR except for the heart rate and the acceptable widths of the QRS complex (complexes wider than 0.12 seconds are acceptable). Sympathetic stimulation does cause certain changes in the appearance of the cardiac complexes electrocardiographically, as mentioned above. Sympathetic stimulation alters the rate of conduction through most tissue by increasing transit times of the cardiac impulse. The P wave amplitude is usually affected one way or the other by this increased transit time. Usually, the amplitude of the P waves is decreased; however, in some cases, the amplitude of the P waves may actually be increased.

Sympathetic discharge also causes faster transit times through the AV node. These faster rates shorten the length of the PR interval considerably. The interval,

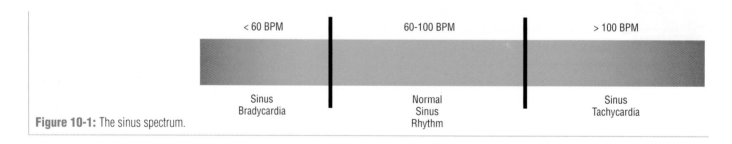

< 60 BPM	60-100 BPM	> 100 BPM
Sinus Bradycardia	Normal Sinus Rhythm	Sinus Tachycardia

Figure 10-1: The sinus spectrum.

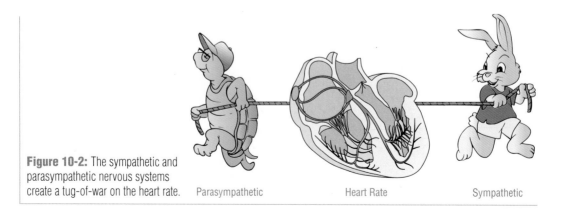

Figure 10-2: The sympathetic and parasympathetic nervous systems create a tug-of-war on the heart rate.

Parasympathetic   Heart Rate   Sympathetic

however, should still be between 0.12 and 0.20 seconds to be considered normal.

The QRS complex is usually not affected by the sinus tachycardia itself. However, there are two separate pathologies associated with any tachycardia that can be seen in sinus tachycardia: rate-related aberrancy and *electrical alternans*.

To quickly review, rate-related aberrancy refers to an aberrantly conducted impulse in the ventricles due to the impulses arriving at a section of the electrical conduction system before the refractory period has completed. The impulse must continue on from this refractory area by direct cell-to-cell transmission, which leads to a slow, abnormal QRS complex. For a complete discussion on this topic, please review Chapter 5.

Electrical alternans is an alteration of the size or amplitude of the QRS complex. This alteration in size can occur either every other beat or over a series of beats (Figure 10-3).

Briefly stated, the most common cause of electrical alternans is a tachycardic rhythm. The rapid mechanical contractions of the heart cause the electrical axis of the ventricles to fluctuate in its orientation (Figure 10-4). This fluctuation makes the size of the complex change as the axis points more directly toward an electrode one moment and more directly away from an electrode the next. Electrical alternans can also be seen in pericardial effusions, pericardial tamponade (a medical emergency), and as a respiratory variation. Complete discussion of this topic is beyond the scope of this book. If you would like a complete discussion of the topic, you may refer to our accompanying text *12-Lead ECG: The Art of Interpretation* by Garcia and Holtz.

The ST segment in many tachycardic strips may be depressed. Some sinus tachycardia strips also show this variant morphology. The ST depression may be due to various reasons: the atrial repolarization wave or Tp wave, *relative* endocardial ischemia, *actual* endocardial

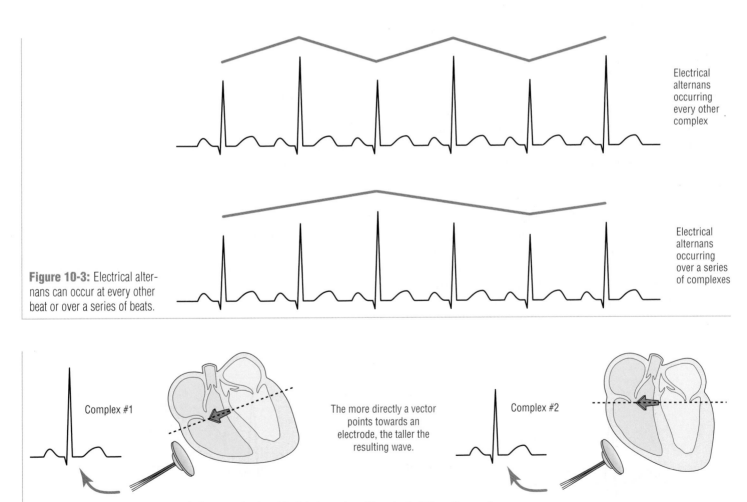

Electrical alternans occurring every other complex

Electrical alternans occurring over a series of complexes

Figure 10-3: Electrical alternans can occur at every other beat or over a series of beats.

Complex #1

The more directly a vector points towards an electrode, the taller the resulting wave.

Complex #2

Figure 10-4: When the electrical axis fluctuates back and forth between two different orientations, the result is an alternating change in the size of the complex—electrical alternans.

ischemia, or a buried P wave, just to name a few possibilities. A word to the wise: Whenever you see any ST depression, get a full 12-lead ECG to evaluate the situation. It could save you and your patient a lot of heartache—literally!

The Tp wave was discussed in Chapter 3 and shown in Figure 10-5. To review, this is a negative wave that is caused by atrial repolarization. It is usually not seen because it is buried in the QRS complex. The electrical forces involved in ventricular depolarization overwhelm the relatively small forces of atrial repolarization, making it electrocardiographically invisible. In tachycardia, the QRS complex comes earlier in time due to a shorter PR interval. The result is that the Tp wave is visible as a slight depression of the ST segment (Figure 10-6).

The endocardium of the heart can be relatively, or actually, underperfused in any tachycardia. This can lead to ST depression. The endocardium can be *relatively* underperfused because tachycardias require the heart to contract forcefully and rapidly. This requires more oxygen stocking. In many cases, the endocardial tissue is receiving adequate amounts of oxygen but not enough to compensate for the increased workload. The result is relative ischemia. The endocardium can also experience *actual* ischemia even though the area is not infarcting. As we shall discuss in greater detail later in this chapter, tachycardias can cause a marked drop in cardiac output. This drop in cardiac output means that the heart is receiving less oxygen during a time when it needs it the most. That results in actual ischemia.

In addition to direct subendocardial injury, an AMI occurring in an area electrocardiographically opposite a lead causes ST depression to appear in those leads. This is called the reciprocal changes of an AMI. (For a full discussion of this topic, see *12-Lead ECG: The Art of Interpretation*.)

As we shall see in later chapters, certain tachycardias have more P waves than QRS complexes. Atrial

flutter is one example. In these tachycardias, the P waves are sometimes buried or superimposed on the QRS, the ST segment, or the T wave. The result of these superimposed waves can vary depending on their orientation and their exact location. A negative P wave that falls directly on the ST segment can present as a downward deflection of the ST segment.

Now, let's get back to the need for an ECG. As you can see, the cause of ST depression can vary from the benign to the life threatening. It is to isolate and identify these life-threatening events that a full 12-lead ECG should be obtained on any patient showing ST depression on a rhythm strip.

The QT interval is also not immune to the sympathetic stimulation with which the heart is being bombarded during periods of stress. The result is a marked shortening of the QT interval during sinus tachycardia. The shortening is directly proportional to the speed of the tachycardia; the faster the rate, the shorter the QT. The variation in the normal measurement of the QT interval with heart rate is the reason that the QTc was created. The QTc is a number that nullifies the effect of heart rate on the length of the interval. For more on this, see Chapter 3.

However, just as in sinus bradycardia, the area that is most affected by the sympathetic stimulation is Phase 4 of the action potential and in its electrocardiographic representation, the TP segment. If you recall, sinus bradycardia caused a slowing of automaticity and a lengthening of the TP segment. In sinus tachycardia, because of the sympathetic stimulation, we see the opposite effect. The time during which Phase 4 completes is greatly shortened and the TP segment follows suit by becoming much shorter (Figures 10-7 and 10-8).

Sinus tachycardia is easily identifiable because it has discrete complexes, which are identical to the NSR complexes but separated by shorter TP segments (Figure 10-8). Once again, notice that the P waves, PR inter-

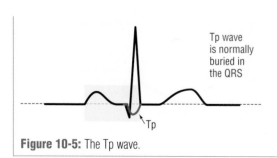

Tp wave is normally buried in the QRS

Figure 10-5: The Tp wave.

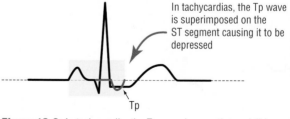

In tachycardias, the Tp wave is superimposed on the ST segment causing it to be depressed

Tp

Figure 10-6: In tachycardia, the Tp wave is sometimes visible as a slight depression of the ST segment.

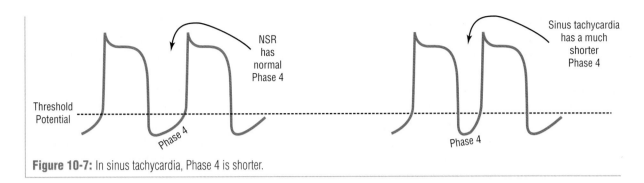

Figure 10-7: In sinus tachycardia, Phase 4 is shorter.

vals, and QRS complexes are all identical (except for the variations noted before).

A Quick Clinical Word

As mentioned before, the heart rate is determined by a constant tug-of-war between the sympathetic and the parasympathetic divisions of the autonomic nervous system. If the parasympathetic dominates, the rhythm is slowed. If the sympathetic dominates, the rhythm is sped up. Sinus tachycardia is, therefore, just a physiologic response to the autonomic stress and should not really be considered a pathological rhythm. Let's clarify that statement.

Cardiac output is maintained by heart rate times stroke volume (amount of blood ejected by the heart during each mechanical contraction). Stroke volume depends on the mechanical filling of the heart, which is both a passive process and an active process. The heart passively fills when the AV valves open and the blood from the atria floods into the ventricular chambers. The atria actively "overfill" the ventricles when the atria mechanically contract. This pushes the remaining atrial contents into the already filled ventricles, the so-called atrial kick.

Tachycardias cause a decrease in cardiac output when their rates become so high as to affect the stroke volume. Tachycardias decrease the amount of passive filling time that is available because of a shorter diastolic phase and they decrease the amount of blood that is expelled during the atrial kick. In other words, as the amount of time needed to fill the ventricles decreases with increasing heart rates, the less the ventricles are filled. This decreased ejection fraction lowers the stroke volume, which in turn drops the cardiac output and blood pressure.

In general, tachycardias are an abnormality of the rhythm that are caused by some inherent problem or set of circumstances in the heart itself. Sinus tachycardia, as we have seen, is not due to some inherent cardiac problem (in the vast majority of cases) but to some general stressor that stimulates sympathetic activity. Therefore, we should treat tachycardia by treating the underlying cause and not the rhythm itself. Put another way, treat what is causing the sinus tachycardia and not the tachycardia itself.

Let's look at a couple of examples. Fevers cause sinus tachycardia. Should you give beta-blocking agents like propranolol to everyone with a fever? Of course not! You can treat it simply by giving acetaminophen

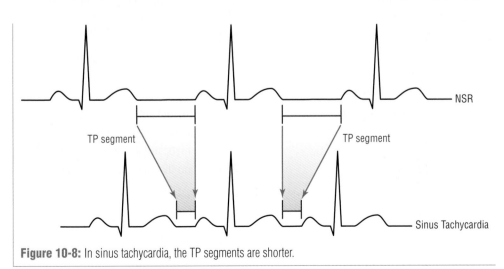

Figure 10-8: In sinus tachycardia, the TP segments are shorter.

and bringing the fever down a bit. Hypoxemia causes sinus tachycardia. How do you treat it? By giving supplemental oxygen. If a person is having a myocardial infarction, should you give beta-blocking agents to slow the heart down? Yes, as long as there are no contraindications! Why? Because tachycardias cause an increase in myocardial oxygen demand that can make the heart deteriorate further in this circumstance. But notice, we give the beta-blockers not as a treatment of the tachycardia but to protect the myocardium. How do you treat the tachycardia? Stop the infarction.

This is an important concept to understand before we go on to discuss the other tachycardic rhythms. Generally, you should focus your clinical attention or treatment directly at the tachycardia. Sinus tachycardia is the exception to the rule. Don't treat the arrhythmia, treat the cause.

Clinical Characteristics

Rate

As mentioned at the beginning of this chapter, the heart rate in sinus tachycardia is greater than 100 BPM. Generally, it is between 101 and 160 BPM in most patients. At this rate, the tachycardia itself does not pose any significant problems. The heart rate of the rhythm can,

however, go up to 200 BPM and maybe even as high as 220 BPM in rare circumstances. At these rates, the rhythm can pose both clinical and diagnostic challenges. We will discuss the differential diagnosis of wide complex tachycardias in Chapter 33. For now, we will concentrate on the typical forms that are not as difficult to identify.

In general, the maximum heart rate that can be considered normal for any individual patient is derived by using the formula:

Maximum Heart Rate = 220 BPM − Age (years)

For example, a 20-year-old man has a maximum heart rate of 200 BPM (220 BPM − 20 years = 200 BPM). Anything above that level would be considered abnormal and would require further evaluation.

The maximum heart rate is usually reached during exercise or forced activity of some kind. Athletes and young people are able to tolerate the high levels without difficulty. Elderly patients or patients with some cardiac pathology cannot tolerate levels near their maximum heart rate without some difficulty. Luckily, many patients never get to their maximum levels because they have some disease in their electrical conduction system that limits the rate they can reach.

ARRHYTHMIA RECOGNITION

Sinus Tachycardia

Rate:	> 100 BPM
Regularity:	Regular
P wave:	Present
Morphology:	Same
Upright in II, III, and aVF:	Yes
P:QRS ratio:	1:1
PR interval:	Normal, consistent
QRS width:	Normal or wide
Grouping:	None
Dropped beats:	None

DIFFERENTIAL DIAGNOSIS

Sinus Tachycardia

1. Exercise
2. Anxiety or stress
3. Fever
4. Hypoxemia or decreased ventilation
5. Hyperthermia (fever)
6. Hypotension
7. Drugs: beta-adrenergic agents, caffeine, alcohol, anticholinergic drugs
8. Anemia
9. Hyperthyroidism
10. Congestive heart failure
11. Acute myocardial infarction
12. Anything that stimulates sympathetic activity

ECG Strips

ECG 10-1

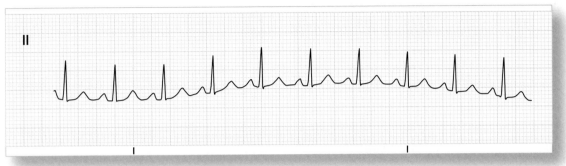

Rate:	About 110 BPM	PR intervals:	Normal, consistent
Regularity:	Regular	QRS width:	Normal
P waves:	Present	Rhythm:	**Sinus tachycardia**

Discussion:

ECG 10-1 has a wandering baseline, but the criteria are all present for the diagnosis of sinus tachycardia. Be careful not to confuse a wandering baseline for electri- cal alternans. Electrical alternans refers to a variation in the amplitude of the QRS complex. In a wandering baseline, the QRS complexes are all the same height.

ECG 10-2

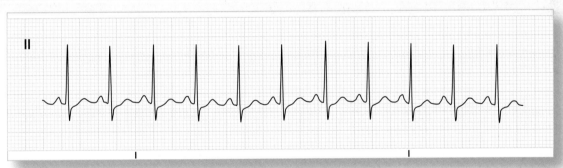

Rate:	About 130 BPM	PR intervals:	Normal, consistent
Regularity:	Regular	QRS width:	Normal
P waves:	Present	Rhythm:	**Sinus tachycardia**

Discussion:

ECG 10-2 is a classic example of sinus tachycardia. Note the slight depression of the ST segment. This could be due to the atrial repolarization wave or Tp wave, a slight amount of endocardial ischemia due to the tachycardia, or to some other cause. Whenever you see any signifi- cant abnormality on a rhythm strip, you should obtain an ECG to further evaluate the possible causes. In this case, the worst-case scenario could be that the ST de- pressions are due to reciprocal changes found in the in- ferior leads during a lateral acute myocardial infarction.

ECG 10-3

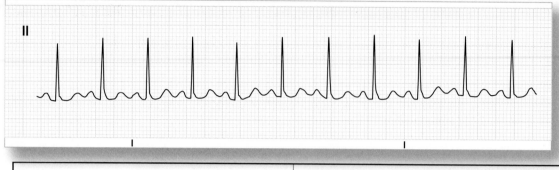

Rate:	About 120 BPM	PR intervals:	Normal, consistent
Regularity:	Regular	QRS width:	Normal
P waves:	Present	Rhythm:	**Sinus tachycardia**

Discussion:

ECG 10-3 is classic for sinus tachycardia. Note the easily identifiable P waves and the very slight irregularities in the morphology of the complexes. The irregularities are enough to be noticeable but not to the degree that you would expect from ectopic pacemakers.

ECG 10-4

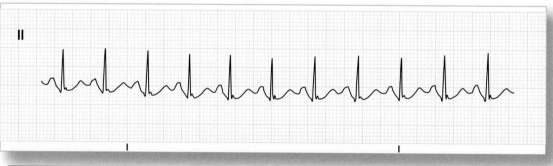

Rate:	About 125 BPM	PR intervals:	Normal, consistent
Regularity:	Regular	QRS width:	Normal
P waves:	Present	Rhythm:	**Sinus tachycardia**

Discussion:

ECG 10-4 is also fairly classic for sinus tachycardia. Note that the T waves and the P waves run into each other because the TP segment is nonexistent. In these cases, you need to use the base of the PR interval as the baseline for the strip. Using this as the baseline, the height of the P waves is dramatic. However, you cannot make the call of atrial enlargement on a rhythm strip—a full 12-lead ECG is needed to make that diagnosis.

ECG 10-5

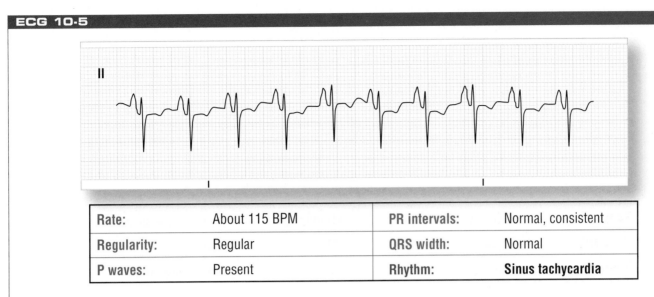

Rate:	About 115 BPM	PR intervals:	Normal, consistent
Regularity:	Regular	QRS width:	Normal
P waves:	Present	Rhythm:	**Sinus tachycardia**

Discussion:

ECG 10-5 is, once again, sinus tachycardia. Note the tall, prominent P waves, the flat ST segment, and the flipped T waves present on the complexes. The combination of flat ST segments and flipped T waves on an ECG would be consistent with ischemia. All you can say about them on a rhythm strip is that they are suggestive of ischemia, and a 12-lead ECG should be obtained for further evaluation. Always be suspicious and you won't get burned!

ECG 10-6

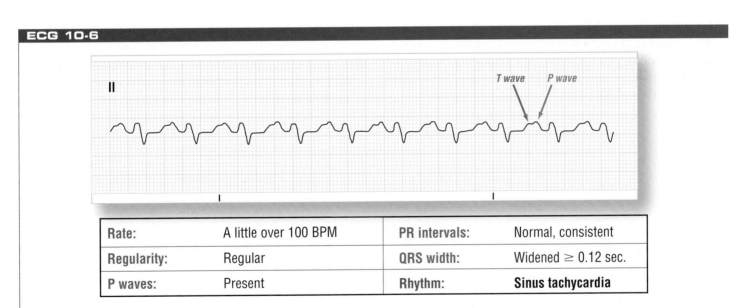

Rate:	A little over 100 BPM	PR intervals:	Normal, consistent
Regularity:	Regular	QRS width:	Widened ≥ 0.12 sec.
P waves:	Present	Rhythm:	**Sinus tachycardia**

Discussion:

ECG 10-6 is a bit more problematic than the previous ones. There are a couple of reasons for this. First, the QRS complexes are wider than 0.12 seconds. This means you have to think about bundle branch blocks, aberrancy, or ventricular complexes as the source of the widened interval. Secondly, the T wave and the P waves run into each other to further complicate issues; however, with a P wave before each complex and a 1:1 ratio of P and QRS complexes, you can pretty well rule out ventricular complexes. A 12-lead ECG verified the fact that this was a patient with sinus tachycardia and a right bundle branch block.

ECG 10-7

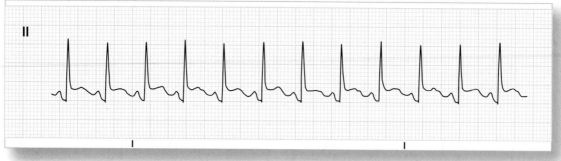

Rate:	A little over 135 BPM	PR intervals:	Normal, consistent
Regularity:	Regular	QRS width:	Normal
P waves:	Present	Rhythm:	**Sinus tachycardia**

Discussion:

ECG 10-7 has clear P waves before each QRS complex and the heart rate is over 100 BPM, making it consistent with sinus tachycardia. Once again, it is not a good idea to make a diagnosis about anything but the rhythm on a rhythm strip, but we can use it to justify some further investigation. Do you notice anything troubling about the strip above? What sticks out the most is the obvious ST segment elevation that is present. Is this an AMI? Should we give thrombolytics? The answer to both of these questions is . . . we need to see a 12-lead ECG. The ST segment elevation that is present could represent an AMI; however, it could also represent pericarditis. Giving thrombolytics to a patient with an AMI is definitely a good idea, provided there are no contraindications and the medication is clinically warranted. Giving throm-

bolytics to someone with pericarditis is NOT a very good idea. It would probably kill the patient by causing a hemorrhagic pericardial tamponade.

A 12-lead ECG, or at least additional leads, would be highly suggested and therapy should be based on the patient's clinical history, physical examination, and ECG. This patient was indeed having an inferior wall MI. Quick and definitive action led to a good outcome.

The take-home point is that rhythm strips can be of more use than just a tool to recognize an arrhythmia. When you look at a rhythm strip, analyze the whole strip and remember that it represents one lead of a whole ECG. Then, put that information together with your history, physical, and other diagnostic tests to formulate your best clinical impression of the entire situation.

CHAPTER **REVIEW**

1. In sinus tachycardia, the heart rate must be above _____ BPM.

2. The heart rate in sinus tachycardia is usually between ___ and ___ BPM. It may, however, reach up to ___ BPM and in some rare circumstances up to ___BPM.

3. Maximum heart rate is equal to ___ BPM − Age (in years).

4. Sinus tachycardia is caused by a predominant effect of the parasympathetic nervous system. True or False.

5. Wide QRS complexes are acceptable in sinus tachycardia. True or False.

6. Sympathetic discharge causes faster transit times through the AV node. This leads to a shortening of the __ interval. However, the interval should still be in the normal range of between 0.12 and 0.20 seconds.

7. Electrical alternans is electrocardiographically represented as a varying _____ of the QRS complex.

8. Electrical alternans must be seen in every other complex in order to make the diagnosis. True or False.

9. The following conditions may lead to electrical alternans:
   A. Tachycardias
   B. Myocardial infarctions
   C. Pericardial effusions
   D. Pericarditis
   E. Both A and C are correct
   F. Both B and D are correct

10. The ST segment can be depressed in tachycardias. Some possible causes include:
    A. Atrial repolarization or Tp wave
    B. Relative endocardial ischemia
    C. Actual endocardial ischemia
    D. Buried P waves
    E. All the above are correct

11. Sinus tachycardia has a much shorter Phase 4 of the action potential. This is electrocardiographically represented by a short ___ segment.

12. Sinus tachycardia should not be considered a pathological rhythm but merely a physiologic response to autonomic stress. True or False.

13. The treatment of sinus tachycardia is to _____.

14. Tachycardias _____ the amount of passive filling time during diastole. This leads to a _____ in the stroke volume which, in turn, leads to a _____ in cardiac output.

15. The differential diagnosis of sinus tachycardia includes:
    A. Exercise
    B. Fevers
    C. Cocaine
    D. Anemia
    E. CHF
    F. All of the above

16. It is common for the TP segment to be completely missing on a strip showing sinus tachycardia. True or False.

17. In an acute myocardial infarction, the tachycardia may lead to further damage because of the increased oxygen demand placed on the myocardium by the tachycardia. In this case, slowing down the heart by using beta-blocking agents, for example, is clinically appropriate (if there are no clinical contraindications or extenuating circumstances). True or False.

18. The main therapy in a sinus tachycardia that is hemodynamically stable in a patient with fever is the beta-blockers. True or False.

19. Sinus tachycardias are always benign hemodynamically. True or False.

20. Treatment for sinus tachycardias includes synchronized cardioversion. True or False.

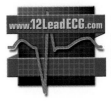

To enhance the knowledge you gain in this book, access this text's website at www.12leadECG.com! This valuable resource provides flashcards, an online glossary, web links, and more. Simply click on the Arrhythmias book cover once at the site.

CHAPTER 11

Sinus Arrhythmia

Under normal circumstances, NSR is a very regular rhythm. The sinus node functions as the body's metronome, keeping an exact and regularly recurring cardiac beat. However, in the field of medicine, there are very few things that are exactly the same among all patients. Normal sinus rhythm is no exception to this rule.

In some patients, the normally occurring sinus complexes can have some slight irregularity in the timing of each of the complexes. That variability should never be by an interval greater than 0.16 seconds, or 4 small boxes, in NSR throughout the entire strip. There are some patients, however, who have normally occurring complexes that originate in the SA node, but the irregularities vary by more than 0.16 seconds. We call this irregular rhythm sinus arrhythmia to differentiate it from normal sinus rhythm.

Generally, sinus arrhythmia is very easily identified because of the gradual widening and narrowing of the interval. Some cases, however, may not be so evident. For those cases, it is a good idea to know the specifics needed to make the diagnosis. The Additional Information box will show you how to be certain you are dealing with sinus arrhythmia.

ADDITIONAL INFORMATION

Identifying Sinus Arrhythmia

The mathematical way to identify a sinus arrhythmia is to make sure that all of the complexes are identical (within reason) and that the P waves are consistent with a sinus pacemaker. Calculate the P-P interval for the two fastest complexes (the ones that are closest to each other), then calculate the P-P interval for the two slowest complexes (the ones that are farthest from each other) (Figure 11-1). The difference between these distances should not exceed 0.16 seconds. If it does, the rhythm is sinus arrhythmia.

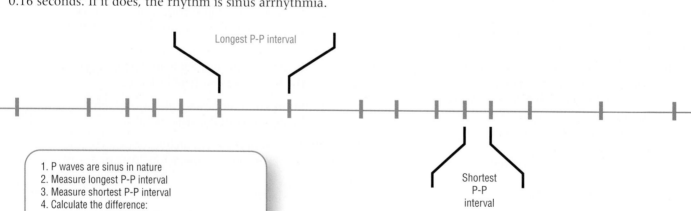

Longest P-P interval

Shortest P-P interval

1. P waves are sinus in nature
2. Measure longest P-P interval
3. Measure shortest P-P interval
4. Calculate the difference:

$$\text{Longest P-P interval} - \text{Shortest P-P interval} = \text{Difference}$$

5. If the difference between the two is greater than 0.16 seconds, then you have sinus arrhythmia

Figure 11-1: Identify sinus arrhythmia by measuring the longest and shortest P-P intervals. If the difference between these distances is greater than 0.16 seconds, it is sinus arrhythmia.

Now that we know a little bit about sinus arrhythmia, let's make matters more interesting. There are two kinds of sinus arrhythmia: the *respiratory* or *phasic* variant, which occurs during normal circumstances, and the *nonrespiratory* or *nonphasic* variant, which is only found in pathological states.

Respiratory Sinus Arrhythmia

When we breathe, our chest wall acts like the bellows that are used by blacksmiths (Figure 11-2). As the lungs expand with inspiration, the intrathoracic pressure (pressure inside the chest cavity) decreases. The laws of physics state that gases and fluids will always try to move from an area of higher pressure to an area of lower pressure. Therefore, air rushes into the lungs when we expand our chest wall because it is going from an area of higher pressure (the outside air) to an area of less pressure (the space within our lungs during inspiration). Notice that the air movement is passive, but the wall motion is active and controlled by the person. In addition to the air, blood from our extremities and abdomen also follows the pressure gradient and moves from our bodies to the right side of the heart.

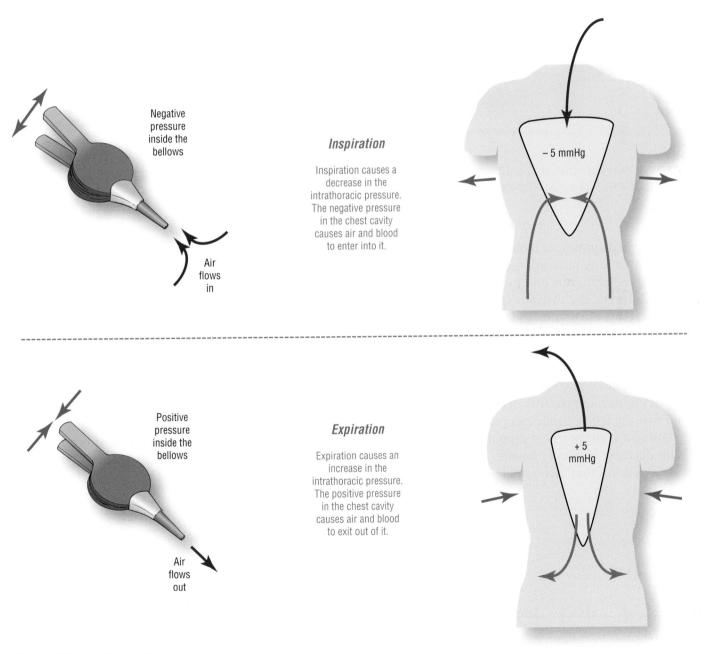

Figure 11-2: Inspiration and Expiration.

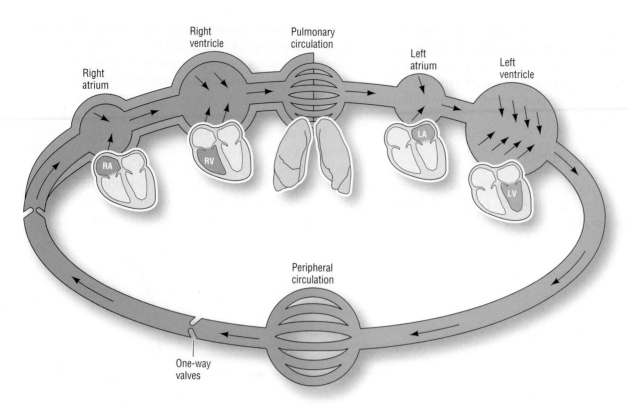

Figure 11-3: The green area represents the additional blood volume in the intrathoracic space due to inspiration. Note that the blood pools in the pulmonary circulation.

The increased amount of blood that comes into the thoracic cavity during inspiration causes the right ventricle to fill more efficiently and pump more blood (Figure 11-3). However, the vascular system in our lungs is very, very large. It can accommodate the extra right-sided cardiac output easily and, since blood wants to stay in an area of low pressure, the additional flow does not make it all the way to the left side of the heart and just sits in the pulmonary vascular bed. This vascular pooling, in essence, temporarily decreases the amount of blood that the left ventricle can pump out into the body, causing a slight transient drop in the blood pressure. This decrease in blood pressure, in turn, triggers some vagal reflexes that increase the heart rate and vascular tone in an effort to equalize the drop in blood pressure. The importance of this discussion is that it is a transient vagal stimulation that causes the heart rate to momentarily speed up during inspiration (Figure 11-4).

All of the changes mentioned above occur in seconds during the respiratory cycle. The transient increase in the heart rate that results from the vagal stimulation can be easily spotted on an ECG or a rhythm strip. This transient speeding up of the rate is especially evident when the underlying heart rate is bradycardic. That is why respiratory sinus arrhythmia is seen more commonly during slower heart rates and in athletes, since they usually have slower rates at baseline.

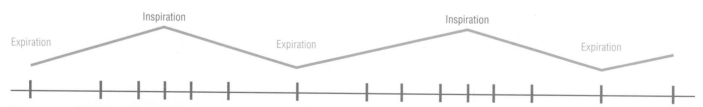

Figure 11-4: The green line represents a baseline on an ECG. The blue lines represent individual complexes. Note the gradual speeding up and slowing down of the heart rate with each respiratory cycle.

Sinus arrhythmia is also very common in young children and disappears as they get older. In general, the rhythm also tends to disappear when the rate increases, as occurs, for example, with atropine or with exercise.

It is important to always remember that respiratory or phasic sinus arrhythmia is a variant of normal and is not a pathological arrhythmia.

Nonrespiratory or Nonphasic Sinus Arrhythmia

The second kind of sinus arrhythmia is the nonrespiratory or nonphasic type. This type of sinus arrhythmia is not associated with the respiratory cycles or any other physiologic events. It occurs spontaneously and has no definite pattern, with the P-P interval varying at random throughout the strip. There is no gradual increase and decrease in the rate.

ADDITIONAL INFORMATION

Changes in the Main Pacemaker Site

Recent information from electrophysiology (EPS) studies has shown that, in some patients, there can be a transient change in the location of the main pacemaker during respiration within the SA node itself. Remember, the SA node is a large, horseshoe-shaped structure. The main pacemaking site can transiently change in these patients because of vagal stimulation from an area in the upper pole to an area in the lower pole. This could account for the small changes seen in the morphology of the P waves and the PR intervals seen in some sinus arrhythmia patients.

In contrast to respiratory sinus arrhythmia, nonrespiratory SA occurs in the elderly and in patients with serious ischemic heart disease or structural abnormalities. Because of its association with pathological states, this type of sinus arrhythmia should be considered a true arrhythmia and should not be considered a variant of normal. This does not mean that it requires treatment, emergent or otherwise, but it does mean that you need to approach those patients with care and a suspicious clinical eye. In other words, if they tell you they are having any symptoms, believe them!

Because of its association with pathological heart disease, consider this type of sinus arrhythmia a true arrhythmia and not a variant of normal.

Some Additional Clinical Points

The biggest problem associated with sinus arrhythmia, and with the nonrespiratory variant in particular, is that it is frequently mislabeled as multiple PACs. The inverse is also true; an ECG with many PACs is frequently considered sinus arrhythmia (Figure 11-5). The possibility of frequent PACs should always be considered before making the diagnosis of SA.

While we are on the topic of PACs . . . sinus arrhythmia is a cardiac rhythm. Just like any other cardiac rhythm, the pattern can be broken by an event, such as a PAC. The event can cause a further deterioration of the baseline irregularity caused by the sinus arrhythmia itself. In certain cases, an event overlying a respiratory variant sinus arrhythmia can look just like a nonrespiratory variant SA (Figure 11-6). As we saw, the difference between the two possibilities can be of critical clinical importance. Always evaluate the P waves for any inconsistencies that could be caused by ectopic or premature complexes!

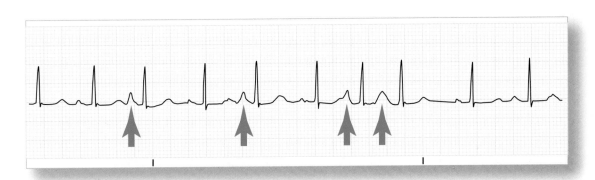

Figure 11-5: Note the irregularity of the rhythm. The P waves identified with the green arrows are PACs.

Respiratory Sinus Arrhythmia:

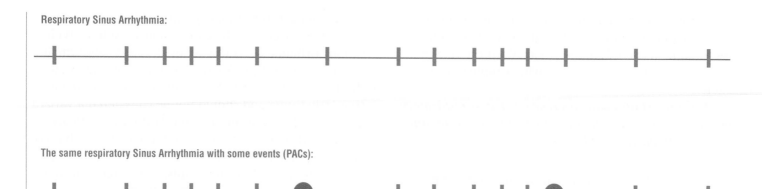

The same respiratory Sinus Arrhythmia with some events (PACs):

Figure 11-6: Notice how just two well-placed events, in this case PACs, can change the appearance of an easily identifiable respiratory variant sinus arrhythmia.

ARRHYTHMIA RECOGNITION

Sinus Arrhythmia

Rate:	Usually around 60 to 100 BPM, but can be slow or fast
Regularity:	Regularly irregular, but can be irregularly irregular
P wave:	Present and sinus in origin
Morphology:	Same throughout
Upright in II, III, and aVF:	Yes
P:QRS ratio:	1:1
PR interval:	Normal, consistent
QRS width:	Normal or wide
Grouping:	None
Dropped beats:	None

NOTE

Because sinus arrhythmia is a relatively slow rhythm and the changes in rate due to respirations may take a few seconds to develop, the ECG strips in this section will be presented in landscape format. Keeping the original size of the rhythm strip is important in correctly learning to identify rhythm abnormalities.

We will continue to do this from time to time as the situation warrants. Next, full-size ECGs will be presented in landscape format to maintain the actual size of the tracing.

ECG Strips

ECG 11-1

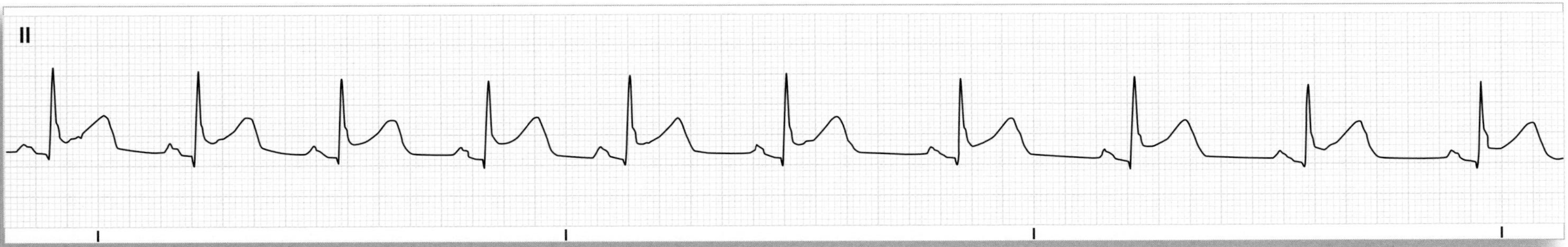

Rate:	50 to 60 BPM		PR intervals:	Normal, consistent
Regularity:	Regularly irregular		QRS width:	Normal
P waves:	Present		Grouping:	None
Morphology:	Normal		Dropped beats:	None
Axis:	Normal			
P:QRS ratio:	1:1		Rhythm:	**Sinus arrhythmia**

Discussion:

ECG 11-1 is classic for the respiratory variant form of sinus arrhythmia. Note the rhythmical speeding up and slowing of the rate throughout the strip (to fully appreciate the respiratory variation completely, a longer strip would be necessary). Note the slight irregularities in the appearance of the P waves throughout the strip. This is commonly seen in SA, and can sometimes be confused with other rhythm abnormalities.

ECG 11-2

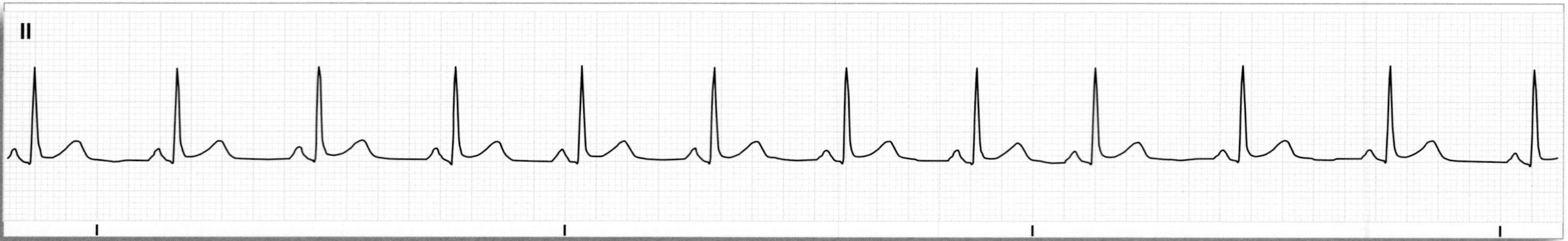

Rate:	Around 60 BPM
Regularity:	Regularly irregular
P waves:	Present
Morphology:	Normal
Axis:	Normal
P:QRS ratio:	1:1
PR intervals:	Normal, consistent
QRS width:	Normal
Grouping:	None
Dropped beats:	None
Rhythm:	**Sinus arrhythmia**

Discussion:

Once again, ECG 11-2 is classic for the respiratory variant form of sinus arrhythmia. In this case, the gradual slowing and speeding up of the heart rate is very obvious at first glance. Notice that we are stating that this rhythm strip is regularly irregular. The reason is that the rhythmical changes in heart rate are continuously recurring and predictable. Hence, the rate changes are regular and very much associated with the normal breathing cycles.

ECG 11-3

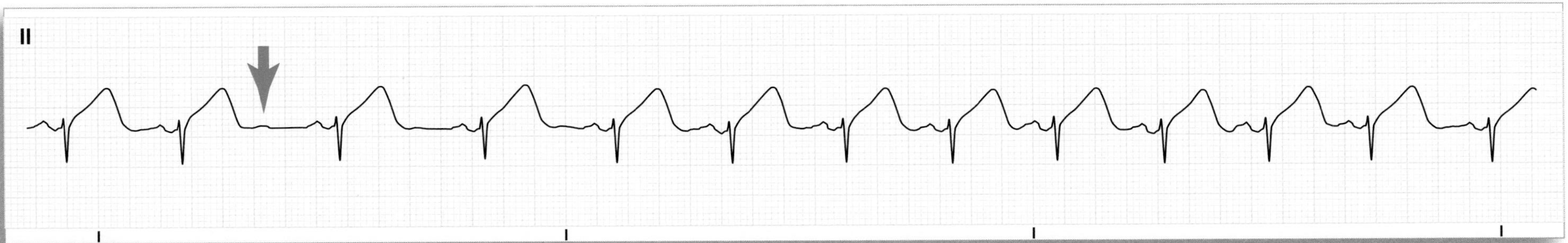

Rate:	Around 65 BPM
Regularity:	Regularly irregular
P waves:	Present
Morphology:	Normal
Axis:	Normal
P:QRS ratio:	1:1
PR intervals:	Normal, consistent
QRS width:	Normal
Grouping:	None
Dropped beats:	None
Rhythm:	**Sinus arrhythmia**

Discussion:

By this time, you should easily be able to identify ECG 11-3 as a respiratory variant sinus arrhythmia. There are some other interesting things to be concerned about on this strip, however. For example, the ST segments are very elevated and very flat. This could possibly represent an inferior wall MI. If you ever see a strip like this one, make sure that you get a full 12-lead ECG to evaluate the possibility of injury or infarction. Remember, using a strip to make a diagnosis about anything but the rhythm is dangerous. Always obtain a full ECG!

Another interesting point to make about this ECG is the small wave right under the green arrow. There are a couple more similar waves after some of the other complexes. What are they? Are they another P wave that is not conducted? The answer is no. Those are U waves, and can occur normally in some patients. Ischemia also causes them to occur and is probably the cause in this patient. Notice that you can only see them between the complexes that are fairly far apart. They are still there on the other complexes but are not visible because they are buried in the P wave of the subsequent complex.

ECG 11-4

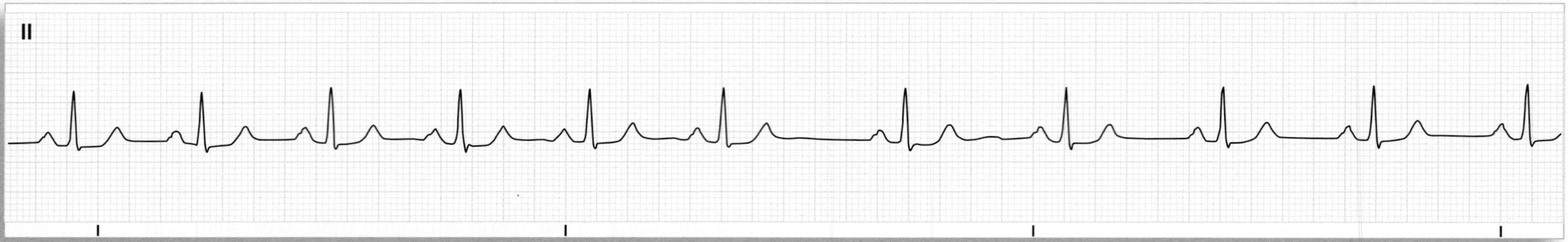

Rate:	Around 55 BPM		PR intervals:	Normal, consistent
Regularity:	Regularly irregular		QRS width:	Normal
P waves:	Present		Grouping:	None
Morphology:	Normal			
Axis:	Normal		Dropped beats:	None
P:QRS ratio:	1:1		Rhythm:	**Sinus arrhythmia**

Discussion:

ECG 11-4 also shows the rhythmical and gradual slow-ing and speeding up of a respiratory variant sinus ar-rhythmia. Notice the longer pause that is present near the middle of the strip. It is common in sinus arrhyth-mia to have longer pauses than usual. This is all part of the rhythm and is not an indication for a pacemaker unless the patient is symptomatic or if the pauses are too long. How long is too long? That is a clinical deci-sion you are going to have to make based on your pa-tient and his or her presentation.

This strip shows some slight depressions on the ST segments, and the depressions are flat. Flat ST changes, either elevations or depressions, can be ischemic. Once again, it would be a good idea to obtain an ECG to eval-uate the problem further.

ECG 11-5

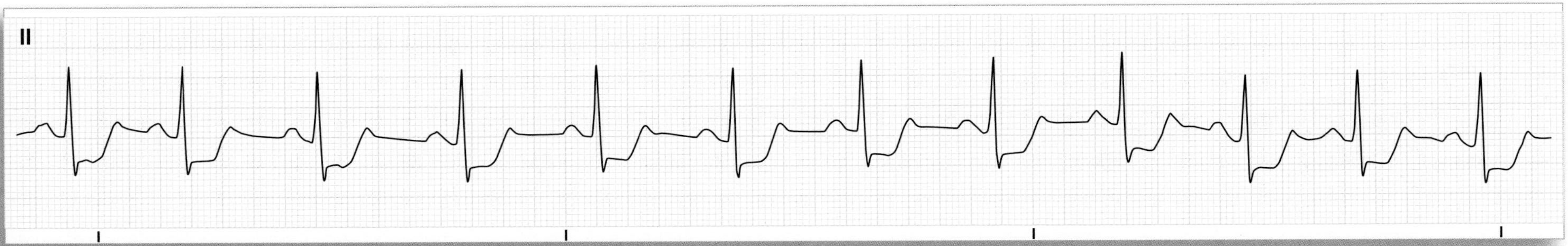

Rate:	Around 60 BPM
Regularity:	Regularly irregular
P waves:	Present
Morphology:	Normal
Axis:	Normal
P:QRS ratio:	1:1
PR intervals:	Normal, consistent
QRS width:	Normal
Grouping:	None
Dropped beats:	None
Rhythm:	**Sinus arrhythmia**

Discussion:

ECG 11-5 is a little tougher to spot by just a quick eyeballing of the rhythm. Here is one place where calipers would come in very handy to spot the gradual slowing and speeding up of the heart rate. This is, however, respiratory variant sinus arrhythmia.

These ST segments are cause for concern. They are depressed, flat, and just plain ugly. A full 12-lead ECG would really be helpful in evaluating this patient further. Be very careful with this patient, who could be having a large MI.

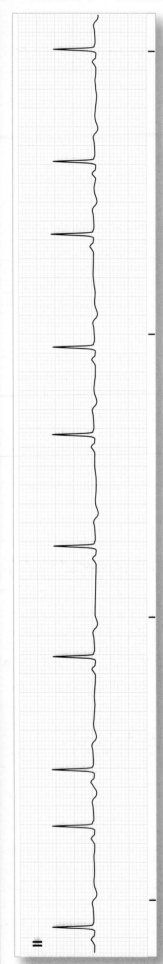

ECG 11-6

Rate:	Around 50 BPM
Regularity:	Regularly irregular
P waves:	Present
Morphology:	Normal
Axis:	Normal
P:QRS ratio:	1:1

PR intervals:	Normal, consistent
QRS width:	Normal
Grouping:	None
Dropped beats:	None
Rhythm:	**Sinus arrhythmia**

Discussion:

ECG 11-6 is a really tough rhythm to figure out! Let's approach it logically, and you'll see that you can do it. It is definitely slow. If you take the number of beats in a 12-second strip and multiply it by 5, you get about 50 BPM. The rhythm is regularly irregular because, if you use your calipers, you have many P-P intervals that are the same throughout the strip (see ECG 11-7).

Next, look at the P waves. Are they all the same? Yes, they are all the same. This removes multiple PACs

as an option. What about the PR intervals? They are all the same. That means that all of the complexes originated in the same pacemaker. The P waves are upright in lead II, so it is less likely that the pacemaker is ectopic.

The irregularity, the same P waves, a normal P wave axis, and the same PR intervals all point to the only possibility: nonrespiratory sinus arrhythmia.

Use your calipers!
All the P-P intervals
marked by the
blue stars are the same.

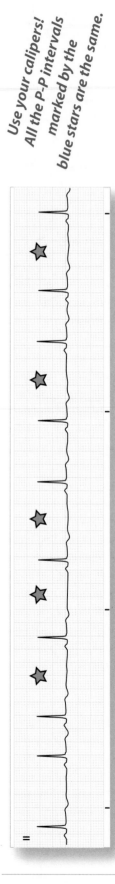

Figure 11-7: P-P intervals are marked by the blue stars.

CHAPTER **REVIEW**

1. Normal sinus rhythm can normally have some slight variability in the regularity of the complexes. However, the difference between the longest and shortest intervals should never be greater than 0.16 seconds. True or False.

2. Sinus arrhythmia refers to a rhythm of sinus origin that has a variability in the regularity of the complexes of greater than 0.16 seconds. True or False.

3. There are two kinds of sinus arrhythmias:
   A. Respiratory or phasic sinus arrhythmia
   B. Circulatory or episodic sinus arrhythmia
   C. Nonrespiratory or nonphasic sinus arrhythmia
   D. A and B are correct
   E. A and C are correct

4. Respiratory sinus arrhythmia is caused by:
   A. Decreased blood pressure to the brain.
   B. Transient vagal stimulation.
   C. Excessive catecholamine upsurge.
   D. Increased blood flow to the left side of the heart during inspiration.
   E. All of the above

5. Respiratory sinus arrhythmia is a variant of normal. True or False.

6. The heart rate normally speeds up during:
   A. Inspiration
   B. Expiration
   C. All of the above
   D. None of the above

7. Respiratory sinus arrhythmia is normally seen in:
   A. Adolescents.
   B. Older patients.
   C. Athletes.
   D. MI patients.
   E. Both A and C are correct
   F. Both B and D are correct

8. You should always consider other possibilities closely before making the diagnosis of sinus arrhythmia because, frequently, multiple PVCs can be mistaken for sinus arrhythmia. True or False.

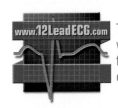

To enhance the knowledge you gain in this book, access this text's website at www.12leadECG.com! This valuable resource provides flashcards, an online glossary, web links, and more. Simply click on the Arrhythmias book cover once at the site.

CHAPTER 12

Sinus Blocks, Pauses, and Arrests

In this chapter we are going to cover three different, but very related, pathological processes involving the SA node proper: Sinus blocks, sinus pauses, and sinus arrest. In these three rhythms, the sinus pacemaker fires but the impulse does not make it to depolarize the atrial tissue. The result is that all three of these arrhythmic events do not form an initial P wave. In addition, since the atrial myocardium and the electrical conduction system are not depolarized, the rest of the heart also fails to depolarize. The result is that there are also no QRS complexes, ST segments, or T waves.

In the case of sinus blocks, the sinus node is completely blocked or obstructed from conducting the impulse. In the case of sinus pauses, the impulse propagation is delayed. Finally, sinus arrest is a combination of both complete block and delay.

These events are relatively uncommon in everyday practice. They are, however, very commonly seen when there is disease around the SA node proper. This condition is known as the *sick sinus syndrome*. We will spend some time reviewing this syndrome at the end of this chapter. For now, let's turn our attention to the events themselves.

Sinus Block

As its name implies, a *sinus block* (SA block) refers to a complete block or failure of the sinus node to capture or depolarize the atrial myocardium. The block can last for one, two, or more cycles, but the hallmark of a sinus block is that the pause is always an exact multiple of the normal P-P interval (Figure 12-1). The block is an exact multiple of the P-P interval because the sinus pacemaker, unaware of the block that is occurring further down the line, continues to fire at its intrinsic rate. Eventually, one of the sinus impulses will be able to get through to capture the atrial myocardium and end the SA block.

Take a look at Figure 12-1. Note that there is a normal sinus rhythm occurring at the intrinsic rate set by the sinus pacemaker. Suddenly, one of the impulses fires (see red X) but that depolarization wave does not reach the atrial tissue and does not form a P, QRS, or T wave (see purple complex). However, the sinus rate or cadence is not interrupted by the block and it continues to fire on schedule. The pause is two times the normal P-P interval. If two complexes were blocked, the pause would be three times the normal P-P interval, and so forth. The key is that the pause is always an exact multiple of the P-P interval (Figure 12-2).

There is one thing that commonly occurs and can mimic a sinus block: a blocked premature atrial contraction (PAC; see Chapter 13). Basically, another sinus pacemaker or an ectopic atrial pacemaker fires earlier than expected. That impulse depolarizes the atria but is blocked by the AV node from ever reaching the ventricles. The net result is that you have a P wave but no

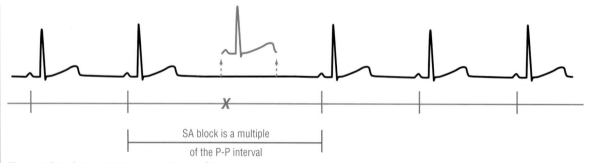

X

SA block is a multiple
of the P-P interval

Figure 12-1: A sinus block occurs when the SA node is completely prevented from conducting the impulse to the atria but the pacemaker itself remains untouched. For this reason, the underlying cadence of the rhythm remains untouched. SA blocks are always some multiple of the P-P interval. In this case, note that the SA block is two times the normal P-P interval.

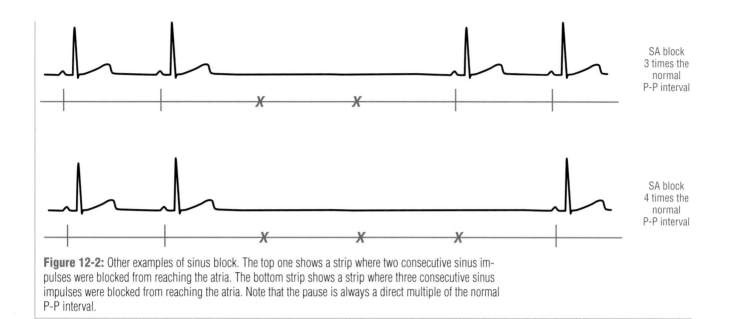

Figure 12-2: Other examples of sinus block. The top one shows a strip where two consecutive sinus impulses were blocked from reaching the atria. The bottom strip shows a strip where three consecutive sinus impulses were blocked from reaching the atria. Note that the pause is always a direct multiple of the normal P-P interval.

QRS or T waves. Sometimes that P wave will fall on and fuse with the previous T wave. ***Note, however, that there is always a P wave in a PAC, blocked or not.*** In sinus blocks, there are no P waves because the impulse never reaches the atria and, therefore, does not depolarize the atrial tissue to form a P wave.

The sinus blocks can occur intermittently on the same strip and can sometimes be mistaken for a severe sinus bradycardia (Figure 12-3). Obtaining a longer strip in these patients will be very helpful in making the diagnosis.

Sinus Pause and Sinus Arrest

A *sinus pause* is caused by a delay in the formation of a sinus impulse in the sinus node itself. The delay is represented on the rhythm strip as a longer pause between the complexes (Figure 12-4). In other words, a sinus pause is represented electrocardiographically as a longer P-P interval.

Sinus pauses do not occur as exact multiples of the normal P-P interval because the delay usually occurs in

the sinus node itself. When the sinus node returns after the pause, it may be set at the same rate as before the pause or it may be a different rate.

A sinus arrest is caused by a longer delay in the formation of an atrial impulse (Figure 12-5). A surface ECG is not accurate enough to adequately interpret if sinus blocks can also be found within the pause of a sinus arrest. One thing is for certain—sinus arrests can be long, but they are never an exact multiple of the normal P-P interval.

Where the cut-off point between a sinus pause and a sinus arrest exactly falls is not clear. There is no clear consensus as to where a sinus pause ends and a sinus arrest begins. Basically, we use this rule of thumb: If the pause is shorter than three times the normal P-P interval (at least two nonconducted complexes), we say that it is a sinus pause. If the pause is greater than three times the normal P-P interval, we say it is a sinus arrest. Is this system correct? Well, no one can say this is right or wrong because no one knows the answer. This system is completely arbitrary, but does work for our purposes.

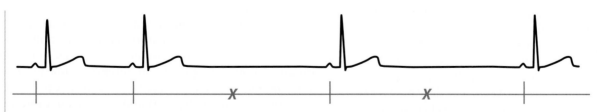

Figure 12-3: Two nonconsecutive sinus blocks on the same strip. Note that the middle and end of this strip could easily be mistaken for a sinus bradycardia. One clue to the presence of block would be that sinus bradycardia is formed slowly by a gradual slowing of the rate and does not occur as abruptly as that seen in Figure 12-2.

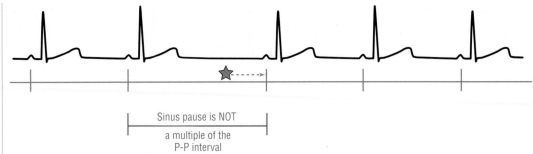

Sinus pause is NOT
a multiple of the
P-P interval

Figure 12-4: A sinus pause refers to a delay or failure of the sinus node to create a depolarization wave. In this figure, the expected firing time for the sinus node is represented by the pink star. Note the delay in the timing of the actual firing. The net result is that the normal P, QRS, and T wave complex is not formed on time. The sinus pause is not found at a direct multiple of the P-P interval.

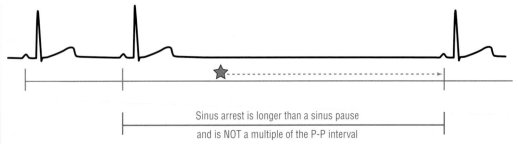

Sinus arrest is longer than a sinus pause
and is NOT a multiple of the P-P interval

Figure 12-5: A sinus arrest refers to a delay or failure of the sinus node to create a depolarization wave, but at an interval much longer than that seen during a sinus pause. The net result is that the normal P, QRS, and T wave complex is not formed on time. The sinus arrest is not found at a direct multiple of the P-P interval.

ADDITIONAL INFORMATION

Sick Sinus Syndrome

It is difficult to cover a topic as complicated as the sick sinus syndrome (SSS) at this point in the book because we have not covered many of the rhythms involved. For that reason, we are placing this section as an Additional Information box. You can skip over this section and return to it later after you have covered some of the sections, or you can turn to Chapter 7 to quickly refresh your memory on those rhythm abnormalities.

The sick sinus syndrome refers to a series of arrhythmias that are frequently seen in patients with diseased sinoatrial nodes. The diseased node can cause severe bradycardias, marked sinus arrhythmias, sinus blocks, pauses, and arrests to develop. The diseased node can also frequently alternate between very slow bradycardias and very fast tachycardias (the so-called tachy-brady syndrome, which is a variant of SSS).

In addition to sinus node dysfunction, the same processes that cause the sinus node to start to malfunc-tion will also affect the AV node and the rest of the conduction system. This can lead to the formation of AV blocks, junctional escape rhythms, and chronic atrial fibrillation.

The arrhythmias can develop in any combination and not every patient will exhibit all of them. Typically, the syndrome is suspected when the patient develops symptoms of fatigue, exercise intolerance, or congestive heart failure and has an ECG or rhythm strip with any of the rhythms mentioned above. Verification of the syndrome and its manifestations is usually made by obtaining a 24-hour ambulatory monitoring study.

The most common treatment for the sick sinus syndrome is to give the patient an antiarrhythmic to prevent the formation and severity of the tachycardias (e.g., procainamide, digoxin) and to place an artificial pacemaker to control the bradycardias and blocks.

ARRHYTHMIA RECOGNITION

Sinus Blocks, Pauses, and Arrests

Rate:	These are either single or multiple events.
Regularity:	Regular with events
P wave:	Nonconducted or delayed
Morphology:	Not applicable
Upright in II, III, and aVF:	Not applicable
P:QRS ratio:	Not applicable
PR interval:	Not applicable
QRS width:	Not applicable
Grouping:	None
Dropped beats:	Yes

DIFFERENTIAL DIAGNOSIS

Sinus Blocks, Pauses, and Arrests

1. Sick sinus syndrome
2. CAD, inferior wall MI
3. Hypersensitive carotid sinus syndrome
4. Drugs: digoxin, antiarrhythmics, etc.
5. Digoxin toxicity
6. Myocarditis
7. Electrolyte disorders
8. Idiopathic and benign

The list above is not inclusive but reflects the most common causes of the rhythm disturbance.

ECG Strips

ECG 12-1

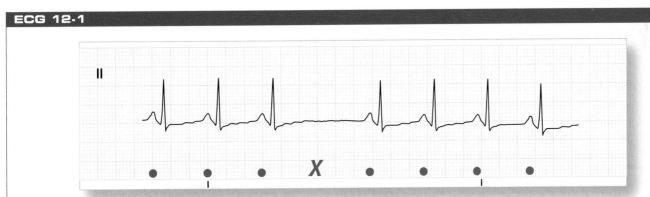

Rate:	About 100 BPM	PR intervals:	Normal, except in event
Regularity:	Regular, with event	QRS width:	Normal
P waves:	Normal, except in event	Grouping:	None
Morphology:	Normal		
Axis:	Normal	Dropped beats:	Yes
P:QRS ratio:	1:1, except in event	Rhythm:	**Sinus tachycardia with a sinus block**

Discussion:

This strip shows a patient with an underlying sinus tachycardia. The patient has a sinus block of one com-plex. Notice that the pause is exactly twice the normal P-P interval found throughout the rest of the strip.

ECG 12-2

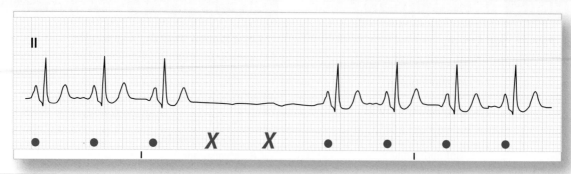

Rate:	About 92 BPM	PR intervals:	Normal, except in event
Regularity:	Regular, except in event	QRS width:	Normal
P waves: Morphology: Axis:	Normal, except in event Normal Normal	Grouping:	None
		Dropped beats:	Yes
P:QRS ratio:	1:1, except in event	Rhythm:	**Sinus rhythm with a sinus block**

Discussion:

ECG 12-2 shows an underlying sinus rhythm. The patient then develops a long pause which, upon measuring, is exactly three times the normal P-P interval. This is an example of a sinus block in which two of the sinus impulses were blocked. Remember, sinus blocks can occur when either one, two, or more sinus impulses are blocked from being conducted to the atria.

ECG 12-3

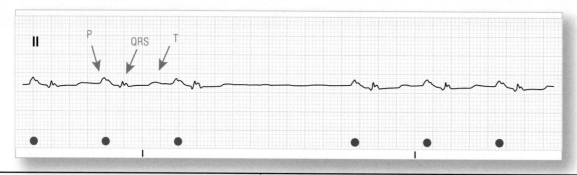

Rate:	About 76 BPM	PR intervals:	Normal, except in event
Regularity:	Regular, except in event	QRS width:	Wide
P waves: Morphology: Axis:	Normal, except in event Normal Normal	Grouping:	None
		Dropped beats:	Yes
P:QRS ratio:	1:1, except in event	Rhythm:	**Sinus rhythm with a sinus pause**

Discussion:

ECG 12-3 shows a sinus rhythm with very small QRS complexes. The P, QRS, and T waves above have been labeled for your convenience. The complexes are wider than 0.12 seconds. Near the middle of the strip, the patient has a prolonged pause which is longer than two times the normal P-P interval. This is an example of a sinus pause.

ECG 12-4

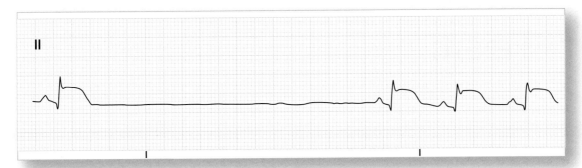

Rate:	About 80 BPM	PR intervals:	Normal, except in event
Regularity:	Regular, except in event	QRS width:	Normal
P waves: Morphology: Axis:	Normal, except in event Normal Normal	Grouping:	None
		Dropped beats:	Yes
P:QRS ratio:	1:1, except in event	Rhythm:	**Sinus rhythm with a sinus arrest**

Discussion:

ECG 12-4 shows a patient with an underlying sinus rhythm. The patient then has a very prolonged pause which was longer than four times the normal P-P interval. This is an example of a sinus arrest. The patient also has some very impressive ST segment elevation. Evalu-ation with a full 12-lead ECG is indicated to evaluate the possibility of an acute MI. Clinical correlation is also indicated to evaluate the patient's hemodynamic status because of the possible MI and the sinus arrest.

CHAPTER REVIEW

1. Sinus blocks, pauses, and arrests all have one big thing in common: the lack of a ___ wave.

2. A sinus block refers to a complete block or failure of the depolarization wave to capture or depolarize the _____ myocardium.

3. SA blocks can never last for three cycles. True or False.

4. The hallmark of a sinus block is that the pause is always an exact multiple of the normal _–_ _____.

5. The sinus pacemaker is reset in the case of a sinus block. True or False.

6. _____ can sometimes be mistaken for sinus blocks. Choose the best one:
   A. Sinus arrhythmias
   B. Sinus tachycardias
   C. Junctional escape rhythms
   D. Premature atrial contractions

7. A sinus _____ is caused by a delay in the formation of a sinus impulse in the SA node itself.

8. A sinus _____ is caused by a longer delay in the formation of an atrial impulse.

9. A sinus arrest can be caused by any combination of sinus pause or block. In any case, it is an extremely long delay. True or False.

10. Neither sinus pauses nor sinus arrests are ever an exact multiple of the normal P-P interval. True or False.

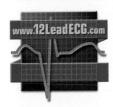
To enhance the knowledge you gain in this book, access this text's website at www.12leadECG.com! This valuable resource provides flashcards, an online glossary, web links, and more. Simply click on the Arrhythmias book cover once at the site.

Self-Test

Test ECG 1

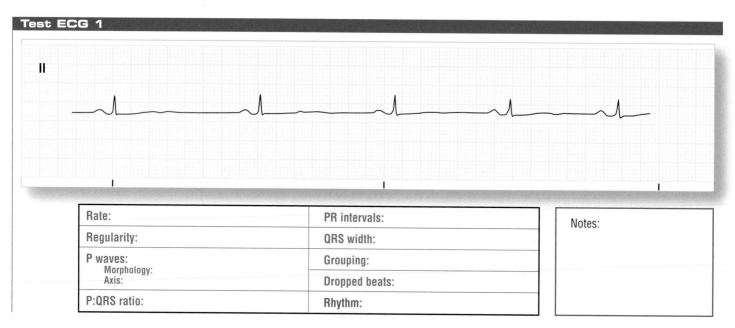

II

Rate:	PR intervals:	Notes:
Regularity:	QRS width:	

P waves:
   Morphology:
   Axis:
	Grouping:	

	Dropped beats:	
P:QRS ratio:	Rhythm:	

Test ECG 2

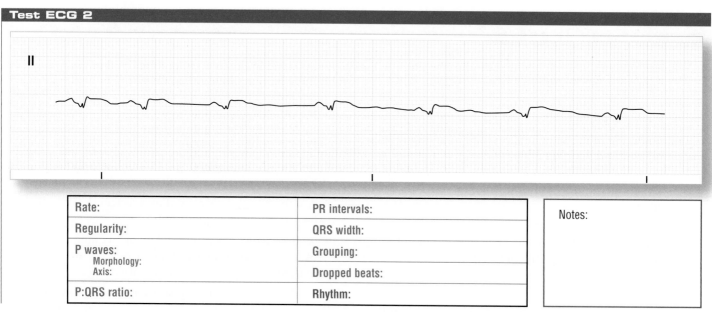

II

Rate:	PR intervals:	Notes:
Regularity:	QRS width:	

P waves:
   Morphology:
   Axis:
	Grouping:	

	Dropped beats:	
P:QRS ratio:	Rhythm:	

Test ECG 3

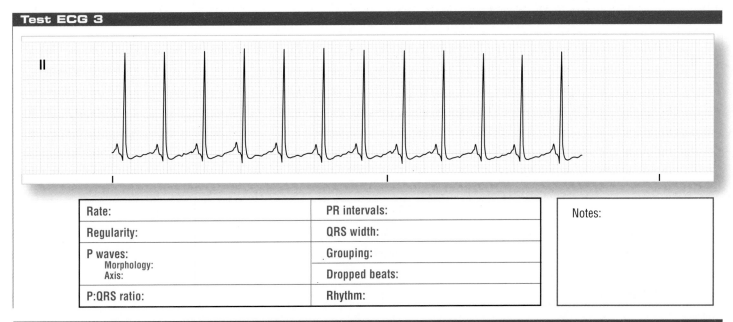

Rate:	PR intervals:	Notes:
Regularity:	QRS width:	

P waves:
    Morphology:
    Axis:
	Grouping:	

	Dropped beats:	
P:QRS ratio:	Rhythm:	

Test ECG 4

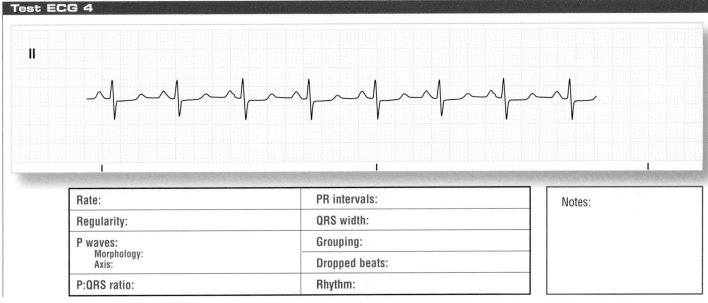

Rate:	PR intervals:	Notes:
Regularity:	QRS width:	

P waves:
    Morphology:
    Axis:
	Grouping:	

	Dropped beats:	
P:QRS ratio:	Rhythm:	

Test ECG 5

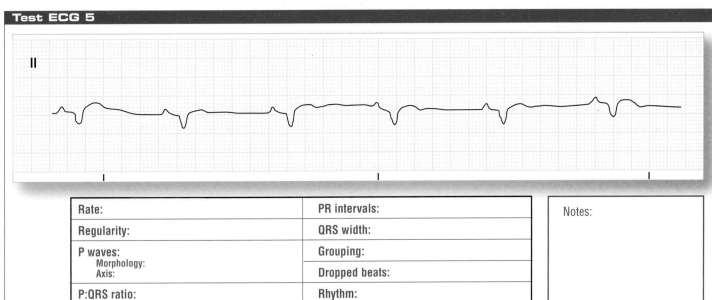

Rate:	PR intervals:	Notes:
Regularity:	QRS width:	

P waves:
    Morphology:
    Axis:
	Grouping:	

	Dropped beats:	
P:QRS ratio:	Rhythm:	

Test ECG 6

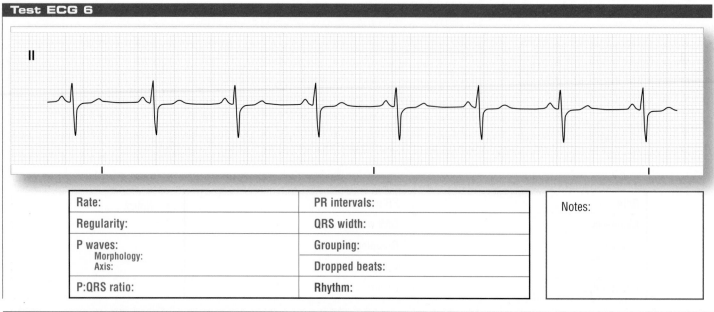

Rate:		PR intervals:		Notes:
Regularity:		QRS width:		
P waves:		Grouping:		
Morphology:				
Axis:		Dropped beats:		
P:QRS ratio:		Rhythm:		

Test ECG 7

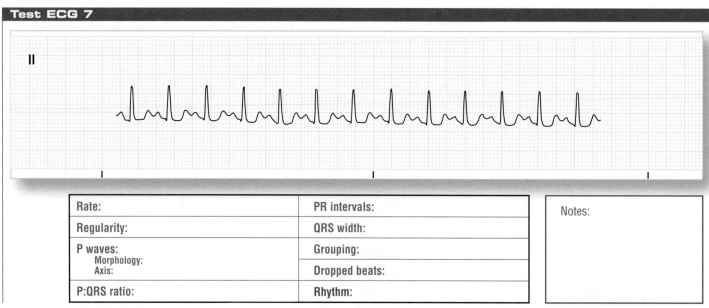

Rate:		PR intervals:		Notes:
Regularity:		QRS width:		
P waves:		Grouping:		
Morphology:				
Axis:		Dropped beats:		
P:QRS ratio:		Rhythm:		

Test ECG 8

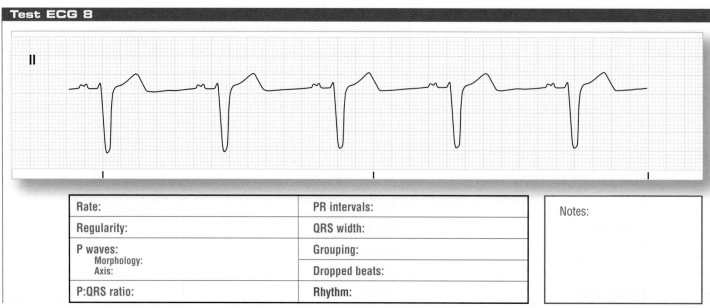

Rate:		PR intervals:		Notes:
Regularity:		QRS width:		
P waves:		Grouping:		
Morphology:				
Axis:		Dropped beats:		
P:QRS ratio:		Rhythm:		

Test ECG 9

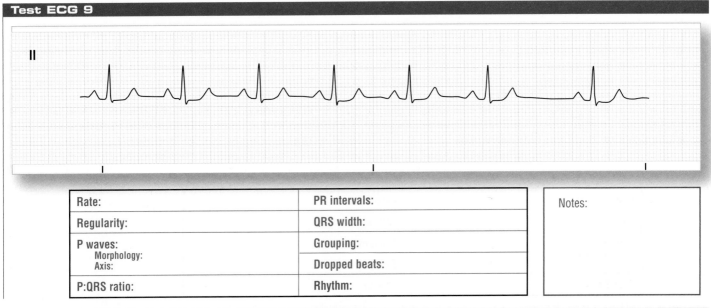

Rate:		PR intervals:	Notes:
Regularity:		QRS width:	
P waves: Morphology: Axis:		Grouping:	
		Dropped beats:	
P:QRS ratio:		Rhythm:	

Test ECG 10

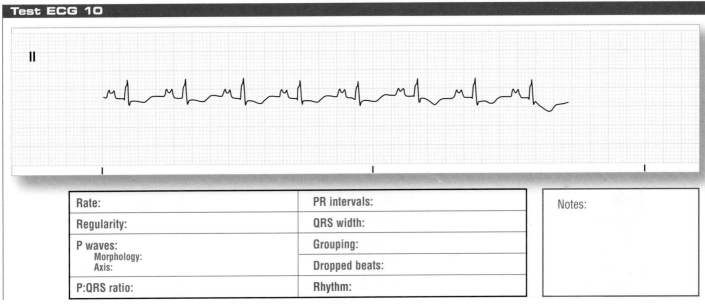

Rate:		PR intervals:	Notes:
Regularity:		QRS width:	
P waves: Morphology: Axis:		Grouping:	
		Dropped beats:	
P:QRS ratio:		Rhythm:	

Test ECG 11

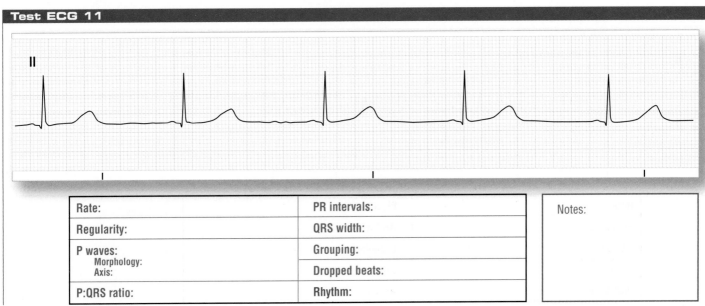

Rate:		PR intervals:	Notes:
Regularity:		QRS width:	
P waves: Morphology: Axis:		Grouping:	
		Dropped beats:	
P:QRS ratio:		Rhythm:	

Test ECG 12

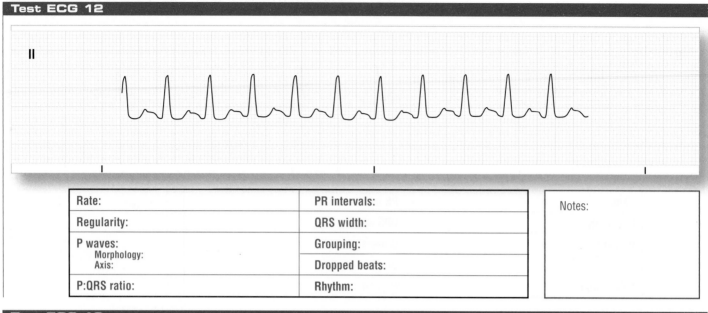

II

Rate:	PR intervals:	Notes:
Regularity:	QRS width:	
P waves:	Grouping:	
Morphology:	Dropped beats:	
Axis:		
P:QRS ratio:	Rhythm:	

Test ECG 13

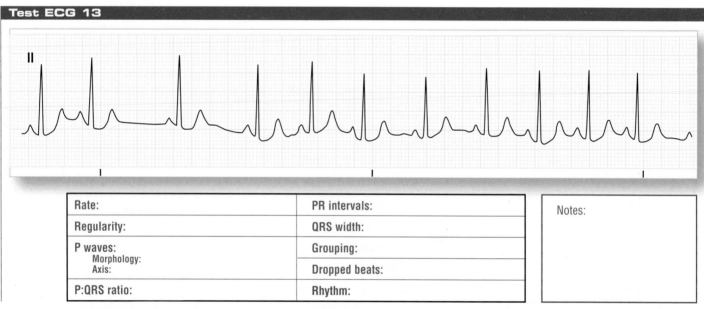

II

Rate:	PR intervals:	Notes:
Regularity:	QRS width:	
P waves:	Grouping:	
Morphology:	Dropped beats:	
Axis:		
P:QRS ratio:	Rhythm:	

Test ECG 14

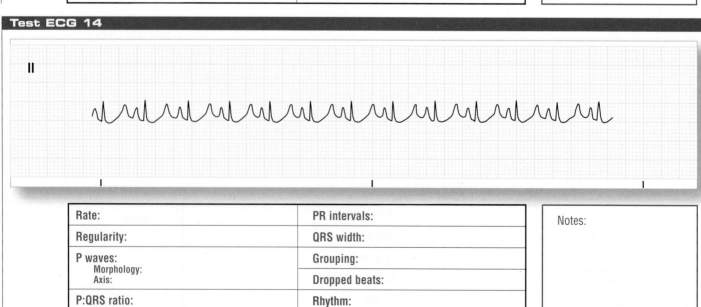

II

Rate:	PR intervals:	Notes:
Regularity:	QRS width:	
P waves:	Grouping:	
Morphology:	Dropped beats:	
Axis:		
P:QRS ratio:	Rhythm:	

Test ECG 15

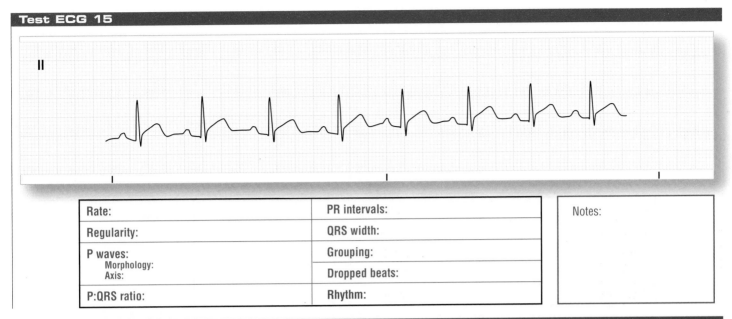

Rate:	PR intervals:	Notes:
Regularity:	QRS width:	
P waves: 　Morphology: 　Axis:	Grouping:	
	Dropped beats:	
P:QRS ratio:	Rhythm:	

Test ECG 16

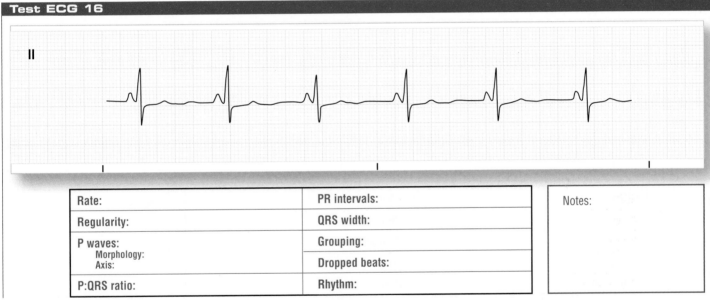

Rate:	PR intervals:	Notes:
Regularity:	QRS width:	
P waves: 　Morphology: 　Axis:	Grouping:	
	Dropped beats:	
P:QRS ratio:	Rhythm:	

Test ECG 17

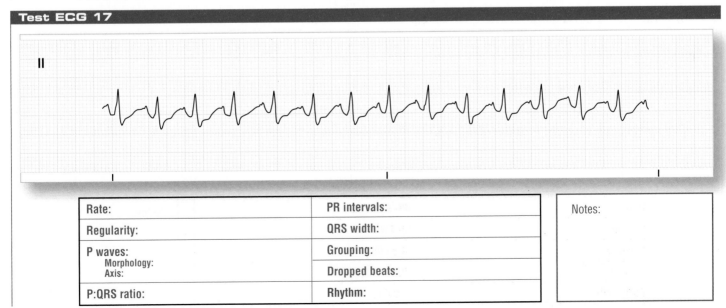

Rate:	PR intervals:	Notes:
Regularity:	QRS width:	
P waves: 　Morphology: 　Axis:	Grouping:	
	Dropped beats:	
P:QRS ratio:	Rhythm:	

Test ECG 18

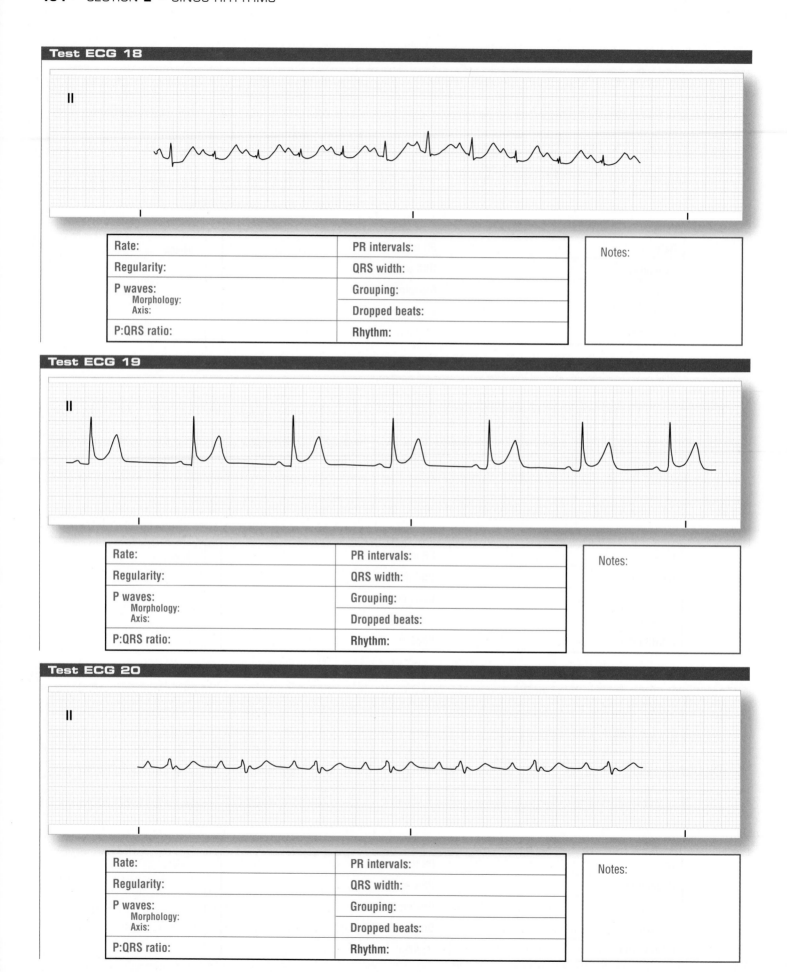

II

Rate:	PR intervals:	Notes:
Regularity:	QRS width:	
P waves: Morphology: Axis:	Grouping:	
	Dropped beats:	
P:QRS ratio:	Rhythm:	

Test ECG 19

II

Rate:	PR intervals:	Notes:
Regularity:	QRS width:	
P waves: Morphology: Axis:	Grouping:	
	Dropped beats:	
P:QRS ratio:	Rhythm:	

Test ECG 20

II

Rate:	PR intervals:	Notes:
Regularity:	QRS width:	
P waves: Morphology: Axis:	Grouping:	
	Dropped beats:	
P:QRS ratio:	Rhythm:	

Section 2 Self-Test Answers

Test ECG 1

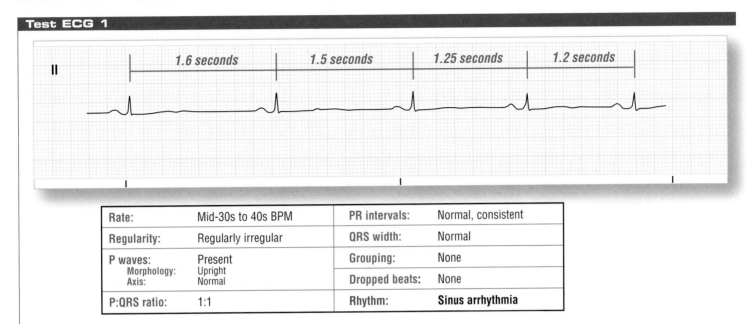

Rate:	Mid-30s to 40s BPM	PR intervals:	Normal, consistent
Regularity:	Regularly irregular	QRS width:	Normal
P waves: Morphology: Axis:	Present Upright Normal	Grouping:	None
		Dropped beats:	None
P:QRS ratio:	1:1	Rhythm:	**Sinus arrhythmia**

Discussion:

This ECG strip is clearly bradycardic. The rate slowly changes between the mid-30s to the upper 40s. It is, however, not just simple sinus bradycardia. If you notice, the R-R intervals are slowly decreasing but the PR intervals are exactly the same. The morphology of the P waves is unchanged throughout the strip. The QRS com-plexes are all the same and within the accepted range for the interval. The diagnosis is sinus arrhythmia.

By the way, a longer rhythm strip taken shortly afterward showed the traditional slowing down and speeding up of the rate, as expected. The patient remained bradycardic but hemodynamically stable.

Test ECG 2

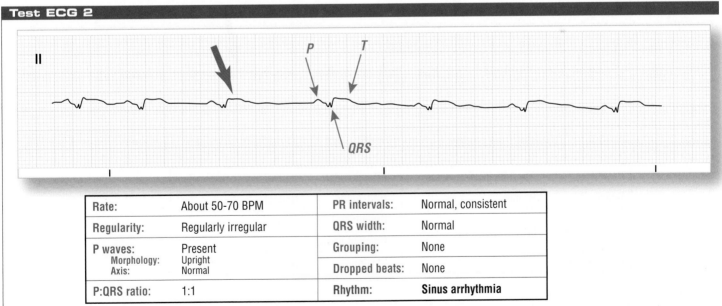

Rate:	About 50-70 BPM	PR intervals:	Normal, consistent
Regularity:	Regularly irregular	QRS width:	Normal
P waves: Morphology: Axis:	Present Upright Normal	Grouping:	None
		Dropped beats:	None
P:QRS ratio:	1:1	Rhythm:	**Sinus arrhythmia**

Discussion:

If you use your calipers on the strip above, you will notice that the rhythm is very irregular. As a matter of fact, it is completely irregularly irregular. The P wave morphology is the same throughout the strip and the PR intervals remain constant. This rules out the most common causes of an irregularly irregular rhythm. Based on these findings, the diagnosis is sinus arrhythmia.

There is an additional finding which is of interest in this strip. If you notice, the ST segments are elevated and flat (see blue arrow). A 12-lead ECG showed that the patient was having an acute myocardial infarction at the time the strip was taken. Remember to always be suspicious!

Test ECG 3

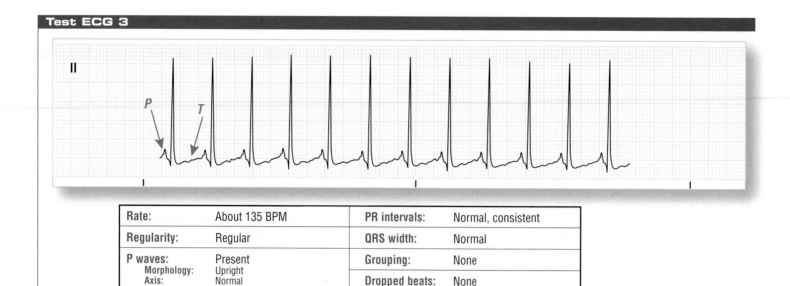

Rate:	About 135 BPM	PR intervals:	Normal, consistent
Regularity:	Regular	QRS width:	Normal
P waves:	Present	Grouping:	None
Morphology:	Upright		
Axis:	Normal	Dropped beats:	None
P:QRS ratio:	1:1	Rhythm:	**Sinus tachycardia**

Discussion:

The rhythm strip above shows a pretty rapid sinus tachycardia. The strip is even more impressive because of the very tall QRS complexes that are found in this patient. These very tall QRS complexes can be found in young people, hypertrophy, and cardiomyopathies, to mention a few possible sources.

The T waves are almost isoelectric in this lead and are almost not visible. The P waves are tall and peaked and the morphology is consistent throughout the strip. The PR interval is also consistent and within the normal range.

Test ECG 4

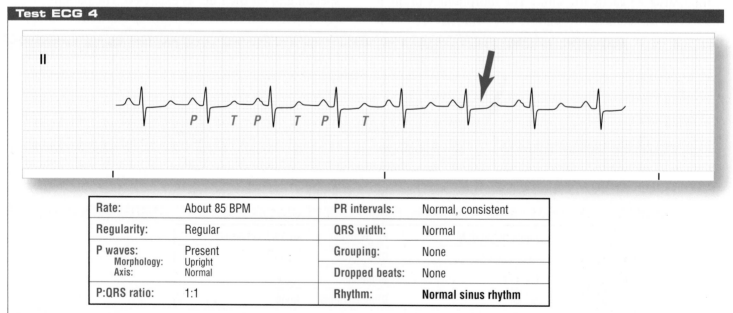

Rate:	About 85 BPM	PR intervals:	Normal, consistent
Regularity:	Regular	QRS width:	Normal
P waves:	Present	Grouping:	None
Morphology:	Upright		
Axis:	Normal	Dropped beats:	None
P:QRS ratio:	1:1	Rhythm:	**Normal sinus rhythm**

Discussion:

You have to be a little careful not to confuse the T waves and the P waves in the strip above. Careful identification of the different waves would be helpful in preventing mistakes that could arise due to mislabeling. Do you notice anything peculiar about the third and seventh P waves? They have a slightly different morphology than the others. They are not ectopic complexes,

however, because the PR intervals are identical and the cadence of the rhythm is not altered by their appearance. Perhaps they represent a slight alteration of the pacemaker site within the SA node itself. In any case, they are of no clinical significance. On the other hand, the ST depressions (see blue arrow) should be evaluated further with a 12-lead ECG.

Test ECG 5

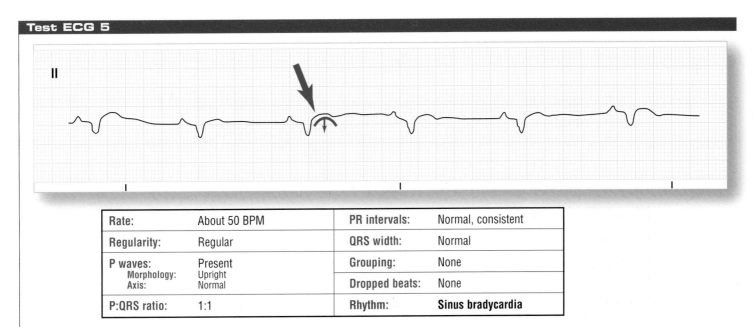

Rate:	About 50 BPM	PR intervals:	Normal, consistent
Regularity:	Regular	QRS width:	Normal
P waves: Morphology: Axis:	Present Upright Normal	Grouping:	None
		Dropped beats:	None
P:QRS ratio:	1:1	Rhythm:	**Sinus bradycardia**

Discussion:

This ECG strip shows sinus bradycardia. There is some slight variation in the cadence of the rhythm, but the variation is well within the accepted upper limit of 0.12 seconds. The P waves all show the same basic morphology with a consistent PR interval. The PR interval is right at the borderline of 0.20 seconds. The slight morphological differences in the appearance of the waves can be accounted for by the baseline which is not exactly straight. The QRS complexes are all within normal ranges and similar in morphology. The ST segments are troubling because they are elevated and concave downward (see blue arrow and diagram). These ST segments can be commonly found in ischemia or infarction and may be the cause of the patient's bradycardia. Further evaluation with a 12-lead ECG is indicated.

Test ECG 6

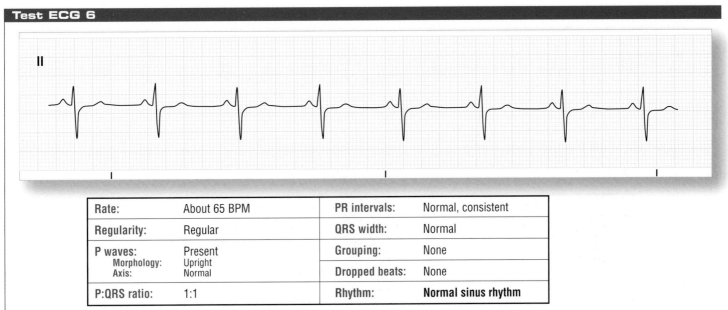

Rate:	About 65 BPM	PR intervals:	Normal, consistent
Regularity:	Regular	QRS width:	Normal
P waves: Morphology: Axis:	Present Upright Normal	Grouping:	None
		Dropped beats:	None
P:QRS ratio:	1:1	Rhythm:	**Normal sinus rhythm**

Discussion:

This is a good example of normal sinus rhythm. Note the consistency in the P wave morphology and the recurrence of the identical PR intervals throughout the strip. The QRS complex is within normal limits for duration and morphology. There is some very slight ST segment depression noted throughout, which could be an abnormality of the rhythm strip itself. As mentioned before, rhythm strips are notorious for the presence of slight abnormalities that are not present on a full 12-lead ECG. If there are any questions or if the patient is exhibiting any symptoms, a full 12-lead can be obtained for further evaluation just to be sure.

Test ECG 7

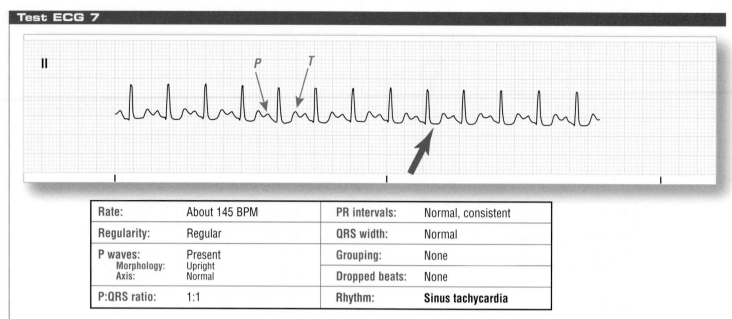

Rate:	About 145 BPM	PR intervals:	Normal, consistent
Regularity:	Regular	QRS width:	Normal
P waves:	Present	Grouping:	None
Morphology:	Upright		
Axis:	Normal	Dropped beats:	None
P:QRS ratio:	1:1	Rhythm:	**Sinus tachycardia**

Discussion:

The rhythm strip above shows a very rapid sinus tachycardia. The P waves are upright and morphologically similar throughout the strip. The PR intervals are consistent and within acceptable limits. There is no evidence for any buried P waves noted on the strip which could confuse the diagnosis. The QRS intervals are within the normal limit and are consistent with the diagnosis of sinus tachycardia.

Note the ST segment depression labeled by the blue arrow above. ST segment depression is common in tachycardias and is not necessarily a sign of ischemia. Clinical correlation with the patient and his or her presentation is indicated, however, to rule out more dangerous causes for the depression.

Test ECG 8

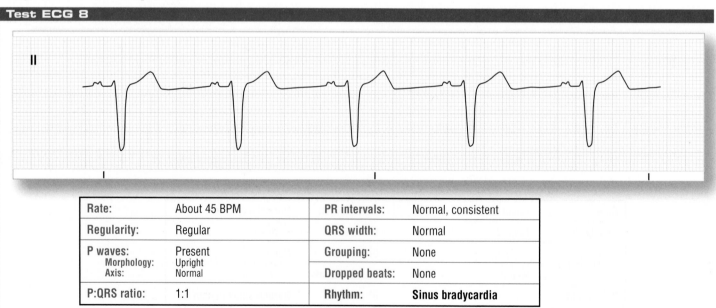

Rate:	About 45 BPM	PR intervals:	Normal, consistent
Regularity:	Regular	QRS width:	Normal
P waves:	Present	Grouping:	None
Morphology:	Upright		
Axis:	Normal	Dropped beats:	None
P:QRS ratio:	1:1	Rhythm:	**Sinus bradycardia**

Discussion:

This rhythm strip shows the characteristics of a typical sinus bradycardia. The P waves all show similar morphology and the PR intervals are within the normal range and consistent. The QRS complexes are wide, which could be due to a bundle branch block; further correlation is indicated with an old strip, or an ECG would be helpful in this evaluation.

The P waves show a double-humped morphology, which could be consistent with a left atrial abnormality if the finding were present on a 12-lead ECG. Once again, you should be very careful about evaluating wave morphology on a rhythm strip.

Test ECG 9

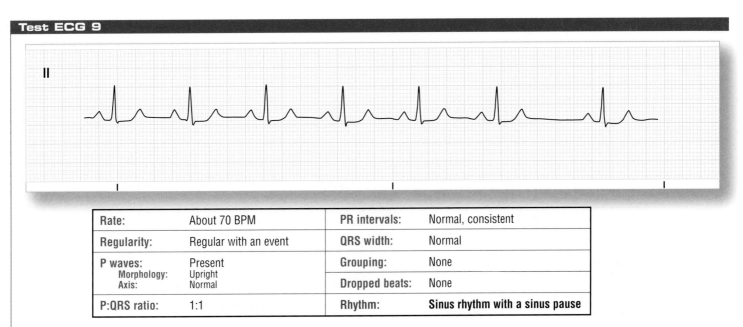

Rate:	About 70 BPM	PR intervals:	Normal, consistent
Regularity:	Regular with an event	QRS width:	Normal
P waves: Morphology: Axis:	Present Upright Normal	Grouping:	None
		Dropped beats:	None
P:QRS ratio:	1:1	Rhythm:	**Sinus rhythm with a sinus pause**

Discussion:

This strip shows a regular rhythm with an event. The rhythm strip has consistent P wave morphology, upright P waves in lead II, and normal, consistent PR intervals. There is some slight discrepancy in the cadence of the rhythm during the first six complexes, which is within acceptable limits, and then there is a much longer pause. The pause is followed by a complex with an identical P wave and PR interval to the rest of the strip. The longer pause is due to a delay in the impulse from exiting the SA node and is consistent with a sinus pause.

Test ECG 10

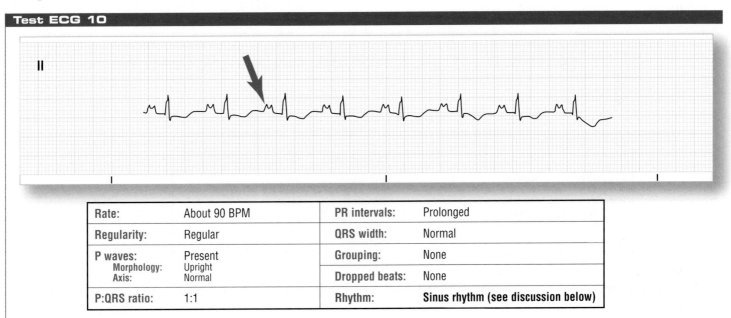

Rate:	About 90 BPM	PR intervals:	Prolonged
Regularity:	Regular	QRS width:	Normal
P waves: Morphology: Axis:	Present Upright Normal	Grouping:	None
		Dropped beats:	None
P:QRS ratio:	1:1	Rhythm:	**Sinus rhythm (see discussion below)**

Discussion:

This strip shows very prominent P waves that are double humped and notched (see blue arrow). The morphology of the P waves is consistent throughout the strip. The PR intervals are slightly over 0.20 seconds and, therefore, slightly prolonged (first-degree AV block will be covered fully in Chapter 35). The QRS complexes are of normal duration. The ST segments are depressed and the T waves are inverted. Clinical correlation of these findings and a full 12-lead ECG are suggested for further evaluation.

For completeness, this rhythm strip cannot be called normal sinus rhythm because of the prolonged PR interval. Instead, we will simply call it sinus rhythm (with a first-degree AV block, for you more advanced students).

Test ECG 11

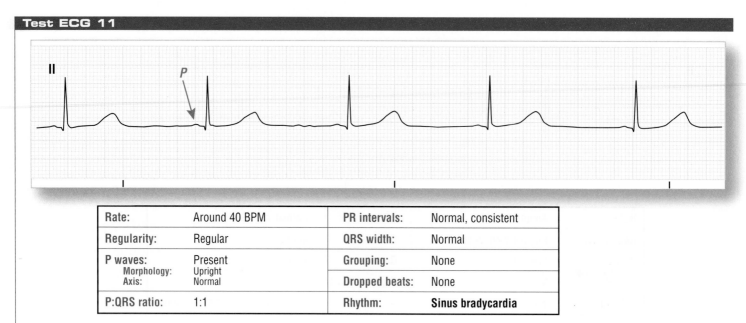

Rate:	Around 40 BPM	PR intervals:	Normal, consistent
Regularity:	Regular	QRS width:	Normal

P waves:
  Morphology:
  Axis:
	Present
	Upright
	Normal
		Grouping:	None

		Dropped beats:	None
P:QRS ratio:	1:1	Rhythm:	**Sinus bradycardia**

Discussion:

The P waves on these complexes are not very prominent. However, they are positive in lead II and are consistent throughout the strip. The PR intervals are also
consistent and within normal limits. The heart rate is
around 40 BPM. Putting it all together, we have a sinus
bradycardia.

Test ECG 12

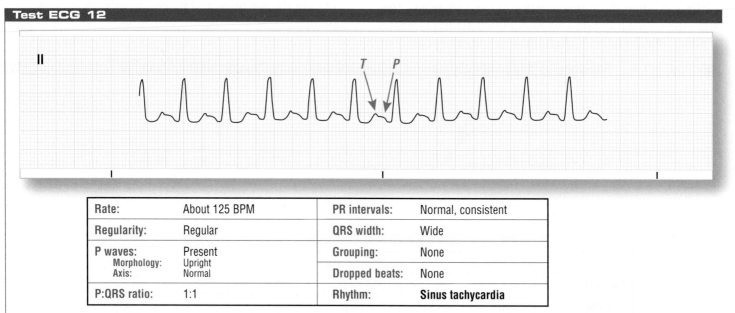

Rate:	About 125 BPM	PR intervals:	Normal, consistent
Regularity:	Regular	QRS width:	Wide

P waves:
  Morphology:
  Axis:
	Present
	Upright
	Normal
		Grouping:	None

		Dropped beats:	None
P:QRS ratio:	1:1	Rhythm:	**Sinus tachycardia**

Discussion:

This rhythm strip can be quite confusing to interpret.
The reason for the confusion is the near fusion of the T
waves and the P waves. There are two main reasons for
this near-fusion to develop: (1) The rhythm is a tachycardia. Tachycardias typically cause the TP segment to
shorten; (2) The patient has a prolonged QT interval because of the wide QRS complexes (preexisting bundle
branch block). The prolongation of the interval causes
the T wave to occur later than would normally be expected. The net result of both of those findings is additive, causing the TP segment to be nonexistent and the
T waves and the P waves to almost become superimposed on each other. Take a look at the waves labeled
on the strip above and imagine a vertical line drawn
right between the two complexes. This will help you see
the individual waves a bit more clearly.

The strip is consistent with sinus tachycardia at
about 125 BPM. The ST segment depressions may be
due to the tachycardia, but clinical and ECG correlation
should be considered.

Test ECG 13

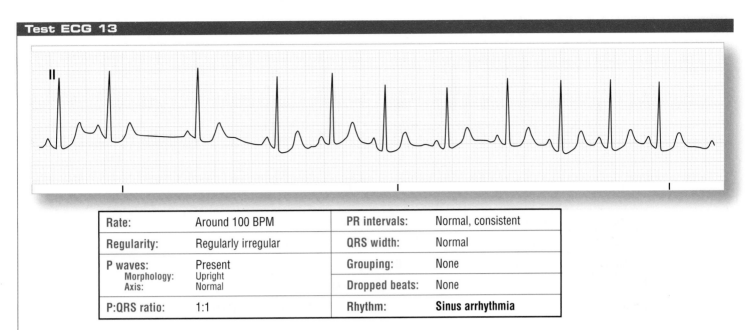

Rate:	Around 100 BPM	PR intervals:	Normal, consistent
Regularity:	Regularly irregular	QRS width:	Normal
P waves:	Present	Grouping:	None
Morphology:	Upright		
Axis:	Normal	Dropped beats:	None
P:QRS ratio:	1:1	Rhythm:	**Sinus arrhythmia**

Discussion:

This strip is obviously irregular. The presence of identical P wave morphology and PR intervals throughout the strip cinch the diagnosis of sinus arrhythmia.

When you have a wandering baseline, always take a few extra seconds to look at the strip a bit closer. Morphological changes of premature or ectopic complexes can be hidden within the wandering baseline or in artifact. If there continue to be questions about the rhythm, obtaining a longer strip or simply readjusting the leads on the patient will often clear the issues right up.

Test ECG 14

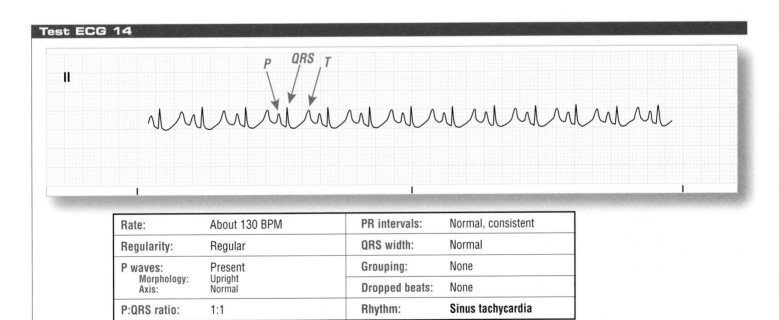

Rate:	About 130 BPM	PR intervals:	Normal, consistent
Regularity:	Regular	QRS width:	Normal
P waves:	Present	Grouping:	None
Morphology:	Upright		
Axis:	Normal	Dropped beats:	None
P:QRS ratio:	1:1	Rhythm:	**Sinus tachycardia**

Discussion:

This strip also shows complexes with fairly prolonged QT intervals. In this example, however, the P waves and the T waves are distinct. Using your calipers to map out the various waves and then marching them through the strip can be quite helpful in these cases.

The relatively low amplitude of the QRS complexes in this strip can also lead to some confusion. Changing leads on the monitor or obtaining a 12-lead ECG will address this potential problem.

Test ECG 15

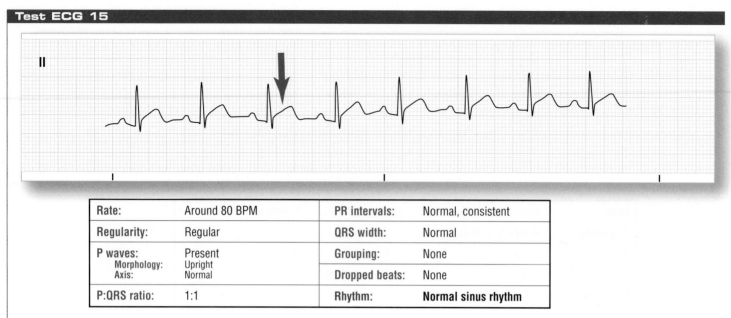

Rate:	Around 80 BPM	PR intervals:	Normal, consistent
Regularity:	Regular	QRS width:	Normal

P waves:
  Morphology:
  Axis:
	Present
	Upright
	Normal
		Grouping:	None

		Dropped beats:	None
P:QRS ratio:	1:1	Rhythm:	**Normal sinus rhythm**

Discussion:

This strip also shows a wandering baseline. In this case, however, it does not affect our interpretation in any way. The P waves are clearly seen and show the same morphology throughout the strip. They are upright in Lead II, as would be expected. The PR interval is consistent throughout the strip as well. The strip is a good example of a normal sinus rhythm.

Did you pick up the ST segment abnormality in this strip (see blue arrow)? Once again, the ST segments are elevated and flat. These are very troublesome and consistent with injury or infarct. Clinical correlation and a full 12-lead ECG should be obtained emergently on this patient.

Test ECG 16

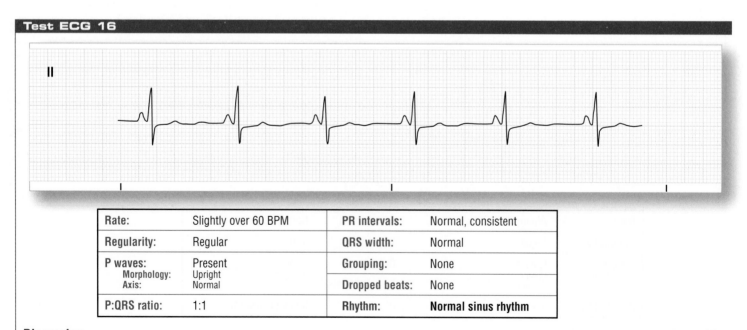

Rate:	Slightly over 60 BPM	PR intervals:	Normal, consistent
Regularity:	Regular	QRS width:	Normal

P waves:
  Morphology:
  Axis:
	Present
	Upright
	Normal
		Grouping:	None

		Dropped beats:	None
P:QRS ratio:	1:1	Rhythm:	**Normal sinus rhythm**

Discussion:

This is another example of normal sinus rhythm. The rate is slightly over 60 BPM, putting it within the normal range. The PR interval gives you the impression of being short. Careful measurement, however, will show you that it is 0.12 seconds long and in the normal range.

Once again, there is some slight ST depression noted on this strip. Clinical and electrocardiographic correlation should be considered.

Test ECG 17

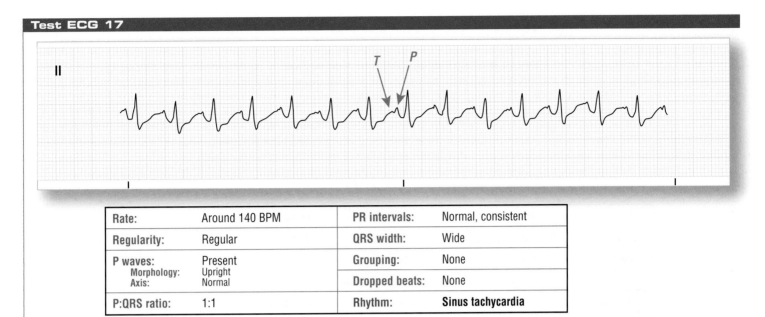

Rate:	Around 140 BPM	PR intervals:	Normal, consistent
Regularity:	Regular	QRS width:	Wide
P waves: Morphology: Axis:	Present Upright Normal	Grouping:	None
		Dropped beats:	None
P:QRS ratio:	1:1	Rhythm:	**Sinus tachycardia**

Discussion:

This is a tough one! Take a close look at the area between the end of the QRS complex and the start of the next one. Use a magnifying glass if you need to see it more clearly. You will notice that there are distinct P waves but, once again, they are nearly buried in the preceding T wave.

The consistent P wave morphology and PR interval, along with a heart rate of around 140 BPM, makes the rhythm a sinus tachycardia. Note that the width of the QRS complexes (greater than 0.12 seconds) does not affect the rhythm in any way; it is still a sinus tachycardia.

Test ECG 18

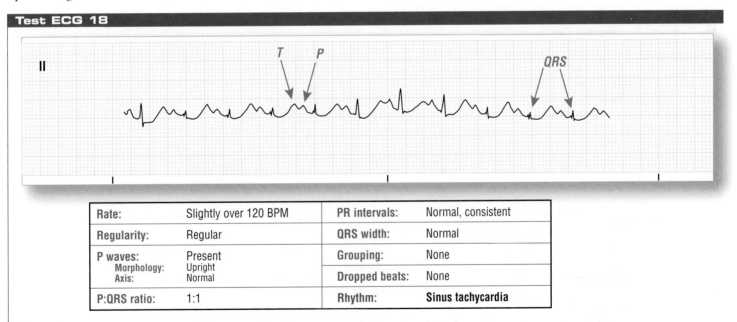

Rate:	Slightly over 120 BPM	PR intervals:	Normal, consistent
Regularity:	Regular	QRS width:	Normal
P waves: Morphology: Axis:	Present Upright Normal	Grouping:	None
		Dropped beats:	None
P:QRS ratio:	1:1	Rhythm:	**Sinus tachycardia**

Discussion:

We are showing you another example of prolonged QT interval with P on T phenomenon because they can be quite confusing. This strip has waves that are a bit more distinct, which helps with evaluation. The P waves are all upright in lead II and the morphology is consistent throughout the strip. The PR intervals are also consistent throughout the strip. The QRS complexes vary in amplitude, demonstrating a common occurrence in tachycardias: electrical alternans. This can normally be seen in many tachycardias. There is some ST segment depression noted on the strip. Clinical and electrocardiographic correlation should be considered in this case for further evaluation of the abnormal findings and to determine the cause of the tachycardia.

Test ECG 19

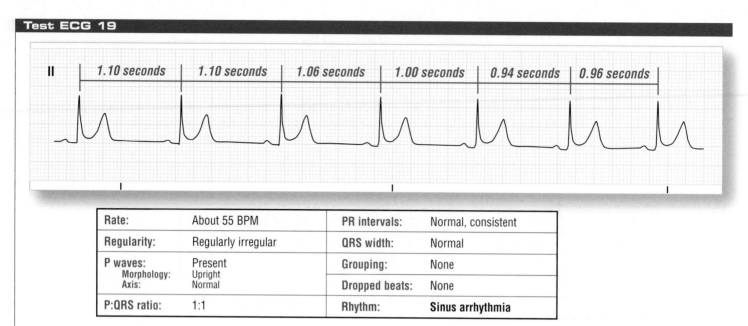

Rate:	About 55 BPM	PR intervals:	Normal, consistent
Regularity:	Regularly irregular	QRS width:	Normal
P waves: Morphology: Axis:	Present Upright Normal	Grouping:	None
		Dropped beats:	None
P:QRS ratio:	1:1	Rhythm:	**Sinus arrhythmia**

Discussion:

Unless you have a very good eye or used your calipers, it would be very difficult to spot the small amount of narrowing that occurs between each of the complexes. The key in this strip is to see the difference between the first two and the last two complexes in the strip. The difference is more than 0.16 seconds, which makes the variation abnormal. On a long rhythm strip, the undu-lation of the distances with the patient's respirations becomes more obvious.

For those who have studied electrocardiography, note the slight PR depressions and the scooping ST segments, which could be an early repolarization pattern or early pericarditis.

Test ECG 20

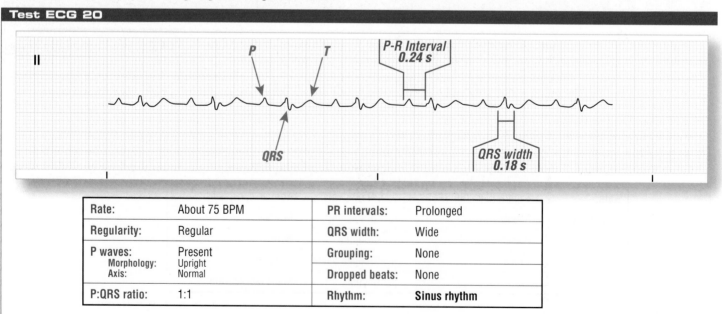

Rate:	About 75 BPM	PR intervals:	Prolonged
Regularity:	Regular	QRS width:	Wide
P waves: Morphology: Axis:	Present Upright Normal	Grouping:	None
		Dropped beats:	None
P:QRS ratio:	1:1	Rhythm:	**Sinus rhythm**

Discussion:

We are throwing a bit of a curve ball with this rhythm strip. There are a couple of reasons for this: (1) The small amplitude and the morphology of the QRS complexes can cause some confusion when examining this rhythm strip; (2) The PR interval is prolonged at 0.24 seconds; (3) The QRS complexes are wider than 0.12 seconds. Recall that part of the criteria for normal sinus rhythm is to have intervals within the normal range. This patient has a prolonged PR interval—which as we shall see later on, makes this a first-degree heart block—and a wide QRS complex. Note that this is still a sinus rhythm, but not normal sinus rhythm. This slight difference in nomenclature is usually overlooked by many clinicians and authors, but is the correct terminology.

Atrial Rhythms

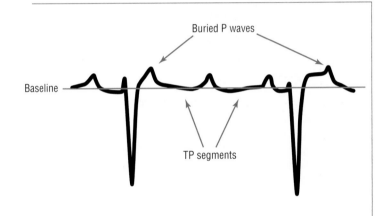

Baseline

Buried P waves

TP segments

CHAPTER 13

Premature Atrial Contraction

A premature atrial contraction (PAC) refers to an impulse or complex that occurs earlier than expected and originates in an atrial focus, not in the SA node (Figure13-1). PACs typically occur when a small area of the atria is more irritable than the rest of the atrial tissue (Figure 13-2). The irritability increases the intrinsic pacing rate for the potential ectopic focus in the area and, eventually, one fires off earlier than the sinus node.

PACs are normally clinically insignificant. Since they occur intermittently, the slight alterations in the timing of the mechanical contractions of the heart that are produced are usually not enough to affect hemodynamics to any great degree. However, under certain circumstances (frequent PACs, valvular disorders, heart failure), the inappropriate filling of the ventricles caused by the early complexes can cause slight, but clinically significant, alterations in the cardiac output and blood pressure. These hemodynamic changes are typically not life threatening but can lead to lightheadedness, palpitations, and a feeling of fluttering in the chest.

Earlier, in Chapter 8, we saw how NSR was formed. The regularity of the rhythm was set by the fastest pacemaker, the SA node (Figure 13-3). The stability of a sinus nodal origin of the impulse creates a consistency in the P-P interval on the ECG. In addition, since the P wave always originates in the sinus node, the P waves in NSR all have the same morphology and are upright in leads II, III, and AVF.

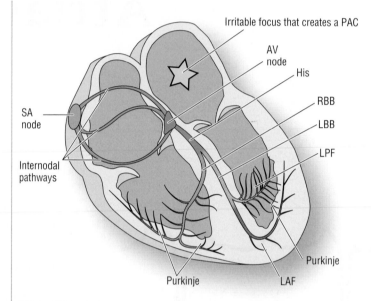

Figure 13-1: An irritable focus, represented by the yellow star, acts as a pacemaker and causes an impulse to occur sooner than would ordinarily be expected. This creates the typical characteristics of a PAC as represented in Figure 13-2.

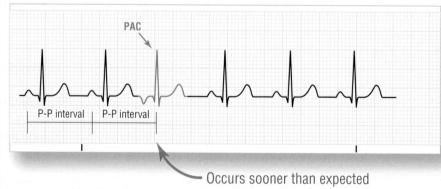

Figure 13-2: Electrocardiographically, the ectopic firing causes an event that breaks up the underlying regular rhythm. The PAC has a P-P interval that is shorter than expected and a different P wave morphology and PR interval because it does not originate in the SA node. Let's see why this occurs.

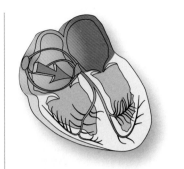
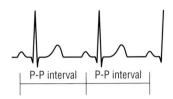

Figure 13-3: The SA node normally sets the rhythm, creating consistent P-P intervals.

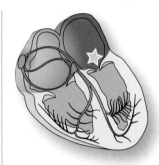
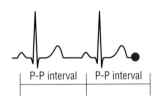

Figure 13-4: The faster SA node usually fires before an ectopic focus gets the chance.

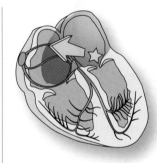
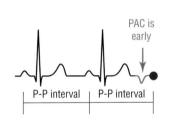

Figure 13-5: When an ectopic focus fires early, the heart contracts early and a PAC results.

We need to clear up a problem with the nomenclature. In today's literature, many terms are used to describe an atrial complex that arrives prematurely. These include premature atrial contractions, premature atrial complexes, atrial premature contractions, and atrial premature depolarizations, just to name a few. Presently, there is no consensus on which is the best label to place on these events. We are going to stick to the old tried and true term premature atrial contraction (PAC). Be aware that all of these terms refer to the same electrocardiographic event. This same nomenclature issue will also apply to premature junctional contractions (PJC) and premature ventricular contractions (PVC).

Normally, the pacemaking function of the atrial tissue is set at a slower rate than that of the SA node (usually around 55–60 BPM). The result is that, as the more frequent sinus impulses wash over the focus represented by the yellow star, the pacemaking function of the focus is continuously reset and it, therefore, never fires (Figure 13-4).

Every once in awhile, however, an ectopic focus in the atria becomes irritable and fires early. This premature impulse leads to an early contraction of the heart and, hence, a PAC (Figure 13-5). Note that the impulse of the PAC moves in a different direction and route than that taken by a sinus impulse. In this case, the depolarization wave travels upward and to the left.

The abnormal vector caused by the depolarization wave from an ectopic focus causes a different P wave morphology to be formed (Figure 3-6). In addition to the P wave, the PR interval also has to be different because of the different route taken by the wave. After

Take Special Note. . .

The ventricular portion of the impulse proceeds normally along the electrical conduction system of the heart once it reaches and leaves the AV node. This gives rise to a normal, narrow QRS complex that is identical to the ones seen in NSR. The only exceptions to the rule occur when there is a preexisting bundle branch block, some electrolyte abnormality, or some aberrancy in conduction because the premature impulse could not get through an area of the conduction system that is still refractory. We will discuss this a bit further when we get to the rhythm strips themselves. For now, just remember that in PACs, the QRS complexes are usually narrow.

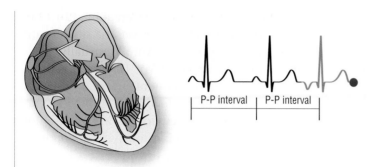

Figure 13-6: The ectopic focus creates a PAC and a different P wave morphology.

the PAC, the SA node should once again take over its primary role as the main pacemaker.

In addition to the information discussed above, the formation of a PAC allows us to examine some basic concepts of arrhythmia recognition in greater detail. These include the P wave axis, the PR interval, the pauses, and aberrancy. These are critical concepts in the analysis of any arrhythmia, and a thorough understanding of these principles is vital to your continued success.

The P Wave Axis

In Chapters 3 and 6, we reviewed the concept of the electrical axis of the heart. If you remember, each myocyte in the ventricles forms its own small electrical vector (Figure 13-7). The electrical axis of the heart is the main vector that remains when all of those individual small vectors are added together.

So, why the big deal about the electrical axis? Well, an ECG machine or monitor does not measure each individual small vector. It only measures the single resultant vector produced during a single instant. In the case of the ventricles, that vector is the electrical axis.

Recall that the electrical leads act like cameras taking individual pictures of a vector from its own individual vantage point (Figure 13-7). That electrode sees a vector traveling toward it as a positive wave. A vector traveling away from it produces a negative wave (Figure 13-8). Since the vector causes the different positive and negative waves to appear on an ECG strip, the direction, amplitude, and duration of the vector are extremely important. These properties of the vector *as seen over time* form the resultant shape of the wave on the ECG tracing.

In the atria, the same process of vector formation occurs during the depolarization of the myocytes. The atrial myocytes each form their own individual vectors that, when added together, form one large vector. That

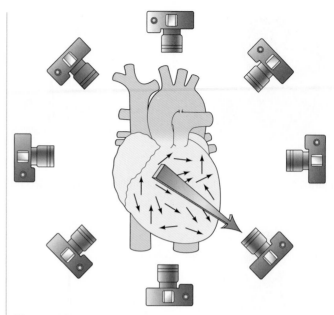

Figure 13-7: Leads are like cameras.

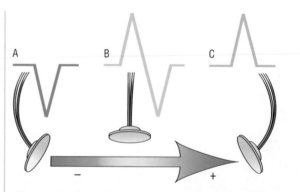

Figure 13-8: A positive wave heading toward an electrode gives rise to a positive deflection. A positive wave heading away from an electrode gives rise to a negative deflection.

large vector is known as the *P wave axis* (Figure 13-9). Calculating the exact P wave axis is more complicated than figuring out the ventricular axis and belongs with the study of 12-lead ECGs; however, the P wave axis remains extremely important to the analysis of any arrhythmia in a way that is very simple and easy to identify: its relation to certain leads.

Remember, the electrocardiographic representation of the P wave in any one lead depends on its own particular vantage point as it views the P wave axis. For example, if the P wave axis is headed inferiorly, backward and to the left, the P wave will be seen in leads I and II as being positive (Figure 13-9). If, on the other hand, the vector is headed superiorly, backward, and to the right, the P wave will be seen in leads I and II as being negative (Figure 13-10). The length or duration of the P wave is dependent on the duration of the atrial depolarization process and, therefore, the length of its vector.

Notice how the number of possible combinations is pretty extensive, and so are the possible morphologies of the P waves. Since each myocyte is in a different three-dimensional position, each one will give rise to its own particular vector, its own way of initiating and propagating a depolarization wave, and, hence, its own particular P wave morphology.

Now, let's get back to PACs. PACs, by definition, originate in an ectopic atrial focus. The P wave morphology in PACs and their PR intervals (as we shall see in the next section) will, therefore, always differ from those complexes that originated in the sinus node. These morphological differences provide some excellent clinical clues to the presence of an ectopic complex. The

P waves can, however, provide another important diagnostic clue: The direction of the P wave in leads I, II, and V$_5$ to V$_6$.

Previously we discussed the fact that a vector heading from the sinus node must travel inferiorly and to the left (Figure 13-11). As we have just seen, this causes the P waves to be upright in leads II, III, and aVF. (To be completely correct, the P waves must be upright in leads I, II, and V$_5$ to V$_6$, if you have a 12-lead ECG.) The P waves have to be upright in those leads because the sinus node is at the high end of the heart and the depolarization wave and its resulting vector has to head inferiorly. This is, therefore, the direction of the normal P wave vector or, more technically, the direction of the P wave axis.

Now, suppose you had an ectopic pacemaker triggering a PAC. The P wave axis of that complex depends on the location of the ectopic pacer. As an example,

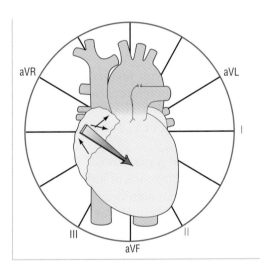
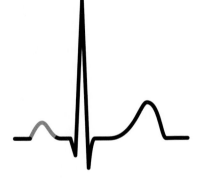

Figure 13-9: In this example, the P wave vector is headed inferiorly, backward, and to the left. Leads I and II see a positive vector headed toward them, and this is represented electrocardiographically as a positive P wave in those leads.

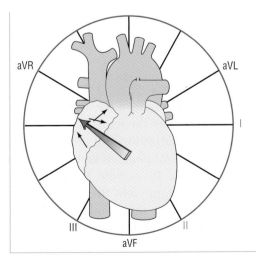
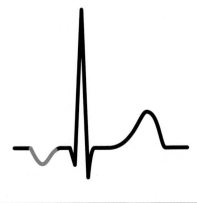

Figure 13-10: In this example, the P wave vector is headed superiorly, backward, and to the right. Leads I and II see a positive vector headed away from them and this is represented electrocardiographically as a negative P wave in those leads.

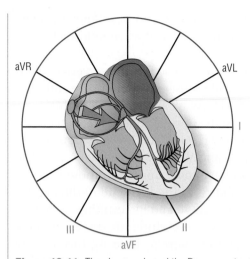

Figure 13-11: The sinus node and the P wave vector. This figure graphically represents the P wave vector as a light blue vector heading inferiorly and to the left. Note that the vector is heading toward the positive poles of leads I and II. Remember, a vector heading toward the positive pole of a lead gives rise electrocardiographically to an upright or positive wave in that lead. Since an impulse that originated in the sinus node can only travel downward and to the left, then the P wave has to be upright in leads I, II, III, aVF, and V_5 to V_6.

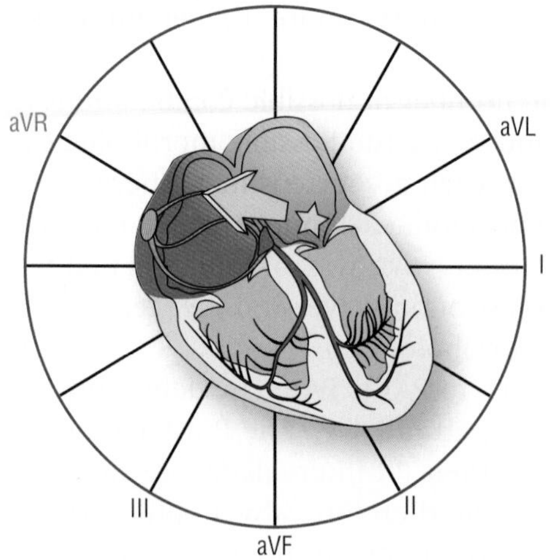

Figure 13-12: An ectopic focus and its P wave vector. This figure graphically represents the P wave vector as a yellow vector heading superiorly and to the right. Note that the vector is heading toward the positive pole of lead aVR only. The P waves would be negative in leads I, II, III, and aVF.

look at Figure 13-12. In this example, the yellow area represents the irritable focus that fires early. As the depolarization wave proceeds outward from this zone, it creates a main P wave vector that proceeds superiorly, anteriorly, and to the right. Would the P wave be positive in leads I, II, III, and aVF? The answer is no. The P waves would be negative because the vector is heading away from those leads.

The main take-home points and the whole reason to discuss the P wave axis can be summed up easily in a couple of sentences. If a complex starts out in the sinus node, the P wave will always be positive in leads I, II, III, and aVF. Likewise, the reverse leads us to one of the most important rules in arrhythmia recognition:

If the P wave is not upright in leads I, II, and V_5 to V_6, then the P wave had to have originated in some ectopic focus.

The ectopic focus could be anywhere in the atria or below (as in the case of retrograde conduction to the atria from the AV node or the ventricles).

Take special note, however, of a very important implication of the statement above. Many times you can still have an ectopic atrial pacemaker with upright P waves in leads II, III, and aVF. This can occur when the ectopic focus is adjacent to the sinus node or somewhere along the superior portions of the right atria.

These ectopic foci will still give you vectors that are directed downward and will, therefore, give rise to upright P waves in lead II of a rhythm strip. BUT, a negative P wave in either leads I, II or V_5 to V_6 *has* to originate in some ectopic focus.

As you can imagine, the P wave axis is a tremendous help in the differential diagnosis of a rhythm abnormality. The presence of an abnormal P wave axis automatically focuses your differential diagnosis into either an ectopic atrial rhythm, or as a rhythm that originated in the AV node or below and is being spread retrogradely to the atria. Please take the time to understand this point completely and thoroughly, as we will refer to this concept over and over again throughout the rest of this book.

PACs and the PR Interval

The PR interval is composed of quite a few components (Figure 13-13). It is composed of the interval of time it takes to complete atrial depolarization and the physiologic block that occurs at the AV node, as well as the transmission time through the His bundle, the bundle branches, and finally, the Purkinje cells themselves. Take a look at Figure 13-13—the time it takes for the depolarization wave to travel from the sinus node to the AV node is represented by the bracketed area. Once the impulse reaches the AV node, the time interval of the physiologic block begins. This is a set interval of time that is innate in the AV tissue; the tissue will not let the impulse travel through until that time is up.

So, what does this have to do with PACs? Well, the time interval in the brackets is affected by the location of the ectopic pacemaker. If the pacemaker site is close to the AV node, the time it takes for the depolarization wave to reach the AV node is shorter. Since that time is shorter, the whole PR interval will be shorter. If the pacemaker site is farther from the AV node than the dis-

tance from the SA node to the AV node, then the depolarization wave takes longer to reach the AV node and the PR interval is longer. Let's look at some examples.

In Figure 13-14, the ectopic pacemaker is in the right atria close to the AV node. Would you expect the PR interval during a PAC to be prolonged or shorter than that seen during a sinus beat in the same patient? Well, since the distance is shorter, the PR interval should be shorter as well. The P wave axis of the PAC is headed superiorly, anteriorly, and to the left. What would you expect the P wave of a PAC from this focus to look like in lead II? It would be negative in lead II.

In Figure 13-15, the ectopic pacemaker is in the left atria and is pretty far from the AV node. You would expect the PR interval of the PAC to be longer than the one seen in NSR, and it is. The P wave of the PAC is positive in lead II, as you would expect. Don't worry about the fact that it is biphasic; that is not important. The important thing is that the P wave is positive in lead II. In this case, the P wave axis didn't help you much, but the early arrival of the PAC, the differing morphology of the P wave, and the different PR interval all point to the presence of a PAC. Note, however, that a strip from lead I or V$_5$ or V$_6$ would have shown negative Ps.

The Pause

Many times during your career you will come face-to-face with a diagnostic dilemma. You will have a complex that has the features of one type of arrhythmia, but with some features that point directly toward another possibility. At times like these, you want to use every tool available to you to help you distinguish between the two possibilities. The type of pause that

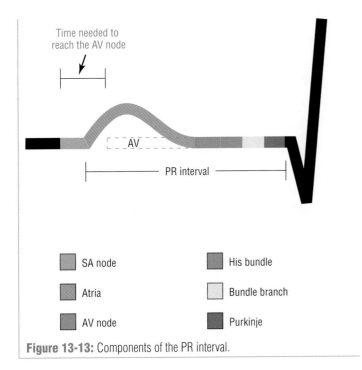

Figure 13-13: Components of the PR interval.

SA node

Atria

AV node

His bundle

Bundle branch

Purkinje

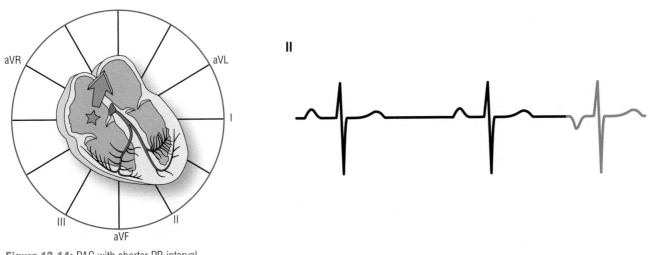

II

Figure 13-14: PAC with shorter PR interval.

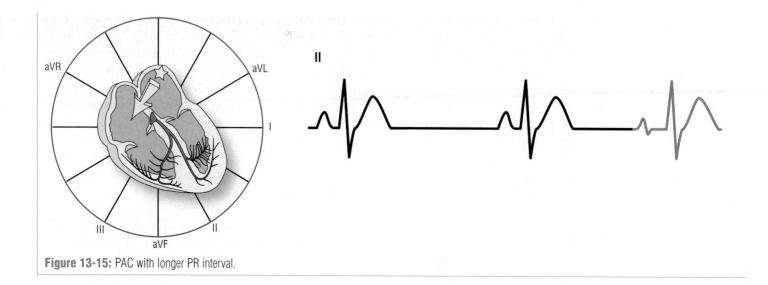

Figure 13-15: PAC with longer PR interval.

occurs immediately after a premature complex is just such a tool. Luckily, there are only two types of pauses that you need to worry about—the compensatory and noncompensatory pauses.

The key to understanding the two types of pauses is to understand the concept of phase 4 repolarization (Figure 13-16) and the resetting of the pacemaker. Recall from Chapter 2 that phase 4 repolarization refers to the slow influx of ions that cause a gradual depolarization of the cell toward the threshold potential. This is the basis of the pacemaking function of the cells of the heart. The rate of the ascent of phase 4 is individual to each type of cell found in the heart, and is responsible for the intrinsic pacing rate for each of those cell types (Figure 13-17).

Now, for the sake of discussion, let's take a look at one cell in the SA node as it is clipping along. The cell goes through a continuous series of phase 4 depolarizations and firing whenever the threshold potential is crossed (see Figure 13-18). Suddenly, there is an unexpected depolarization wave that causes the cell to fire sooner than expected (e.g., a PAC, represented by the green star). As long as the cell is not in its absolute refractory phase, it will fire immediately. After the premature depolarization has occurred, the cell will continue with its phase 4 depolarization as before. But, notice that the regularity of the rhythm has been altered. The pacemaker was *reset* by the premature impulse. The new rate may be the same as before or it may be different (faster or slower).

To think about it another way, let's consider a very common occurrence in our everyday lives. Have you ever been counting something, such as money, and someone calls out a different number? Suddenly, you are confused and can't remember what number you

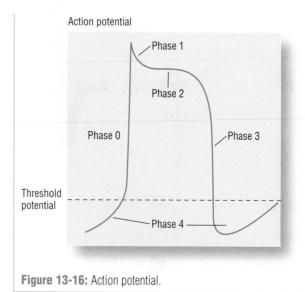

Figure 13-16: Action potential.

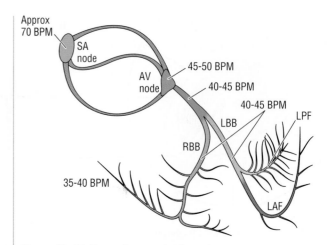

Figure 13-17: Pacemaker rates for the various areas.

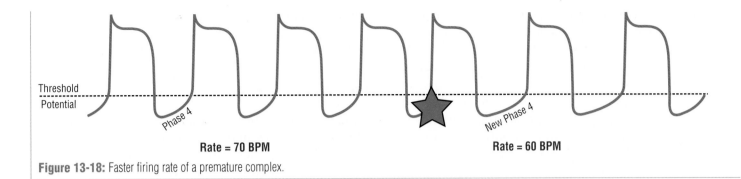

Threshold
Potential

Phase 4

New Phase 4

Rate = 70 BPM

Rate = 60 BPM

Figure 13-18: Faster firing rate of a premature complex.

were on. What is it that most of us do at this point? We start all over again. That is exactly what the SA node does. It is pacing and minding its own business, when suddenly a PAC comes along and confuses it with an early discharge. The SA node then resets and starts a new count (Figure 13-19).

Electrocardiographically, the same thing is happening. First, we see a nice, regular sinus rhythm. Then a PAC occurs, which resets the pacer. A new sinus rate emerges. The pause that includes the PAC and the time immediately after the PAC is the diagnostic point that we will focus on in this section. Notice that if the SA node were depolarized and reset, the time frame during which the PAC and the pause occurred would not be an exact multiple of the normal P-P interval. That type of pause is known as a *noncompensatory pause*. If the SA node were not reset, the pause would be an exact multiple of the regular P-P interval, and then you know that the SA node was not reset. That type of pause is known as a *compensatory pause*.

First, let's take a closer look at the noncompensatory pause. In a noncompensatory pause, the pause is not a multiple of the normal P-P interval (Figure 13-20). This is because the resetting of the SA node causes a variable time period to occur before it starts up again. The key to this type of pause is that the SA node was reset. The SA node is usually reset with a PAC. (PJCs and PVCs can also cause noncompensatory pauses if there is some retrograde conduction of the impulse back

through the AV node to depolarize the atria. However, this doesn't occur all the time.) The take-home message is that a noncompensatory pause usually points you in the direction of a PAC.

Now, let's switch our attention over to a compensatory pause (Figure 13-21). In a compensatory pause, the SA node is not reset. It continues clipping along at its normal pace, oblivious to the premature impulse that

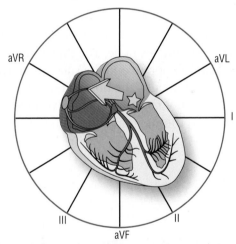

aVR

aVL

I

III

aVF

II

Figure 13-19: The rushing depolarization wave from the PAC causes the SA node to immediately depolarize. This resets the pacemaker, which can either take up the same rate, go a little faster, or go a little slower than before.

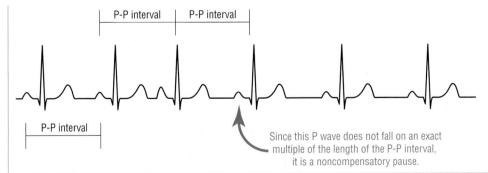

P-P interval | P-P interval

P-P interval

Since this P wave does not fall on an exact multiple of the length of the P-P interval, it is a noncompensatory pause.

Figure 13-20: Noncompensatory pause.

occurred. It would be very unusual for an atrial depolarization wave to avoid the SA node entirely. However, an impulse that originated in the AV node or in the ventricles could have occurred with no retrograde conduction to the atria.

It is important to remember, when dealing with compensatory pauses, that the atria and the ventricles live in two different worlds with their only source of contact being the AV node. The AV node functions as a gatekeeper between the atria and the ventricles. As such, the AV node was created to allow antegrade conduction; it was not created to allow retrograde conduction. It allows impulses to pass easily to the ventricles. However, retrograde conduction back to the atria is a different matter. Retrograde conduction is only allowed to pass through once in awhile.

If the AV node does not allow a ventricular impulse to be spread retrogradely to the atria, then the atria would never know about it. Think of it as an event that occurred in another country. We would only be aware of it if we heard of it in the news. If you don't hear about it, you can't react to it. The same is true with the SA node. If it does not get depolarized by the impulse, it will not reset and will keep clipping along at its regular uninterrupted pace (Figure 13-22).

A compensatory pause occurs when a premature impulse fails to reset the SA node. The time interval involving the premature impulse and the subsequent pause will, therefore, be a multiple of the normal P-P interval because the SA node was not reset. Frequently, you will see the sinus P marching through or fusing with the premature complex. Compensatory pauses usually occur with premature junctional or ventricular complexes, not with PACs. Not a bad diagnostic tool to have in your arsenal.

The PAC and Aberrancy

We covered aberrancy in Chapter 5 in some detail, but a few reminders wouldn't hurt at this point. PACs are usually not associated with any aberrancy of the QRS complexes. The main reason is that most PACs allow ample time for the electrical conduction system in the ventricles to completely repolarize and thus avoid issues with refractoriness. However, occasionally you will get some PACs that come extra early, and these are the ones that cause the problem.

The most common pattern of aberrancy is a right bundle branch block pattern (Figure 13-23). This is because the right bundle branch has the longest refractory period. Once an impulse hits an area of refractoriness, it needs to continue its march through the ventricles by the slow cell-to-cell means of conduction. This slow conduction means that the QRS is wider and, therefore, more aberrant (Figures 13-24 and 13-25).

Left bundle branch block pattern is encountered less often, but does occur. It is usually associated with patients who have some structural or ischemic heart disease.

The Hidden PAC

PACs, like every other wave or complex on an ECG strip, can sometimes occur at such a point that they

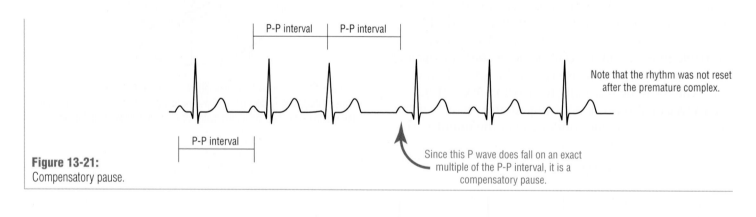

Figure 13-21: Compensatory pause.

Note that the rhythm was not reset after the premature complex.

Since this P wave does fall on an exact multiple of the P-P interval, it is a compensatory pause.

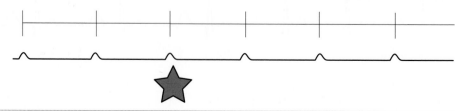

Figure 13-22: This is a strip isolating atrial activity only. Note that there is no break in the regularity of the rhythm. The premature complex, represented by the green star, did not influence the SA node in any way.

overlap another wave or complex. When this occurs, they may be difficult to spot. Let's go over some of these possible pitfalls in diagnosis.

P Falling on a T

Every once in awhile the P wave of a PAC will fall right over the T wave of the previous complex. Most of the time, the two waves will be easily distinguishable (Figure 13-26). Occasionally, however, the presence of the P wave makes the T wave appear to be double humped or biphasic (Figure 13-27). At other times, the P wave and the T wave can be indistinguishable because they fuse. In these cases, the presence of the P can only be inferred from the added height or width that the P wave gives to the underlying T wave due to the fusion (Figure 13-28).

The key to spotting hidden or partially hidden P waves is to look closely at your strip. Look over each wave and see if any of them has a big difference in their morphology when compared to their brothers and sisters in the other complexes. If you do spot something

that is unusual, spend the time to evaluate that area closely. When interpreting ECGs or arrhythmias, the key lies with the abnormality.

Blocked PACs

When a PAC fails to cause ventricular depolarization, it is known as a *blocked* or *nontransmitted PAC*. On some occasions, the transmission of an atrial impulse from a PAC can be blocked at the AV node. As you can imagine, blocked PACs can be very difficult to diagnose. Once again, careful evaluation of the waves of a complex preceding a pause may yield the diagnosis. (See Figures 13-29 to 13-31.)

Blocked PACs, if frequent, may lead to hemodynamic compromise. Careful monitoring and removing or treating the offending cause is critical in these cases. In extreme cases, transcutaneous and transvenous pacing may be needed if the hemodynamic compromise cannot be controlled.

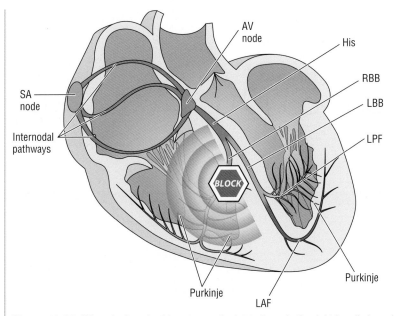

Figure 13-23: When the impulse hits an area of refractoriness in the right bundle branch, the impulse is forced to continue by direct cell-to-cell transmission throughout the rest of the right ventricle.

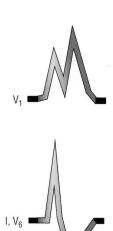

Figure 13-24: The right bundle branch block pattern is caused by the slow conduction through the right ventricle.

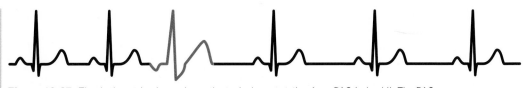

Figure 13-25: The rhythm strip above shows the typical presentation for a PAC in lead II. The PAC causes the formation of an aberrancy with an RBBB morphology.

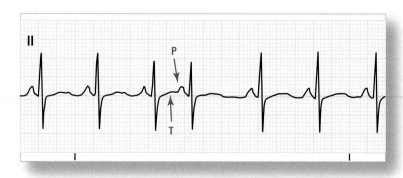

Figure 13-26: P wave superimposed on previous T wave. In this example, the P is easily identifiable and is obviously superimposed on the T wave of the previous complex.

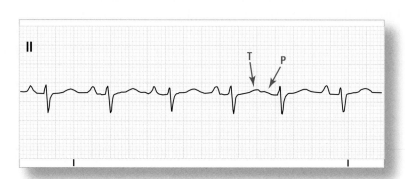

Figure 13-27: P wave superimposed on previous T wave. In this example, the P wave appears to be blending into the T wave of the previous complex. Note that this is the only T wave in the strip which shows a double-humped appearance. These PACs are difficult to pick up and a keen eye is needed to make the definitive diagnosis.

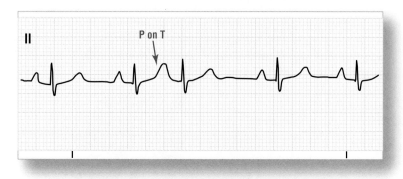

Figure 13-28: P wave superimposed on previous T wave. In this example, the P wave amplitude has been added to the T wave amplitude of the previous complex to create an extra-high and wide T wave. This is a common occurrence and is often confused with PJCs. Always be aware of the possibility of the fusion of two waves when you are evaluating an arrhythmia.

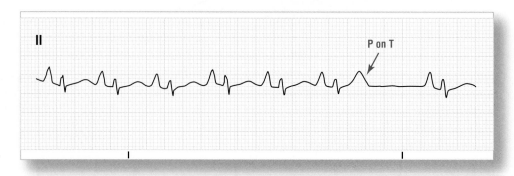

Figure 13-29: Blocked P wave. In this example, the T wave and P wave have fused into one larger combination wave. Notice the pause that follows due to the lack of ventricular depolarization.

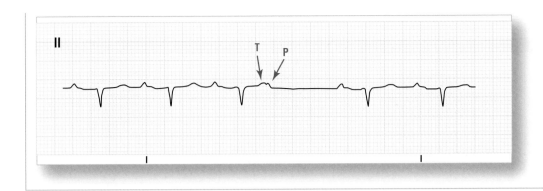

Figure 13-30: Blocked P wave. This strip shows a distinct double-humped quality to the labeled T wave. Evaluation of the subsequent pause leads us to take a closer look at the T wave. Notice how that T wave is different from the others. This is a combination of T and P wave due to a blocked PAC.

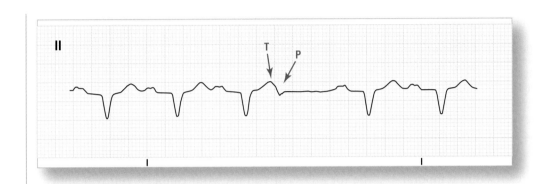

Figure 13-31: Blocked P wave. Here we clearly see a pause with a morphologically different T wave preceding it. This morphological difference is due to an inverted P wave. The PAC is nonconducted.

ARRHYTHMIA RECOGNITION

Premature Atrial Contractions

Rate:	Single complexes
Regularity:	Regular with an event
P wave:	Present
Morphology:	Different in event
Upright in II, III, and aVF:	Variable in event
P:QRS ratio:	1:1
PR interval:	Different in event
QRS width:	Normal
Grouping:	None
Dropped beats:	None

DIFFERENTIAL DIAGNOSIS

Premature Atrial Contractions

1. Idiopathic and benign
2. Anxiety
3. Fatigue
4. Drugs: Nicotine, alcohol, caffeine, etc.
5. Enlarged atria
6. Heart disease
7. Electrolyte disorders

The list above is not inclusive, since the causes of PACs are extensive. Normally, PACs are benign and cause no hemodynamic compromise. However, hemodynamic compromise can rarely occur.

ECG Strips

ECG 13-1

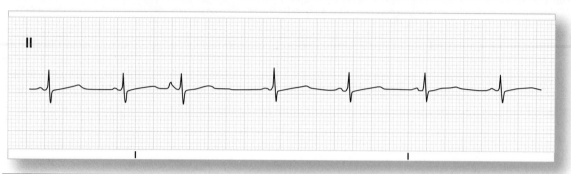

Rate:	About 75 BPM	PR intervals:	Different in event
Regularity:	Regular with an event	QRS width:	Normal
P waves:	Present	Grouping:	None
Morphology:	Normal		
Axis:	Normal	Dropped beats:	None
P:QRS ratio:	1:1	Rhythm:	**Sinus rhythm with a PAC**

Discussion:

This strip shows a nice, regular sinus rhythm temporarily broken by one PAC. Notice that the third complex arrives earlier than expected and has a different P wave morphology and PR interval. This meets all of the criteria for a PAC. If you use your calipers, you will notice that this is one of those instances when a PAC is associated with a full compensatory pause.

ECG 13-2

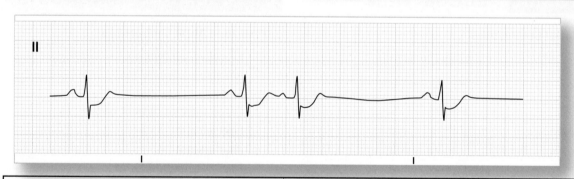

Rate:	About 30 BPM	PR intervals:	Different in event
Regularity:	Regular with an event	QRS width:	Normal
P waves:	Present	Grouping:	None
Morphology:	Normal		
Axis:	Normal	Dropped beats:	None
P:QRS ratio:	1:1	Rhythm:	**Sinus bradycardia with a PAC**

Discussion:

In this strip we have a pretty intense sinus bradycardia as the underlying rhythm. The third complex is a PAC. This is easily identifiable by the different P wave morphology, the different PR interval, the early arrival, and the noncompensatory pause. The cause for the serious bradycardia is probably infarct related. Notice the severe, flat ST depressions present in the complexes. You should get an ECG immediately on this patient and get ready to do some emergency pacing.

ECG 13-3

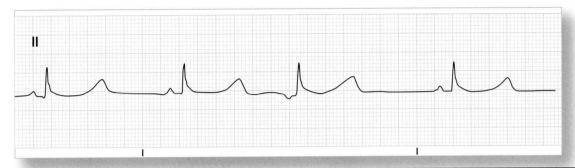

Rate:	About 40 BPM	PR intervals:	Different in event
Regularity:	Regular with an event	QRS width:	Normal
P waves: Morphology: Axis:	Present Inverted in event Abnormal in event	Grouping:	None
		Dropped beats:	None
P:QRS ratio:	1:1	Rhythm:	**Sinus bradycardia with a PAC**

Discussion:

The rhythm strip above shows a sinus bradycardia with a single PAC. The PAC is the third complex on the strip. Notice the inverted P wave and the early timing of this complex. This PAC is associated with a full compensatory pause.

ECG 13-4

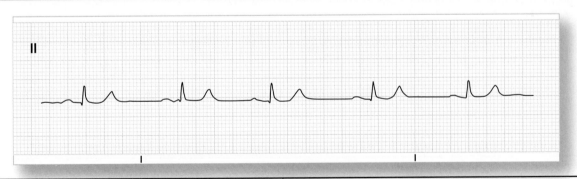

Rate:	About 55 BPM	PR intervals:	Different in event
Regularity:	Regular with an event	QRS width:	Normal
P waves: Morphology: Axis:	Present Different in event Normal	Grouping:	None
		Dropped beats:	None
P:QRS ratio:	1:1	Rhythm:	**Sinus bradycardia with a PAC**

Discussion:

This strip also shows a sinus bradycardia associated with one PAC; however, the findings are much more subtle. At first glance, it appears to be a regular rhythm, but using your calipers, it soon becomes apparent that the third complex is a PAC. Note the differing morphology and PR interval of this complex. The pause is also a noncompensatory pause, as would be expected. Do not confuse this rhythm with a sinus arrhythmia. A longer strip would be helpful in isolating the abnormality.

ECG 13-5

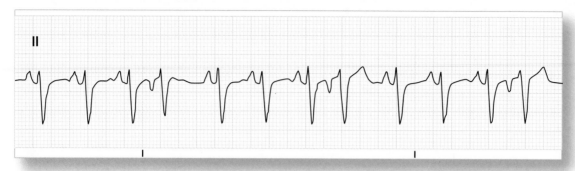

Rate:	About 120 BPM	PR intervals:	Normal, consistent
Regularity:	Regular with multiple events	QRS width:	Normal
P waves:	Present	Grouping:	None
Morphology:	Inverted in event		
Axis:	Abnormal in event	Dropped beats:	None
P:QRS ratio:	1:1	Rhythm:	**Sinus tachycardia with frequent PACs**

Discussion:

This strip shows a sinus tachycardia at about 120 BPM associated with frequent PACs. They actually occur every fourth beat, making this a supraventricular quadrigeminy, to be exact. Either terminology is correct with this type of rhythm. Notice the inverted P waves associated with the PACs and the noncompensatory pauses (only slightly off the mark).

ECG 13-6

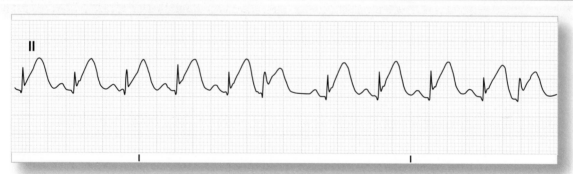

Rate:	A little over 100 BPM	PR intervals:	Different in event
Regularity:	Regular with multiple events	QRS width:	Normal
P waves:	Present	Grouping:	None
Morphology:	Different in event		
Axis:	Not applicable	Dropped beats:	None
P:QRS ratio:	1:1	Rhythm:	**Sinus tachycardia with frequent PACs**

Discussion:

This poor patient is having one heck of an AMI with that much ST elevation! The underlying rhythm is sinus tachycardia associated with frequent PACs. The PACs are probably due to the myocardial irritability from the AMI, but other possibilities need to be ruled out. For example, drugs, hypoxemia, and congestive heart failure must be ruled out and treated accordingly. Remember, you need to treat the underlying cause of the PACs, not the PACs themselves, in this case.

ECG 13-7

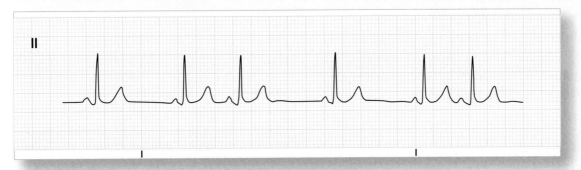

Rate:	A bit over 60 BPM	PR intervals:	Different in event
Regularity:	Regular with multiple events	QRS width:	Normal
P waves:	Present	Grouping:	None
Morphology:	Different in event		
Axis:	Normal	Dropped beats:	None
P:QRS ratio:	1:1	Rhythm:	**Sinus rhythm with frequent PACs**

Discussion:

The strip above shows a normal sinus rhythm with frequent PACs. This is, in actuality, supraventricular trigeminy with every third beat being a PAC. Once again, be careful of calling this a sinus arrhythmia or, as we shall study later on, a second-degree AV block.

ECG 13-8

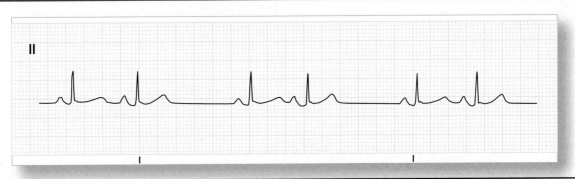

Rate:	Slightly over 60 BPM	PR intervals:	Different in event
Regularity:	Regular with multiple events	QRS width:	Normal
P waves:	Present	Grouping:	None
Morphology:	Different in event		
Axis:	Normal	Dropped beats:	None
P:QRS ratio:	1:1	Rhythm:	**Sinus rhythm with frequent PACs**

Discussion:

What do you call this rhythm? Every other beat is a PAC. You can easily call it sinus rhythm with frequent PACs and be perfectly correct. But, the more appropriate diagnosis is sinus rhythm with supraventricular bigeminy due to PACs. When you are confronted with this type of rhythm, you obtain the rate by multiplying the number of complexes in a 6-second strip by 10.

CHAPTER **REVIEW**

1. The pacemakers responsible for the PACs are found in the _____.

2. PACs are usually clinically significant and require immediate attention. True or False.

3. The basic pacemaking rate of atrial tissue is usually set at:
   A. 70–80 BPM
   B. 65–70 BPM
   C. 60–65 BPM
   D. 55–60 BPM
   E. 50–55 BPM

4. After a PAC, the sinus node takes over as the pacemaker. However, the rhythm may be reset at a different rate. True or False.

5. The P wave is an electrocardiographic representation of atrial depolarization. Each myocyte is responsible for its own small vector. When these vectors are added together, they form the _____.

6. A P wave vector heading toward the AV node (inferiorly) makes the P waves appear _____ in leads II, III, and aVF.

7. A P wave vector heading away from the AV node (superiorly) makes the P waves appear _____ in leads II, III, and aVF.

8. A premature junctional contraction with retrograde conduction to the atria will give you upright P waves in lead II. True or False.

9. Whenever you see inverted P waves in lead II, it should make you think of ectopic pacemakers in either the atria, AV node, or the ventricles. True or False.

10. In a PAC, the PR intervals are:
    A. Shorter than expected
    B. Longer than expected
    C. Can be either shorter or longer than expected

11. The longer the distance to the AV node that the depolarization wave has to travel, the longer the PR interval. True or False.

12. The pacemaking function of any cardiac tissue is dependent on the rate of phase 4 depolarization that it intrinsically possesses. True or False.

13. A PAC causes the sinus node to _____ its pacemaking rate by depolarizing the tissue early.

14. A pause that is an exact multiple of the P-P interval and is associated with premature complexes is known as a:
    A. Compensatory pause
    B. Competitive pause
    C. Noncompensatory pause
    D. Noncompetitive pause
    E. None of the above

15. A pause that is not an exact multiple of the P-P interval and is associated with premature complexes is known as a:
    A. Compensatory pause
    B. Competitive pause
    C. Noncompensatory pause
    D. Noncompetitive pause
    E. None of the above

16. PACs are usually associated with noncompensatory pauses because the SA node is reset by the premature atrial depolarization wave. True or False.

17. Aberrantly conducted PACs generally have QRS complexes that show:
    A. Left bundle branch block pattern
    B. Right bundle branch block pattern
    C. Intraventricular conduction delay
    D. None of the above

18. The P waves in a PAC will always be clearly identifiable. True or False.

19. The T waves and P waves of adjacent complexes sometimes appear together, forming unusual shapes or actually fusing. True or False.

20. Sometimes the conduction to the ventricles from a PAC may actually be blocked. This makes the P wave of the PAC visible, but the QRS and T waves are not. When this occurs, it is known as a blocked PAC. True or False.

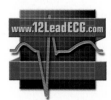

To enhance the knowledge you gain in this book, access this text's website at www.12leadECG.com! This valuable resource provides flashcards, an online glossary, web links, and more. Simply click on the Arrhythmias book cover once at the site.

CHAPTER 14

Ectopic Atrial Rhythm

An ectopic atrial rhythm is a rhythm where an ectopic atrial focus functions as the main pacemaker of the heart temporarily. The rate set by this ectopic pacemaker must be below 100 BPM, and the PR interval is within the normal range or slightly prolonged. The QRS interval and morphology should be identical to that found in normal sinus rhythm, unless some aberrancy in the conduction of the impulse through the AV node or ventricles is encountered, there is an electrolyte abnormality present, or there is a preexisting bundle branch block.

Usually, ectopic atrial rhythms are hemodynamically insignificant because the rates are within the normal range. The atria contract fairly well and the PR interval is normal or slightly prolonged, as mentioned above. These factors allow the ventricles to overfill and the sequence of systole and diastole are kept within acceptable limits.

The rhythm can be found in patients with or without significant structural heart disease and is usually transient. Recurrences can occur and are commonly found. In general, ectopic atrial rhythm is commonly found in patients on routine Holter monitoring. Treatment should be based on symptoms and on the hemodynamic status of the patient. As usual, even though this rhythm is usually benign, these patients should be referred for further evaluation.

Diagnostic Challenges

In Figure 14-1, making the diagnosis of an ectopic P wave was simplified by the presence of an inverted P wave in lead II. Many times, as we saw in Chapter 13, the morphological difference between an ectopic P and the sinus P is minimal. Take, for example, Figure 14-2. If you were handed this strip, wouldn't you call it normal sinus rhythm? It meets all of the criteria for NSR, doesn't it? Clearly making the definitive diagnosis would be quite a diagnostic challenge.

In many cases, it is truly impossible to make the diagnosis of ectopic atrial rhythm without some addi-

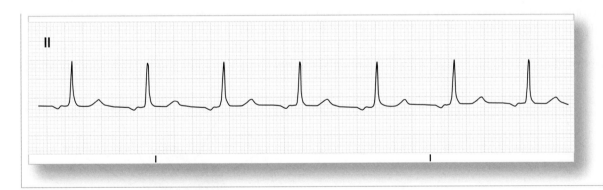

Figure 14-1: This rhythm strip shows the typical changes found in an ectopic atrial rhythm: An ectopic P-wave morphology, rate less than or equal to 100 BPM, normal or slightly prolonged PR interval, and normal QRS morphology.

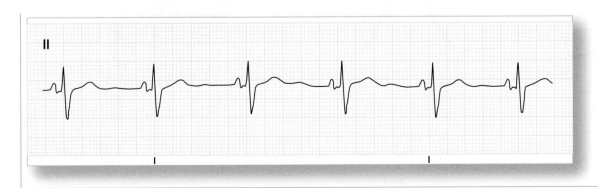

Figure 14-2: This example of an ectopic atrial rhythm would be impossible to correctly diagnose if it were not for the previous strip shown in Figure 14-1. Note the difference in P-wave morphologies and PR intervals.

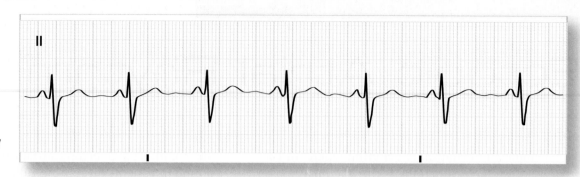

Figure 14-3: This rhythm strip is representative of the patient's P-wave morphology and PR intervals while in normal sinus rhythm.

tional clinical or electrocardiographic information. Sometimes, it just takes some plain good old-fashioned luck. However, there are some clues to help you along the way. The rest of this chapter is devoted to those clues and how to recognize them.

Hint #1: Always try to compare your new strip to an old ECG or rhythm strip.

As you can imagine, the P-wave morphology in an ectopic atrial rhythm will differ from that found in normal sinus rhythm. (We discussed the origins of these morphological differences in the ectopic P waves in Chapter 13. Quickly review these concepts again if you need to.) Many times the P waves are obviously ectopic in nature and easily identified. In some cases, however, the P-wave morphology can be very close to that of the normal sinus P wave. In these cases, an old ECG or a strip showing the transition from NSR to the ectopic atrial pacemaker may be the only way to correctly identify this rhythm.

Take a look at Figure 14-2. This rhythm strip could easily be mistakenly diagnosed as normal sinus rhythm if

viewed alone. Luckily, an old strip taken earlier of the same patient (Figure 14-3) was available. Notice the subtle, but significant, differences in the morphology of the P waves and the PR intervals between the two strips (Figure 14-4). Without the ability to compare the two strips, making the diagnosis would have been next to impossible.

Hint #2: Always evaluate the P wave morphology and the PR interval.

Inverted P waves can be found in two circumstances: (1) Low or distal ectopic foci in the atria, and (2) P waves with retrograde conduction to the atria from the AV node or ventricles. We presented the concept of low or distal ectopic foci in the atria before in Chapter 13, and we will give you a short review here. In this chapter, we will introduce the concept of retrograde conduction of P waves from the AV node. This topic will be covered in much greater detail later in the book.

If you remember, a low ectopic focus near the AV septum will cause a depolarization wave to develop that must primarily spread upward toward the upper poles of

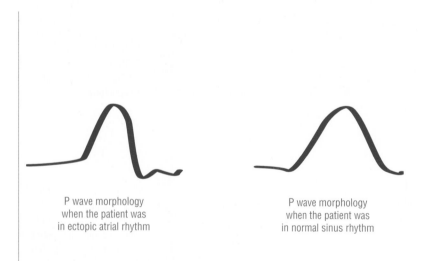

P wave morphology when the patient was in ectopic atrial rhythm

P wave morphology when the patient was in normal sinus rhythm

Figure 14-4: When the P-wave morphologies of Figure 14-2 and Figure 14-3 are magnified, the differences become obvious.

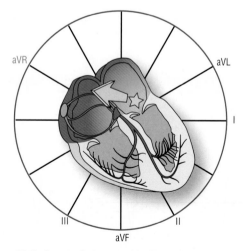

Figure 14-5: An ectopic focus and its P-wave vector. This figure graphically represents the P-wave vector as a yellow vector heading superiorly and to the right. Note that the vector is heading toward the positive pole of lead aVR only. P waves produced by this focus would be negative and inverted in leads I, II, III, and aVF.

the atria (Figure 14-5). This depolarization wave gives rise to a vector that heads away from leads II, III, and aVF, causing a negative P wave to appear on the strip in those leads. Since the depolarization wave must still cross the physiologic block produced by the AV node, the PR interval would be normal or slightly different than a sinus complex. This concept, a normal or near normal PR interval, is critical in your differential diagnosis of the origins of a rhythm with an inverted P wave.

Now that we understand how a low ectopic atrial pacemaker gives rise to inverted P waves, let's turn our attention to retrograde conduction through the AV node. Remember, any tissue in the heart can act as a primary pacemaker if the circumstances are just right. The AV node is no exception to this rule. There are many cases in which the AV node functions as a primary pacemaker. If the AV node functions as a primary pacemaker, we call the rhythm a *junctional rhythm*. We will spend quite a bit of time talking about junctional rhythms starting in Chapter 21, but for now, let's just look at retrograde conduction from the AV node.

Picture in your mind a complex originating in the AV node. In which direction would the depolarization wave spread? The answer is that the impulse would spread in a circular fashion radiating outward from the primary focus (Figure 14-6). In the case of the ventricles, it would proceed down the electrical conduction system as it normally should. This gives you a nice, tight QRS complex. How about the atria? Well, the impulse would radiate upward and outward through the atria, giving you a vector that is directed superiorly away from leads II, III, and aVF (Figure 14-7).

So, why did we introduce the concept of junctional complexes and their inverted P waves at this time? Because it is almost impossible to tell whether an inverted P wave originated in the atria or the AV node based on its morphology alone. To make the correct diagnosis, we need to look at "the company it keeps." We need to look at the PR interval. *By convention, if the PR interval is equal to or greater than 0.12 seconds in a complex with an inverted P wave, it is considered to be atrial in origin. If the PR interval is less than 0.12 seconds, then the complex is considered to have originated in the AV node.* This is critical information that you will need to use over and over again.

In Chapter 1, we talked about the concept of the AV node being like a guardhouse causing the physiologic block (Figure 14-8). Continuing with this analogy, let's suppose that an impulse originated in the atria. That impulse would have to undergo the physiologic block

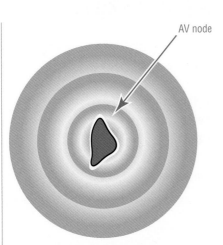

Figure 14-6: Depolarization wave originating in the AV node. An impulse originating in the AV node creates a depolarization wave that moves outward in all directions.

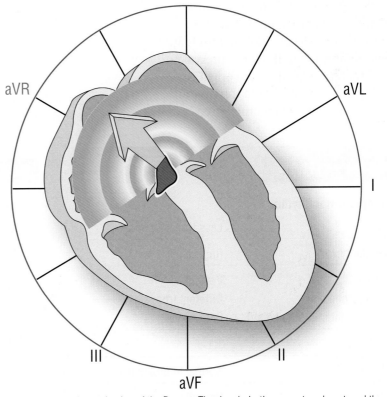

Figure 14-7: Retrograde conduction of the P wave. The depolarization wave travels outward through the atria by direct cell-to-cell transmission, giving rise to a vector directed upward. This causes a negative deflection on the rhythm strip in leads II, III, and aVF. Since the impulse travels backward from the AV node through the atria, it is called retrograde conduction. The impulse progresses normally (antegrade) through the ventricles via the electrical conduction system.

imposed by the AV node before moving on to the ventricles. The physiologic block would make the PR interval fall into the normal or slightly prolonged range.

Now, suppose that the impulse originated in the AV node itself, as occurs in a junctional complex. Would the impulse have to undergo the physiologic block? In most cases, the answer is no. The impulse would spread almost instantaneously to the atria and the ventricles (Figure 14-9). The impulse would spread by direct cell-to-cell transmission through the atria and through the electrical conduction system to the ventricles. The result is that the physiologic block would be completely or partially bypassed, making the PR interval shorter than normal or causing it to be buried within the QRS complex itself.

The take-home point of this discussion is that if you have an inverted P wave in leads II, III, or aVF, you need to look at the PR interval for some additional information before assigning a name to the rhythm in question. If the PR interval is normal or prolonged (≥ 0.12 seconds), then the origin of the impulse can be assigned to the atria and the rhythm is an ectopic atrial rhythm. If the PR interval is shorter than normal, then the origin is probably in the AV node and the rhythm is junctional until proven otherwise.

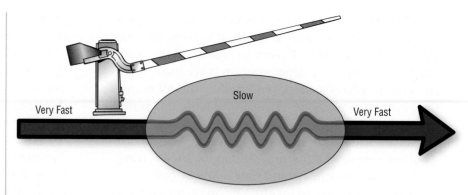

Figure 14-8: The AV node functions as a gatekeeper between the atria and the ventricles. An atrial impulse would have to undergo the physiologic block imposed by the AV node before moving on to the ventricles.

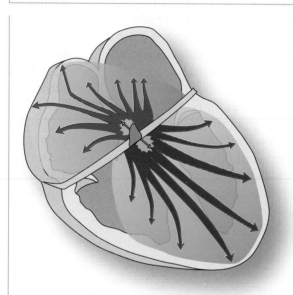

Figure 14-9: An impulse that originates in the AV node bypasses most or all of the physiologic block, making the PR interval much shorter or nonexistent.

ARRHYTHMIA RECOGNITION

Ectopic Atrial Rhythm

Rate:	Less than 100 BPM
Regularity:	Regular
P wave:	Present
Morphology:	Different from sinus
Upright in II, III, and aVF:	Sometimes
P:QRS ratio:	1:1
PR interval:	Normal to prolonged
QRS width:	Normal
Grouping:	None
Dropped beats:	None

DIFFERENTIAL DIAGNOSIS

Ectopic Atrial Rhythm

1. Idiopathic and benign
2. Anxiety
3. Drugs: nicotine, alcohol, caffeine, etc.
4. Structural heart disease
5. Electrolyte disorders

The list above is not all-inclusive.

ECG Strips

ECG 14-1

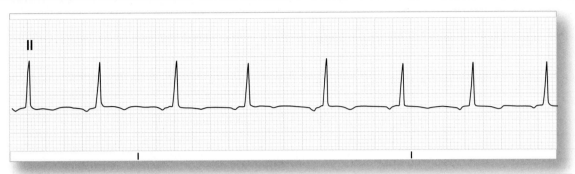

Rate:	About 75 BPM	PR intervals:	Normal, consistent
Regularity:	Regular	QRS width:	Normal
P waves: Morphology: Axis:	Present Inverted Abnormal	Grouping: Dropped beats:	None None
P:QRS ratio:	1:1	Rhythm:	**Ectopic atrial rhythm**

Discussion:

This rhythm strip is a typical example of ectopic atrial rhythm. First, let's look at the rate. In this case it is about 75 BPM. Next, look at the P wave morphology. In this case, it is easy to see that the P waves are inverted in lead II, which is grossly abnormal. The inverted P waves rule out the possibility of a normal sinus rhythm.

Since inverted P waves can be seen in both junctional rhythms and ectopic atrial rhythms, we have a decision to make. To help us with this decision, we look at the PR interval. In this case, the PR interval is within the normal range, making the diagnosis of ectopic atrial rhythm likely.

ECG 14-2

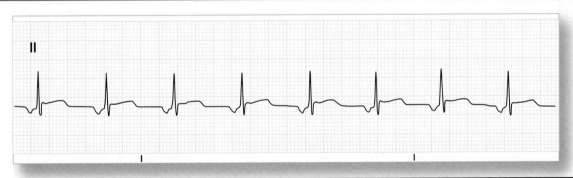

Rate:	About 80 BPM	PR intervals:	Normal, consistent
Regularity:	Regular	QRS width:	Normal
P waves: Morphology: Axis:	Present Inverted Abnormal	Grouping: Dropped beats:	None None
P:QRS ratio:	1:1	Rhythm:	**Ectopic atrial rhythm**

Discussion:

This rhythm strip is also a good example of an ectopic atrial rhythm. Following the same logic as above, the inverted P waves and the normal PR intervals clinch the diagnosis. Should you get a regular 12-lead ECG on this patient? Yes, you should because of the presence of a rhythm abnormality and the ST segment elevation. Remember, it is better to be safe than sorry!

ECG 14-3

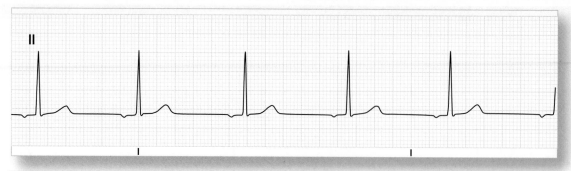

Rate:	About 50 BPM	PR intervals:	Normal, consistent
Regularity:	Regular	QRS width:	Normal
P waves:	Present	Grouping:	None
Morphology:	Inverted		
Axis:	Abnormal	Dropped beats:	None
P:QRS ratio:	1:1	Rhythm:	**Ectopic atrial rhythm**

Discussion:

This strip poses more problems than the previous ones. Why? Because the rate is so slow. It is about 50–55 BPM. This rate could very easily fit with a junctional rhythm, which is usually about this range. Once again, our saving grace is the presence of a normal PR interval.

The normal PR interval makes the diagnosis of ectopic atrial rhythm more likely. Medications can often cause a significant bradycardia, and you should evaluate this and other possibilities as well for your patient.

ECG 14-4

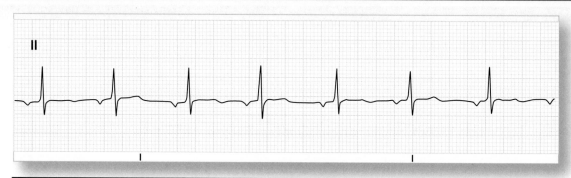

Rate:	About 75 BPM	PR intervals:	Normal, consistent
Regularity:	Regular	QRS width:	Normal
P waves:	Present	Grouping:	None
Morphology:	Inverted		
Axis:	Abnormal	Dropped beats:	None
P:QRS ratio:	1:1	Rhythm:	**Ectopic atrial rhythm**

Discussion:

The inverted P waves and the normal PR interval make the diagnosis in this strip. By now, you should be feeling a bit more comfortable with the possibility of an

ectopic atrial rhythm. Remember, however, to always try to obtain an old ECG to verify your suspicions and confirm your diagnosis.

ECG 14-5

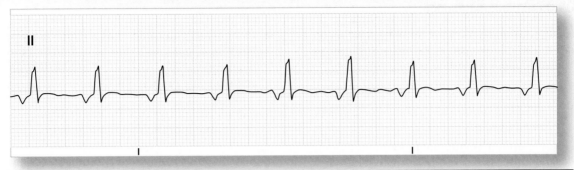

Rate:	About 85 BPM	PR intervals:	Normal, consistent
Regularity:	Regular	QRS width:	Normal
P waves:	Present	Grouping:	None
Morphology:	Inverted		
Axis:	Abnormal	Dropped beats:	None
P:QRS ratio:	1:1	Rhythm:	**Ectopic atrial rhythm**

Discussion:

This strip is a bit troubling because the QRS complexes appear to be wider. But, are they? Using your calipers and some careful measuring, you will note that the QRS complexes are not wider than 0.12 seconds. Therefore, the inverted P waves, normal PR interval, and normal QRS complexes make the diagnosis of ectopic atrial rhythm the correct diagnosis. Comparison to an old ECG or rhythm strip would be, as always, very helpful in confirming your suspicions.

Now, suppose that the QRS complexes were wider than 0.12 seconds. What should you do differently if that were the case? The first thing to check is if the patient had a bundle branch block of some sort in the past. The next possibility would be aberrancy in the conduction of the impulse to or through the ventricles. The aberrancy could be rate related, and a long rhythm strip may show the aberrancy coming and going as the patient's heart rate changes. The aberrancy can also be caused by ischemia or a diseased portion of the conduction system, which causes longer refractory periods in that area. Electrolyte imbalances can often cause aberrancy or rhythm abnormalities to develop. After you have exhausted these possibilities, there could be some other rhythms that can cause a similar picture, but that is for later on in the book.

CHAPTER **REVIEW**

1. In an ectopic atrial rhythm, the primary pacemaker is found in the inferior part of the atria. It is always near the AV node. True or False.

2. The P wave morphology in an ectopic atrial rhythm is always inverted in leads II, III, and aVF. True or False.

3. In an ectopic atrial rhythm, the P wave morphology in leads II, III, and aVF can be:
   A. Inverted
   B. Upright
   C. Always different from the morphology of the sinus P wave
   D. All of the above

4. For simplicity, the PR interval in an ectopic atrial rhythm is:
   A. Greater than or equal to 0.12 seconds
   B. Always less than 0.12 seconds
   C. May be prolonged
   D. Both A and C

5. The QRS morphology and the interval involved should be exactly the same when the patient is in an ectopic atrial rhythm as when they are in normal sinus rhythm. In some cases, however, rate-related aberrancy may develop. True or False.

6. If the patient normally has a wide QRS complex because of either a left or right bundle branch block, an ectopic atrial rhythm will also show the same bundle branch block pattern. True or False.

7. Ectopic atrial rhythms are easily diagnosed based on P wave morphology. True or False.

8. Which are useful in determining an ectopic atrial rhythm?
   A. The PR segment
   B. P wave morphology
   C. QT interval
   D. PR interval
   E. Both B and D

Find the correct match:

9. Inverted P wave, PR interval of 0.20 seconds
   A. Ectopic atrial rhythm
   B. Junctional rhythm
   C. Normal sinus rhythm

10. Inverted P wave, PR interval of 0.10 seconds
   A. Ectopic atrial rhythm
   B. Junctional rhythm
   C. Normal sinus rhythm

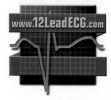

To enhance the knowledge you gain in this book, access this text's website at www.12leadECG.com! This valuable resource provides flashcards, an online glossary, web links, and more. Simply click on the Arrhythmias book cover once at the site.

CHAPTER 15

Ectopic Atrial Tachycardia

Until electrophysiologic testing became widely available, ectopic atrial tachycardia (EAT) was always a bit of a dilemma for clinicians. There was some spirited debate between two camps of clinicians as to the cause of the arrhythmia. One side believed that the arrhythmia was triggered by a reentry loop that did or did not involve the SA node. The other side believed that the rhythm was due to increased automaticity of an ectopic focus. The result of this debate was that there were a lot of descriptive terms used to describe this arrhythmia. These terms included paroxysmal atrial tachycardia, intra-atrial reentrant supraventricular tachycardia, sinus nodal reentry SVT, and automatic atrial tachycardia, to name a few. This has led to continued confusion about the rhythm and its nomenclature.

It turned out that both camps were right. The rhythm is sometimes caused by a reentry mechanism, and sometimes caused by increased automaticity of an ectopic pacemaker. Electrocardiographically, however, the difference is essentially nonexistent. For our purposes, we will group all of the different terms above under one heading: ectopic atrial tachycardia.

Traditionally, ectopic atrial tachycardia accounts for about 15% of all regular, narrow supraventricular tachycardias in adults and the numbers are a bit higher in children. If the causative mechanism is known, reentry beats automaticity as the main cause. It is found equally among males and females.

Basically, an ectopic atrial tachycardia (EAT) is an ectopic atrial rhythm that is over 100 BPM. All of the characteristics that we covered in the chapter on ectopic atrial rhythms apply to these tachycardias (Figure 15-1). A quick summary of the important points is as follows:

1. The atrial rates are usually between 100 and 180 BPM, although rates up to 250 BPM are possible.

2. Ectopic P waves are present, differing in morphology from the normal sinus P wave.

3. There is a ratio of one P wave to one QRS complex.

4. The PR intervals are normal or slightly prolonged.

5. The rhythm is regular.

6. The QRS complex is of normal width and looks like the ones found in normal sinus rhythm, unless aberrancy or bundle branch block is present.

7. Secondary ST and T wave abnormalities can occur because of the tachycardia.

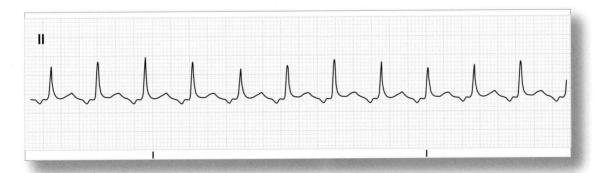

Figure 15-1: The ectopic atrial tachycardia above demonstrates all of the typical characteristics of the rhythm: an ectopic P-wave morphology, rate greater than or equal to 100 BPM, normal or slightly prolonged PR interval, and normal QRS morphology. In addition, a slight alteration in the QRS amplitude is noted (electrical alternans), which can normally be found in many tachycardias.

The rhythm can be transient, sustained, or incessant. Transient episodes occur when three or more complexes are noted for a very brief period of time. If the rhythm lasts for longer than 30 seconds, it is considered to be sustained. If the rhythm does not terminate, or is present most of the time, it is considered incessant.

Transient episodes are fairly common in the general population, usually involve heart rates about the 150 BPM range, and are relatively benign. Incessant rhythms are rare, and can lead to serious congestive heart failure or cardiomyopathies if left untreated. As usual, all abnormal rhythms should be referred for further evaluation and possible treatment. Any hemodynamically significant rhythm should be emergently treated with medication and/or cardioversion/defibrillation.

The tachycardia is usually regular. We say "usually" because the onset of most tachycardias has some irregularity associated with it. This is found in many, many types of tachycardias. Think of it like an engine that is just starting up. It usually needs a slight warm-up period before it can really clip along at its normal pace. The heart, and the ectopic focus in particular, need the same type of warm-up period. At the onset of the ectopic atrial tachycardia, you will usually find a PAC followed by a series of complexes, which occur at faster and faster rates, until they reach the "cruising speed" of the tachycardia.

As mentioned in the first paragraph, the P wave morphology will always be different from that normally seen with sinus rhythm. In the case of an inverted P wave in leads I, II, III, and aVF, the diagnosis will be clear and easy to make (inverted P waves in leads II, III, and aVF that are associated with normal or prolonged PR intervals are considered ectopic atrial until proven otherwise). However, sometimes the morphological differences between an ectopic and a sinus P wave may only be very slight. Indeed, there will be many times that a skilled clinician will find it difficult, if not impossible, to distinguish the morphology of a P wave on an isolated strip as ectopic, unless an old strip or ECG is available for comparison. When an old strip is available, you will *always* notice that the ectopic P waves will be either wider, taller, notched, or biphasic, or somehow different in many leads when compared to the sinus P.

A final word about P-wave morphology. If you are lucky enough to catch the onset of the tachycardia, you will note that it is usually initiated by a PAC. The morphology of the P wave that triggered the PAC, and the ones found within the tachycardia itself, are usually the same or very, very similar (Figure 15-2). This occurs because the irritable ectopic focus in both cases is the same. The morphology of the P wave in the initiating complex is a very useful tool in helping you to identify the correct rhythm in a case of supraventricular tachycardia.

Conduction through the AV node will be either normal or prolonged during the tachycardia. But note that this does not directly translate into a normal or prolonged PR interval in all cases. As we discussed in Chapters 13 and 14, the location of the ectopic focus, or circus loop, also affects the length of the PR interval. If the focus or loop is near the AV node, then the PR interval would be shorter than expected, and vice versa. Therefore, depending on the combination of various factors, the PR interval in the ectopic complexes may be either shortened, the same, or prolonged when compared to the sinus complexes in any one patient.

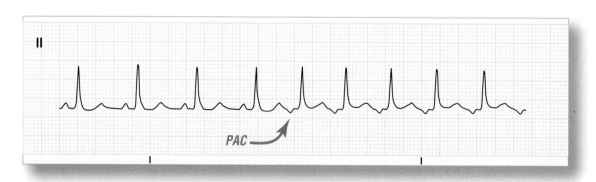

Figure 15-2: The strip above starts off with a normal sinus rhythm. The PAC labeled in the diagram shows an inverted P-wave morphology. The PAC triggers an ectopic atrial tachycardia that has the same P-wave morphology as the PAC. The similarity of the P-wave morphology between the triggering PAC and those present in the tachycardia itself is typical for this arrhythmia.

Occasionally, the rate of the tachycardia will exceed the rate at which the AV node can transmit the impulse. When this occurs, the AV node may block some of the impulses from reaching the ventricles. When this occurs, we say that an AV block exists. (We will discuss AV blocks in great detail later.) In the case of ectopic atrial tachycardia, we can have a rhythm with an atrial tachycardia but the ventricular rate may be within the normal range. Traditionally, an ectopic atrial tachycardia with AV nodal block is called a paroxysmal atrial tachycardia with block. We will review this particular entity in depth in the next chapter. For now, just be aware that it exists.

The QRS complex is normal in both appearance and duration. The only exception is when a rate-related aberrancy develops because of the tachycardia or there is a preexisting bundle branch block. Electrolyte abnormalities can often cause widening of the QRS complexes as well. Electrical alternans may also be seen occasionally. This is typically due to the tachycardia and not to some other underlying pathologic problem.

The ST segment may frequently be depressed, sometimes up to 2 mm, and may appear ischemic. Resolution of the ST segments back to baseline should occur on termination of the tachycardia. Remember to always have a high index of suspicion when approaching any ST segment changes. As always, the clinical presentation and hemodynamic status of the patient are critical elements to keep in mind as you evaluate the ECG.

Clinically, the rhythm is usually well tolerated. This is because the ventricular rates are usually slower than many tachycardias. AV block is often present at very high atrial rates, which helps to maintain tolerable hemodynamic parameters. Recurrences tend to occur in adults and may need to be referred for catheter ablation for permanent control.

ARRHYTHMIA RECOGNITION

Ectopic Atrial Tachycardia

Rate:	Between 100 to 180 BPM, although rates up to 250 BPM are possible
Regularity:	Regular
P wave:	Present
Morphology:	Different
Upright in II, III, and aVF:	Sometimes
P:QRS ratio:	1:1; AV block can occur
PR interval:	Normal, prolonged
QRS width:	Normal
Grouping:	None
Dropped beats:	None

DIFFERENTIAL DIAGNOSIS

Ectopic Atrial Tachycardia

1. Idiopathic
2. Cardiomyopathy
3. Valvular heart disease
4. Myocardial infarction
5. COPD and lung disease
6. Digitalis toxicity
7. Other drugs: theophylline
8. Post-catheter ablation and surgery

The list above represents the common causes of EAT, but is not complete.

ECG Strips

ECG 15·1

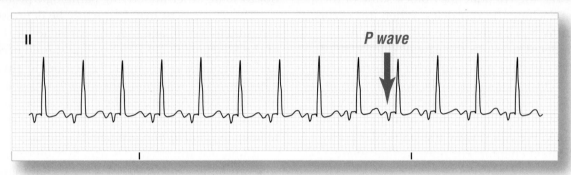

P wave

Rate:	About 135 BPM	PR intervals:	Normal, consistent
Regularity:	Regular	QRS width:	Normal
P waves:	Present	Grouping:	None
Morphology:	Inverted		
Axis:	Abnormal	Dropped beats:	None
P:QRS ratio:	1:1	Rhythm:	**Ectopic atrial tachycardia**

Discussion:

The strip above shows an inverted P wave in lead II in a patient with obvious tachycardia. These findings are consistent with ectopic atrial tachycardia. Note that the QRS complex is of normal duration and that there is some slight ST segment depression. The ST depression is consistent with the presence of a tachycardia, but clinical correlation should be obtained to assure that ischemia is not the underlying cause of the tachycardia. Remember, AMI can cause an EAT to develop in an adult patient.

ECG 15·2

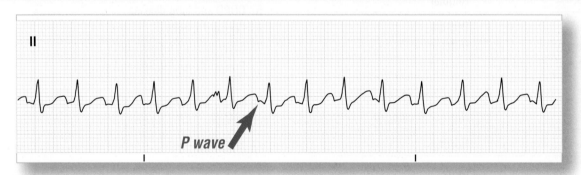

P wave

Rate:	About 140 BPM	PR intervals:	Normal, consistent
Regularity:	Regular	QRS width:	Normal
P waves:	Present	Grouping:	None
Morphology:	Inverted		
Axis:	Abnormal	Dropped beats:	None
P:QRS ratio:	1:1	Rhythm:	**Ectopic atrial tachycardia**

Discussion:

The P waves in this strip are difficult to spot. If you notice, at the end of the T wave there is a sudden drop-off and a small inverted segment. This is an inverted P wave buried in the T wave. It is especially visible in some of the complexes, for example, the last one. The regularity of the rhythm and the consistency of the inverted notch are indicative of an ectopic atrial tachycardia. Comparison with a normal sinus strip in this patient confirmed the P-wave morphology change present above.

ECG 15-3

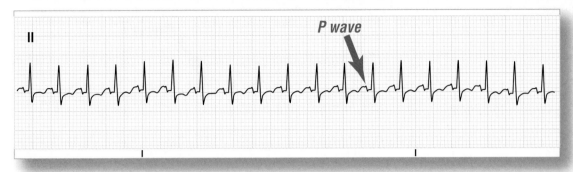

Rate:	About 190 BPM	PR intervals:	Normal, consistent
Regularity:	Regular	QRS width:	Normal
P waves: Morphology: Axis:	Present Inverted Abnormal	Grouping:	None
		Dropped beats:	None
P:QRS ratio:	1:1	Rhythm:	**Ectopic atrial tachycardia**

Discussion:

This is a very fast tachycardia! The rate is so fast that the P waves are almost lost in the T waves once again. These P waves, however, are biphasic. (It is a good idea to use a magnifying glass to evaluate these complexes.) This rapid rate is rare to find in an EAT because, as the rate speeds up, the AV node usually causes some block to develop. As we shall see in the next chapter, rapid atrial rates that are blocked at the AV node to give you slower ventricular rates are more the norm in rapid EAT.

ECG 15-4

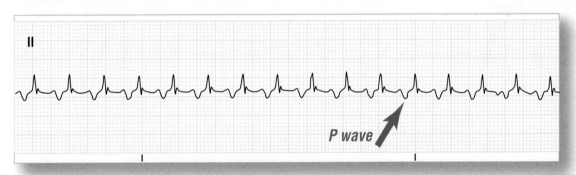

Rate:	About 155 BPM	PR intervals:	Normal, consistent
Regularity:	Regular	QRS width:	Normal
P waves: Morphology: Axis:	Present Inverted Abnormal	Grouping:	None
		Dropped beats:	None
P:QRS ratio:	1:1	Rhythm:	**Ectopic atrial tachycardia**

Discussion:

This EAT also shows a rapid rate at about 155 BPM. In this case, the P waves are inverted. The positive wave just prior to the P waves is a truncated T wave. As a side note, buried P waves become much more common as the rates of a tachycardia increase. An additional cause of buried P wave is the presence of a prolonged PR interval.

ECG 15-5

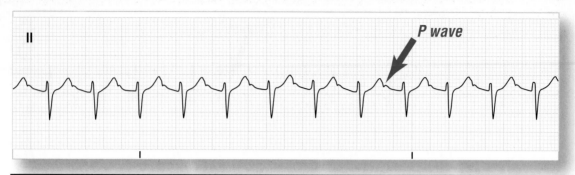

Rate:	About 120 BPM	PR intervals:	Normal, consistent
Regularity:	Regular	QRS width:	Normal
P waves:	Present	Grouping:	None
Morphology:	Inverted		
Axis:	Abnormal	Dropped beats:	None
P:QRS ratio:	1:1	Rhythm:	**Ectopic atrial tachycardia**

Discussion:

ECG 15-5 shows a tachycardia with narrow-complex QRSs. There are no obvious P waves but, on close examination, there is a small inverted notch at the end of the previous T waves. These are buried P waves. The PR intervals are normal.

ECG 15-6

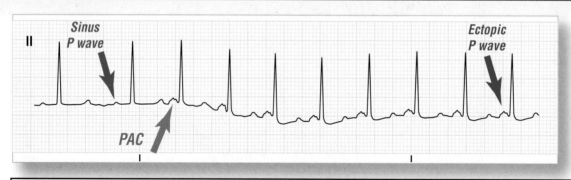

Rate:	About 115 BPM	PR intervals:	Normal, consistent
Regularity:	Regular	QRS width:	Normal
P waves:	Present	Grouping:	None
Morphology:	Inverted		
Axis:	Abnormal	Dropped beats:	None
P:QRS ratio:	1:1	Rhythm:	**Ectopic atrial tachycardia**

Discussion:

This strip shows the onset of an ectopic atrial tachycardia. Note the P wave morphology of the normal sinus beats at the start of the strip (green arrow). Then there is a PAC (pink arrow) that triggers off the tachycardia. Note that the ectopic P waves in the tachycardia (blue arrow) have the same morphology as the PAC. This is a common occurrence in EAT that can help you to identify the rhythm, if you are lucky enough to capture the onset of the tachycardia on paper.

CHAPTER **REVIEW**

1. Ectopic atrial tachycardias are maintained by:
   A. The sinus node
   B. The ectopic atrial focus
   C. The AV node
   D. Circus movement
   E. Both B and D

2. Ectopic atrial tachycardias are usually triggered by a premature atrial contraction. Typically, the morphology of the P wave in the PAC and the P waves in the tachycardia itself are the same. True or False.

3. Paroxysmal atrial tachycardia is another term used to describe this same rapid rhythm caused by an ectopic atrial pacemaker. True or False.

4. Ectopic atrial tachycardias account for about _____% of supraventricular tachycardias.
   A. 5
   B. 10
   C. 15
   D. 20

5. If the atrial rate is over 230 BPM, the rhythm cannot be caused by an ectopic atrial pacemaker. True or False.

6. At the onset, EAT can be slightly irregular. True or False.

7. Secondary ST-segment depression can occur in an ectopic atrial tachycardia. True or False.

8. ST segment depression is always due to the tachycardia and is not indicative of possible ischemia. True or False.

9. Ectopic atrial tachycardias are always benign and never need emergent therapy. True or False.

10. The following circumstances may lead to the formation of an ectopic atrial tachycardia:
    A Digoxin overdose
    B. Myocardial infarction
    C. Cardiomyopathies
    D. COPD and lung disease
    E. All of the above

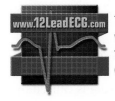

To enhance the knowledge you gain in this book, access this text's website at www.12leadECG.com! This valuable resource provides flashcards, an online glossary, web links, and more. Simply click on the Arrhythmias book cover once at the site.

CHAPTER 16

Ectopic Atrial Tachycardia with Block

This chapter will actually be a continuation of the previous one. Why did we elect to separate out two aspects of the same topic? We split them up because, even though they are both variations on a theme, they are different in many respects, especially in recognition. In particular, they are very lead dependent and the P waves are sometimes unrecognizable in lead II. EAT with blocks are also often misdiagnosed as atrial flutters or other supraventricular tachycardias, and these arrhythmias have totally different treatment strategies. Correctly identifying an EAT with block may save your patient's life by making you think of the various precipitating factors that cause it to develop.

Traditionally, EAT with block was known as paroxysmal atrial tachycardia with block. This terminology is still very much in use today by many clinicians. Why has the term stuck where other nomenclature has changed? We feel that it's because the term *PAT with block* rolls off the tongue a bit smoother than *EAT with block*. Get used to hearing it both ways and understand that it refers to the same clinical entity. However, whenever you hear either term, think about the possibility that the patient is digoxin toxic. This is a classic arrhythmia that is almost exclusively found in this patient population. For this reason, it is critical for every clinician, beginner or advanced, to recognize it.

In this chapter, we are not going to discuss the criteria for an ectopic atrial tachycardia. If you would like to review these criteria, refer to the previous chapter. In this chapter, we are going to concentrate on the block and on arrhythmia recognition.

Diagnostic Criteria

The diagnostic criteria for ectopic atrial tachycardia with block (Figure 16-1) are as follows:

1. *An ectopic atrial tachycardia between 150 and 250 BPM (can be faster in rare instances).*
2. *A return to an isoelectric baseline between the ectopic P waves in all leads.*
3. *AV block, either second or third degree.*

We know that ectopic atrial tachycardia is caused by a rapid atrial impulse going about 100 to 180 BPM (can go as high as 250 BPM or, very rarely, even higher). Ectopic atrial tachycardia with block is at the faster end

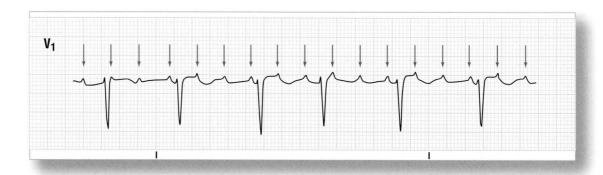

Figure 16-1: Ectopic atrial tachycardia with variable block. The P waves have been marked with a blue arrow for easy identification.

of that spectrum, at about 150 to 250 BPM or higher in rare circumstances. So far, however, we have only seen strips where each P wave triggered off a QRS. Now, we are going to address those times where it takes more than one P wave to trigger an individual QRS.

As we discussed in Chapter 5, it is a proven fact that the heart does not like very fast rates, ventricular rates to be exact. Why? At very fast ventricular rates, the ventricles do not have time to adequately fill. Remember from physiology that the largest amount of ventricular filling occurs during diastole, when the atrioventricular valves open up and a rush of blood floods the ventricular chamber (Figure 16-2, A and B). This is known as the *rapid filling phase of diastole*. Near the end of diastole, when the ventricles are almost full, the atria contract and push a little extra blood into the ventricles to overfill them (Figure16-2C). This overfilling stretches the cardiac muscle and helps to improve contractility. The net result is a strong ejection of blood into the aorta that is needed to maintain blood pressure. This mechanical process takes time—time that is missing in a rapid tachycardia.

So, how do the ventricles protect themselves from the rapid onslaught of the atrial impulses coming at them from above? They use their built-in gatekeeper, the AV node, to block some of the impulses from reaching them. The extra time created by the blocked atrial impulses allows the ventricles to fill appropriately, thereby maintaining cardiac output. Do the extra atrial impulses superfill the ventricles? No. The reason is that the atria are not filling to maximal capacity themselves, so the amount of blood they eject into the ventricles is minimal. So, as we can see, the AV block is quite protective in cases of rapid ectopic atrial tachycardia and is a survival tool for the body.

EAT with block is always associated with either second- or third-degree AV blocks. Type I blocks just wouldn't allow the time needed by the ventricles to adequately fill. Wenckebach, type I second-degree AV block, or type II second-degree AV block can be seen.

Describing an EAT with block verbally is a bit more complex than, say, describing a sinus tachycardia. The AV block creates a different atrial rate and ventricular rate. In addition, either the atrial or ventricular cadence can be regular or irregular. The correct way to describe these complex rhythms is to first describe the atrial events and then the ventricular events. We would describe the strip by saying that there is an ectopic atrial tachycardia at a rate of _____ BPM associated with a (second/third/variable) degree AV block with (2:1/3:1, etc.) conduction causing a (regular/irregular) ventricular response at _____ BPM. (For further discussion on the AV blocks, see Chapter 35.)

P Waves in EAT with Block

Take a look at Figures 16-1 and 16-3, looking closely at the P waves. You will see that each P wave is a very discrete entity. The P waves are surrounded by segments that are at the baseline for the strip. The only exception to this rule is when they are buried within another wave. They can be buried in the QRS complex, the ST segment, or the T waves.

Let's repeat this critically important diagnostic point. ***The P waves in EAT with block are discrete entities with a return of the baseline to normal between each wave.*** The importance of this point will become clear when we discuss atrial flutter and how to tell them apart.

When evaluating P waves, it is also critical to keep in mind that they vary in morphology based on each lead's vantage point for viewing the P wave vector. The clinical implication of this statement is that you never know which is the best lead to view the P waves for any one particular patient. Each patient, and each P wave vector, is different. In one patient, the P waves may be upright and clearly visible in lead I and isoelectric and electro-

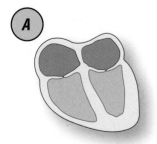
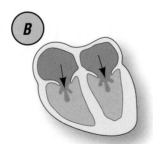
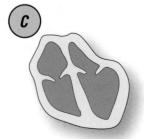

Figure 16-2: Rapid filling phase and the overfilling caused by atrial contraction.

cardiographically invisible in aVF. In another patient, they may be upright and visible in lead aVF and isoelectric and invisible in lead I. In general, however, the best single lead to identify and evaluate P waves is in lead V$_1$. Let's take a closer look at this problem.

The Problem with Lead II

Take a look at Figure 16-4. Can you recognize the rhythm? Notice that there are no discernible P waves that repeat throughout the strip. The rhythm is irregularly irregular and in the normal range for rate. The QRS complexes are normal and there are minimal nonspecific changes in the ST segments. Those of you with some previous arrhythmia recognition background may say that the rhythm is atrial fibrillation and, based on this strip alone, you could be right. But is that the right answer?

Now, take a look at the strip below taken from the same patient (Figure 16-5). Can you figure out why the

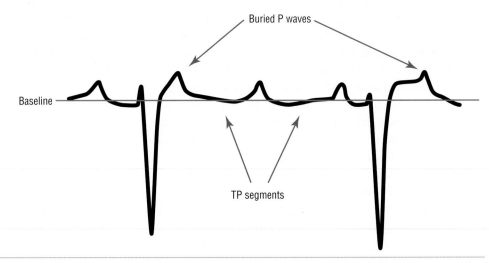

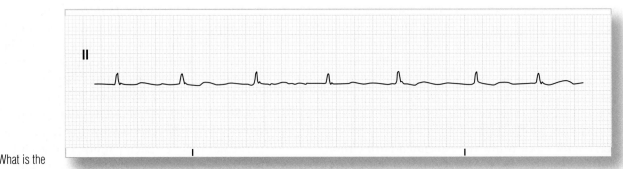

Figure 16-3: The P waves in EAT with block. Note that the P waves are discrete entities and there is a return to the baseline during the P-P intervals. There are two buried P waves in the example shown. One occurs immediately after the QRS complex and the other is well within the ST segment.

Figure 16-4: What is the rhythm?

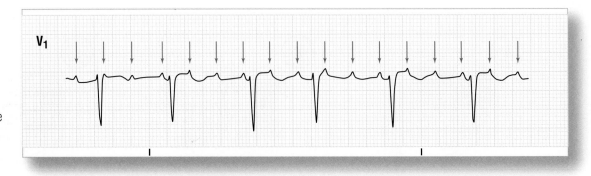

Figure 16-5: What is the rhythm? The P waves are obvious in lead V$_1$ (see blue arrows) when compared to lead II.

rhythms appear to be so clearly different? The answer lies in the leads that were used. In Figure 16-4, lead II was used. In Figure 16-5, lead V₁ was used. In the strip taken from lead V₁, we see clearly that there are some P waves. They are recurrent, reproducible, and consistent. That knocks out the theory that this is atrial fibrillation.

So, what is the rhythm? Let's go over the information slowly and methodically. As we mentioned, the P waves are regular. In addition, they are occurring at a very fast rate. This is definitely an atrial tachycardia. Now, are the P waves consistent with sinus P wave morphology? You need an old strip or ECG to correctly answer that question beyond a reasonable doubt, but we can make an educated guess, looking at the strip, that they are not. Let's keep going.

How fast are the atria going? The atrial rate is about 200 BPM! Remember, the normal rate for a sinus tachycardia is between 100 and 160 BPM, although rates as high as 220 BPM have been documented. This is at the higher end of the sinus tachycardia spectrum. Ectopic atrial tachycardias are usually between 100 and 180 BPM, but rates as high as 250 BPM are not uncommon. Therefore, it is more likely that an ectopic atrial tachycardia is the answer, but we can't be sure.

Are the P waves upright in lead II? Remember, P waves are normally upright in lead II because the normal atrial repolarization wave travels toward leads I and II (Figure16-6). In Figure 16-1, the P waves are isoelectric in lead II. That means that, at the very least, the P wave axis of the atria is not normal. In other words, there is a very high possibility that the P waves are starting at an ectopic focus. Putting this together with the rate information makes ectopic atrial tachycardia the most likely culprit. Once again, a previous strip showing the sinus P wave morphology would be confirmatory.

To close out our discussion of problems with lead II in EAT with block, let's go over an important clinical point. Usually, the ventricular response to the atrial tachycardia is regular. In Figures 16-4 and 16-5, the ventricular response was irregular. This occurred because of a variable AV block (see Chapter 35 for a full discussion). If the P waves in lead II are isoelectric or of small amplitude, the appearance of the strip could easily be misdiagnosed as atrial fibrillation by an experienced clinician. You need to have a high index of suspicion when approaching any rhythm abnormality, especially EAT with block.

Another clinical point to keep in mind is that EAT with block is quite often associated with digitalis toxicity. What is the primary use today for digitalis? It is primarily used to control chronic atrial fibrillation. If you have a strip like Figure 16-4, you may diagnose it quickly as atrial fibrillation and not think twice about your diagnosis. As part of your treatment, you may actually give the patient more digitalis. As you can imagine, this could be a fatal mistake if the patient's rhythm was actually an EAT with block caused by dig toxicity. Giving more digitalis to a toxic patient would be like adding fuel to a fire.

The take-home message in this section is that lead II alone is not always dependable to make the diagnosis in many rhythms, and especially in EAT with block. If the P waves are isoelectric or of small amplitude, the chance of missing the diagnosis could be very high. Whenever you see a change in a patient's rhythm, especially in someone taking digoxin, you should obtain a full 12-lead ECG and look at all of the leads to evaluate the rhythm correctly.

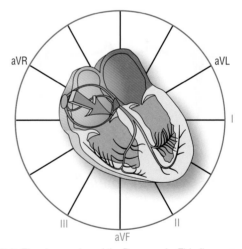

Figure 16-6: The sinus node and the P wave axis. This figure graphically represents the P wave axis as a light blue vector heading inferiorly and to the left. Note that the vector is heading toward the positive poles of leads I and II. Remember, a vector heading toward the positive pole of a lead gives rise electrocardiographically to an upright or positive wave in that lead. Since an impulse that originated in the sinus node can only travel downward and to the left, then the P wave has to be upright in leads I, II, III, aVF, V₅, and V₆.

ARRHYTHMIA RECOGNITION

Ectopic Atrial Tachycardia with Block

Rate:	Atrial 150 to 250 BPM; variable ventricular rate
Regularity:	Regular or regularly irregular
P wave:	Present
Morphology:	Different
Upright in II, III, and aVF:	Sometimes
P:QRS ratio:	Variable due to type of AV block
PR interval:	Variable due to type of AV block
QRS width:	Normal
Grouping:	Usually none
Dropped beats:	Yes

DIFFERENTIAL DIAGNOSIS

Ectopic Atrial Tachycardia with Block

1. Digitalis toxicity
2. Advanced heart disease: Ischemic cardiomyopathy, etc.
3. Total body potassium depletion
4. COPD

CLINICAL PEARL

If you ever see a P wave near the midpoint between two QRS complexes, look for a buried P wave. Very long PR intervals are much less common than arrhythmias containing a 2:1 block!

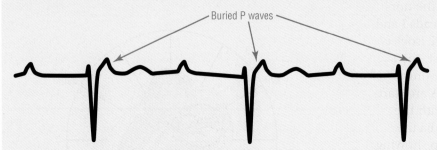

Buried P waves

Figure 16-7: This is not a sinus rhythm with a first-degree AV block!

Here is an easy way to do it...

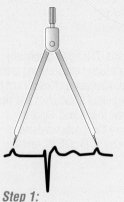

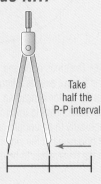

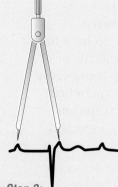

Take half the P-P interval

Step 1:
Use your calipers to measure the P-P interval.

Step 2:
Use your ECG paper to calculate half the distance.

Step 3:
See if there is a buried P wave!

Figure 16-8: Identifying a buried P wave.

ECG Strips

ECG 16-1

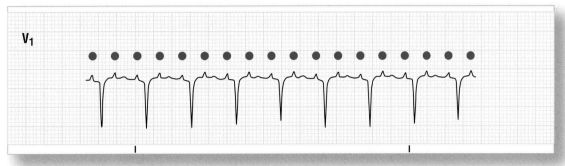

Rate:	Atrial: About 240–250 BPM Ventricular: About 120 BPM	PR intervals:	Variable
		QRS width:	Normal
Regularity:	Regular	Grouping:	None

P waves:
  Morphology:
  Axis:
	Present
	Upright in lead V₁
	Unknown
		Dropped beats:	Yes

		Rhythm:	**Ectopic atrial tachycardia with block**
P:QRS ratio:	2:1		

Discussion:

The ECG strip above was taken in lead V_1. Lead II was useless in this patient. This is an ectopic atrial tachycardia with a 2:1 AV block. The atrial and ventricular cadence is regular throughout the strip. The QRS complexes are normal morphology and there is some slight alteration in amplitude consistent with tachycardia-related electrical alternans. The blue dots represent P waves.

ECG 16-2

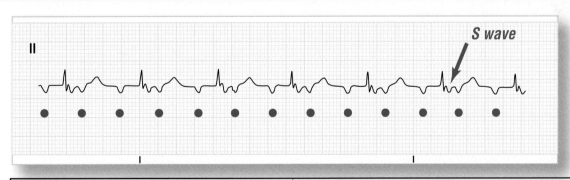

S wave

Rate:	Atrial: About 145 BPM Ventricular: About 72 BPM	PR intervals:	Regular
		QRS width:	Normal; 0.11 seconds
Regularity:	Regular	Grouping:	None

P waves:
  Morphology:
  Axis:
	Present
	Inverted
	Abnormal
		Dropped beats:	Yes

		Rhythm:	**Ectopic atrial tachycardia with block**
P:QRS ratio:	2:1		

Discussion:

At first glance, this strip appears to be a sinus rhythm with a very prolonged PR interval. However, notice that the P waves (represented by the blue dots) are inverted. That means that the P waves are ectopic. As mentioned in the Clinical Pearl, when the PR interval is very prolonged you should look for a buried P wave. There definitely is a buried P wave right after the terminal S wave of the QRS complex. Notice that, in this case, lead II was the best lead to see the P waves.

ECG 16-3

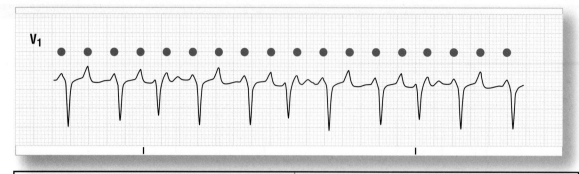

Rate:	Atrial: Slightly over 200 BPM Ventricular: About 120 BPM	PR intervals:	Variable
		QRS width:	Normal
Regularity:	Regularly irregular	Grouping:	None
P waves: 　Morphology: 　Axis:	Present Upright in lead V₁ Unknown	Dropped beats:	Yes
		Rhythm:	**Ectopic atrial tachycardia with block**
P:QRS ratio:	Variable		

Discussion:

The ECG strip above was taken in lead V₁. The P waves occur with a regular cadence, but the ventricular response is irregular due to the variable AV block. There is a return to the baseline in the segments between the P waves, as expected in an EAT with block. There is some electrical alternans noted, most probably due to the tachycardia itself. Note that the QRS morphology is altered slightly because of the fusion that is occurring with the P waves.

ECG 16-4

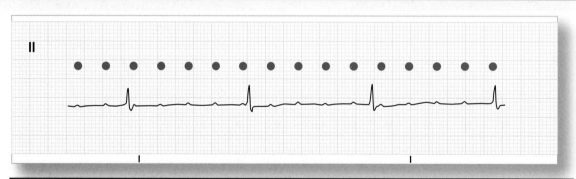

Rate:	Atrial: About 200 BPM Ventricular: About 45 BPM	PR intervals:	Variable
		QRS width:	Normal
Regularity:	Regular	Grouping:	None
P waves: 　Morphology: 　Axis:	Present Upright Normal	Dropped beats:	Yes
		Rhythm:	**Ectopic atrial tachycardia with block**
P:QRS ratio:	Variable		

Discussion:

This ECG is the first one we have shown you with a third-degree heart block. Up to now, the strips have shown either Type II second-degree or variable AV block. The way you can tell is that the QRS complexes are regular and narrow but completely dissociated from the P waves. You would describe this strip as follows: This is an ectopic atrial tachycardia at a rate of about 200 BPM associated with a complete third-degree heart block and a junctional escape rhythm at a rate of about 45 BPM.

ECG 16-5

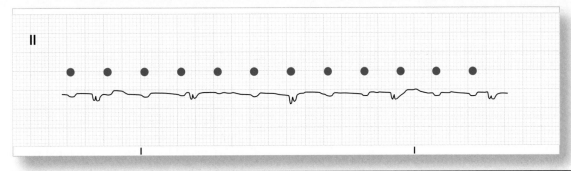

Rate:	Atrial: About 150 BPM Ventricular: About 55 BPM	PR intervals:	Variable
		QRS width:	Normal
Regularity:	Regular	Grouping:	None

P waves:
    Morphology:
    Axis:
	Present
	Upright
	Normal
		Dropped beats:	Yes

		Rhythm:	**Ectopic atrial tachycardia with block**
P:QRS ratio:	Variable		

Discussion:

This strip also shows a complete third-degree heart block with a regular ventricular response. The QRS complexes are within acceptable limits for width in lead II, so a junctional escape rhythm is likely. However, to be completely sure that these are not ventricular complexes, you will need to measure the width of the complexes in the other leads. If any exceed 0.12 seconds, then you would have a ventricular escape rhythm.

ECG 16-6

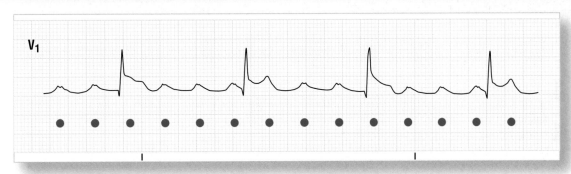

Rate:	Atrial: About 160 BPM Ventricular: About 45 BPM	PR intervals:	Variable
		QRS width:	Normal
Regularity:	Regular	Grouping:	None

P waves:
    Morphology:
    Axis:
	Present
	Upright
	Unknown
		Dropped beats:	Yes

		Rhythm:	**Ectopic atrial tachycardia with block**
P:QRS ratio:	Variable		

Discussion:

This is an EAT with a third-degree heart block and a junctional escape. Take special notice of the ST segment elevation in lead V_1. This is grossly abnormal. It is not due to the buried P waves, as they are buried in the ST segments only in the first and third QRS complexes.

Notice that the second and fourth T waves are pointier and taller than the others due to the fusion with the P waves. The cause of the arrhythmia in this patient is probably an acute myocardial infarction. Get a 12-lead ECG . . . *stat!*

CHAPTER REVIEW

1. Another common term used interchangeably with ectopic atrial tachycardia with block is:
   A. Rapid atrial tachycardia with block (RAT with block)
   B. Multiple atrial thyrotoxic tachycardia with block (MATT with AV block)
   C. Juvenile atrial coronary killer with block (JACK with block)
   D. Paroxysmal atrial tachycardia with block (PAT with block)

2. EAT with block is usually a benign rhythm. True or False.

3. The heart rate in EAT with block is usually:
   A. Atrial rate of 100–150 BPM
   B. Atrial rate of 150–250 BPM
   C. Ventricular rate of 80–120 BPM
   D. Variable rate depending on amount of AV block
   E. B and D

4. Ectopic P waves in EAT with block can be easily missed in some leads. They are characterized by a return to baseline during the intervening P-P intervals. True or False.

5. Buried P waves are rare in EAT with block. True or False.

6. Which of the following statements is incorrect?
   A. EAT with block can be associated with a first-degree AV block.
   B. EAT with block can be associated with a type I second-degree AV block.
   C. EAT with block can be associated with a type II second-degree AV block.
   D. EAT with block can be associated with a third-degree AV block.
   E. EAT with block can be associated with variable AV block.

7. Sometimes AV blocks can be protective to the heart. True or False.

8. In EAT with block, the atrial impulses will always be regular or pretty close to regular. The ventricular response may be either regular or irregular depending on the type of AV block seen. True or False.

9. Buried P waves can always be seen clearly in an EAT with block in lead V_1. True or False.

10. You can always count on lead II to get you through any rhythm abnormality! True or False.

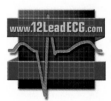

To enhance the knowledge you gain in this book, access this text's website at www.12leadECG.com! This valuable resource provides flashcards, an online glossary, web links, and more. Simply click on the Arrhythmias book cover once at the site.

CHAPTER 17

Wandering Atrial Pacemaker

In Chapter 13, we saw some strips that showed multiple or frequent PACs. The underlying theme to these strips was that there was an underlying rhythm (either NSR, sinus bradycardia, or sinus tachycardia) as the baseline and PACs were occasional "events" that broke up the underlying regularity.

In this chapter, we review the first of two irregularly irregular rhythms that are composed entirely of randomly occurring ectopic atrial complexes. The two rhythms are wandering atrial pacemaker (WAP) and multifocal atrial tachycardia (MAT).

Before we start talking about wandering atrial pacemaker in depth, we should clarify a nomenclature issue. There is some confusion between how WAP is classically defined and what occurs in true clinical practice. We are going to be discussing these two "variations on a theme" separately because it is easier to understand each on its own merits. Just be aware that the same term, wandering atrial pacemaker, is used to describe both types of electrocardiographic presentations.

Wandering Atrial Pacemaker: The Classical Definition

Traditionally, wandering atrial pacemaker was considered to be a rhythm created when the pacemaking function of the heart swung back and forth between the sinus node and some ectopic site. The resulting rhythm strips showed a variation in P-wave morphology, along with a slight variation in the regularity of the complexes This presentation was very similar to a sinus arrhythmia but with varying P-wave morphology.

In reality, we now know that this type of WAP is due to a swinging of the pacemaking site within the sinus node itself. Remember on page 174, we discussed the fact that the P waves in normal sinus rhythm can vary by a slight amount morphologically because of some slight variations in the exact point of origin of the atrial impulse (Figure 17-1). Well, the traditional definition of a wandering atrial pacemaker is an exaggeration of this mechanism.

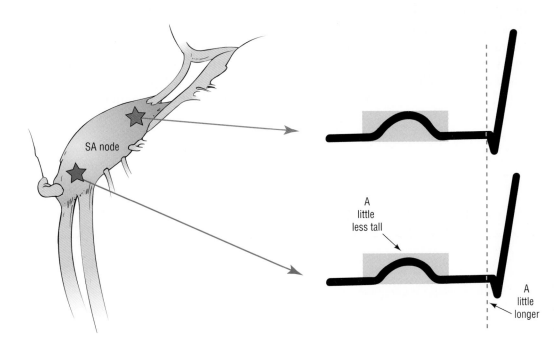

SA node

A little less tall

A little longer

Figure 17-1: P waves in normal sinus rhythm can vary by a slight amount morphologically because of some slight variations in the exact point of origin of the atrial impulse.

The sinus node is an elongated structure within the atria. Respiratory variation and metabolic changes that occur as a result of respiration can cause a temporary fluctuation of the main pacemaking area that actually stimulates the impulse. During those periods when the heart rate is faster on the rhythm strip (inspiration), the pacing area is at the higher end of the node and the resulting P wave on the strip is taller with a longer PR interval. During slower parts of the rhythm (expiration), the pacing area is lower down on the node and the resulting P wave is shorter, with a shorter PR interval. This explains why the wandering atrial pacemaker rhythm, classically defined, is very similar to sinus arrhythmia (Figure 17-2). It is basically just an exaggerated response of the same processes.

Wandering Atrial Pacemaker: A Clinical Variation

In addition to the cases that meet the traditional definition of the wandering atrial pacemaker that was given above, there is another variation that occurs more commonly in everyday clinical medicine but has never, to our knowledge, been given an official title. Clinically, wandering atrial pacemaker also refers to an irregularly irregular rhythm created by multiple (three or more) ectopic atrial pacemakers each firing at its own rate. The resulting rhythm has no underlying regularity and is completely chaotic. Note, however, that the heart rate for WAP is always less than 100 BPM.

This entity or presentation is more common than the classical presentation because it is found in patients with enlarged atria and pulmonary disease (e.g., COPD). Because these clinical scenarios are relatively common in everyday practice, this rhythm abnormality is encountered more frequently. Since clinicians were forced to call this arrhythmia by some name, they chose to call it wandering atrial pacemaker.

How does this rhythm develop, and what does it look like on a rhythm strip? We went over some of the information already when we discussed regularity in Chapter 5, but it is worthwhile to review these concepts again.

This variation of wandering atrial pacemaker develops when at least three atrial pacemaking sites are involved in the production of the rhythm. As we saw in Chapter 13, each atrial pacemaker has its own intrinsic three-dimensional location on the atria. Because of this location, its P wave morphology, and the PR interval associated with it, form an electrocardiographic pattern that is unique (Figure 17-3).

In addition to its appearance, each site also has a characteristic rate associated with it. Now, suppose we took a tracing from each of our three pacemakers above individually. In Figure 17-4, each complex is represented by a small rectangle filled with its own individual color for simplicity. Notice how the three pacemakers each have an individual rate. But, in real time and in real life, the complexes would sometimes cancel each other out. The combined strip at the bottom of Figure 17-4 would be the result.

Notice that we have not even included two other factors that add to the complete chaos that is represented in this type of wandering atrial pacemaker: irritability and fusion. In addition to its own intrinsic pacemaking rate, the ectopic atrial foci in the clinical scenarios associated with this presentation are typically irritable. As we have seen, irritability leads to premature complexes, which could further alter the regularity of the rhythm. Fusion of the various components of the complexes or the complexes themselves also occurs, leading to frequent aberrancy and bizarre fused morphologies of the waves in WAP.

The final strip in Figure 17-5 shows the typical pattern of this presentation of WAP. For this type of presentation, therefore, the definition of wandering atrial

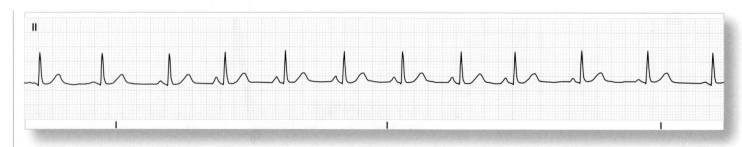

Figure 17-2: Wandering atrial pacemaker.

pacemaker becomes: *A wandering atrial pacemaker is an irregularly irregular rhythm with a ventricular rate less than 100 BPM, characterized by at least three different P-wave morphologies on the same strip, each* associated with their own PR interval. Note that, contrary to a tracing with just frequent PACs, there is no underlying regular rhythm associated with it.

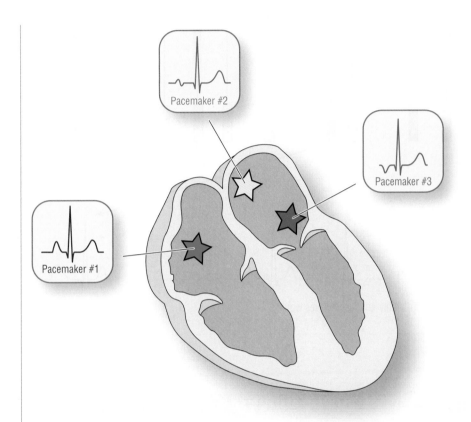

Figure 17-3: At least three individual pacemaker sites are at work in creating this presentation of wandering atrial pacemaker. Each site is associated with an individual P-wave morphology and PR interval.

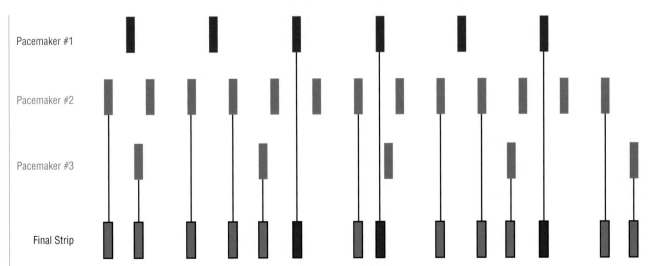

Figure 17-4: Individual rates of three ectopic pacemakers being electrocardiographically represented as one rhythm.

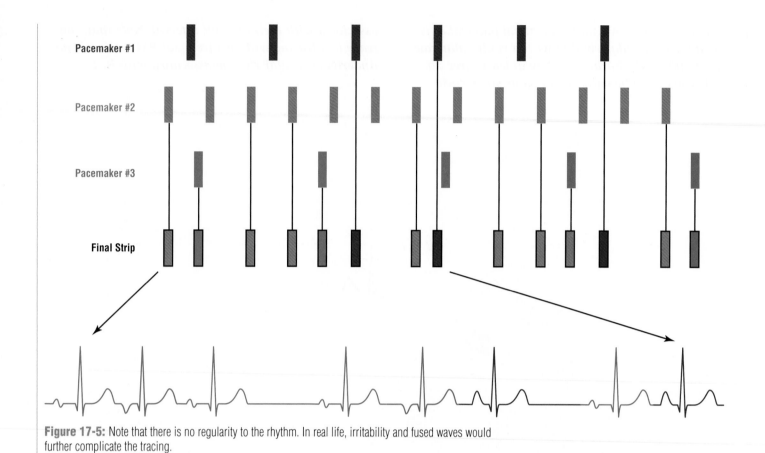

Figure 17-5: Note that there is no regularity to the rhythm. In real life, irritability and fused waves would further complicate the tracing.

ARRHYTHMIA RECOGNITION

Wandering Atrial Pacemaker

Rate:	Less than 100 BPM
Regularity:	Irregularly irregular
P wave:	Present
Morphology:	Variable
Upright in II, III, and aVF:	Sometimes
P:QRS ratio:	1:1
PR interval:	Variable
QRS width:	Normal or wide
Grouping:	None
Dropped beats:	Sometimes

DIFFERENTIAL DIAGNOSIS

Wandering Atrial Pacemaker

1. COPD
2. Respiratory failure
3. Atrial enlargement
4. Electrolyte abnormalities
5. Drugs: nicotine, alcohol, caffeine, etc.

The list above is not all-inclusive.

ECG Strips

ECG 17·1

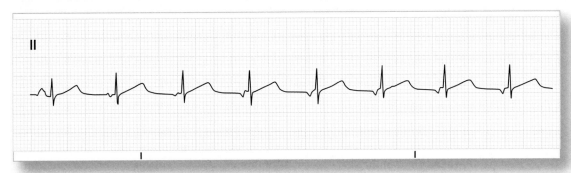

Rate:	Around 85 BPM	PR intervals:	Variable
Regularity:	Irregularly irregular	QRS width:	Normal
P waves: Morphology: Axis:	Present Variable Variable	Grouping:	None
		Dropped beats:	None
P:QRS ratio:	1:1	Rhythm:	**Wandering atrial pacemaker**

Discussion:

This ECG strip shows the classic changes of a wandering atrial pacemaker. Notice the slow, gradual transition of the P waves from upright to inverted. Longer strips show the transition occurring back and forth between the pacemakers. Notice that the QRS complexes and T waves are identical in this strip. There is no evidence of any aberrant conduction, as can sometimes occur with faster rates.

ECG 17·2

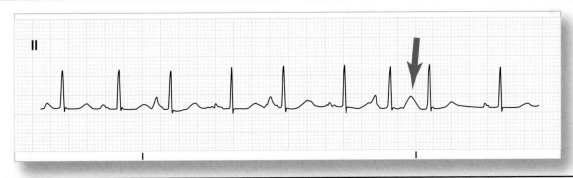

Rate:	Upper 90s BPM	PR intervals:	Variable
Regularity:	Irregularly irregular	QRS width:	Normal
P waves: Morphology: Axis:	Present Variable Variable	Grouping:	None
		Dropped beats:	None
P:QRS ratio:	1:1	Rhythm:	**Wandering atrial pacemaker**

Discussion:

The strip above shows an irregularly irregular rhythm with at least three P-wave morphologies. As a matter of fact, just the first three complexes show differing P-wave morphologies and PR intervals. This is a typical example of a wandering atrial pacer. Note the area highlighted by the blue arrow. This is a fusion between the T wave of the preceding complex with the P wave of the complex that follows, the buried P-wave phenomenon we discussed before.

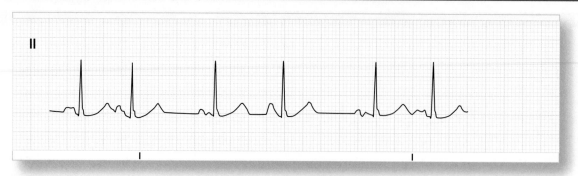

ECG 17-3			
Rate:	Around 70 to 80 BPM	PR intervals:	Variable
Regularity:	Irregularly irregular	QRS width:	Normal
P waves:	Present	Grouping:	None
Morphology:	Variable		
Axis:	Variable	Dropped beats:	None
P:QRS ratio:	1:1	Rhythm:	**Wandering atrial pacemaker**

Discussion:

It is very easy to identify the different P-wave morphologies and PR intervals in the strip above. The irregularly irregular rhythm, along with at least three different P-wave morphologies that are present, clinch the diagnosis as WAP.

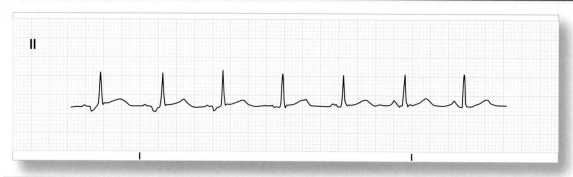

ECG 17-4			
Rate:	Around 90 BPM	PR intervals:	Variable
Regularity:	Irregularly irregular	QRS width:	Normal
P waves:	Present	Grouping:	None
Morphology:	Variable		
Axis:	Variable	Dropped beats:	None
P:QRS ratio:	1:1	Rhythm:	**Wandering atrial pacemaker**

Discussion:

The strip above shows the classic changes of a wandering atrial pacemaker. Note the slow transition from the negative P-wave morphologies at the onset of the strip to the more normal-appearing P waves found at the end of the strip. Be careful though; you cannot state that any of the P waves above resemble sinus P waves unless you have old strips to compare, in which the patient was in normal sinus rhythm.

ECG 17-5

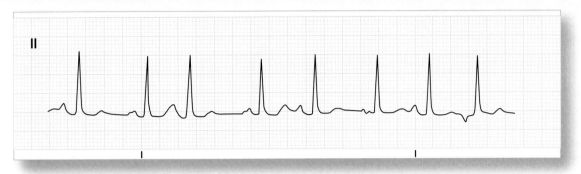

Rate:	Around 90 BPM	PR intervals:	Variable
Regularity:	Irregularly irregular	QRS width:	Normal

P waves:
    Morphology:
    Axis:
	Present
	Variable
	Variable
		Grouping:	None

		Dropped beats:	None
P:QRS ratio:	1:1	Rhythm:	**Wandering atrial pacemaker**

Discussion:

Once again, note the irregularly irregular rhythm with the differing P-wave morphologies and PR intervals. There are at least three differing P-wave morphologies, which makes the diagnosis a wandering atrial pace-maker. There is a fusion of the T wave of the second complex with the P wave of the third complex. Always think about a buried P wave when you see a single abnormal T wave on a strip.

ECG 17-6

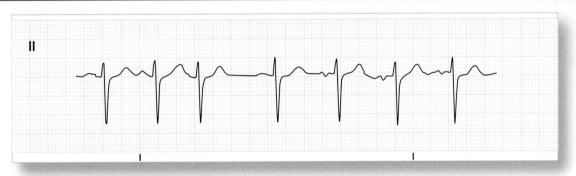

Rate:	Around 90 BPM	PR intervals:	Variable
Regularity:	Irregularly irregular	QRS width:	Normal

P waves:
    Morphology:
    Axis:
	Present
	Variable
	Variable
		Grouping:	None

		Dropped beats:	None
P:QRS ratio:	1:1	Rhythm:	**Wandering atrial pacemaker**

Discussion:

The strip above shows a wandering atrial pacemaker rhythm very clearly. Once again, the third P wave is buried in the T wave of the second complex.

CHAPTER **REVIEW**

1. Wandering atrial pacemaker is one of three _____ _____ rhythms.

2. The three irregularly irregular rhythms include (pick all that apply):
   A. Wandering atrial pacemaker
   B. PAC
   C. Multifocal atrial tachycardia
   D. Atrial fibrillation
   E. Accelerated junctional

3. Respiratory variations and metabolic changes that occur during respiration can cause a temporary fluctuation of the main area that actually stimulates the impulse within the SA node itself. True or False.

4. Clinically, wandering atrial pacemaker can also refer to an irregularly irregular rhythm created by multiple (_____ or more) ectopic atrial pacemakers each firing at its own pace.

5. The following entity is commonly associated with WAP:
   A. Young patients
   B. Elderly patients
   C. COPD
   D. AV nodal dysfunction
   E. Sick sinus syndrome

6. Classic WAP can be frequently confused with sinus arrhythmia. True or False.

7. There are always only three ectopic atrial pacemaking sites associated with WAP. True or False.

8. Which of the following parts of the complexes are different from complex to complex in WAP?
   A. P wave
   B. QRS waves
   C. PR intervals
   D. QT intervals
   E. Both A and C

9. WAP is a completely_____ rhythm.

10. The average atrial rate in MAT is _____ _____ 100 BPM.

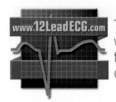

To enhance the knowledge you gain in this book, access this text's website at www.12leadECG.com! This valuable resource provides flashcards, an online glossary, web links, and more. Simply click on the Arrhythmias book cover once at the site.

CHAPTER 18

Multifocal Atrial Tachycardia

Now that you understand the basic principles of a wandering atrial pacemaker, let's turn our attention to its closely related family member: multifocal atrial tachycardia (MAT). Remember when we were discussing normal sinus rhythm and sinus tachycardia, we mentioned that NSR and ST were basically the same rhythm but at different points along a heart rate or beats per minute spectrum. The same is true of wandering atrial pacemaker and multifocal atrial tachycardia. They are basically the same rhythm but with different ranges of rates: WAP is below 100 BPM and MAT is over 100 BPM.

Basically, multifocal atrial tachycardia is a rapid tachycardia usually with heart rates between 100 and 150 BPM (but can be as high as 250 BPM) that is caused by the chaotic firing of at least three different ectopic atrial pacemaking sites (Figure 18-1). The result is an irregularly irregular or chaotic rhythm with varying P-wave morphology, PR intervals and P-P or R-R intervals (Figure 18-2). Due to the increased rate of firing of the pacemakers in this tachycardic rhythm, fusions and aberrancy are much more common than in WAP.

While we are on the topic of heart rates in the irregularly irregular rhythms, since wandering atrial pace-

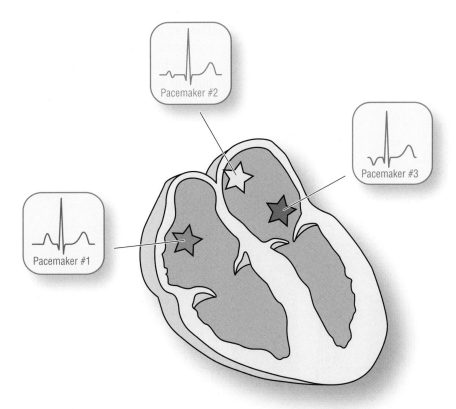

Figure 18-1: At least three individual pacemaker sites are at work in creating a completely chaotic and tachycardic rhythm. Each site is associated with an individual P-wave morphology and PR interval just as in WAP.

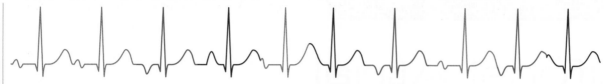

Figure 18-2: The ECG strip in MAT shows multiple P-wave morphologies, PR, P-P, and R-R intervals throughout the strip. There are more fusions of the P waves with the previous T waves and an increase in aberrantly conducted QRS complexes because of the tachycardia.

maker and multifocal atrial tachycardia are both chaotic rhythms, their rates may momentarily cross from the normal to the tachycardic ranges and vice versa. For example, a strip that contains mostly P-P intervals in the 60 to 80 BPM range may have one or two complexes that are being transmitted at a rate of 120 BPM. This strip would still be considered WAP and not MAT just because of the few variations noted. Likewise, a strip with the majority of the complexes occurring in the 100 to 120 BPM range does not mean that it should be called a WAP due to a momentary slowdown in the rate.

When you are considering WAP or MAT, you need to consider the overall rate of the rhythm strip and the presentation of the majority of the complexes. If the overall rate of the strip (as discussed in Chapter 4), obtained by multiplying the number of complexes in a 6-second strip by 10 is over 100 BPM, then the rhythm is MAT. If the overall rate is below 100 BPM, then the rhythm is WAP.

Fusion of the complexes, mostly the P and T waves, is very common in multifocal atrial tachycardia. As you can imagine, three or more pacemakers firing chaotically and rapidly causes a lot of overlap between the cycles. The net result is an increased number of buried P waves, P waves occurring on T waves, P waves occurring on QRS complexes, and even blocked P waves (Figure 18-3).

In addition to the fusions mentioned above, aberrancy in the morphology of the QRS complex is also very commonly encountered in MAT. This occurs because the chaotic tachycardia causes many impulses to fall on the absolute and relative refractory period of the conduction system. As we mentioned, the right bundle branch block has an especially long refractory period and is very susceptible to block the impulse from being transmitted normally down to the ventricles (Figures 18-4 and 18-5). The net result is a wide QRS complex with a morphology consistent with a right bundle branch block pattern. Left bundle branch block pattern can also occur in aberrancy, but it is less common than RBBB.

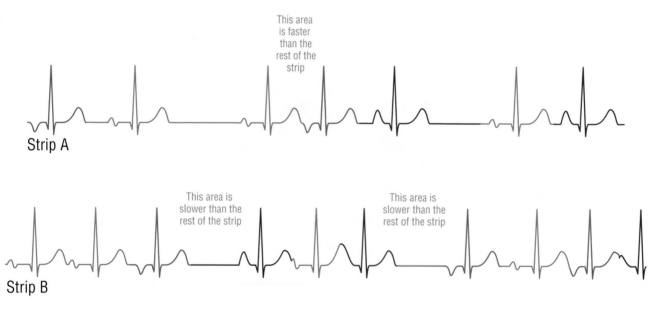

Figure 18-3: ECG strip A is an example of a wandering atrial pacemaker. The slight area of tachycardia is not enough to bring the overall rate above 100 BPM, nor are the majority of the complexes in the tachycardic range. ECG strip B is an example of an MAT. Note that the majority of the strip is tachycardic and that the overall rate of the strip is above 100 BPM.

Clinical Scenario

Almost all of the patients who develop MAT are elderly and have some sort of respiratory compromise or failure. The rhythm is commonly found in patients with chronic obstructive pulmonary disease (COPD), especially during an exacerbation of their symptoms. Drugs used to treat COPD exacerbations, such as beta-adrenergic agonists (e.g., albuterol), frequently cause the rhythm to develop. The rhythm usually resolves when the underlying condition is treated and corrected. Additional treatment strategies are beyond the scope of this book.

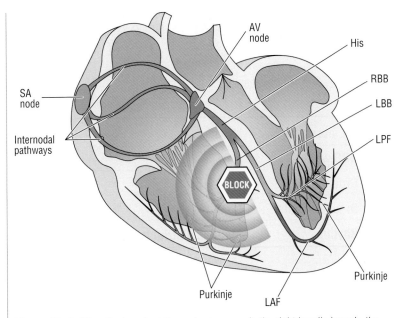

Figure 18-4: When the impulse hits a refractory area in the right bundle branch, the impulse is forced to continue by direct cell-to-cell transmission throughout the rest of the right ventricle.

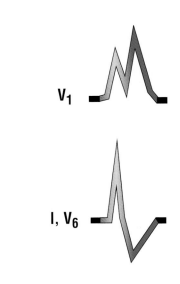

Figure 18-5: The right bundle branch block pattern is caused by the slow conduction through the right ventricle.

ARRHYTHMIA RECOGNITION

Multifocal Atrial Tachycardia

Rate:	100 to 150 BPM (can be as high as 250 BPM)
Regularity:	Irregularly irregular
P wave:	Present
Morphology:	Different
Upright in II, III, and aVF:	Sometimes
P:QRS ratio:	1:1
PR interval:	Variable
QRS width:	Normal or aberrantly conducted
Grouping:	None
Dropped beats:	Blocked PACs are possible

DIFFERENTIAL DIAGNOSIS

Multifocal Atrial Tachycardia

1. COPD
2. Respiratory failure
3. Electrolyte abnormalities
4. Drugs: nicotine, alcohol, caffeine, etc.

ECG Strips

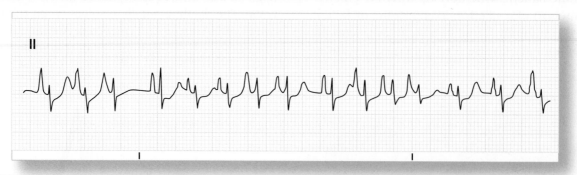

Rate:	140 to 150 BPM		PR intervals:	Variable
Regularity:	Irregularly irregular		QRS width:	Normal

P waves:
  Morphology:
  Axis:
	Present
	Normal
	Normal
			Grouping:	None

			Dropped beats:	None
P:QRS ratio:	1:1		Rhythm:	**Multifocal atrial tachycardia**

Discussion:

This is a great ECG to start our review of actual strips because the P waves are so easy to identify. Note that the P waves vary in morphology and that the PR intervals are different as well. The rhythm is irregularly irregular. Putting it all together, it screams out: MAT! A couple of extra points: Note the differing QRS morphology. This is due to fusion in some cases, aberrancy in others. The varying heights of the QRS complex are due to electrical alternans, which is common in many tachyarrhythmias.

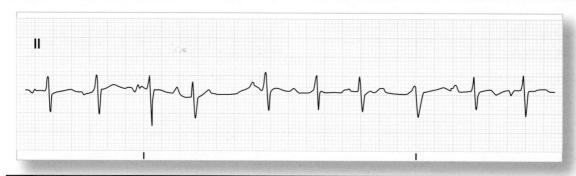

Rate:	100 to 110 BPM		PR intervals:	Variable
Regularity:	Irregularly irregular		QRS width:	Normal or aberrancy

P waves:
  Morphology:
  Axis:
	Present
	Normal
	Normal
			Grouping:	None

			Dropped beats:	Blocked PACs are present
P:QRS ratio:	1:1		Rhythm:	**Multifocal atrial tachycardia**

Discussion:

This strip also shows an irregularly irregular rhythm with varying P-wave morphology and PR intervals. Once again, it is classic for MAT or WAP. Taking into account that the vast majority of the complexes occur at P-P intervals that place them in the tachycardic range, and that the overall rate of the strip is over 100 BPM, MAT is the correct diagnosis for this rhythm.

ECG 18-3

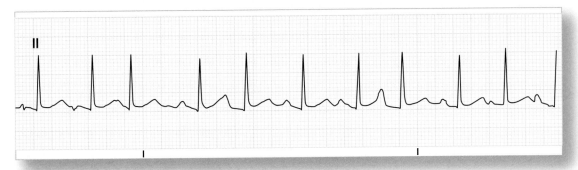

Rate:	100 to 110 BPM	PR intervals:	Variable
Regularity:	Irregularly irregular	QRS width:	Normal
P waves:	Present	Grouping:	None
Morphology:	Normal	Dropped beats:	None
Axis:	Normal		
P:QRS ratio:	1:1	Rhythm:	**Multifocal atrial tachycardia**

Discussion:

The strip above shows a wide variation in P-wave morphology, each with a different PR interval. The rhythm is tachycardic and irregularly irregular, making the diagnosis of this rhythm MAT. There are some buried P waves and P-on-T phenomena, that are fairly evident on closer examination of the strip. The buried P waves belong to complexes 3, 5, and 8, when you count from the left.

ECG 18-4

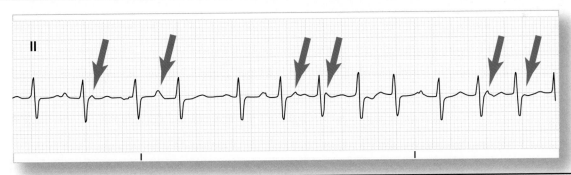

Rate:	110 to 140 BPM	PR intervals:	Variable
Regularity:	Irregularly irregular	QRS width:	Normal
P waves:	Present	Grouping:	None
Morphology:	Normal	Dropped beats:	Blocked PAC is present
Axis:	Normal		
P:QRS ratio:	1:1	Rhythm:	**Multifocal atrial tachycardia**

Discussion:

This chaotic, tachycardic rhythm also shows all of the characteristics that make a perfect MAT. Note that there are some buried P waves that have very long PR intervals associated with them. These buried P waves are identified by the blue arrows. The waves that immediately follow these P waves are actually the T waves of the preceding complexes.

ECG 18-5

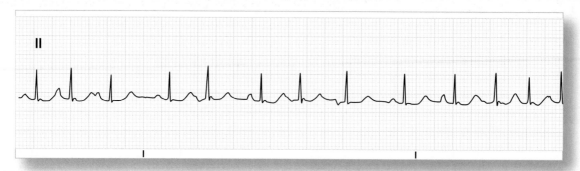

Rate:	110 to 120 BPM	PR intervals:	Variable
Regularity:	Irregularly irregular	QRS width:	Normal
P waves:	Present	Grouping:	None
Morphology:	Normal		
Axis:	Normal	Dropped beats:	None
P:QRS ratio:	1:1	Rhythm:	**Multifocal atrial tachycardia**

Discussion:

This ECG strip shows a chaotic rhythm that is tachycardic and associated with multiple P-wave morphologies and PR intervals consistent with MAT. Once again, the presence of buried P waves is noted in a few complexes. Can you identify them? They are the 2nd, 5th, 7th, 11th and 12th complexes from the left. The third P wave is not buried, but is at the tail end of the preceding T wave.

ECG 18-6

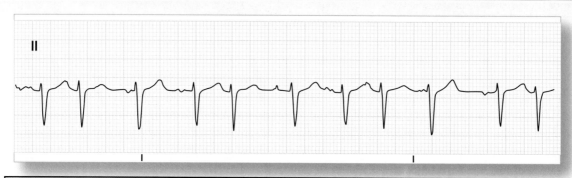

Rate:	100 to 120 BPM	PR intervals:	Variable
Regularity:	Irregularly irregular	QRS width:	Normal
P waves:	Present	Grouping:	None
Morphology:	Normal		
Axis:	Normal	Dropped beats:	None
P:QRS ratio:	1:1	Rhythm:	**Multifocal atrial tachycardia**

Discussion:

At the risk of sounding redundant, this strip also shows an irregularly irregular tachycardia with multiple P-wave morphologies and PR intervals. There are some buried P waves in this strip as well. As we mentioned before, this type of fusion is very common in MAT. Note the presence of the negative QRS complexes on this ECG. You should definitely obtain a 12-lead ECG on any patient with a complex arrhythmia to fully evaluate the electrocardiographic pathology.

CHAPTER **REVIEW**

1. There are three rhythms that are always irregularly irregular. These are _____ _____, _____ _____ _____, and _____ _____ _____.

2. MAT is caused by at least three ectopic atrial pacemakers and has a rate of greater than 100 BPM. True or False.

3. The rates in MAT never go above 150 BPM. True or False.

4. Fusion often occurs in MAT between P waves and T waves. Occasionally, fusion between P waves and QRS complexes can also occur. True or False.

5. Aberrantly conducted complexes are rarely seen in MAT. True or False.

6. A rhythm strip shows MAT with a heart rate that is variable throughout. In one section, the rate is 80 BPM. In another, the rate is about 225 BPM. Most of the strip is about 150 BPM. Which is the overall rate of the strip?
  A. 80 BPM
  B. 120 BPM
  C. 150 BPM
  D. 225 BPM

7. Aberrancy is usually of a _____ bundle branch block morphology.

8. MAT is usually found in patients with COPD or respiratory failure. True or False.

9. MAT is only found in patients with COPD or respiratory failure. True or False.

10. MAT usually resolves when the underlying condition is corrected. True or False.

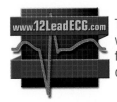

To enhance the knowledge you gain in this book, access this text's website at www.12leadECG.com! This valuable resource provides flashcards, an online glossary, web links, and more. Simply click on the Arrhythmias book cover once at the site.

CHAPTER 19

Atrial Flutter

General Overview

Atrial flutter refers to a very rapid, very regular atrial tachycardia, occurring at rates between 200 and 400 BPM, which typically have no associated isoelectric segments between the atrial complexes. The lack of an isoelectric or baseline segment between the atrial waves, and the smooth, biphasic P wave morphology, gives the atrial baseline a "saw-tooth" appearance on the ECG (Figure 19-1). That saw-tooth appearance is the most distinctive, and unique, feature of atrial flutter.

The saw-tooth appearance of the atrial rhythm is intermittently broken up by the QRS complexes of the ventricular response. The ventricular response rates are usually slower than the atrial rates, typically occurring between 140 and 160 BPM. The ventricular response can occur at either regular or variable intervals.

The slower ventricular rates develop when the AV node "blocks" conduction of the supraventricular impulses, to safeguard the ventricles from the very fast atrial rates. We say "block" because this is not a true AV block caused by a pathologic obstruction to conduction. It is, instead, a normal protective mechanism of the AV node to the constant bombardment it faces from the rapid supraventricular impulses which makes it intermittently refractory to further conduction. More on this later.

The Making of the Saw-Tooth Pattern

As mentioned in Figure 19-1, the saw-tooth pattern of the atrial complexes is pathognomonic for atrial flutter. That means that, whenever you see an underlying saw-tooth pattern that is constantly undulating with no discrete isoelectric segment in between the atrial complexes, the patient has atrial flutter. Let's take a closer look at how this classic saw-tooth pattern is made.

The leading theory on how atrial flutter is formed involves the formation of a macroreentry circuit inside of an enlarged or scarred right atria. This is our first exposure to reentry, and we need to understand this important concept before we move on to examine macroreentry.

As the term implies, reentry involves the reentry of an impulse back to an area of the heart that was previously depolarized during any one complex. Suppose you had a group of cells laid down side-to-side on a plate, forming a circle pattern (Figure 19-2). Let's make another rule: The impulse can only travel in one direction. Depolarizing any one cell will begin a cascade of cell-to-cell depolarization that will quickly spread throughout the entire circle. This spread is so fast that by the time the impulse makes its way back around to the first depolarized cell, the cell would still be refractory and would not be able to "refire" (Figure 19-3).

Now, suppose we add one more ingredient to this mix. Suppose that somewhere along the circle there

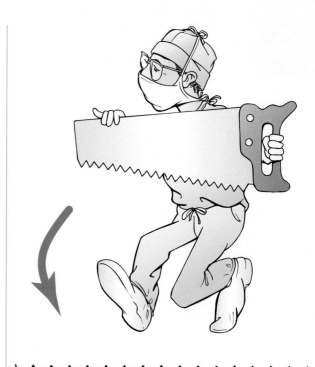

Figure 19-1: The atrial complexes in atrial flutter appear in a saw-tooth pattern that is pathognomonic, or found only in this rhythm. The difficulty comes when ventricular complexes are superimposed on the saw-tooth pattern, as they often fuse with, and thus partially obscure, the underlying atrial pattern.

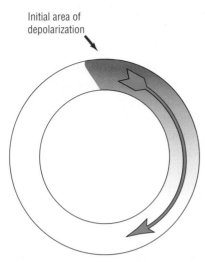

Figure 19-2: The original impulse site fires and triggers a depolarization wave that spreads throughout the rest of the cells in the direction shown.

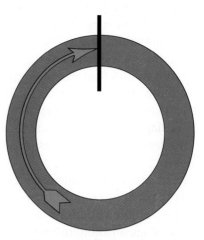

Figure 19-3: By the time the depolarization wave reaches the original site (represented by the black line) the original site is still refractory and cannot accept the new impulse. The depolarization wave essentially dies at this point.

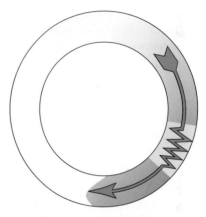

Figure 19-4: The area in yellow represents an area of slow conduction. The depolarization wave slows down as it traverses this area.

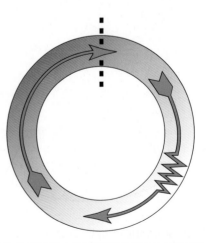

Figure 19-5: By the time the depolarization wave reaches the original site (represented by the dotted black line) the original site is now ready to receive a new impulse. The result is a circus movement that is self-perpetuating.

was an area that did not conduct the impulse as quickly as the rest of the cells (Figure 19-4); a kind of a bioelectrical speed trap where the depolarization wave would be slowed down substantially. What would happen to the overall rate of transmission of the depolarization wave when it reached this point? It would slow it down dramatically. Now, due to the slower conduction of the impulse, would the initial site still be refractory to accepting a new impulse by the time the depolarization wave got there? Probably not. The initial site would be ready to accept a new impulse (Figure 19-5). Note that the new impulse, in this case, would actually be the first depolarization wave after finishing its travel through the entire circle. This is the way a reentry or circus movement is created in the heart. The impulse would just travel around and around, self-propagating itself every time it made a circuit around the "track."

We have seen how a reentry circuit can perpetuate a *circus movement,* causing the heart to depolarize over and over. There is no size limit to the reentry circuit. The circuit can be small and isolated to a small area of the heart, like the AV node, and this type is referred to as a microreentry circuit. It can also involve a large amount of tissue in either the ventricles or the atria. These larger types of circuits are known as macroreentry circuits.

Atrial flutter is caused by just such a macroreentry circuit occurring in the right atria. The slow area of conduction in the circuit may be due to surgical scarring, ischemic cardiac disease, structural heart disease, or normal barriers to transmission in an enlarged right atria. The subsequent macroreentry circuit causes the repeated depolarization of the right and left atria.

It is important at this point to note that the macroreentry circuit can occur in either a clockwise or counterclockwise direction. This is exactly what can occur in real life, and the direction of the rotation of the circuit will give rise to different morphology and direction of the saw-tooth pattern on the ECG. The morphological differences caused by the direction of the circus movement are a major criterion helping to separate atrial flutter into various classifications (see Additional Information box).

There are exact anatomical pathways known to occur in various types of atrial flutter. To go into those pathways and the possible variations that can occur is beyond the scope of an introductory/intermediate book on arrhythmia recognition. If you are interested, consult some advanced books on arrhythmias and electrophysiology (EPS) for that information. For simplicity, and since most of us do not have access to an EPS lab, we will only mention the pertinent clinical information needed for basic arrhythmia recognition.

Every time the depolarization wave completes a turn around the macroreentry circuit, it stimulates the left atria. The direction of the vector created by the left atria determines the direction of the "teeth" in the saw-tooth pattern. In Figure 19-6, the direction is negative in leads II, III, and aVF. In addition, just as the macroreentrant circuit is self-perpetuating without any breaks in the depolarization wave, there are no isoelectric segments between the "teeth" on the ECG. It is a continuously self-perpetuating series of atrial depolarizations. This is how the saw-tooth pattern of atrial depolarization develops on an ECG in a patient with atrial flutter.

Now, a word about correct nomenclature. As you can imagine, "teeth" and "saw-tooth" are not the correct clinical terms for these waves. A new series of terms was created specifically to describe the electrocardiographic findings in atrial flutter. The "teeth" are technically not P waves, since they are a form of aberrant conduction found only in atrial flutter. To differentiate them from normally occurring P waves, they are referred to as **F** or **_flutter waves_**. As mentioned before, it is worthwhile to point out the fact that there are no isoelectric segments between the flutter waves. This is a critical piece in diagnosing atrial flutter. Instead, the F waves blend together continuously in a constant undulating pattern at a rate between 200 and 400 BPM.

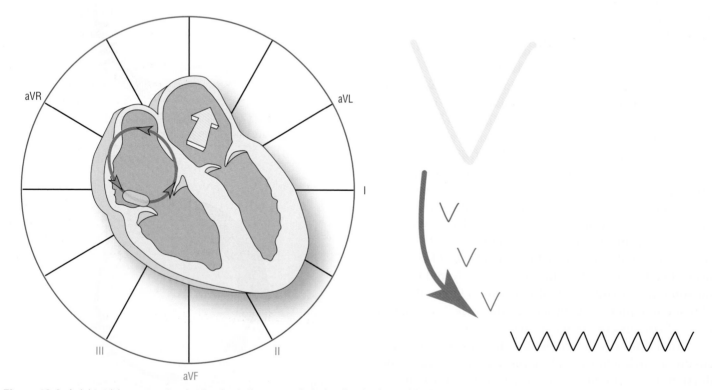

Figure 19-6: A right atrial macroreentry circuit going in the counterclockwise direction is noted in the figure. This gives rise to a depolarization vector in the left atrium that is headed superiorly and to the left in leads II, III, and aVF (see purple vector). This vector causes the morphological appearance of the saw-tooth in the inferior leads to be negative. Each time the cycle repeats, a new "tooth" is added.

Classification of Atrial Flutter

Classification of atrial flutter into different subcategories is very useful for assigning the various available advanced treatment strategies to prevent and treat the arrhythmia. It is an electrophysiological classification and is not overly useful for surface electrocardiography. We mention this here for those of you who are interested, even though it is an advanced concept. Refer to an advanced text on arrhythmias for a more complete discussion.

The major categories include:

1. Typical or type I atrial flutter
   a. Counterclockwise rotation of the macroreentrant circuit
   b. Clockwise rotation of the macroreentrant circuit
2. True atypical or type II atrial flutter
3. Incisional reentrant atrial tachycardia

AV Nodal Conduction Rates

We have mentioned on previous occasions that the AV node functions as the gatekeeper for the ventricles. This function is very obvious in atrial flutter. Normally, the AV node senses the atrial depolarization, holds the impulse for a few milliseconds, and then allows the depolarization wave to proceed forward to stimulate the ventricles. In atrial flutter, and in many supraventricular tachycardias, this gatekeeping function is extended to include a selective transmission of impulses in order to not overwhelm the ventricles with a very fast, very dangerous tachycardia.

Under normal, nontachycardic atrial rates, the AV node transmits the impulses at a 1:1 (1 to 1) conduction rate. The first number before the colon sign is the number of atrial complexes that are occurring. The number after the colon sign refers to the number of impulses conducted to the ventricles to allow ventricular depolarization to occur. Putting it all together, this type of notation refers to the number of atrial depolarizations that have to occur for the AV node to allow conduction through its tissues to allow one ventricular contraction. A number of 2:1 refers to 2 atrial contractions to 1 ventricular contraction; 3:1 means 3 atrial contractions to 1

ventricular contraction, and so on. You can also have other rates of conduction through the AV node. For example, a rate of 3:2 conduction refers to 3 atrial contractions for 2 ventricular contractions. As you can see, there are many possible combinations.

Now, we need to clarify a very important point in electrocardiographic terminology. The AV node can cause a block to the supraventricular impulses as either a protective mechanism or due to a pathological process. This dual meaning, one good and one bad, leads to some serious confusion since they both use the word *block*. In addition, a block and a conduction ratio are not the same thing. For example a 3:2 block means that for every three P waves created, two are blocked. Only one is conducted. However, a 3:2 conduction ratio means that for every three P waves, two are conducted to the ventricles. In order to avoid confusion, and to adhere to the more clinically useful method, we will strictly be using the conduction ratio.

Another reason to use the term conduction rather than block is to remind us of those times when the block is protective, as in atrial flutter. In other words, blocks are pathological and conduction is not. Thinking about the issues will quickly remind us of the treatment options available to us clinically. When the conduction is protective, we need to stop or slow down the supraventricular reentry circuits or automatic foci. When the block itself is the problem, we need to address it by increasing conduction through the node or completely bypassing it with an artificial pacemaker. Remember, you can't get it if you don't think about it. Using the term "conduction" makes you think about it.

Atrial flutter can actually have both types of "block" present at the same time, a physiologic one to prevent the tachycardia from getting out of control and a pathological one secondary to some other reason. The pathological block can be present because of ischemia, drug effect, increased parasympathetic activity, or just underlying AV nodal disease. We will revisit this issue after we have studied the pathological AV blocks in detail in Chapter 35.

Atrial and Ventricular Rates

Now that we have reviewed the concept of AV conduction, let's take a look at how conduction affects rates. Atrial rates in atrial flutter can vary between 200 and 400 BPM. The most common rate is 300 BPM. Notice that this means that the peaks (either positive or negative) will be exactly 0.20 seconds (one big block) apart on an ECG strip (Figure 19-7). Clinically, that means

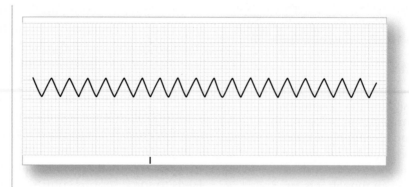

Figure 19-7: Atrial rate at 300 BPM. Note that the peaks fall exactly 0.20 seconds (one big block) apart.

that if you ever have a strip with a small peak that repeats exactly every 0.20 seconds or one big block, you need to think of the possibility of atrial flutter.

So far we have purposely stayed away from adding in the QRS complexes in order to explain the basic mechanisms involved in the atrial component of atrial flutter. Now, let's start adding in the ventricular response to the tachycardia. If the atrial rates are from 200 to 400 BPM, the ventricular rates are typically 100 to 200 BPM (Figure 19-8). However, the most common range is 140 to 160 BPM. Let's take this a huge step clinically: *Since the most common atrial rate is 300 BPM and the most common conduction ratio is 2:1, the most common ventricular rate is 150 BPM.* ***Whenever you see a ventricular rate at exactly 150 BPM (or close to it), think of atrial flutter!*** This is a very important clinical pearl that

you need to remember the rest of your clinical life. You will see this come up again and again when you are evaluating rhythm strips and ECGs.

Recognizing Atrial Flutter

We have reviewed many of the important points related to atrial flutter, but there is still one that needs to be looked at a bit more closely: arrhythmia recognition. Atrial flutter is very easy to pick out when there are higher rates of conduction and the ventricular response is at the lower end. The problem comes in when you have a fast ventricular response with 1:1 or 2:1 conduction. We will start with 2:1 conduction.

When you see a rapid ventricular response with 2:1 conduction, the flutter waves have to be buried in

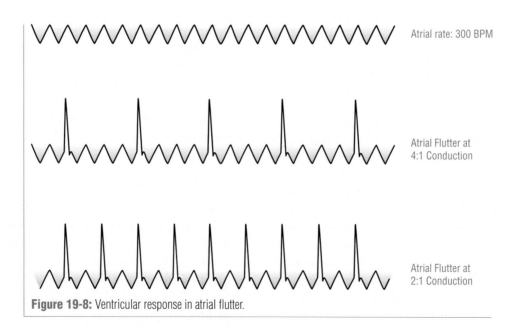

Atrial rate: 300 BPM

Atrial Flutter at 4:1 Conduction

Atrial Flutter at 2:1 Conduction

Figure 19-8: Ventricular response in atrial flutter.

Atrial Flutter with Variable Block

The atrial rhythm in atrial flutter is always regular. But, because most AV conduction in atrial flutter occurs at either odd or even ratios (with even ratios being the most common), the ventricular response is usually either regular or regularly irregular.

Regular ventricular responses occur when the ratios remain stable throughout the strip. For example, suppose you had an atrial rate at 300 BPM with 2:1 conduction. The ventricular response would occur regularly at a rate of 150 BPM. Likewise, an atrial rate at 350 BPM

with a 3:1 rate would lead to a regular ventricular response.

Regularly irregular ventricular response occurs when the conduction ratios vary throughout the strip (Figure 19-9). An example of this would be an atrial flutter with an atrial rate of 300 BPM with a 3:1 and 4:1 intermittent conduction. When the conduction ratio varies, the regularity varies. But, note that the ratio of conduction is always some multiple of the underlying atrial rate. In other words, it will always be some exact multiple of the distance between the F waves.

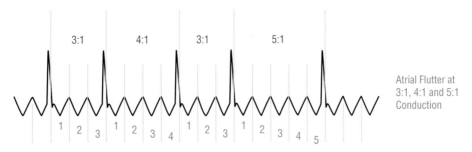

Atrial Flutter at 3:1, 4:1 and 5:1 Conduction

Figure 19-9: Regularly irregular atrial flutter.

In addition to the odd and even ratios of AV conduction previously discussed, AV conduction can occur haphazardly throughout the strip, giving rise to an irregularly irregular atrial flutter (Figure 19-10). This type of conduction is usually due to some intrinsic AV nodal disease that does not allow the AV node to function normally. This is an unusual presentation for atrial flutter, but one that you should be aware of because it

can easily lead you astray of the correct diagnosis. As we mentioned before, almost all irregularly irregular rhythms are either atrial fibrillation, wandering atrial pacemaker, or multifocal atrial tachycardia. Atrial flutter with variable block is one of those uncommon exceptions to the rule. Note that the term we used was variable block instead of variable conduction, implying that there is some pathological process at work here.

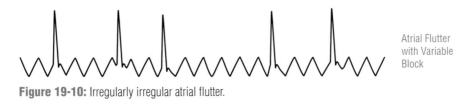

Atrial Flutter with Variable Block

Figure 19-10: Irregularly irregular atrial flutter.

either the QRS or ST-T wave areas of the complexes in question (Figure 19-11). Recognizing the traditional saw-tooth pattern of atrial flutter becomes more difficult at that point. In addition, sometimes the flutter waves are not too deep or are a bit asymmetrical, and recognizing them requires a very high index of suspicion (Figure 19-12). Finally, and more important, is the lead that is used to evaluate the rhythm.

The best leads for trying to evaluate atrial flutter include leads II, III, aVF, and V_1. The most common type of atrial flutter has negative F waves in leads II, III, and aVF and positive F waves in lead V_1. Many times, we are lucky and can easily spot the negative F waves in lead II. Other times, we will need to switch the lead to V_1 to see the F waves more clearly (Figure 19-13), or will need to get a full 12-lead ECG and take a look at the various presentations that are very lead specific.

A clinical word of caution: Whenever you have a ventricular rate of 140 to 160 BPM, think carefully and try to see if there could be an underlying atrial flutter. This is especially true if the ventricular rate is 150 BPM. As far as we are concerned, a ventricular rate of 150 BPM is atrial flutter until proven otherwise. Always remember to use your calipers and map any possible imperfections throughout the strip to see if there can be any buried F waves.

Atrial Flutter and Wide-Complex Tachycardias

We should point out in this section that atrial flutter can be associated with wide QRS complexes for other reasons than an accessory pathway. The QRS complexes can also be wide during episodes of aberrant conduction. In these cases, the ventricular rate could exceed the upper limits of normal transmission for a particular individual who may have some abnormality in his or her conduction system, for example, due to ischemia or regional structural heart disease.

Electrolyte abnormalities can also lead to the presence of wide complexes

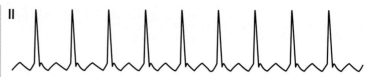

Figure 19-11: Lead II rhythm strip. Note that the QRS complexes are partially obstructing the view of the flutter waves and the traditional saw-tooth pattern.

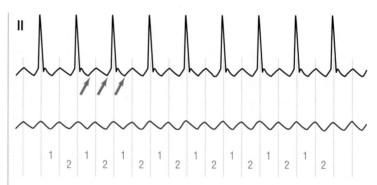

Figure 19-12: This is the same strip as in Figure 19-11, but with the QRS complexes removed. The saw-tooth pattern is clearly visible at this point. The red arrows indicate the trigger points that should make you suspect atrial flutter. Mapping these points throughout the strip with your calipers will show the repetitive nature of the F waves.

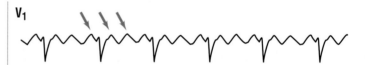

Figure 19-13: Lead V_1 in the same patient. The flutter waves and saw-tooth pattern are more clearly seen in this lead. The red arrows show the tips of the F waves.

ADDITIONAL INFORMATION

1:1 Conduction

One of the most dangerous rhythms covered in this book is atrial flutter with 1:1 conduction. The problem with this conduction ratio is that, since the usual atrial rates are between 200 and 400 BPM, the ventricular rates will match the atrial rate. The net result is a catastrophic drop in blood pressure due to decreased stroke volume. As we saw in Chapter 1, the drop in stroke volume is due to the lack of ventricular filling and the loss of the atrial kick that typically occur in very rapid tachycardias.

When do we get 1:1 conduction of atrial flutter? The answer is variable. It can definitely occur with a normal AV node when the atrial rate is slow. During episodes of slow atrial beating, the AV node can transmit the impulse routinely and does not need to block any of the impulses. Sometimes drugs, like the catecholamines, can stimulate conduction through the AV node to the point that rapid tachycardias can ensue. The most common

mechanism, however, is due to the presence of an accessory pathway. This information is a bit advanced, but the life-threatening quality of this complication and the frequency in which it is clinically found makes review of this topic mandatory for all clinicians.

If you remember from Chapter 1, the only area of communication between the atria and the ventricles involves the AV node in almost all patients. There are, however, a certain few patients that have a second (or multiple) tract that traverses the atrioventricular septum (Figure 19-14). The result is that an electrical impulse can travel back and forth repeatedly through this bypass tract, avoiding the gatekeeping control of the AV node.

The net result of the loss of control created by these bypass tracts is that the atrial rates and the ventricular rates can be identical in these patients. If the atrial rate is 100 BPM, the bypass tract may or may not function. In either case, the net result is the same: the ventricular rate is 100 BPM. If the atrial rate is 300 BPM, the AV node functions as a gatekeeper but the bypass tract does not, and the net result is that the ventricular rate is 300 BPM. This same process can continue for even faster rates, including atrial fibrillation, which we will cover in the next chapter. The lack of AV nodal control can lead to some very serious life-threatening tachycardias (Figure 19-15).

Since the ventricular depolarizations occur through a bypass tract in these cases, the QRS complexes will be wide and aberrantly conducted. This occurs because the normal electrical conduction system is not used at all to transmit the impulse through the ventricles. Instead, the impulse is transmitted throughout the ventricles by the slow direct cell-to-cell transmission route. The morphology of the complexes will depend on the location of the bypass tract and the route taken by the depolarization wave as it makes its way throughout the ventricles.

A clinical pearl to remember is this: Think about a bypass tract on any strip or ECG with a ventricular rate over 250 BPM. These are very rapid rates and are well above the normal ranges for the standard electrical conduction system. The higher the rate, the greater the chance of an accessory pathway.

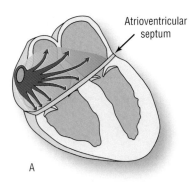
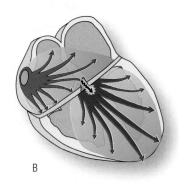
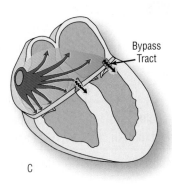

Figure 19-14: The AV septum represents a nonconductive wall between the atria and the ventricles. If the AV septum did not have any communication between the atria and the ventricles, the impulse would never reach the ventricles (A). The AV node provides a normal pathway through the AV septum and provides the gatekeeping function critically needed to maintain AV synchronization (B). An accessory pathway provides a bypass tract that allows an additional area of communication between the atria and the ventricles (C). The problem is that the bypass tract does not have a gatekeeping function and allows unlimited and unhindered communication between the atria and the ventricles. The result could be catastrophic arrhythmias, which could be life threatening in many cases.

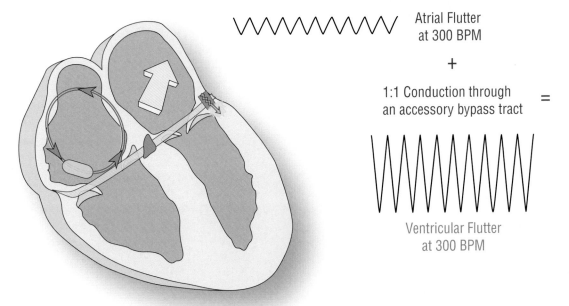

Figure 19-15: 1:1 conduction.

by altering the intracellular transmission of the impulse. It is also associated with increased aberrancy due to alterations in the refractoriness of the bundle branches.

The last, and most common, cause for a wide-complex atrial flutter is the presence of a preexisting bundle branch block. If the person had a preexisting bundle branch block and suddenly developed an episode of atrial flutter, the result would be a wide QRS complex atrial flutter. These two possibilities should always be kept in mind when approaching a wide-complex tachycardia at a rate between 140 and 160 BPM, and especially if the ventricular rate is exactly 150 BPM. However, clinically speaking, a wide-complex tachycardia should always be considered ventricular tachycardia until proven otherwise.

ARRHYTHMIA RECOGNITION

Atrial Flutter

Rate:	Atrial: 200 to 400 BPM
	Ventricular: 100 to 300 BPM
Regularity:	May vary with presentation
P wave:	F or flutter waves present
Morphology:	Not applicable
Upright in II, III, and aVF:	Not applicable
P:QRS ratio:	May vary; usually 2:1 or 4:1
PR interval:	Not applicable
QRS width:	Normal or wide
Grouping:	May occur with advanced block
Dropped beats:	Present

DIFFERENTIAL DIAGNOSIS

Atrial Flutter

Myocardial infarction
Atherosclerosis
Drugs: digoxin

Rheumatic heart disease
Alcoholic holiday heart
Thyrotoxicosis

Pulmonary emboli
Pericarditis
Pneumonia: Right middle lobe

MAD RAT PPP is a mnemonic used to remember the most common causes of atrial flutter. This list is not all-inclusive.

ECG Strips

ECG 19-1

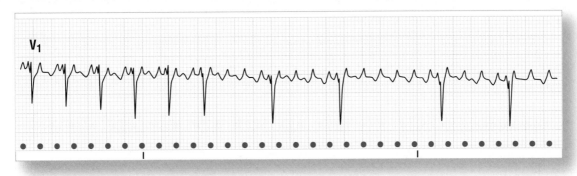

Rate:	Atrial: About 320 BPM Ventricular: Variable	PR intervals:	Not applicable
Regularity:	Regularly irregular	QRS width:	Normal

P waves:
  Morphology:
  Axis:
	F waves present
	Not applicable
	Not applicable
		Grouping:	None

		Dropped beats:	Present
P:QRS ratio:	2:1, 4:1, and 6:1	Rhythm:	**Atrial flutter**

Discussion:

The rhythm strip above shows atrial flutter with varying conduction rates of 2:1, 4:1, and 6:1. The P waves are upright in lead V_1 making them easy to spot. The area with 2:1 conduction shows partial fusion of the QRS complexes and ST segments with the F waves. Notice how much easier it is to identify the rhythm at the higher conduction rates. As is usually the case, the R-R interval is an exact variable of the F-F interval.

ECG 19-2

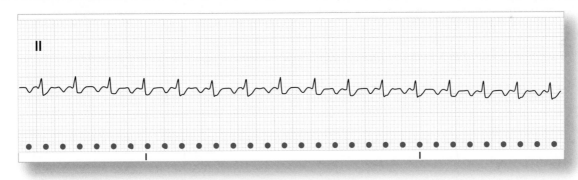

Rate:	Atrial: About 320 BPM Ventricular: About 160 BPM	PR intervals:	Not applicable
Regularity:	Regular	QRS width:	Normal

P waves:
  Morphology:
  Axis:
	F waves present
	Not applicable
	Not applicable
		Grouping:	None

		Dropped beats:	Present
P:QRS ratio:	2:1	Rhythm:	**Atrial flutter**

Discussion:

This rhythm strip is one taken from the same patient as ECG 19-1, but in lead II. The patient was in consistent 2:1 conduction. Notice how the diagnosis is not as evident as in lead V_1. The key to making the diagnosis in this lead is that the presumed PR interval is fairly wide and the presumed "P" waves are inverted. Taking half of this "P-P" interval demonstrates another inverted "P" wave at the exact halfway point. The rate and regularity makes this atrial flutter and the "P" waves are actually F waves.

ECG 19-3

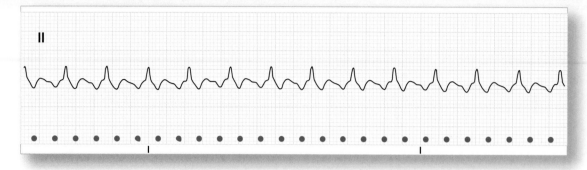

Rate:	Atrial: About 270 BPM Ventricular: About 135 BPM	PR intervals:	Not applicable
Regularity:	Regular	QRS width:	Normal
P waves: Morphology: Axis:	F waves present Not applicable Not applicable	Grouping:	None
		Dropped beats:	Present
P:QRS ratio:	2:1	Rhythm:	**Atrial flutter**

Discussion:

The rhythm strip above shows an atrial flutter with 2:1 conduction. The fusion of the QRS complex and ST segment with the saw-tooth pattern of the F waves makes the rhythm difficult to identify. Use your mind's eye to remove the QRS complexes from the strip. The result-ing saw-tooth pattern is evident. Once again, as in ECG 19-2, the key to the diagnosis is the rate, the inverted "P" waves, and the buried F waves found exactly halfway between the visible F waves. Use your calipers often!

ECG 19-4

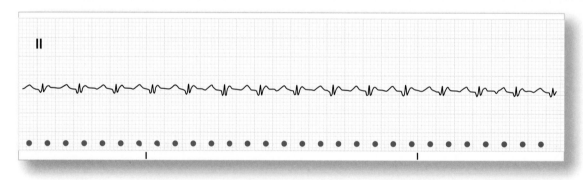

Rate:	Atrial: About 300 BPM Ventricular: About 150 BPM	PR intervals:	Not applicable
Regularity:	Regular	QRS width:	Normal
P waves: Morphology: Axis:	F waves present Not applicable Not applicable	Grouping:	None
		Dropped beats:	Present
P:QRS ratio:	2:1	Rhythm:	**Atrial flutter**

Discussion:

This strip is very difficult to correctly identify. A little extra care and some mental manipulation of the strip should help you make the diagnosis. The ventricular rate is 150 BPM. That rate should immediately raise a red flag in favor of atrial flutter. Mentally removing the QRS complexes will show you the saw-tooth pattern of the underlying F waves. Take your calipers and measure the "F-F" interval. Divide that distance in half and map the rhythm strip. The buried F waves should be fairly easy to spot now.

ECG 19-5

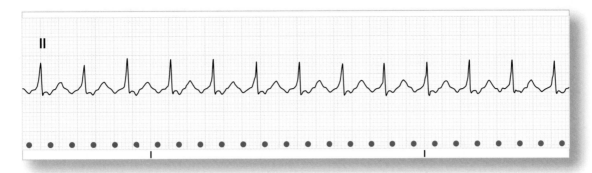

Rate:	Atrial: About 260 BPM Ventricular: About 130 BPM	PR intervals:	Not applicable
Regularity:	Regular	QRS width:	Normal
P waves: Morphology: Axis:	F waves present Not applicable Not applicable	Grouping:	None
		Dropped beats:	Present
P:QRS ratio:	2:1	Rhythm:	**Atrial flutter**

Discussion:

This rhythm strip shows an atrial flutter with a very shallow saw-tooth pattern. It is difficult to see the constant undulation of the flutter waves on this ECG, but it is there. The key to identifying the undulation is the slow rise of the QRS complex, the very prominent T waves, and the apparent ST depression. The slow upstroke of the R wave and the prominent T waves are caused by a fusion of the positive end of the flutter waves. The ST depression is caused by the negative F waves.

ECG 19-6

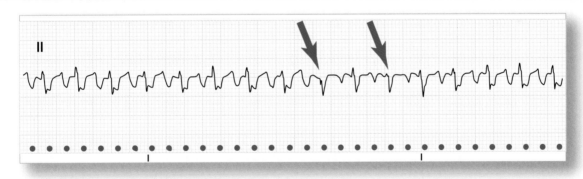

Rate:	Atrial: About 320 BPM Ventricular: About 160 BPM	PR intervals:	Not applicable
Regularity:	Regular with 2 events	QRS width:	Normal
P waves: Morphology: Axis:	F waves present Not applicable Not applicable	Grouping:	None
		Dropped beats:	Present
P:QRS ratio:	2:1	Rhythm:	**Atrial flutter**

Discussion:

This strip shows an atrial flutter with 2:1 conduction. There are two events visible on the strips, which we have highlighted with blue arrows. Can you figure out what they are? They occur later than expected, so they would have to be escape beats. They are narrow and follow the general morphology of the other QRS complexes, so they need to be atrial or junctional escape complexes. The less-than-prominent R waves in those beats are due to fusion with the underlying F waves.

ECG 19-7

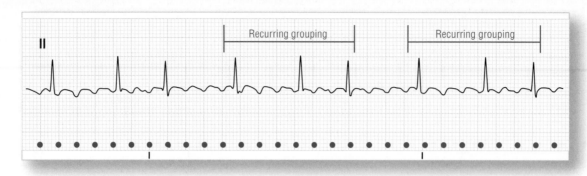

Rate:	Atrial: About 300 BPM Ventricular: Around 80 BPM	PR intervals:	Not applicable
Regularity:	Regularly irregular	QRS width:	Normal
P waves: Morphology: Axis:	F waves present Not applicable Not applicable	Grouping:	Present
		Dropped beats:	Present
P:QRS ratio:	Variable	Rhythm:	**Atrial flutter**

Discussion:

These next two strips have some information for advanced students. The first thing to note is the very obvious atrial saw-tooth pattern consistent with atrial flutter. The atrial rate is 300 BPM, which is a common rate for atrial flutter. The rhythm is regularly irregular, with associated grouping of the ventricular complexes. The regularity of the ventricular response means that this strip is not a true variable block. The grouping and the irregularity are instead classic for Wenckebach grouping (see Chapter 35).

ECG 19-8

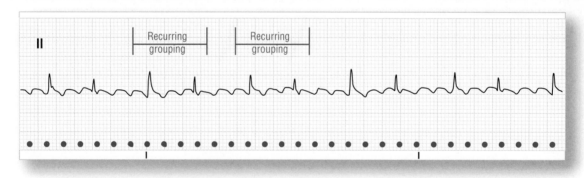

Rate:	Atrial: About 300 BPM Ventricular: About 110 BPM	PR intervals:	Not applicable
Regularity:	Regularly irregular	QRS width:	Normal
P waves: Morphology: Axis:	F waves present Not applicable Not applicable	Grouping:	None
		Dropped beats:	Present
P:QRS ratio:	Variable	Rhythm:	**Atrial flutter**

Discussion:

Once again, the saw-tooth pattern of atrial flutter is obvious on this strip. The QRS morphology of every other beat is slightly different than the others. Some grouping recurs throughout the strip. This could be consistent with Wenckebach grouping. In addition, the varying QRS morphology may be due to aberrancy, or fusion with the F waves, or they could represent escape complexes. Clinical correlation and a longer strip for study are indicated.

CHAPTER **REVIEW**

1. Atrial flutter always has a regular, recurrent atrial rhythm. True or False.

2. The atrial rate is usually between:
   A. 100 and 300 BPM
   B. 200 and 300 BPM
   C. 200 and 400 BPM
   D. 140 and 160 BPM

3. The ventricular response is usually between:
   A. 100 and 300 BPM
   B. 200 and 300 BPM
   C. 200 and 400 BPM
   D. 140 and 160 BPM

4. The atrial complexes in atrial flutter are known by two names: _____ or _____.

5. The baseline between the F waves can be isoelectric for short periods of time. True or False.

6. Atrial flutter involves the formation of a _____ circuit in the _____ atrium.

7. Part of the criteria for any reentry circuit is an area of slower conduction. This area slows the impulse just enough to allow the original depolarization site time to repolarize and be ready to fire again. True or False.

8. Normal AV nodal conduction rates in atrial flutter include:
   A. 2:1
   B. 3:1
   C. 4:1
   D. 6:1
   E. All of the above

9. When discussing atrial flutter, we usually use the term block rather than conduction to signify that the AV node is functioning normally but blocking the impulse from going through to the ventricles. True or False.

10. Most of the direct causes of atrial flutter can be summed up in the mnemonic ____ ____ ____.

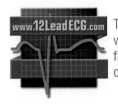

To enhance the knowledge you gain in this book, access this text's website at www.12leadECG.com! This valuable resource provides flashcards, an online glossary, web links, and more. Simply click on the Arrhythmias book cover once at the site.

CHAPTER 20

Atrial Fibrillation

General Information

Atrial fibrillation (Afib) is one of the most common arrhythmias you will run across in your clinical practice. Afib affects millions of people. In addition to the hemodynamic consequences of the arrhythmia, atrial fibrillation is a leading cause of debilitating and deadly strokes. The prevalence in our society increases with age, making Afib even more of a health concern as the "baby boomer" generation continues to age.

Atrial fibrillation is an irregularly irregular rhythm that is marked by an absence of observable P waves (Figure 20-1). Atrial activity in atrial fibrillation is electrocardiographically represented by a continuous, randomly occurring series of oscillations known as *fibrillatory* or *f waves*. These waves are best seen in lead V_1. The f wave rates are typically between 400 and 700 BPM, and the ventricular response can be variable, involving the entire spectrum from bradycardia to very fast tachycardias. Clinically, atrial fibrillation is characterized by a lack of organized atrial activity and the accompanying loss of the atrial kick. The arrhythmia can be further classified as either paroxysmal, persistent, or permanent.

Paroxysmal atrial fibrillation occurs acutely. The patient's episodes are usually very short lived, lasting anywhere from a few seconds to a few days. In many cases, the rhythm may actually spontaneously convert back and forth between atrial fibrillation and sinus rhythm. The symptoms of paroxysmal atrial fibrillation are usually more pronounced, compared with the persistent or permanent subtypes, because compensatory mechanisms are usually not in play during acute episodes. The sudden hemodynamic compromise and rapid pulmonary fluid buildup associated with paroxysmal episodes cause the patient to experience acute shortness of breath, congestive heart failure, light-headedness, palpitations, syncope, and other disabling complications. In many cases, these symptoms spontaneously resolve with termination of the arrhythmia.

Persistent atrial fibrillation refers to a chronic form of the arrhythmia, but one that can still be converted using either pharmacologic means or cardioversion. Permanent atrial fibrillation, on the other hand, is a chronic, stable form of the arrhythmia that does not lend itself to conversion by any means, or once converted, spontaneously reverts back to a fibrillatory pattern.

How f Waves Are Created

Let's take a closer look at how f waves are made. Figure 20-2 shows a section of atrial myocardium during atrial fibrillation. Typically, there are multiple ectopic pacemakers all firing at the same time. The typical number of ectopic foci can be anywhere from the single digits to many tens of sites. These sites are in a constant struggle over which one will dominate.

It is important to make a distinction between F waves and f waves. F waves are the flutter waves seen in *atrial flutter*. The f waves we are talking about in this chapter refer to fibrillatory waves that are found in *atrial fibrillation*.

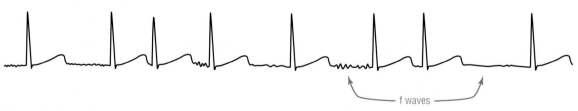

Figure 20-1: Atrial fibrillation.

As each focus fires, it causes the surrounding area of atrial myocardium to depolarize. Slowly, a localized depolarization *wavelet* begins to develop. They are called wavelets because they are very small and never become larger waves. These localized depolarization wavelets never make it big because they crash into the refractory areas created by the surrounding wavelets from other foci. Since each wavelet affects only a small amount of myocardium, they barely make a blip on the ECG strip. These wavelets, therefore, are the source of

the vectors that are represented on the ECG strip as the f waves.

As you can imagine, the amount of atrial tissue involved dictates the size of the vector produced by any one wavelet. If there are only a few ectopic pacemakers causing the atrial fibrillation, then the amount of tissue involved (and their resulting vectors) will be bigger. The larger vectors cause larger f waves to appear on the ECG, resulting in a type of fibrillation known as *coarse atrial fibrillation* (Figure 20-3). If there are many ectopic

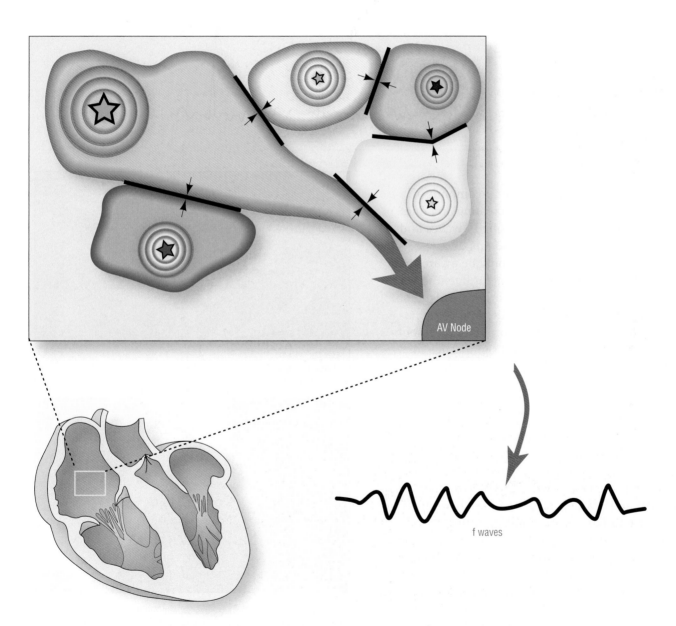

Figure 20-2: In the atrial tissue there could be many, many individual ectopic foci acting as pacemakers at the same time. Most of these small islands of depolarization throughout the atria cancel each other out. These depolarization "wavelets," however, create a small vector that shows up on the ECG strip as minimal deflections from the baseline. Since there are between 400 and 700 wavelets per minute, the resulting electrocardiographic changes are very small waves, known as f waves, which occur completely at random throughout the baseline.

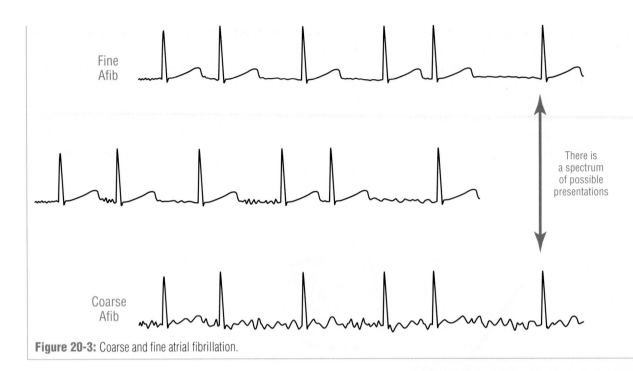

Fine Afib

Coarse Afib

There is a spectrum of possible presentations

Figure 20-3: Coarse and fine atrial fibrillation.

pacemakers causing the rhythm, then the amount of tissue (and their vectors) involved in creating any one wavelet will be smaller. This leads to small f waves and *fine atrial fibrillation*. Some authors also talk about medium atrial fibrillation, but you should be aware that fibrillation can be anything from a straight line to a very aggressive random f wave pattern. In other words, there can be an entire spectrum of possibilities and combinations that can develop with f wave morphology. Present-day thought is that there is no clinical significance to the type of f waves involved.

Ventricular Response

As we saw, the atrial rate is actually somewhere between 400 and 700 BPM. If the ventricles responded on a 1:1 conduction (as can occur in someone with an accessory pathway), the result would be catastrophic. Luckily, the AV node cannot respond in a 1:1 conduction to the constant barrage of impulses hitting it from the atrial wavelets. Figure 20-3 showed a small section of atrial tissue with various wavelets competing for control. In that example, the red wavelet was able to weave its way through the quagmire of refractory tissue and eventually reached the AV node. That red depolarization wave, however, is not going to trigger a ventricular depolarization. Can you figure out why?

Each depolarization wavelet that manages to survive has to compete for control over the AV node (Figure 20-4). Remember, there can be any number of depolarization wavelets hitting the AV node at any one

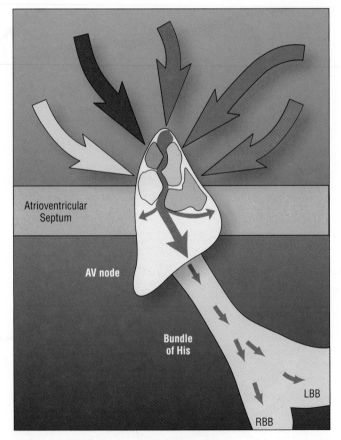

Atrioventricular Septum

AV node

Bundle of His

LBB

RBB

Figure 20-4: This diagram shows five depolarization waves headed toward the AV node at the same time. Each of the waves enters the AV node and begins to depolarize the node. The blue, pink, green, and yellow waves cancel each other out. They cancel each other out because they hit a "wall" of refractory tissue caused by one of the other waves. The red wave hits the AV node, and is able to weave its way through the refractory tissue and effectively depolarizes the distal node. The impulse is then conducted through the rest of the electrical conduction system as usual, leading to a normal-width QRS complex.

time. When these wavelets reach the AV node, they will depolarize a small area of AV nodal tissue, causing their own little refractory sections. Eventually, one wavelet will manage to weave its way through and reach the main area of the AV node. Then, and only then, will the AV node fire and trigger off a ventricular response. This process is variable, and which wavelet will eventually reach the main area of the AV node will be completely random. This randomness reflects exactly how the ventricular response will occur—completely at random.

Other factors also affect the conduction of the impulse through the AV node. The most common problem is intrinsic disease of the AV node itself or the electrical conduction system. Almost all patients with atrial fibrillation have some form of structural heart disease. Age and time-related wear-and-tear on the heart are the most common precipitating factors in the arrhythmia. Left atrial enlargement is another major precipitating factor in the formation and stability of the arrhythmia.

The state of the autonomic nervous system will also greatly affect conduction rates and the irritability of the AV node. Sympathetic stimulation increases the ventricular response and parasympathetic stimulation slows the ventricular response. Finally, drugs can greatly affect conduction through the AV node. Amiodarone, digitalis, beta-blockers, and calcium channel blockers all slow the ventricular response to atrial fibrillation.

The average ventricular response in the *untreated* patient is between 100 and 200 BPM. The term *uncontrolled* or *decompensated* atrial fibrillation is commonly used to describe patients with rates between 100 and 200 BPM, to differentiate this state from the *controlled* state. Ventricular responses that are below 100 BPM are referred to as controlled. Treatment, advanced AV nodal disease, and the chronic state of the arrhythmia all help to slow down ventricular response to the clinically preferred controlled rates.

Clinical Implications

Due to the large amount of wavelets occurring in the atria, there is no organized contraction of the atrial tissue. In fact, a visual inspection of a fibrillating atria resembles a mold made of Jell-O™ in the shape of the atria. The atrial myocardium is just simply trembling uncontrollably, or fibrillating, and does not add the atrial kick to super fill the ventricles. Acutely, as mentioned before, many patients cannot compensate for this drop in stroke volume. This alteration in the stroke volume can lead to clinical symptoms and some level of hemodynamic compromise, ranging from mild to severe.

Since cardiac output is equal to stroke volume times the rate, you can imagine what happens when the ventricular rate is also affected. The faster the rate, the less the filling time. The less the filling time, the lower the stroke volume. The lower the stroke volume, the lower the cardiac output.

As you can imagine, the hemodynamic compromise that can be seen in uncontrolled Afib is multifactorial. The rapid ventricular rates, the irregularity of the ventricular response, the loss of the atrial kick, and the presence of significant structural heart disease, either singly or cumulatively, will affect the hemodynamic status of your patient. Uncontrolled rates in Afib can pose a serious, and sometimes deadly, problem for you and your patient. Rate control is essential to clinical management.

We will not be covering treatment in this book in any great detail, but we highly encourage you to study the clinical management of atrial fibrillation, and its inherent complications and implications, quite thoroughly. Management of these patients can be quite difficult and difficult to maintain. If your patient is in life-threatening hemodynamic compromise, electrical cardioversion or defibrillation may need to be attempted. If the patient converts to sinus rhythm, that's great—just be aware that he could revert back into Afib at any time. If your unstable patient does not convert with cardioversion, then pharmacologic means of controlling the rate and blood pressure may be your only option.

If your patient is somewhat hemodynamically competent, converting the patient to sinus rhythm is still an admirable goal; however, unless the patient is definitely in the acute phase, there is a danger of breaking off an atrial clot and causing a catastrophic stroke to develop. It is like jumping from the frying pan into the fire. Slowing or controlling the ventricular response should actually be your primary goal in these cases. If you slow the rate and control the hemodynamic response, you can have some time to thoroughly assess your patient and determine the best course of further action. Chemical or electrical cardioversion can then be approached logically, and sequentially, once appropriate anticoagulation has been established and the threat of embolic stroke is reduced.

Regular Ventricular Response in Atrial Fibrillation

What happens when you see definite f waves and you have a regular ventricular response? Well, it could be a junctional rhythm (discussed in the next section) with some artifact or it could still be atrial fibrillation. Could Afib be regular? The answer is yes. However, this would not be just simple atrial fibrillation. It would be atrial fibrillation with either pharmacologically, autonomically, anatomically, or ischemically created AV block. We will be addressing the various AV blocks in detail in Chapter 35, but you already possess the knowledge necessary to figure out the problem. Let's go through it and try to reason out this clinical possibility.

What would happen if the AV node completely shut down conduction and communication between the atria and the ventricles? Some junctional or ventricular pacemaker would take over pacemaking functions and the result would be an escape rhythm. The escape rhythm would have either a junctional or ventricular morphology and would be *regular* and slow. That is exactly what happens in these patients. You have the presence of f waves and atrial fibrillation with a regular ventricular response due to either a junctional or ventricular escape rhythm.

Figure 20-5 is an example of an atrial fibrillation with a junctional escape rhythm. Note the presence of a coarse atrial fibrillation between the taller QRS complexes. The QRS complexes are less than 0.12 seconds, making them a supraventricular complex. The rate is around 53 BPM, which is compatible with a junctional pacemaker.

Whenever you see a regular ventricular response in a patient with atrial fibrillation, you need to think of the possible causes for this abnormal response. These include:

1. Atrioventricular block: Pathological, ischemia related, or due to drugs
2. Enhanced automaticity of the Purkinje system
3. Flutter-fibrillation pattern

We have already reviewed how an AV block can cause normalization of the ventricular response. Now, let's turn our attention to the other two causes.

If the Purkinje system is stimulated by any means (e.g., sympathetic activity, drugs), the Purkinje system may fire at a rate above the rate at which the atrial fibrillation is being conducted through the AV node. The result would be that the Purkinje system would be faster and would take over the primary pacemaking function for the heart. Now, when an impulse was normally conducted through the AV node, it would find the conduction system and the ventricle in a refractory state and the conducted depolarization wave would simply fizzle out. This "over-drive" by the Purkinje system could normalize the ventricular response in the presence of the atrial fibrillation.

Flutter-fibrillation pattern refers to the fact that atrial flutter will frequently convert spontaneously into atrial fibrillation and vice versa. This is especially true in patients who are having a paroxysmal or persistent pattern of atrial fibrillation. Many strips will show a patient waxing and waning back and forth between the two arrhythmias, with normalization of the regularity during periods of atrial flutter.

The Morphology of the Complexes in Atrial Fibrillation

The QRS Complex in Atrial Fibrillation

The QRS complex is usually a normal width in patients with atrial fibrillation. This is because the conduction of the impulse occurs normally from the AV node and beyond. The conduction down the electrical conduction system leads to nice, tight QRS complexes with normal morphology.

Wide complexes can occur in atrial fibrillation because of an underlying chronic bundle branch block, aberrancy, or electrolyte abnormalities. In addition, we saw how escape rhythms can develop in patients with AV nodal block and how enhanced automaticity of the Purkinje system can normalize the ventricular response. Remember, if the complex originated in a ventricular foci, including the Purkinje system, the result would be an aberrant, wide QRS complex.

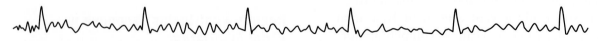

Figure 20-5: Atrial fibrillation with a junctional escape rhythm. In order for this to occur, there has to be no communication present between the atria and the section of the AV node that is acting as the primary pacemaker in this case.

Ashman's Phenomenon

While we're on the topic of regularity, irregularity, and the morphology of the QRS complex, we should review a particular set of circumstances that alters the appearance of an occasional QRS complex in a patient with Afib. It is a situation known as *Ashman's phenomenon*.

As we saw in Chapter 5, when comparing the two bundle branches, the right bundle branch has a longer period of time during which it remains refractory to a subsequent impulse. Therefore, the right bundle branch is the one that will probably "be caught with its pants down" when a premature impulse comes along. That is why most aberrantly conducted complexes have a right bundle branch block pattern.

What we did not mention before, however, is that this refractory period is even longer when the complexes are farther apart on the ECG, that is, they occur at a slower rate. To understand what we mean by that statement, let's go back to the "caught with its pants

down" comment. When the rate of conduction is slow, the right bundle branch lets its guard down, climbs up on the hammock, and begins to take a snooze. It does this because it knows that it has awhile to go before the next impulse arrives and it is forced to go back to work. Suddenly, a premature impulse comes along ahead of schedule. The right bundle branch has to wake up and climb off the hammock before it can even begin to put its pants back on and conduct the impulse. That is just too long for a complex to wait. Instead, the electrical impulse moves around the right bundle branch and the aberrancy in conduction develops.

Ashman's phenomenon refers to the process by which a premature complex is more likely going to be transmitted aberrantly immediately after a long pause with a long R-R interval (Figure 20-6). To put it another way, if you have a long interval followed immediately by a short interval (a premature complex), the premature complex will more likely be conducted aberrantly.

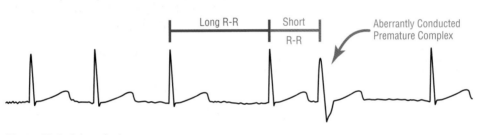

Figure 20-6: Ashman's phenomenon.

QRS morphology may vary slightly throughout a strip of atrial fibrillation because of fusion with the underlying f waves and aberrancy. This problem is especially noticeable in coarse Afib, where the larger vectors produced by larger wavelets will affect the appearance of the complexes.

ST Segments and T Waves

The ST segments and T waves in Afib usually follow their normal pattern. The fusion with the underlying f waves, however, is more pronounced. In fact, there are many strips of coarse Afib where the ST segments and/or the T waves are completely obscured.

A D D I T I O N A L   **I N F O R M A T I O N**

Digitalis Effect

There is one specific kind of ST segment change that we should review at this point because of the frequency with which it occurs in Afib—that is the changes caused by digitalis. Digitalis, and its family of medications, is frequently used for rate control in Afib. Toxicity is associated with various forms of arrhythmias, most notably ectopic atrial tachycardia with block (although this is not the most commonly seen arrhythmia in dig toxicity) and a variety of clinical signs and symptoms. The ST-T wave changes that we will be discussing here appear even in the absence of toxicity.

Digitalis commonly causes a scooping or ladle-like appearance to the ST segments. Traditionally, the term "scooped-out" appearance is used because the ST segments look like the indentation made when you scoop out some ice cream (Figure 20-7). It also looks like a ladle (Figure 20-8). Whatever your preference, the key thing is that when you see a scooped out segment on someone in Afib, you should think of *digitalis effect*.

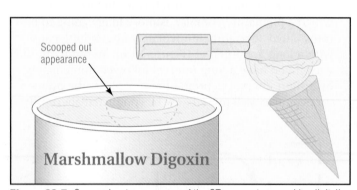

Figure 20-7: Scooped-out appearance of the ST segments caused by digitalis effect.

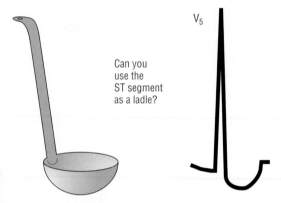

Figure 20-8: Ladle-like appearance of the ST segments caused by digitalis effect.

ARRHYTHMIA **RECOGNITION**

Atrial Fibrillation

Rate:	f waves: 400 to 700 BPM
	Ventricular: Variable
Regularity:	Irregularly irregular
P wave:	Absent!
Morphology:	Not applicable
Upright in II, III, and aVF:	Not applicable
P:QRS ratio:	Not applicable
PR interval:	Not applicable
QRS width:	Normal
Grouping:	None
Dropped beats:	None

DIFFERENTIAL **DIAGNOSIS**

Atrial Fibrillation

1. Atrial enlargement (especially left)
2. Age
3. MAD RAT PPP (see mnemonic below)
4. Idiopathic (or lone atrial fibrillation)

Atrial fibrillation is very dependent on left atrial size. When the left atrial mass exceeds a certain limit, the arrhythmia is more common. Likewise, maintenance of the rhythm and chronicity is based on left atrial size. Age is the next determinant. The list above is not inclusive of all possible causes.

Atrial Fibrillation/Flutter:

Myocardial infarction	**R**heumatic heart disease
Atherosclerosis	**A**lcoholic holiday heart
Drugs: digoxin	**T**hyrotoxicosis

Pulmonary emboli
Pericarditis
Pneumonia: Right middle lobe

ECG Strips

ECG 20-1

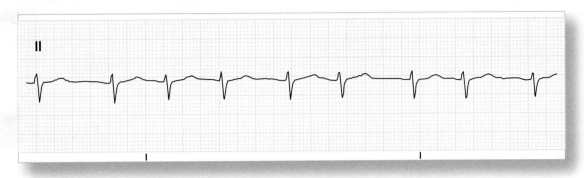

Rate:	Atrial: None Ventricular: About 90 BPM	PR intervals:	Not applicable
Regularity:	Irregularly irregular	QRS width:	Normal

P waves:
  Morphology:
  Axis:
	f waves present
	f waves
	Not applicable
		Grouping:	None

		Dropped beats:	Not applicable
P:QRS ratio:	Not applicable	Rhythm:	**Atrial fibrillation**

Discussion:

The strip above shows the typical changes of atrial fibrillation: lack of P waves and an irregularly irregular ventricular response. Note that the f waves are present but they are very fine, almost a straight line in appearance. Perhaps the f waves would be more easily demonstrated in another lead. The QRS complexes are normal in appearance and narrow, well within the normal limits for the QRS interval. The ST segments and T waves all appear normal.

ECG 20-2

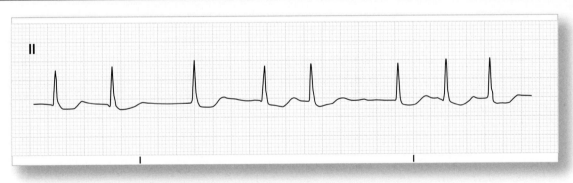

Rate:	Atrial: None Ventricular: About 90 BPM	PR intervals:	Not applicable
Regularity:	Irregularly irregular	QRS width:	Normal

P waves:
  Morphology:
  Axis:
	f waves present
	f waves
	Not applicable
		Grouping:	None

		Dropped beats:	Not applicable
P:QRS ratio:	Not applicable	Rhythm:	**Atrial fibrillation**

Discussion:

This strip shows an irregularly irregular rhythm and no visible P waves. This is another typical example of atrial fibrillation. Some slight morphological differences between the QRS complexes are frequently seen in Afib. The ST segments are depressed and have some scooping visible. However, they are not your typical digitalis-effect scooping ST segments. Ischemia is another dangerous possibility. Clinical correlation is indicated.

ECG 20-3

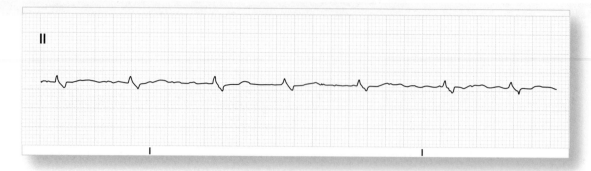

Rate:	Atrial: None Ventricular: About 80 BPM	PR intervals:	Not applicable
Regularity:	Irregularly irregular	QRS width:	Wide
P waves: Morphology: Axis:	f waves present f waves Not applicable	Grouping:	None
		Dropped beats:	Not applicable
P:QRS ratio:	Not applicable	Rhythm:	**Atrial fibrillation**

Discussion:

The strip above shows a more defined f wave pattern and no obvious or recurrent changes that could be interpreted as P waves. The ventricular rhythm is irregularly irregular making this an atrial fibrillation rhythm. What about the ventricular response—do you notice anything unusual? The QRS complexes are wider than 0.12 seconds. The rate is not too fast, so aberrancy is probably not likely. Ventricular escape would result in a regular rhythm; this is also unlikely. A preexisting bundle branch block is your best reason for the wide complexes.

ECG 20-4

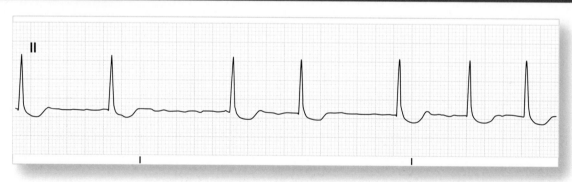

Rate:	Atrial: None Ventricular: About 70 BPM	PR intervals:	Not applicable
Regularity:	Irregularly irregular	QRS width:	Normal
P waves: Morphology: Axis:	f waves present f waves Not applicable	Grouping:	None
		Dropped beats:	Not applicable
P:QRS ratio:	Not applicable	Rhythm:	**Atrial fibrillation**

Discussion:

The rhythm strip above is for the classic patient in atrial fibrillation with the rate controlled by digitalis. The digitalis effect is obvious and appears to be the classic scooped-out or ladle-like appearance. There is a fine f wave pattern visible on the strip, and the irregularly irregular ventricular response is evident.

ECG 20-5

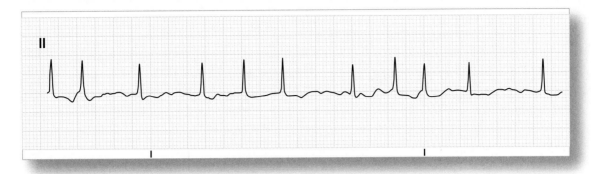

Rate:	Atrial: None Ventricular: About 100 BPM	PR intervals:	Not applicable
Regularity:	Irregularly irregular	QRS width:	Normal

P waves:
  Morphology:
  Axis:
	f waves present
	f waves
	Not applicable
		Grouping:	None

		Dropped beats:	Not applicable
P:QRS ratio:	Not applicable	Rhythm:	**Atrial fibrillation**

Discussion:

This rhythm strip shows the changes expected in atrial fibrillation. In addition, you will notice the QRS, ST segment, and T wave morphological variations we mentioned before due to fusion. In this case, it is not only fusion with the f waves but fusion with each other. The f waves are present in a coarser pattern than we have seen so far in the other strips

ECG 20-6

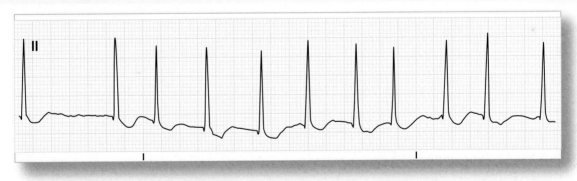

Rate:	Atrial: None Ventricular: About 110 BPM	PR intervals:	Not applicable
Regularity:	Irregularly irregular	QRS width:	Normal

P waves:
  Morphology:
  Axis:
	f waves present
	f waves
	Not applicable
		Grouping:	None

		Dropped beats:	Not applicable
P:QRS ratio:	Not applicable	Rhythm:	**Atrial fibrillation**

Discussion:

This strip also shows your typical atrial fibrillation pattern with an irregularly irregular pattern and no visible P waves. There is some pretty wide variation in the R-R intervals throughout the strip. This makes the rate a bit more troublesome to calculate. Remember, take the number of complexes in a 6-second strip and multiply that number by 10 to get your answer. Some authors simply give the ranges from the slowest to the fastest rates. Either way is OK, and each has its merits.

ECG 20·7

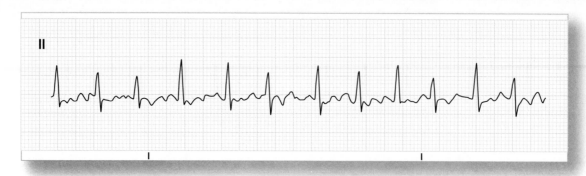

Rate:	Atrial: None Ventricular: About 130+ BPM	PR intervals:	Not applicable
Regularity:	Irregularly irregular	QRS width:	Normal

P waves:
    Morphology:
    Axis:
	f waves present
	f waves
	Not applicable
		Grouping:	None

		Dropped beats:	Not applicable
P:QRS ratio:	Not applicable	Rhythm:	**Atrial fibrillation**

Discussion:

The strip above shows an irregularly irregular rhythm with an uncontrolled, coarse Afib pattern. There is a bit more variation in the QRS morphology in this strip. This could be due to fusion of the QRS complexes with the coarse Afib or aberrancy (rate-related or an atypical Ashman's phenomenon). Coarse Afib is more difficult to evaluate than fine Afib because many of the randomly occurring f waves may appear to be P waves or T waves. Calipers are an invaluable tool in these cases.

ECG 20·8

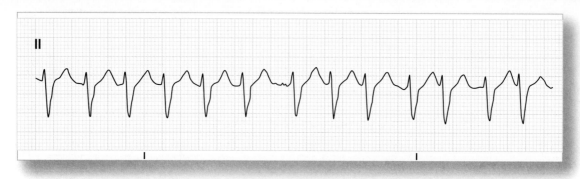

Rate:	Atrial: None Ventricular: About 140 BPM	PR intervals:	Not applicable
Regularity:	Irregularly irregular	QRS width:	Wide

P waves:
    Morphology:
    Axis:
	f waves present
	f waves
	Not applicable
		Grouping:	None

		Dropped beats:	Not applicable
P:QRS ratio:	Not applicable	Rhythm:	**Atrial fibrillation**

Discussion:

Is this uncomplicated Afib? There is some normalization of the QRS rate at the onset of the rhythm, and this breaks down into a random pattern as the strip continues. This patient has typical flutter-fibrillation pattern. At the onset of the strip, the patient has a recurrent R-R interval at about 140 BPM. There are no visible flutter waves, but you can assume they are there. The rhythm breaks down into Afib as the arrhythmia continues. Strips from other leads may help tremendously in diagnosing the rhythm.

ECG 20-9

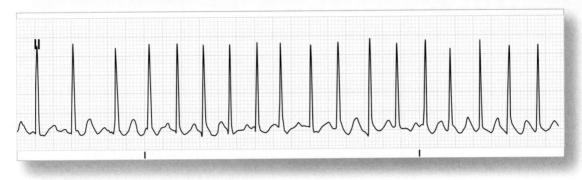

Rate:	Atrial: None Ventricular: About 200+ BPM	PR intervals:	Not applicable
Regularity:	Irregularly irregular	QRS width:	Normal

P waves:
  Morphology:
  Axis:
	f waves present
	f waves
	Not applicable
		Grouping:	None

		Dropped beats:	Not applicable
P:QRS ratio:	Not applicable	Rhythm:	**Atrial fibrillation**

Discussion:

This is one fast arrhythmia! It is a narrow-complex tachycardia above 200 BPM. The most important thing in the differential diagnosis is the irregularity of the rhythm. As a matter of fact, it is completely irregularly irregular.

This is uncontrolled atrial fibrillation. The faster an Afib becomes, the greater the chance of an accessory pathway being involved. You always need to consider that possibility in any patient with Afib over 200 BPM.

ECG 20-10

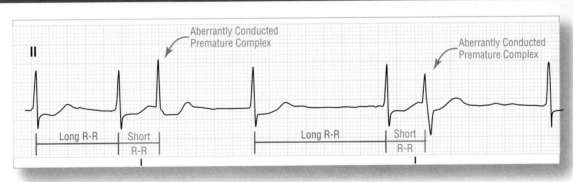

Rate:	Atrial: None Ventricular: About 70 BPM	PR intervals:	Not applicable
Regularity:	Irregularly irregular	QRS width:	Normal

P waves:
  Morphology:
  Axis:
	f waves present
	f waves
	Not applicable
		Grouping:	None

		Dropped beats:	Not applicable
P:QRS ratio:	Not applicable	Rhythm:	**Atrial fibrillation**

Discussion:

The rhythm is atrial fibrillation. There are no obvious P waves throughout the strip, a fine f wave pattern, and irregularly irregular pattern. There is some aberrancy caused by Ashman's phenomenon present on the ECG, with the third and sixth complexes being aberrantly conducted. Note that there is the classic Ashman's pattern of a long cycle followed by aberrancy during the short cycle. The two aberrant complexes have different morphologies because the refractory area was different in both cases.

CHAPTER REVIEW

1. Atrial fibrillation is an _____ _____ rhythm (refers to cadence) and is marked by an absence of _____.

2. In atrial fibrillation, electrical activity in the atria is referred to as (circle all that are correct):
   A. F waves
   B. f waves
   C. Flutter waves
   D. Fibrillatory waves

3. The rates for the f waves in Afib are between:
   A. 100 and 200 BPM
   B. 150 and 350 BPM
   C. 300 and 500 BPM
   D. 400 and 700 BPM

4. In atrial fibrillation, the atrial tissue has many ectopic foci firing at the same time. The result is the formation of small depolarization areas or wavelets that each give rise to their own small vector. These vectors form the pattern of the f waves on the ECG strip. True or False.

5. Clinically speaking, the type of f wave pattern (fine or coarse) is critical to treatment. True or False.

6. In the AV node during atrial fibrillation, there are multiple depolarization waves striking the surface at any one time. These sometimes cancel each other out, leaving only one to conduct the impulse to the ventricles. True or False.

7. Uncontrolled Afib usually occurs at a ventricular rate of _____ and _____ BPM.

8. The ventricular response to atrial fibrillation is *always* irregularly irregular. True or False.

9. Complete AV block can occur in patients with Afib. True or False.

10. Ashman's phenomenon refers to a pattern where a premature complex is transmitted aberrantly if it occurs after a long cycle. In other words, if you have a _____ cycle length, followed by a _____ cycle length, the complex that belonged to the short cycle will usually be conducted aberrantly.

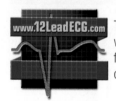

To enhance the knowledge you gain in this book, access this text's website at www.12leadECG.com! This valuable resource provides flashcards, an online glossary, web links, and more. Simply click on the Arrhythmias book cover once at the site.

Self-Test

Test ECG 1

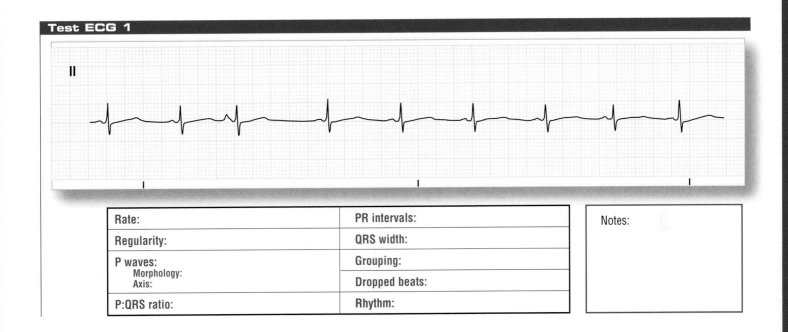

Rate:	PR intervals:
Regularity:	QRS width:

P waves:
    Morphology:
    Axis:
	Grouping:
	
	 Dropped beats:

P:QRS ratio:	Rhythm:

Notes:

Test ECG 2

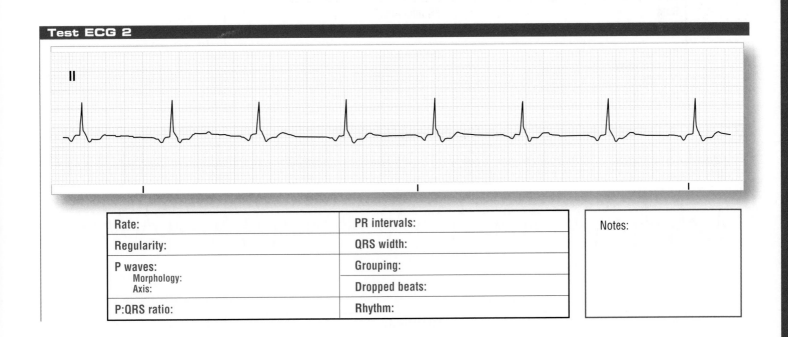

Rate:	PR intervals:
Regularity:	QRS width:

P waves:
    Morphology:
    Axis:
	Grouping:
	
	 Dropped beats:

P:QRS ratio:	Rhythm:

Notes:

Test ECG 3

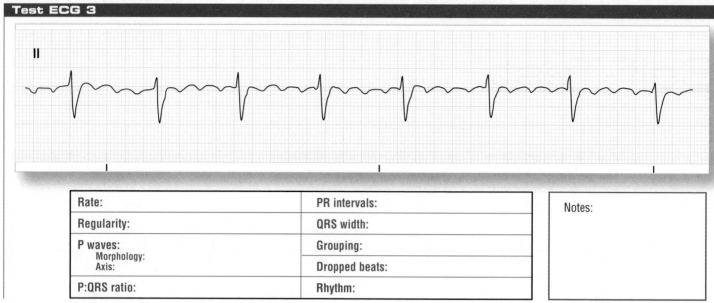

Rate:		PR intervals:	Notes:
Regularity:		QRS width:	
P waves:		Grouping:	
Morphology:			
Axis:		Dropped beats:	
P:QRS ratio:		Rhythm:	

Test ECG 4

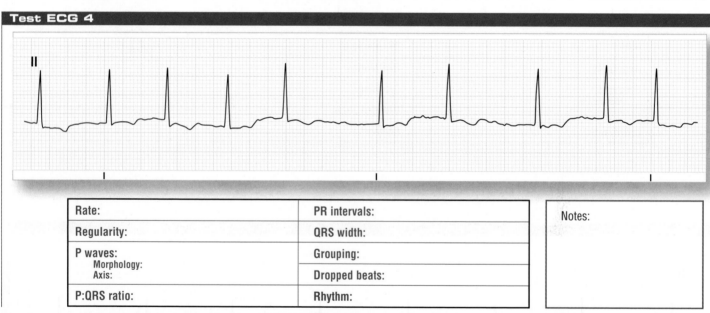

Rate:		PR intervals:	Notes:
Regularity:		QRS width:	
P waves:		Grouping:	
Morphology:			
Axis:		Dropped beats:	
P:QRS ratio:		Rhythm:	

Test ECG 5

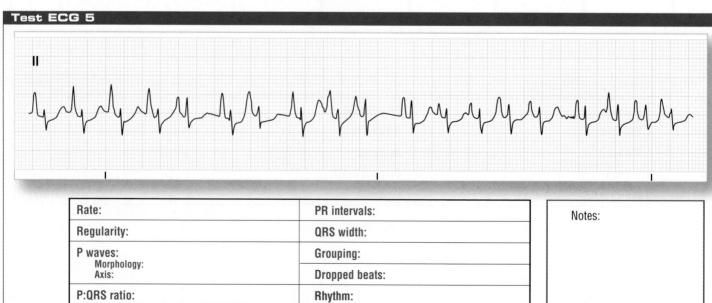

Rate:		PR intervals:	Notes:
Regularity:		QRS width:	
P waves:		Grouping:	
Morphology:			
Axis:		Dropped beats:	
P:QRS ratio:		Rhythm:	

Test ECG 6

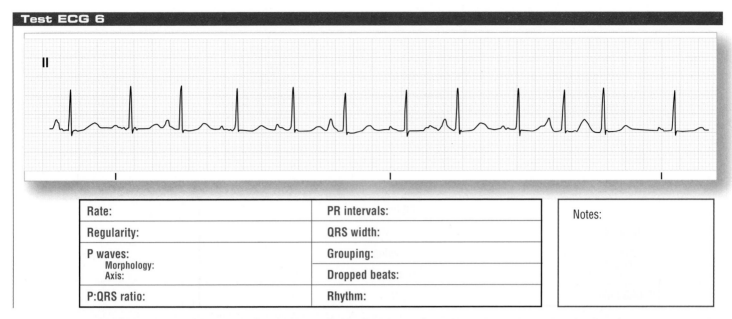

Rate:	PR intervals:	Notes:
Regularity:	QRS width:	
P waves:	Grouping:	
Morphology:		
Axis:	Dropped beats:	
P:QRS ratio:	Rhythm:	

Test ECG 7

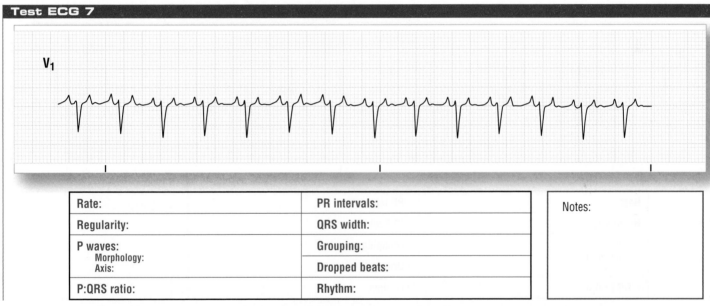

Rate:	PR intervals:	Notes:
Regularity:	QRS width:	
P waves:	Grouping:	
Morphology:		
Axis:	Dropped beats:	
P:QRS ratio:	Rhythm:	

Test ECG 8

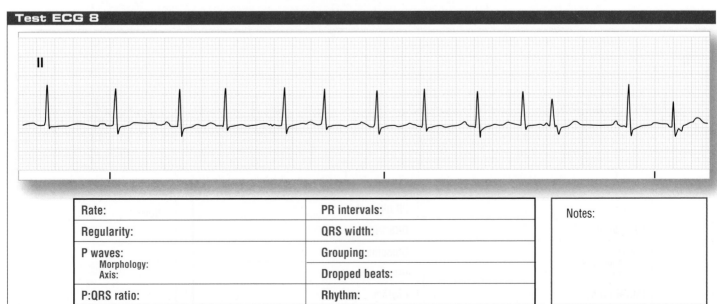

Rate:	PR intervals:	Notes:
Regularity:	QRS width:	
P waves:	Grouping:	
Morphology:		
Axis:	Dropped beats:	
P:QRS ratio:	Rhythm:	

Test ECG 9

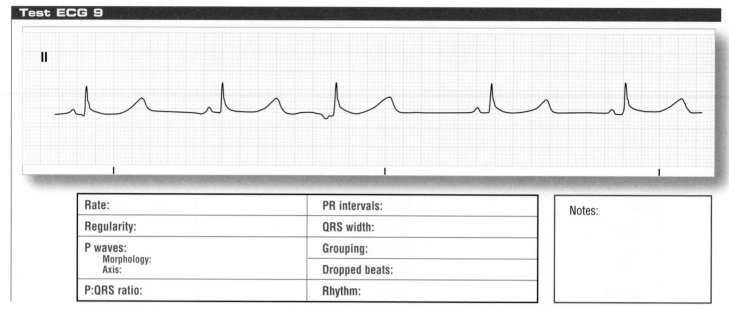

Rate:		PR intervals:
Regularity:		QRS width:
P waves:		Grouping:
Morphology:		Dropped beats:
Axis:		
P:QRS ratio:		Rhythm:

Notes:

Test ECG 10

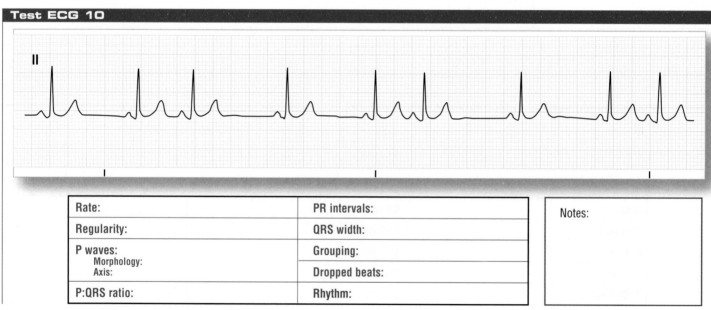

Rate:		PR intervals:
Regularity:		QRS width:
P waves:		Grouping:
Morphology:		Dropped beats:
Axis:		
P:QRS ratio:		Rhythm:

Notes:

Test ECG 11

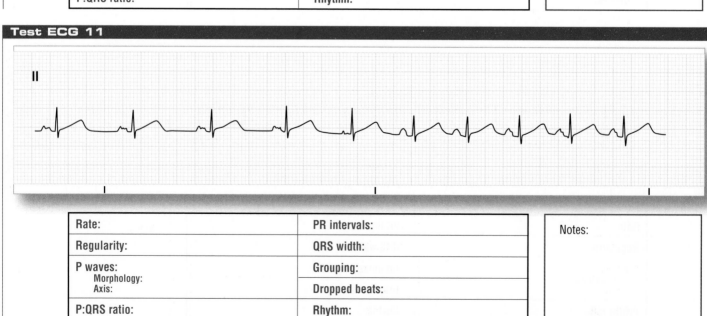

Rate:		PR intervals:
Regularity:		QRS width:
P waves:		Grouping:
Morphology:		Dropped beats:
Axis:		
P:QRS ratio:		Rhythm:

Notes:

Test ECG 12

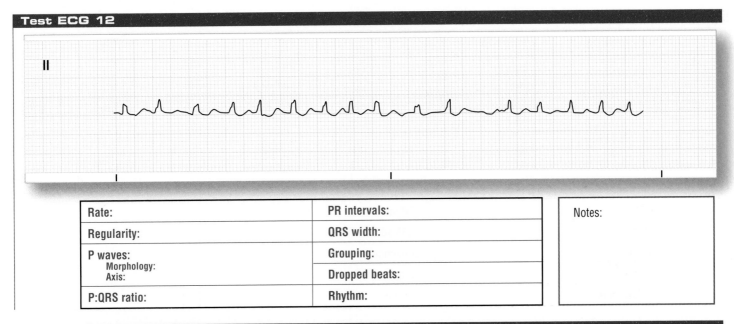

Rate:	PR intervals:	Notes:
Regularity:	QRS width:	

P waves:
    Morphology:
    Axis:
	Grouping:	

	Dropped beats:	
P:QRS ratio:	Rhythm:	

Test ECG 13

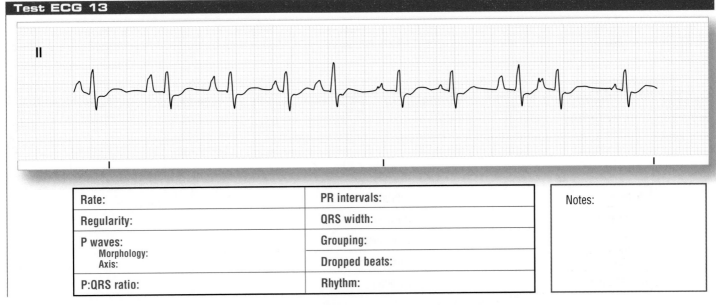

Rate:	PR intervals:	Notes:
Regularity:	QRS width:	

P waves:
    Morphology:
    Axis:
	Grouping:	

	Dropped beats:	
P:QRS ratio:	Rhythm:	

Test ECG 14

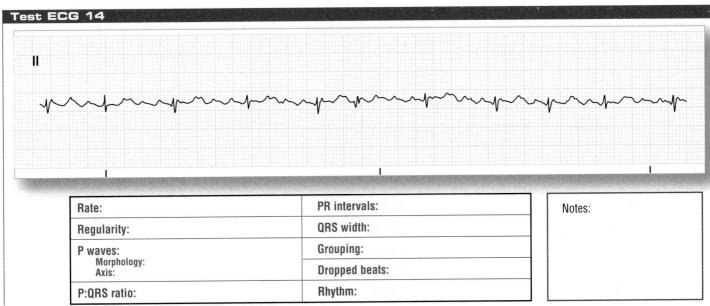

Rate:	PR intervals:	Notes:
Regularity:	QRS width:	

P waves:
    Morphology:
    Axis:
	Grouping:	

	Dropped beats:	
P:QRS ratio:	Rhythm:	

Test ECG 15

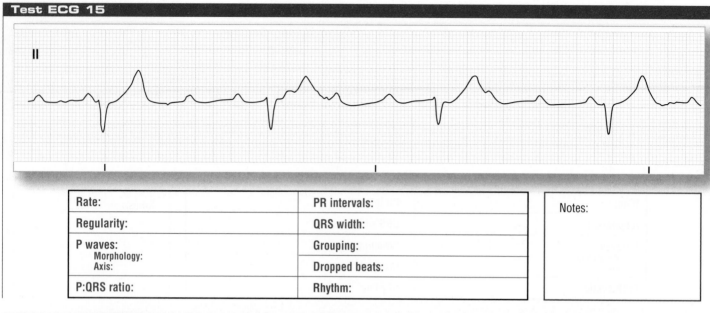

Rate:	PR intervals:	Notes:
Regularity:	QRS width:	
P waves:	Grouping:	
Morphology:		
Axis:	Dropped beats:	
P:QRS ratio:	Rhythm:	

Test ECG 16

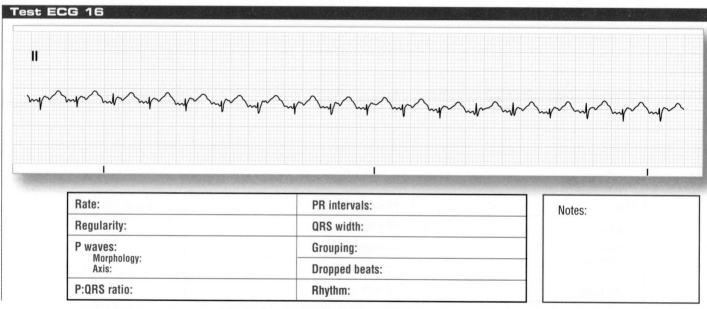

Rate:	PR intervals:	Notes:
Regularity:	QRS width:	
P waves:	Grouping:	
Morphology:		
Axis:	Dropped beats:	
P:QRS ratio:	Rhythm:	

Test ECG 17

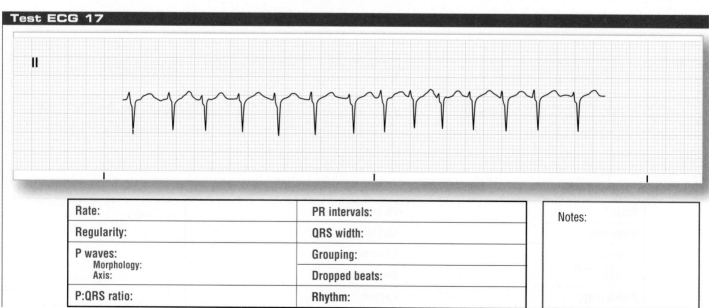

Rate:	PR intervals:	Notes:
Regularity:	QRS width:	
P waves:	Grouping:	
Morphology:		
Axis:	Dropped beats:	
P:QRS ratio:	Rhythm:	

Test ECG 18

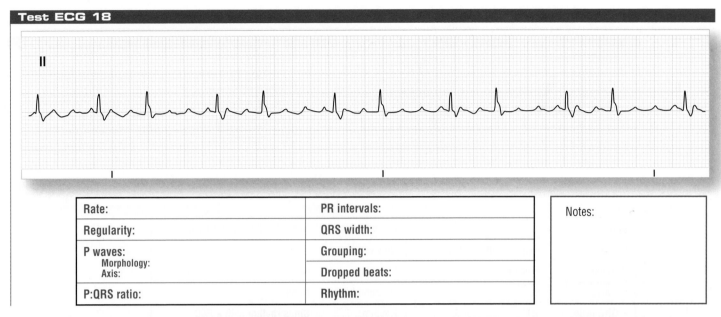

Rate:		PR intervals:		Notes:
Regularity:		QRS width:		

P waves:
    Morphology:
    Axis:
		Grouping:		

		Dropped beats:		
P:QRS ratio:		Rhythm:		

Test ECG 19

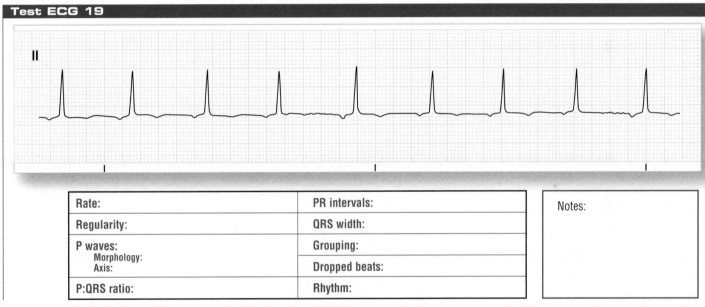

Rate:		PR intervals:		Notes:
Regularity:		QRS width:		

P waves:
    Morphology:
    Axis:
		Grouping:		

		Dropped beats:		
P:QRS ratio:		Rhythm:		

Test ECG 20

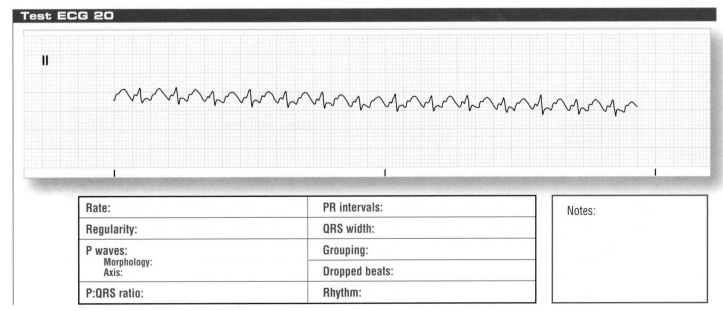

Rate:		PR intervals:		Notes:
Regularity:		QRS width:		

P waves:
    Morphology:
    Axis:
		Grouping:		

		Dropped beats:		
P:QRS ratio:		Rhythm:		

Section 3 Self-Test Answers

Test ECG 1

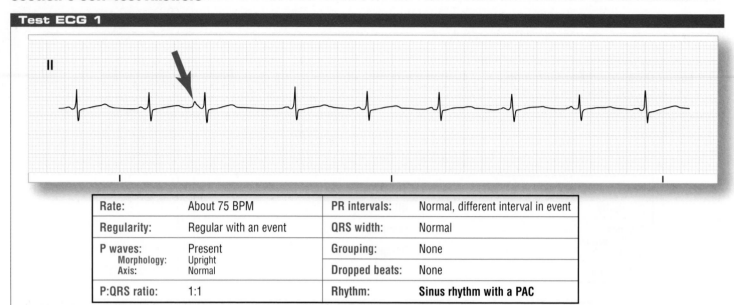

Rate:	About 75 BPM	PR intervals:	Normal, different interval in event
Regularity:	Regular with an event	QRS width:	Normal

P waves:
   Morphology:
   Axis:
	Present
	 Upright
	 Normal
		Grouping:	None

		Dropped beats:	None
P:QRS ratio:	1:1	Rhythm:	**Sinus rhythm with a PAC**

Discussion:

Test ECG 1 shows an underlying sinus rhythm with one PAC (see blue arrow). Note that the morphology of the ectopic P wave is different from the other sinus P waves. The cadence of the underlying sinus rhythm is not affected by the PAC. This happens when the sinus node is not reset by the ectopic beat. This pause, therefore, is a full compensatory pause and is two times the R-R interval of the preceding complexes. It is interesting to note that most PACs are associated with noncompensatory pauses, making this particular case a bit unusual.

Test ECG 2

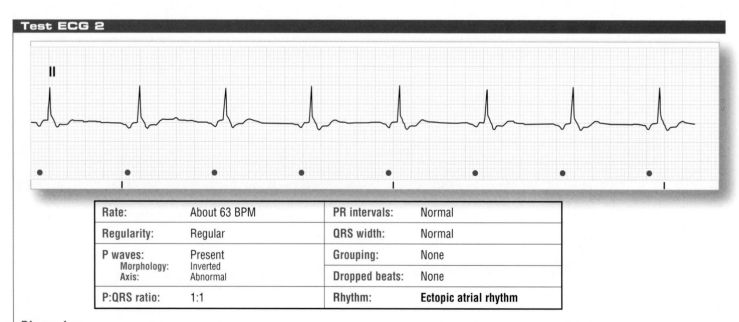

Rate:	About 63 BPM	PR intervals:	Normal
Regularity:	Regular	QRS width:	Normal

P waves:
   Morphology:
   Axis:
	Present
	 Inverted
	 Abnormal
		Grouping:	None

		Dropped beats:	None
P:QRS ratio:	1:1	Rhythm:	**Ectopic atrial rhythm**

Discussion:

The P waves are where the money is on this strip (see blue dots). The P waves are inverted in lead II, which means that the P wave axis is grossly abnormal. The rhythm is about 63 BPM and regular. There is no grouping or dropped beats and the QRS complexes are within the normal range. In these cases, you have one major difficulty: Is this an ectopic atrial rhythm or a junctional rhythm? The main deciding factor that many people use to distinguish between the two is the length of the PR interval. If the PR interval is normal, it is suggestive of an ectopic atrial pacemaker. If the PR interval is short, then a junctional rhythm is more likely. In this case, the PR interval is normal, making the final diagnosis an ectopic atrial rhythm.

Test ECG 3

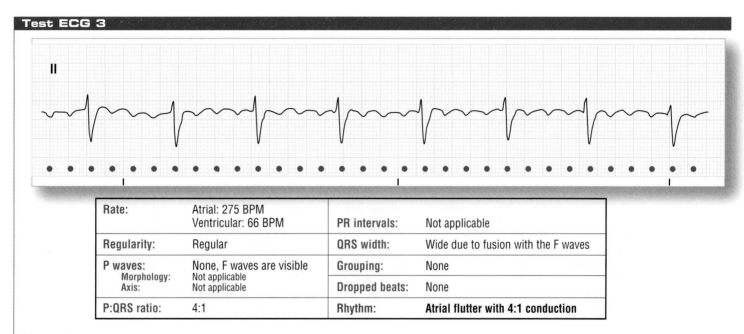

Rate:	Atrial: 275 BPM Ventricular: 66 BPM	PR intervals:	Not applicable
Regularity:	Regular	QRS width:	Wide due to fusion with the F waves

P waves:
    Morphology:
    Axis:
	None, F waves are visible
	Not applicable
	Not applicable
		Grouping:	None

		Dropped beats:	None
P:QRS ratio:	4:1	Rhythm:	**Atrial flutter with 4:1 conduction**

Discussion:

Test ECG 3 shows an obvious flutter wave pattern at the baseline. The F waves are occurring at a rate of about 275 BPM and the ventricular response is about 66 BPM. The conduction ratio is 4:1. Here is an easy way to calculate the conduction ratio in atrial flutter: Take the number of visible F waves and add one to that figure (there is always going to be one F wave buried in the QRS complex). In this case, the morphology of the QRS complex is widened because of an underlying right bundle branch block. But, be careful! The QRS complexes, in some strips, may be widened because of fusion with the underlying F waves, aberrancy, or because of a ventricular escape rhythm. A full 12-lead ECG will help answer the question of bundle branch block or aberrancy, and an old ECG would be invaluable in these cases.

Test ECG 4

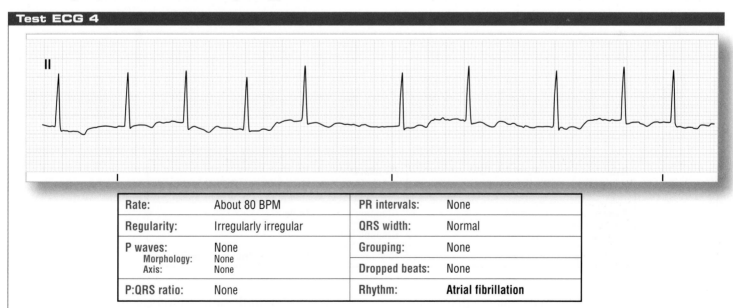

Rate:	About 80 BPM	PR intervals:	None
Regularity:	Irregularly irregular	QRS width:	Normal

P waves:
    Morphology:
    Axis:
	None
	None
	None
		Grouping:	None

		Dropped beats:	None
P:QRS ratio:	None	Rhythm:	**Atrial fibrillation**

Discussion:

This rhythm strip shows an irregularly irregular rhythm occurring at a rate of about 80 BPM. There are no visible P waves anywhere on the strip. Remember, the three main irregularly irregular rhythms are atrial fibrillation, wandering atrial pacemaker, and multifocal atrial tachycardia. WAP and MAT both have P waves. By a process of elimination, the answer is controlled atrial fibrillation. Other possibilities for irregularly irregular rhythms exist, but are not commonly found. These include variable conduction atrial flutter, very frequent premature complexes (usually regularly irregular), and the initial period at the onset of many tachycardias, just to name a few. Other clues will help you out to make the final diagnosis in those cases.

Test ECG 5

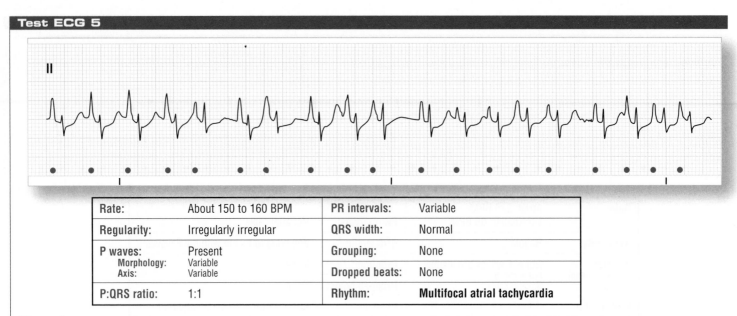

Rate:	About 150 to 160 BPM	PR intervals:	Variable
Regularity:	Irregularly irregular	QRS width:	Normal
P waves: Morphology: Axis:	Present Variable Variable	Grouping:	None
		Dropped beats:	None
P:QRS ratio:	1:1	Rhythm:	**Multifocal atrial tachycardia**

Discussion:

This strip shows some pretty impressive P waves (see blue dots)! They are actually taller than the R wave of the QRS complex. We included this strip to make a point. Sometimes the morphology of a part of the complex will be very unusual and will distract you from the evaluation of the rest of the strip. Just remember, a P wave is a P wave is a P wave. The same applies to the other waves in the complex, as well. In this strip, the rhythm is irregularly irregular and there are varying P wave morphologies (at least three) and PR intervals throughout the entire strip. These criteria are compatible with either multifocal atrial tachycardia or wandering atrial pacemaker. Since the rhythm is a tachycardia, the correct answer is MAT.

Test ECG 6

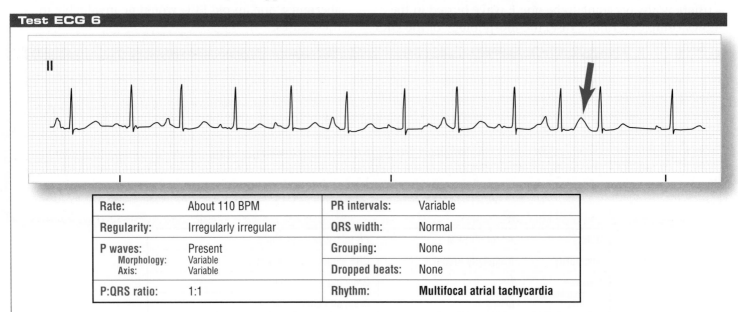

Rate:	About 110 BPM	PR intervals:	Variable
Regularity:	Irregularly irregular	QRS width:	Normal
P waves: Morphology: Axis:	Present Variable Variable	Grouping:	None
		Dropped beats:	None
P:QRS ratio:	1:1	Rhythm:	**Multifocal atrial tachycardia**

Discussion:

Test ECG 6 shows a series of complexes that each contain a P wave and a QRS complex with a 1:1 conduction ratio. The P wave morphology and the PR intervals, however, are constantly changing and there are at least three different P wave morphologies and PR intervals. The cadence of the rhythm is completely irregularly irregular. As we have mentioned before, there are three main irregularly irregular rhythms to consider: Atrial fibrillation, multifocal atrial tachycardia, and wandering atrial pacemaker. Since there are P waves present, we can throw out Afib. The other two rhythms have the same criteria except for the rate. The strip shows a tachycardic rhythm with a rate a little over 110; this means that it has to be multifocal atrial tachycardia. Note the blue arrow, which is pointing out a buried P wave.

Test ECG 7

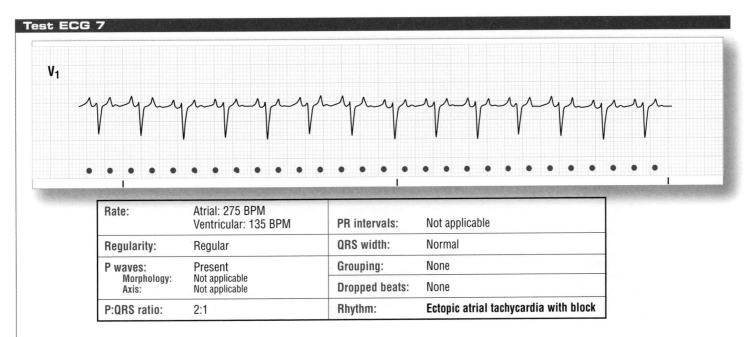

Rate:	Atrial: 275 BPM Ventricular: 135 BPM	PR intervals:	Not applicable
Regularity:	Regular	QRS width:	Normal

P waves:
  Morphology:
  Axis:
	Present
	Not applicable
	Not applicable
		Grouping:	None

		Dropped beats:	None
P:QRS ratio:	2:1	Rhythm:	**Ectopic atrial tachycardia with block**

Discussion:

The rhythm strip above shows a rapid atrial tachycardia at a rate of about 275 BPM. Notice that there is a flat baseline between the atrial complexes in this lead. There is a 2:1 conduction ratio throughout the strip. So, is this atrial flutter with 2:1 block? Flutter waves are in constant motion due to the macroreentry circuit that creates them in the right atria. The baseline in atrial flutter is never flat. Sometimes, however, the baseline may be a little flatter, but there should still be a constant undulation present. Lead II, in this case, also showed a flat baseline, which is inconsistent with atrial flutter. Technically, even though this is above the usual atrial range for EAT with block (150 to 250 BPM), this is the correct answer. Subsequent clinical information did confirm that diagnosis in this patient.

Test ECG 8

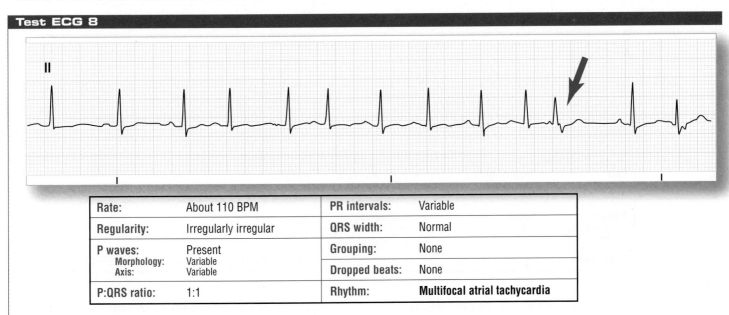

Rate:	About 110 BPM	PR intervals:	Variable
Regularity:	Irregularly irregular	QRS width:	Normal

P waves:
  Morphology:
  Axis:
	Present
	Variable
	Variable
		Grouping:	None

		Dropped beats:	None
P:QRS ratio:	1:1	Rhythm:	**Multifocal atrial tachycardia**

Discussion:

The cadence of this strip is irregularly irregular and there are P waves present throughout the strip. The P waves are dissimilar to each other and they have different PR intervals. The rhythm is also tachycardic. Putting this information together, we have a multifocal atrial tachycardia. Note the presence of some mild aberrancy throughout the strip and one complex (see blue arrow) with gross aberrancy. This is a common finding in multifocal atrial tachycardia, and it usually occurs because of fusion between the components of surrounding complexes. Another frequent cause is aberrancy due to refractoriness of some part of the electrical conduction system. The most frequent culprit is the right bundle branch, but any section of the system may be at risk.

Test ECG 9

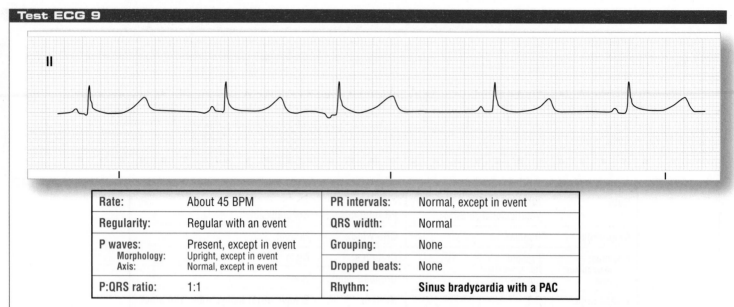

Rate:	About 45 BPM	PR intervals:	Normal, except in event
Regularity:	Regular with an event	QRS width:	Normal

P waves:
    Morphology:
    Axis:
	Present, except in event
	Upright, except in event
	Normal, except in event
		Grouping:	None

		Dropped beats:	None
P:QRS ratio:	1:1	Rhythm:	**Sinus bradycardia with a PAC**

Discussion:

This strip shows a regular rhythm that is markedly bradycardic with one event that occurs prematurely. The P waves and PR intervals are all the same, except for the ones in the premature complex. The premature complex has a shorter PR interval (but still within the normal range) and an inverted P wave. These findings are consistent with a premature atrial contraction. The interval is close to being compensatory and the rate subsequent to the PAC is almost the same. This is a borderline compensatory pause, but you can also argue in favor of a noncompensatory pause. It really doesn't matter too much in this case because the complex is obviously a PAC.

Test ECG 10

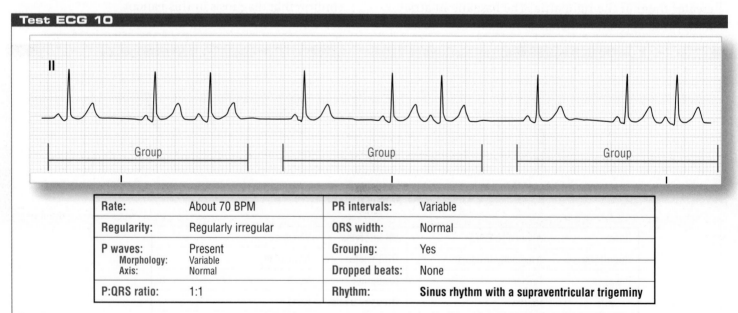

Rate:	About 70 BPM	PR intervals:	Variable
Regularity:	Regularly irregular	QRS width:	Normal

P waves:
    Morphology:
    Axis:
	Present
	Variable
	Normal
		Grouping:	Yes

		Dropped beats:	None
P:QRS ratio:	1:1	Rhythm:	**Sinus rhythm with a supraventricular trigeminy**

Discussion:

This strip can be a little troubling at first glance. The frequent PACs are easy to spot but the grouping can be a little tougher to pick out. If you notice, there is a recurrent pattern of sinus-sinus-PAC that is found throughout the strip. The first thought in your mind when you see grouping should be: Is there an AV block of some kind? Well, the answer is no (AV blocks are covered in Chapter 35; for now, just take our word for it). The third complex is simply a PAC. The rhythm can either be called a sinus rhythm with frequent PACs or, more specifically, a supraventricular trigeminy (a PAC every third complex). The actual description of the strip should be sinus rhythm with an overlying supraventricular trigeminy, to be exact.

Test ECG 11

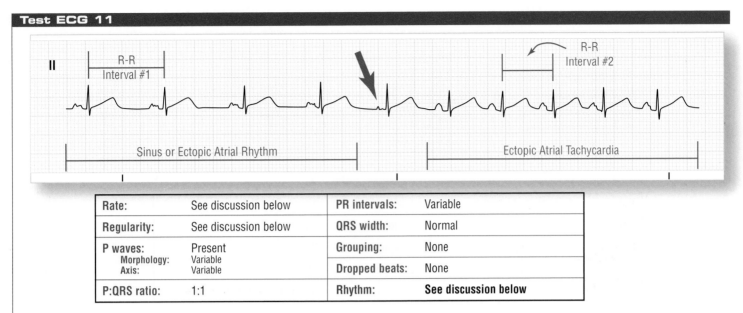

Rate:	See discussion below	PR intervals:	Variable
Regularity:	See discussion below	QRS width:	Normal
P waves: Morphology: Axis:	Present Variable Variable	Grouping:	None
		Dropped beats:	None
P:QRS ratio:	1:1	Rhythm:	**See discussion below**

Discussion:

Even though there are three different P wave morphologies on this strip, this is not a wandering atrial pacemaker. The reason is that the rhythm is not irregularly irregular. It is regularly irregular. Notice that the first four complexes are a sinus or an ectopic atrial rhythm (need an old ECG to compare) firing at a rate of 70 BPM. Then, there is a premature atrial complex (marked by the blue arrow) that triggers a different pacemaker to begin to fire. This pacemaker is obviously an ectopic pacemaker because of the completely different morphology and PR interval from the first one on the strip. The last pacemaker is firing at a tachycardic rate of 105 BPM, making this section of the strip an ectopic atrial tachycardia. The PAC merely acted as the trigger for the new rhythm.

Test ECG 12

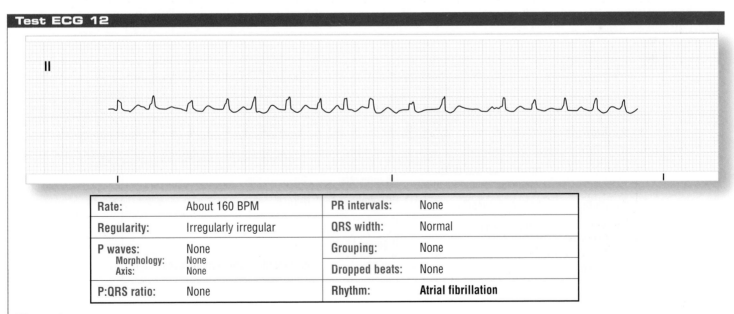

Rate:	About 160 BPM	PR intervals:	None
Regularity:	Irregularly irregular	QRS width:	Normal
P waves: Morphology: Axis:	None None None	Grouping:	None
		Dropped beats:	None
P:QRS ratio:	None	Rhythm:	**Atrial fibrillation**

Discussion:

Test ECG 12 shows an example of an uncontrolled atrial fibrillation. The rate is very fast at about 160 BPM, and is completely random or irregularly irregular. There are no P waves visible throughout the strip. There are a couple of fluctuations in the baseline, which could be interpreted as an occasional P wave, but there is no consistency and these are simply fluctuations in the baseline. The QRS morphology also varies throughout the strip, which could lead to some incorrect diagnoses. This variation is caused by aberrancy and possibly fusion with other waves, including the f waves. A full 12-lead ECG and a longer rhythm strip would be very helpful in evaluating this patient further. The ST segments in the strip appear somewhat scooped, raising the possibility of digitalis effect.

Test ECG 13

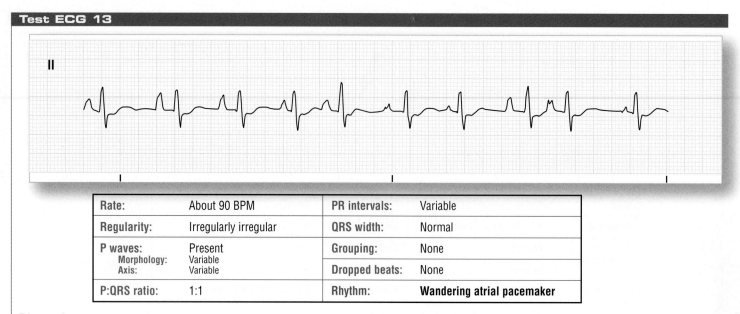

Rate:	About 90 BPM	PR intervals:	Variable
Regularity:	Irregularly irregular	QRS width:	Normal
P waves:	Present	Grouping:	None
Morphology:	Variable		
Axis:	Variable	Dropped beats:	None
P:QRS ratio:	1:1	Rhythm:	**Wandering atrial pacemaker**

Discussion:

Test ECG 13 shows an irregularly irregular rhythm with P waves of at least three different morphologies. The rate is mostly within the normal range, with a few complexes occurring more rapidly. These criteria are consistent with wandering atrial pacemaker. The slight discrepancies in the morphologies of the QRS complexes is consistent with the fusion and aberrancy that is commonly seen in both wandering atrial pacemaker and multifocal atrial tachycardia. A 12-lead ECG should be obtained to evaluate the slight ST depression that is evident throughout the strip.

Test ECG 14

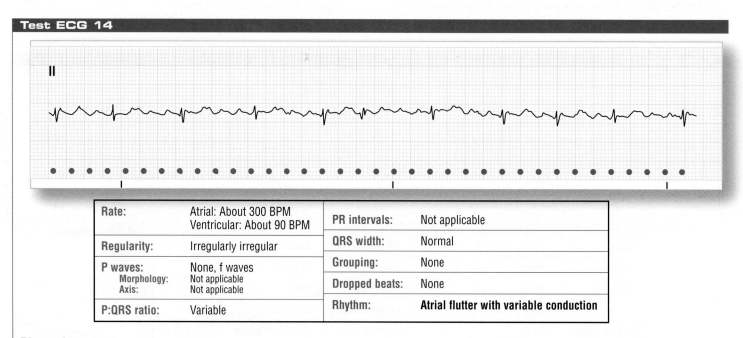

Rate:	Atrial: About 300 BPM Ventricular: About 90 BPM	PR intervals:	Not applicable
Regularity:	Irregularly irregular	QRS width:	Normal
P waves:	None, f waves	Grouping:	None
Morphology:	Not applicable		
Axis:	Not applicable	Dropped beats:	None
P:QRS ratio:	Variable	Rhythm:	**Atrial flutter with variable conduction**

Discussion:

Test ECG 14 shows an irregularly irregular rhythm. Are there any visible P waves? No. What is visible are flutter waves with a continuously undulating baseline at a rate of 300 BPM. This is atrial flutter. The randomness of the ventricular response is because of the variable conduction of the impulses through the AV node. This is not a common presentation for atrial flutter, but does occur often enough that you have to be ready to spot it clinically. The key to the diagnosis is the presence of the flutter waves. The morphological differences in the QRS complexes comes from aberrancy and fusion with the underlying flutter waves. A high index of suspicion would be needed if the flutter waves were not so obvious. Additional leads would greatly aid in the diagnosis in those cases.

Test ECG 15

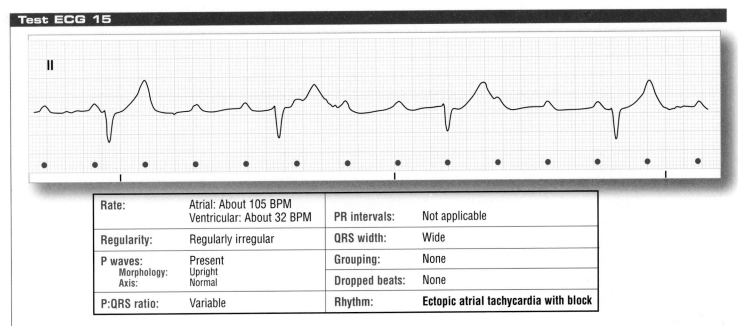

Rate:	Atrial: About 105 BPM Ventricular: About 32 BPM	PR intervals:	Not applicable
Regularity:	Regularly irregular	QRS width:	Wide

P waves:
  Morphology:
  Axis:
	Present
	Upright
	Normal
		Grouping:	None

		Dropped beats:	None
P:QRS ratio:	Variable	Rhythm:	**Ectopic atrial tachycardia with block**

Discussion:

Test ECG 15 shows a variation in the rate of the atria and the ventricles. The atrial complexes are easily identified and are at a rate of 105 BPM. The ventricular complexes are wider than 0.12 seconds and at a rate of about 32 BPM. The ventricular rate and the width of the complexes are compatible with a ventricular origin. The ventricular rhythm is actually a ventricular escape rhythm. In order for the atria and the ventricles to vary so widely, and to not exert any influence on each other, there has to be a complete lack of communication between them. That is exactly what occurs in a complete heart block (see Chapter 35). The final diagnosis for this rhythm strip is ectopic atrial tachycardia with a complete heart block and a ventricular escape rhythm.

Test ECG 16

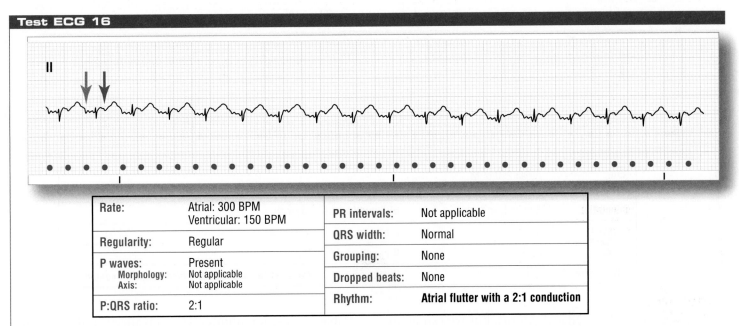

Rate:	Atrial: 300 BPM Ventricular: 150 BPM	PR intervals:	Not applicable
Regularity:	Regular	QRS width:	Normal

P waves:
  Morphology:
  Axis:
	Present
	Not applicable
	Not applicable
		Grouping:	None

		Dropped beats:	None
P:QRS ratio:	2:1	Rhythm:	**Atrial flutter with a 2:1 conduction**

Discussion:

This rhythm strip is rather deceptive. What is the rate of the ventricular complexes? 150 BPM. That rate should immediately spark a question: Am I dealing with atrial flutter? Remember, the most common rate for atrial flutter is 300 BPM with a 2:1 conduction, giving you a ventricular response of 150 BPM. Looking closely at the complexes, we see a deflection a little bit before the QRS complex (see red arrow) and a deflection buried in the ST segment (see blue arrow). These deflections occur at a rate of 300 BPM and are the flutter waves for this patient. Additional leads would be very helpful in confirming your suspicions. In addition, vagal maneuvers such as carotid massage or having the patient Valsalva (push down like they are having a bowel movement) or a little IV adenosine would slow the ventricular response and uncover the flutter waves.

Test ECG 17

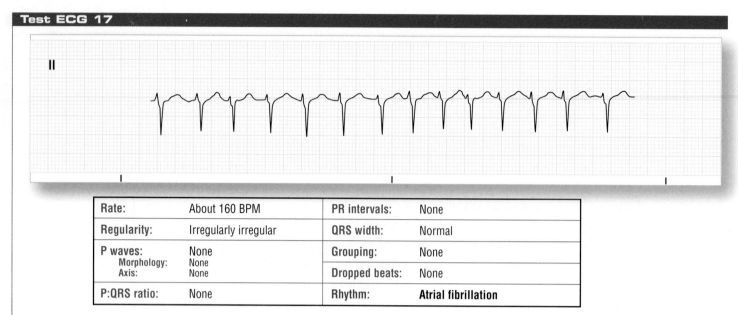

Rate:	About 160 BPM	PR intervals:	None
Regularity:	Irregularly irregular	QRS width:	Normal
P waves:	None	Grouping:	None
Morphology:	None		
Axis:	None	Dropped beats:	None
P:QRS ratio:	None	Rhythm:	**Atrial fibrillation**

Discussion:

This ECG strip shows an uncontrolled atrial fibrillation at a rate of about 160 BPM. Be careful of just quickly eyeballing a rhythm strip and calling it regular, especially a rapid atrial fibrillation. The faster the rate in an uncontrolled Afib, the less the variability that exists from beat to beat. In this case, there are a couple of wider R-R intervals that let you get away with a quick eyeball, but you should get into the habit of using your calipers. After all, what would you rather do: Use your calipers or spend a few months in court discussing issues of malpractice?

Test ECG 18

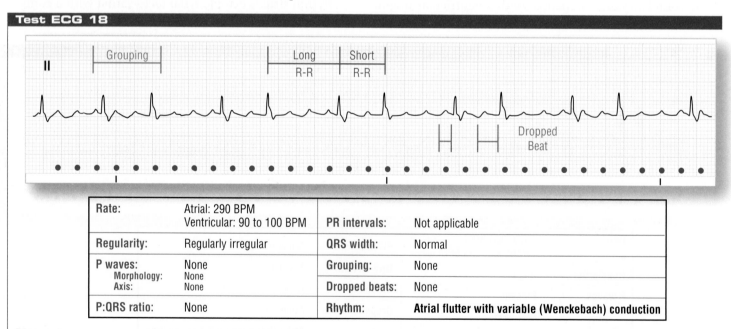

Rate:	Atrial: 290 BPM Ventricular: 90 to 100 BPM	PR intervals:	Not applicable
Regularity:	Regularly irregular	QRS width:	Normal
P waves:	None	Grouping:	None
Morphology:	None		
Axis:	None	Dropped beats:	None
P:QRS ratio:	None	Rhythm:	**Atrial flutter with variable (Wenckebach) conduction**

Discussion:

This is a fairly advanced arrhythmia, but we can figure it out. There are obvious F waves present. What is the cadence of the strip? It is regularly irregular. Once again, calipers are invaluable. Using the distance between the complexes, we see that every other complex is long and every other one is short. This phenomenon recurs throughout the strip. This is a variation of a vari- able conduction aflutter. (For advanced students: Looking at the F waves and their relation to the QRSs, we see that the FR distance increases between the long complex and the short one. The long pause is caused by the dropping of one of the QRS complexes. This type of conduction is called Wenckebach conduction—See Chapter 35.)

Test ECG 19

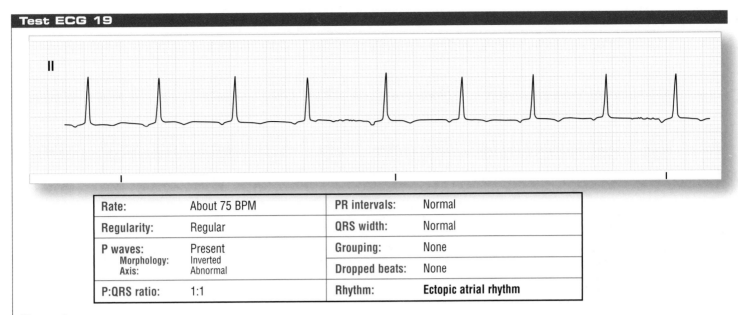

Rate:	About 75 BPM	PR intervals:	Normal
Regularity:	Regular	QRS width:	Normal
P waves: Morphology: Axis:	Present Inverted Abnormal	Grouping:	None
		Dropped beats:	None
P:QRS ratio:	1:1	Rhythm:	**Ectopic atrial rhythm**

Discussion:

This strip shows a regular rhythm at about 75 BPM with inverted P waves in lead II. The inverted P waves and the rate of 75 BPM make the diagnosis ectopic atrial rhythm.

Test ECG 20

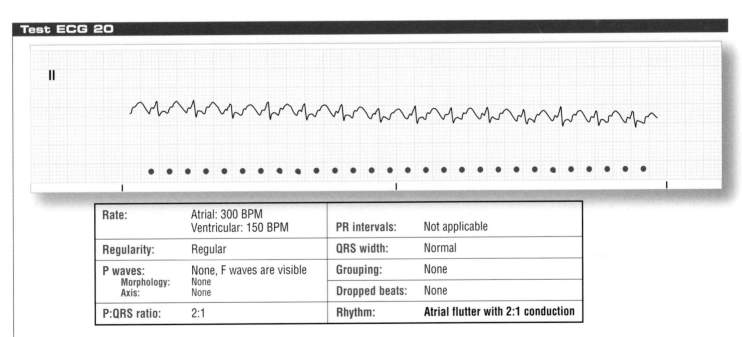

Rate:	Atrial: 300 BPM Ventricular: 150 BPM	PR intervals:	Not applicable
Regularity:	Regular	QRS width:	Normal
P waves: Morphology: Axis:	None, F waves are visible None None	Grouping:	None
		Dropped beats:	None
P:QRS ratio:	2:1	Rhythm:	**Atrial flutter with 2:1 conduction**

Discussion:

This strip is similar to Test ECG 16 that we saw a few strips back. There is an F wave right before the QRS complex and one buried in the ST segment. The key to diagnosis is to realize that the ventricular rate is 150 BPM. Once you hear that number, you should instantly think of atrial flutter with 2:1 conduction and begin looking for the F waves. Remember, if you can't see them in lead II, get another lead, preferably lead V$_1$ because it will show positive F waves and they will be much easier to pick out. Once again, vagal maneuvers and IV adenosine may unmask the F waves in questionable cases and should be attempted if no contraindications to using them exist.

Junctional Rhythms

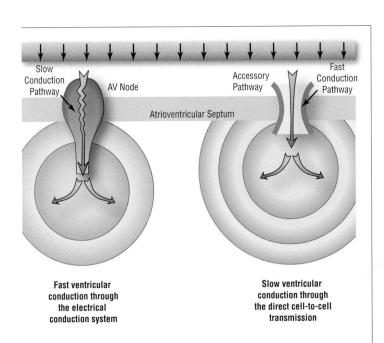

Slow Conduction Pathway

AV Node

Accessory Pathway

Fast Conduction Pathway

Atrioventricular Septum

Fast ventricular conduction through the electrical conduction system

Slow ventricular conduction through the direct cell-to-cell transmission

CHAPTER 21

Introduction to Junctional Rhythms

A Closer Look at the AV Node

We have seen how the AV node functions as a gate-keeper between the atria and the ventricles. In this section, we are going to look at rhythms that origi-nate primarily in the AV node. In order to do this, we need to look at the anatomy of the AV node and its sur-rounding structures in closer detail. Physiologically and arrhythmogenically (ability of the tissue to generate ar-rhythmias), the area around the AV node is just as im-portant as the AV node itself. This distinction is so im-portant that most clinicians have given this area a name, the *AV junction*, and refer to rhythms formed in this area as *junctional* rhythms.

The AV junction is actually not a homogenous structure, but instead is composed of three different zones along with one or two main *approaches* or *tracts* separated by nonconductive fibrous tissue. Each of the tracts and zones has its own particular histologic make-up and arrhythmogenic and conductive properties. The junctional area is located at the base of the right atria near the meeting place of the interatrial and interven-tricular septum. Figure 21-1 is a graphic representation of the AV junctional area and its approaches or tracts.

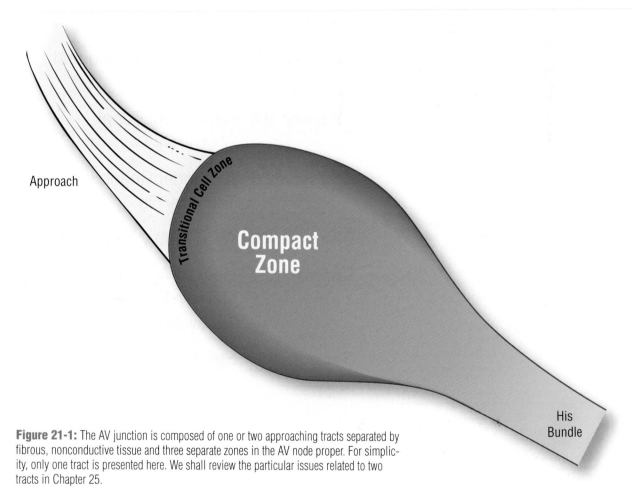

Figure 21-1: The AV junction is composed of one or two approaching tracts separated by fibrous, nonconductive tissue and three separate zones in the AV node proper. For simplic-ity, only one tract is presented here. We shall review the particular issues related to two tracts in Chapter 25.

All of us have either one or two main approaches or tracts leading to the AV nodal area proper. When there are two tracts, these are named the *anterosuperior* and the *posteroinferior* approaches. These approaches are separated from the rest of the myocardium, and each other, by fibrous and other nonconductive tissues. They functionally resemble specialized conduction tracts (most people use the term "tracts" even though this is technically incorrect, so for the sake of conformity, we will be doing the same).

Each of these two tracts has its own individual conductive properties. The anterosuperior tract conducts impulses very rapidly, and so, it is also known as the "fast" tract. The posteroinferior tract is slower in conducting the impulses and is, therefore, also known as the "slow" tract. Most clinicians use the terms "fast tract" and "slow tract" exclusively to keep things simple. As we shall see in Chapter 25, the physiologic characteristics of the two tracts will be a critical factor in forming the rapid circus movements leading up to some pretty fast supraventricular tachyarrhythmias.

Now, let's turn our attention to AV node proper and its surrounding areas. A good way to think about the zones is to envision the AV node like a Q-tip. As you first arrive at the AV node from the atria, you encounter a small area of tissue that surrounds the tip of the node known as the *transitional cell zone* (see Figure 21-1). This is equivalent to the cotton part that is always found at the end of the Q-tip. This zone is full of autonomic fibers and is very arrhythmogenic.

The center or core of the AV node is also called the *compact zone*. This area is composed of cells very similar in histologic appearance and function to those cells found in the sinoatrial node. As you can imagine, the compact zone is prone to function as a primary pacemaker. Whether autonomic fibers influence the compact zone directly is debatable but the influence of autonomic innervation is definitely felt through the adjoining zones.

The final zone we will look at is the area extending from the compact zone to the bifurcation (splitting) of the His bundle. This area is insulated from the rest of the myocardium and penetrates the membranous septum. The main function of this zone is to conduct the impulse rapidly to the bundle branches.

In about 90% of people, the blood supply to the AV node is derived from the right coronary artery system. The remaining 10% usually have the circulation of the node originating in the circumflex artery. The dominance of the right coronary artery as the leading supplier of blood and nutrients to the AV junction is the main reason that myocardial infarctions involving the inferior wall are usually associated with AV nodal blocks and bradyarrhythmias. (The inferior wall of the heart is also primarily supplied by the right coronary artery system, and the inferior descending artery in particular.)

The Junction as a Pacemaker

Now, let's turn our attention to the events that occur when the AV node functions as the primary pacemaker. When an impulse originates in the junctional area, the exact location of the ectopic focus strongly influences the resultant electrocardiographic representation of the complex, particularly the P wave. To examine this more closely, let's go back to the water model we introduced you to in Chapter 5. Take a look at Figure 21-2. If you were to fill up the AV node area with water and then open up both floodgates, the result would be instantaneous flow of water into both the atria and the ventricles. The wave would travel against the expected flow in the atria (from inferior to superior) and would, therefore, stimulate the atria retrogradely. The ventricles would flood in the usual way (using the electrical conduction system) and would be identical to a normally conducted atrial impulse producing a nice, tight QRS complex.

As we saw in Chapter 13, the result of the retrograde conduction of the impulse back to the atria would be an inverted P wave in leads II, III, and aVF. The result of the forward conduction through the normal electrical conduction system throughout the ventricles would be to produce a nice, tight supraventricular QRS

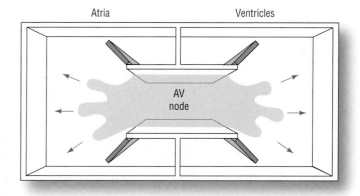

Figure 21-2: If the lock in the middle of the container were filled with water and both gates were opened, the water would flow into both the atria and the ventricles. The water would spread evenly throughout both sides of the container simultaneously.

complex. In the above example, the P wave and the QRS complex would occur at exactly the same time and the P wave would be buried inside the QRS complex. The net result on the ECG strip is that the P wave would either be invisible or would only account for a small amount of variation in the QRS complex (Figure 21-3). This is a very common presentation for a junctional complex on an ECG strip.

Now, let's complicate the issue a little bit further. Suppose that you have an ectopic foci in the lower right atria (represented by the pink star in Figure 21-4). In Chapter 13 we saw that such an ectopic foci would form an ectopic atrial P wave which would be inverted in leads II, III, and aVF and the complex would have a normal PR interval because forward flow would take it through the AV node and it would have to endure the normal physiologic delay.

Now, suppose that the ectopic pacemaker was just a little farther along and just crossed into the transitional zone of the AV node (red star in Figure 21-4). What path would the depolarization wave now have to take? The answer is that this junctional depolarization wave would almost have to travel the same path as the lower atrial ectopic pacemaker! The only difference would be that the physiologic block would be shorter. The P wave

would still be retrogradely spread backward into the atria and the forward depolarization wave would still have to undergo *most* of the normal physiologic block.

What would the resulting complex look like electrocardiographically? The P wave would not be buried in the QRS complex, as it was in the last junctional example we looked at. The P wave would occur before the QRS complex, but the PR interval would be short. *Thus, we see that not all complexes that originate in the junctional area look the same. The location of the ectopic pacemaker site along the AV junction dictates the location of the P wave in relation to its QRS complex.*

We've seen the appearance of the complexes resulting from ectopic pacers firing in the transitional zone and in the compact zone. Now, let's take a look at what happens if the ectopic pacer is in the area of the bundle of His. In these cases, the depolarization wave is already past the sections that cause the physiologic block. In addition, the impulse is immediately transmitted to the ventricles. In order for the impulse to reach the atria, the impulse has to travel a much longer distance retrogradely through the other areas of the AV junction. Where would you expect the P wave to be in these cases? That's right, the inverted P wave would come immediately after the QRS complex in the ST segment (Figure 21-5).

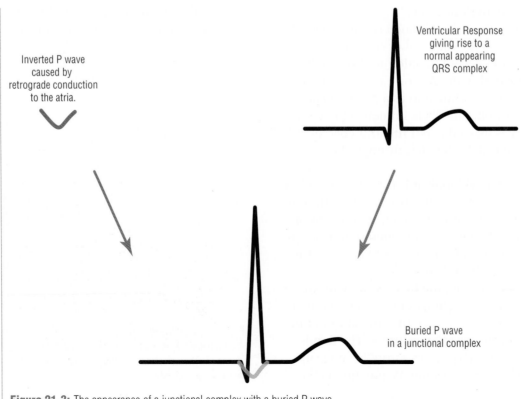

Figure 21-3: The appearance of a junctional complex with a buried P wave.

Inverted P wave caused by retrograde conduction to the atria.

Ventricular Response giving rise to a normal appearing QRS complex

Buried P wave in a junctional complex

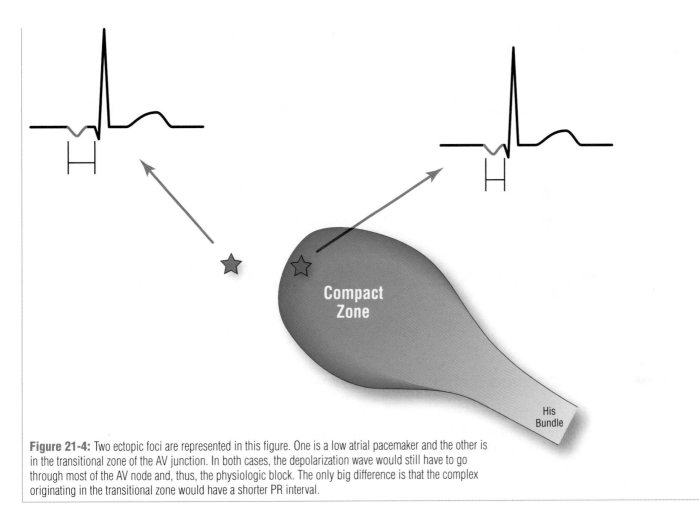

Figure 21-4: Two ectopic foci are represented in this figure. One is a low atrial pacemaker and the other is in the transitional zone of the AV junction. In both cases, the depolarization wave would still have to go through most of the AV node and, thus, the physiologic block. The only big difference is that the complex originating in the transitional zone would have a shorter PR interval.

Figure 21-5: The appearance of a junctional complex originating in the distal AV junction or bundle of His. Note that the P wave is found after the QRS complex.

RP Interval

When the P wave is retrogradely spread to the atria and comes after the QRS complex, we speak of the *RP inter-*

val instead of the PR interval (Figure 21-6). The RP interval is measured from the tip of the QRS complex to the beginning of the next conducted P wave.

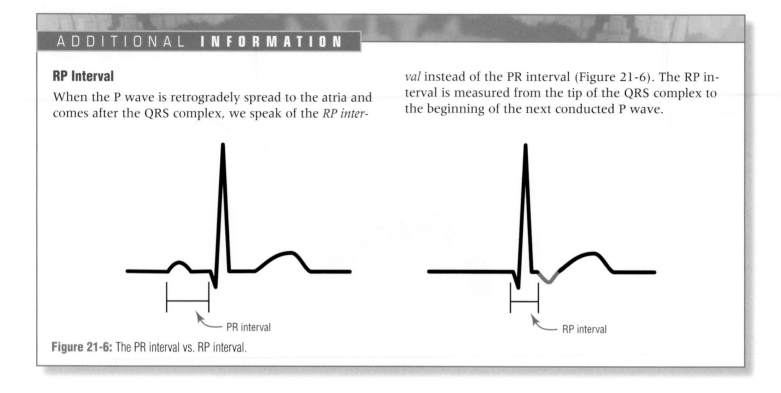

Figure 21-6: The PR interval vs. RP interval.

When you think about the appearance of the P wave in a junctional beat or rhythm, think of a continuum. This continuum is based on the exact location of the ectopic pacemaker and its relation to the rest of the AV junction, to the atria, and to the ventricles. Figure 21-7 is a graphic representing a clear slider with a P wave superimposed on it. As you move the slider along the color gradient representing the AV junction, you will see the placement of the P wave and its relationship to the QRS complex.

Remember, when you see an inverted P wave in front of the QRS complex, take a look at the PR interval. If the PR interval is normal or prolonged, you should consider it an ectopic atrial complex. If the PR interval is short, you are probably dealing with a junctional complex. If you follow these rules, you will be correct in most cases. Exceptions do occur, and you should be aware of their possibilities to be completely correct.

Junctional Rhythms: An Overview

As mentioned in Chapter 1, the intrinsic rate of the AV junctional area is between 40 and 50 BPM. However, we can clinically see junctional rhythms ranging from the 30s to over 300. Clinically, the junctional rhythms can be broken down into the intrinsic rhythms that originate somewhere in the AV junction and the reentrant tachycardias. The intrinsic rhythms include junc-

tional escape complexes and rhythms, junctional premature complexes, accelerated junctional tachycardia, and junctional tachycardia. The two main reentrant tachycardias that we will cover include AV nodal reentry tachycardia and AV reentry tachycardia.

As a failsafe or back-up pacemaker in case of sinus node malfunction, the junctional area performs its job admirably. For this reason, junctional escape complexes are quite common. Any slowing down of the atrial rate, for whatever reason, triggers a junctional escape complex. Many times the junctional escape complex depolarizes the SA node and causes a prolonged wait, which can stimulate another junctional escape, and so on. This type of cycle can easily stimulate a junctional escape rhythm, which is self-perpetuating and will persist until the SA node eventually speeds up. Generally, junctional escape rhythms will be between 40 and 60 BPM. They are easily spotted because of the rate and most importantly because of the presence of narrow, supraventricular QRS complexes with no observable P waves.

Increased automaticity will lead to junctional premature complexes and junctional rhythms that are above 60 BPM. Since this rate is above the intrinsic rate of the AV junction, these rhythms are known as *accelerated junctional rhythms*. If the rates of a junctional rhythm are above 100 BPM, they are referred to as junctional tachycardias. This spectrum is graphically represented by Figure 21-8.

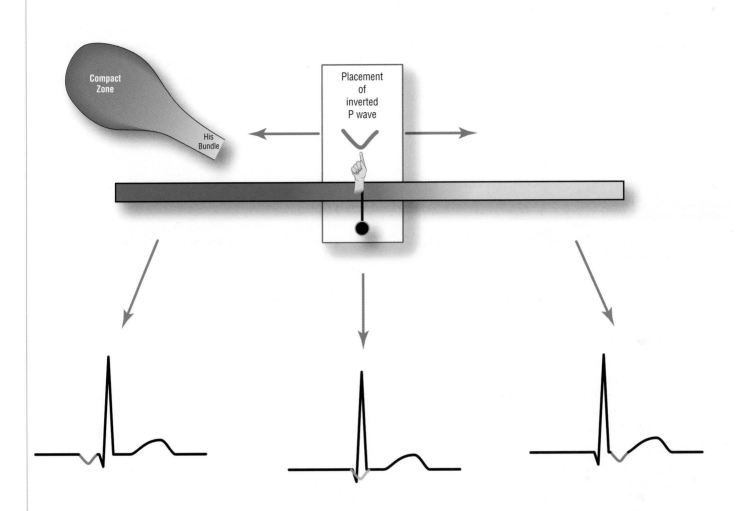

Figure 21-7: The relationship of the inverted P wave to the QRS complex is represented as a continuum. The P waves could be anything from before the QRS complex with a shortened PR interval, to buried within the QRS complex, to occurring slightly after the QRS complex.

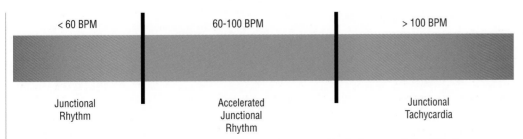

Figure 21-8: The spectrum of the junctional rhythms caused by increased intrinsic automaticity within the AV node and junctional area.

As mentioned, the presence of narrow supraventricular complexes is important in identifying a junctional rhythm. There are some cases in which the complexes will be wide and aberrant. These include patients with pre-existing bundle branch blocks, rate-related or ischemia-related aberrancy, and electrolyte abnormalities, to name a few. When wide supraventricular complexes are noted, it may be very difficult to differentiate the rhythm from a rhythm of ventricular origin such as ventricular tachycardia. If there is ever any question as to a possible ventricular origin of the complexes, they should be treated as if they are ventricular rhythms. Remember, the ventricles control the blood pressure. You should always treat for the worst-case scenario until proven otherwise!

CHAPTER REVIEW

1. The AV node and the AV junction are basically the same thing. True or False.

2. Rhythms that originate in the AV junction are known as _____ rhythms.

3. P waves that originate in the AV junction are always inverted. True or False.

4. The P wave in a junctional rhythm can be found:
   A. Immediately before the QRS complex
   B. Buried within the QRS complex
   C. Immediately after the QRS complex
   D. All of the above

5. If the P wave is ever found in front of the QRS complex, the PR interval would be _____ than normal.

6. When the P wave is found after the QRS complex, we do not talk about the PR interval. Instead, we talk about the ____ interval.

7. When you see an inverted P wave in front of the QRS complex, take a look at the PR interval. If the PR interval is normal or prolonged, you should consider it to be a(n) _____ complex. If the PR interval is short, you are probably dealing with a(n) _____ complex.

8. A junctional rhythm occurs at rates below ____ BPM.

9. An accelerated junctional rhythm occurs at rates between ____ and ____ BPM.

10. A junctional tachycardia occurs at rates above ____ BPM.

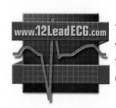

To enhance the knowledge you gain in this book, access this text's website at www.12leadECG.com! This valuable resource provides flashcards, an online glossary, web links, and more. Simply click on the Arrhythmias book cover once at the site.

CHAPTER 22

Junctional Rhythm

In this chapter, we are going to look at how the AV nodal area functions as an escape pacemaker for the heart. The escape pacemaker can trigger off a single escape beat, if that is all that is needed; or it can trigger off an entire escape rhythm, essentially taking over if the SA node completely fails. The pacemaking function of the AV node is critical in maintaining a viable ventricular response in cases of sinus failure for whatever reason.

Junctional Escape Complexes and Rhythms

Remember in Chapter 1 we mentioned that the pacemaking function of all of the cardiac cells is occurring in all of the cells of the heart at the same time. The SA node, being the fastest, usually wins and sets the rate. Next in line would be the atrial myocardium itself. This ectopic pacemaker would give us an ectopic atrial rhythms. The next pacemaker in succession would be the AV node and the AV junctional area. In many cases, the atrial myocardium does not take over pacemaking function when the SA node fails and the pacing function skips right to the AV node directly.

Electrocardiographically, a junctional escape complex looks exactly like a sinus complex except that it doesn't have a normal P wave, if it has any at all. Some

minor variations may be present but, in most cases, the QRS complex, the ST segments, and the T waves are identical to the normally conducted sinus complexes. Take a look at Figure 22-1. Notice how the sinus node suddenly fails to fire. An AV nodal pacemaker then fires, rescuing the ventricles from standstill. Then, the sinus node picks back up again continuing with a sinus rhythm. This is the usual presentation when there is a single solitary junctional escape complex.

Many times, the rate or the rhythm immediately after the junctional escape complex is different than the one before it. A rate change is more commonly seen, but sometimes a different ectopic pacemaker may take over altogether.

Another common sequence is that the junctional escape complex depolarizes the SA node. The SA node then resets, taking a little longer to fire its next impulse. That extra time may be just long enough so that another junctional escape complex is triggered. This cycle is repeated over and over again, essentially creating a *junctional escape rhythm* or simply a *junctional rhythm*. When at least three consecutive complexes are junctional escape complexes, the rhythm is referred to as a junctional rhythm.

Figure 22-2 is an example of a junctional escape rhythm. The usual rate for a junctional rhythm is between 40 and 60 BPM. This rate is usually caused by

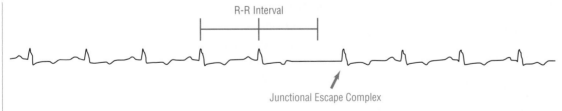

R-R Interval

Junctional Escape Complex

Figure 22-1: Sinus rhythm with a sinus pause leading to a junctional escape complex.

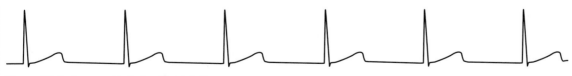

Figure 22-2: An example of a junctional rhythm.

an escape mechanism because it is too slow to be due to increased automaticity of a site (usually greater than 60 BPM). So, in general, even though a junctional rhythm is presumed to be due to escape, the word "escape" is usually presumed and the term shortened to junctional rhythm. The only time escape is explicitly used when describing a junctional rhythm is in the presence of an atrioventricular block.

The baseline in a junctional rhythm can be completely flat, can have some minor irregularities, or as seen in Figure 22-3, can be completely erratic. The erratic baselines are usually caused by some sort of artifact. These sources of artifact can include tremors, outside electrical sources, moving lead wires, and so on.

Cases with erratic baselines may be impossible to differentiate from atrial fibrillation with complete AV dissociation leading to a normalized junctional escape rhythm. It is difficult on a surface ECG to tell the difference between these two with any degree of certainty, and you need to maintain a high index of suspicion in these cases. Obtaining additional information, for example, by ruling out the possibility of digoxin toxicity, is critical. Remember, when interpreting any rhythm, always look at the company the rhythm keeps.

Junctional rhythms also commonly develop when there is no communication between the atria and ventricles. When this occurs, the atrial impulses die off before they ever reach the AV node and the ventricles. In these cases, the AV node takes over primary function as the pacemaker for the ventricles and, hence, a junctional rhythm is formed. We will be reviewing this occurrence in great detail in Chapter 35 when we talk about AV dissociation and complete heart block.

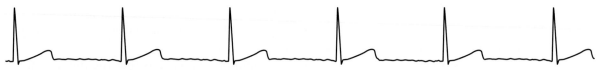

Figure 22-3: The same junctional rhythm but with an erratic baseline.

ARRHYTHMIA RECOGNITION

Junctional Rhythm

Rate:	Between 40 and 60 BPM
Regularity:	Regular
P wave:	Absent or inverted
Morphology:	Abnormal
Upright in II, III, and aVF:	No
P:QRS ratio:	Not applicable
PR interval:	Not applicable
QRS width:	Normal or wide
Grouping:	None
Dropped beats:	None

DIFFERENTIAL DIAGNOSIS

Junctional Rhythm

1. Primary SA node dysfunction
2. AV dissociation
3. Increased parasympathetic activity
4. Drugs: digoxin, beta-blockers, calcium-channel blockers
5. Myocardial ischemia
6. Sick sinus syndrome
7. Electrolyte disorders
8. CNS events
9. Idiopathic

The list above is not all-inclusive.

ECG Strips

ECG 22-1

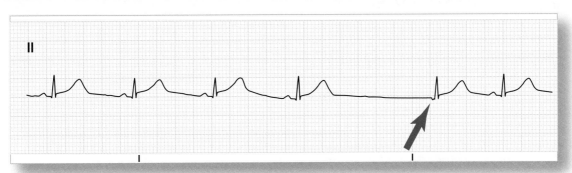

Rate:	About 67 BPM	PR intervals:	Normal, except in event
Regularity:	Regular with an event	QRS width:	Normal

P waves:
  Morphology:
  Axis:
	Present, except in event
	Inverted in event
	Abnormal in event
		Grouping:	None

		Dropped beats:	Present
P:QRS ratio:	1:1, except in event	Rhythm:	**Sinus rhythm with a junctional escape complex**

Discussion:

The underlying rhythm in the strip above is sinus rhythm. The SA node then fails to pace and there is a prolonged pause leading to a junctional escape complex. Notice that the P wave for the junctional escape complex is inverted and found before the QRS complex (see blue arrow). This signifies retrograde conduction of the junctional impulse backward to the atria.

ECG 22-2

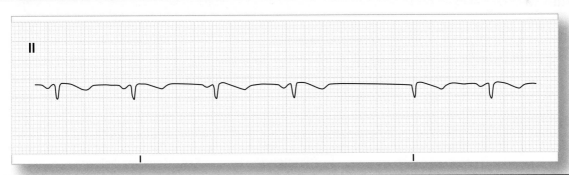

Rate:	About 68 BPM	PR intervals:	Normal, except in event
Regularity:	Regular with an event	QRS width:	Normal

P waves:
  Morphology:
  Axis:
	Present, except in event
	Inverted; none in event
	Abnormal; none in event
		Grouping:	None

		Dropped beats:	Present
P:QRS ratio:	1:1, except in event	Rhythm:	**Ectopic atrial rhythm with a junctional escape complex**

Discussion:

The strip above shows inverted P waves with normal PR intervals all throughout the rhythm. Therefore, the underlying rhythm is an ectopic atrial rhythm. The event that occurs is related to the prolonged pause leading to the formation of a junctional escape complex. Note that the P wave is not visible in the junctional escape complex because it is either missing or buried in the QRS complex.

ECG 22-3

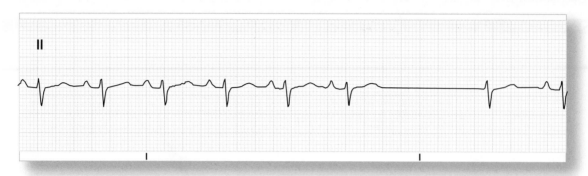

Rate:	About 90 BPM	PR intervals:	Normal, except in event
Regularity:	Regular with an event	QRS width:	Normal

P waves:
    Morphology:
    Axis:
	Present, except in event
	Normal; none in event
	Normal; none in event
		Grouping:	None

		Dropped beats:	Present
P:QRS ratio:	1:1, except in event	Rhythm:	**Sinus rhythm with a junctional escape complex**

Discussion:

This strip shows a normal sinus rhythm with a sinus pause leading to a junctional escape complex. The normal sinus pacemaker appears to take over the pacing functions again after the junctional escape complex. The P wave is either missing or buried within the QRS complex of the junctional escape beat.

ECG 22-4

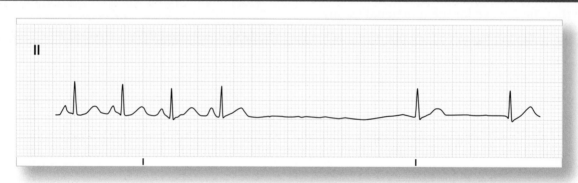

Rate:	About 110 BPM	PR intervals:	See discussion below
Regularity:	Regularly irregular	QRS width:	Normal

P waves:
    Morphology:
    Axis:
	See discussion below
	See discussion below
	See discussion below
		Grouping:	None

		Dropped beats:	Present
P:QRS ratio:	See discussion below	Rhythm:	**Sinus tachycardia, sinus arrest, and a junctional escape rhythm**

Discussion:

This strip starts off with what appears to be a sinus tachycardia. Then the strip shows a fairly long interval with no electrical activity. This is compatible with a sinus arrest followed by a rescue junctional escape rhythm occurring at a rate of about 58 BPM. The P waves are not visible in the junctional rhythm signifying either the absence of P waves or buried P waves.

ECG 22-5

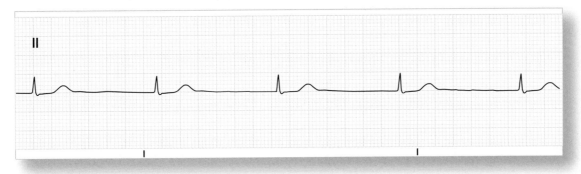

Rate:	About 45 BPM	PR intervals:	Not applicable
Regularity:	Regular	QRS width:	Normal
P waves:	None	Grouping:	None
Morphology:	None		
Axis:	None	Dropped beats:	None
P:QRS ratio:	Not applicable	Rhythm:	**Junctional rhythm**

Discussion:

This strip shows a junctional rhythm at a rate of about 45 BPM. Notice the absence of P waves, the regularity of the rhythm, and the normal-looking supraventricular complexes.

ECG 22-6

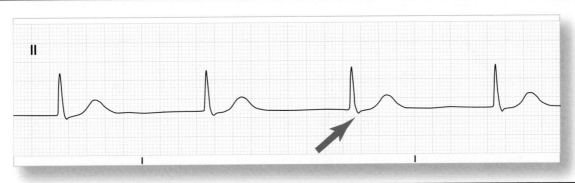

Rate:	About 38 BPM	PR intervals:	Not applicable
Regularity:	Regular	QRS width:	Normal
P waves:	None	Grouping:	None
Morphology:	None		
Axis:	None	Dropped beats:	None
P:QRS ratio:	Not applicable	Rhythm:	**Junctional rhythm**

Discussion:

This strip shows a junctional rhythm with a rate that is slightly lower than expected for the AV nodal area. Drugs, ischemia, or a CNS event may be the culprit behind the slower rate. Notice the slight depression immediately after the QRS complex. This negative wave could represent a retrograde P wave occurring immediately after the QRS complex. An old ECG strip would be helpful to see if this finding was present during a period of normal sinus rhythm.

ECG 22·7

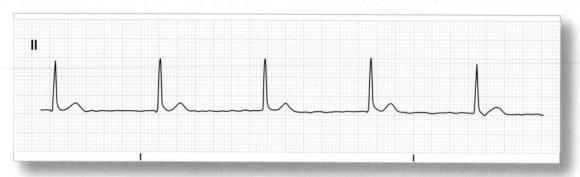

Rate:	About 52 BPM	PR intervals:	Not applicable
Regularity:	Regular	QRS width:	Normal
P waves:	None	Grouping:	None
Morphology:	None		
Axis:	None	Dropped beats:	None
P:QRS ratio:	Not applicable	Rhythm:	**Junctional rhythm**

Discussion:

The strip above is also a textbook example of a junctional rhythm. There are no discernible P waves anywhere along the strip. The QRS complexes are narrow and obviously of supraventricular origin. Finally, the rate of 52 BPM is definitely consistent with a junctional rhythm.

ECG 22·8

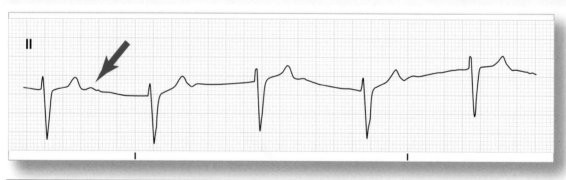

Rate:	About 51 BPM	PR intervals:	Not applicable
Regularity:	Regular	QRS width:	Normal
P waves:	None	Grouping:	None
Morphology:	None		
Axis:	None	Dropped beats:	None
P:QRS ratio:	Not applicable	Rhythm:	**Junctional rhythm**

Discussion:

The strip above is also a great example of a junctional rhythm. The wandering baseline is due to movement of the patient or one of the leads. The blue arrow is pointing toward a positive wave immediately after the T wave. This deflection is not a P wave but an example of a typical U wave. The U wave has no special clinical sig- nificance in the evaluation of this arrhythmia, except that it could raise the possibility of a pathological process, especially an electrolyte abnormality (hypokalemia). Typically, however, U waves are seen in the absence of pathology.

CHAPTER **REVIEW**

1. Junctional escape complexes and junctional rhythms are typically a normal response to the SA node failing its function as the primary pacemaker. True or False.

2. Junctional rhythms are of critical importance in maintaining _____ and _____ during a failure of an SA nodal or atrial pacemaker. (Please pick the correct answers to the statement above.)
   A. Atrial response
   B. Ventricular response
   C. Atrial kick
   D. Hemodynamic stability

3. Electrocardiographically, junctional rhythms have the following characteristics:
   A. Inverted, buried P wave
   B. Absence of P wave
   C. Narrow supraventricular complex
   D. Regular rate between 40 and 60 BPM
   E. All of the above

4. Junctional rhythms are typically formed as _____ rhythms.

5. Junctional rhythms are typically greater than 60 BPM but less than 100 BPM. True or False.

6. A wandering, random baseline is always a sign of atrial fibrillation with a regular response. True or False.

7. Part of the differential diagnosis for a randomly erratic baseline with a regular supraventricular response between 40 and 60 BPM is atrial fibrillation with complete AV block and a junctional escape rhythm. True or False.

8. Junctional rhythms are always benign. True or False.

9. _____ is a drug that is frequently associated with a regularization of atrial fibrillation mimicking a junctional rhythm.

10. Possible causes of a junctional rhythm include:
    A. Myocardial ischemia
    B. CNS events
    C. Electrolyte abnormalities
    D. Sick sinus syndrome
    E. All of the above

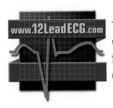

To enhance the knowledge you gain in this book, access this text's website at www.12leadECG.com! This valuable resource provides flashcards, an online glossary, web links, and more. Simply click on the Arrhythmias book cover once at the site.

CHAPTER 23

Premature Junctional Contraction

As you can imagine, premature junctional contractions (PJCs) are junctional complexes that occur earlier than expected and are interspersed in the underlying rhythm for one or more cycles (Figure 23-1). The PJCs have the morphological characteristics expected from any junctional complex (absent or buried P wave, inverted P waves in leads II, III, and aVF, and narrow supraventricular QRS complexes). PJCs are usually associated with a noncompensatory pause because the retrogradely conducted atrial impulse typically depolarizes and resets the SA node (discussed in Chapter 13). However, the pause may be fully compensatory when there is no retrograde conduction back toward the atria.

PJCs are a fairly common electrocardiographic phenomenon and can be found in people with and without structural and ischemic heart disease. They are typically caused by increased automaticity of the AV junction. They can occur singly or can be recurrent.

The coupling interval—the distance from the PJC to the previous QRS complex—can be fixed or variable. A fixed coupling interval (Figure 23-2) is commonly found in PACs and PVCs, and represents an identical distance between the normal complex and the premature beat. PJCs typically do not have a fixed coupling interval and the R-R interval between complexes is usually variable (Figure 23-3).

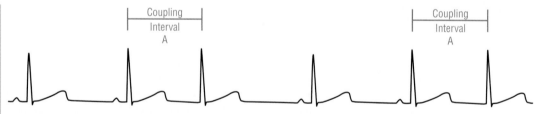

Figure 23-1: A premature junctional contraction.

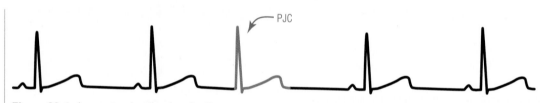

Figure 23-2: The coupling interval refers to the distance between the premature complex and the preceding normal beat found in the underlying rhythm. A fixed coupling interval is the same whenever an individual ectopic focus fires.

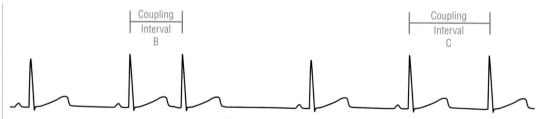

Figure 23-3: A variable coupling interval refers to a variability in the coupling distance every time that the same ectopic focus fires.

The supraventricular complexes of the PJCs typically have narrow QRS complexes associated with them. If the QRS complex is wider than 0.12 seconds, the usual causes include a pre-existing bundle branch block, aberrantly conducted beats, electrolyte abnormalities, and fusion complexes with the T waves of the previous complexes.

ADDITIONAL **INFORMATION**

PAC with Aberrancy vs. PJC with Aberrancy

We are going to look at the differential diagnosis of wide, aberrant complexes very closely in Chapter 27, but certain points would be very helpful to discuss now. How can you tell if a complex is actually an aberrantly conducted PAC or an aberrantly conducted PJC? The answer is to look at the company it keeps. The events and appearance of the waves around it will be your best clue.

1. *Always look for morphological variation in the preceding T wave.*

   We have studied buried P waves before, but this topic deserves reinforcement. Start by looking at the T waves of the preceding complexes that are normally transmitted for that patient. The morphology of the T wave will most likely be identical from complex to complex. Mild variations may exist, but there should never be any gross differences. A gross difference in morphological appearance, especially when associated with a premature complex, almost always signifies the presence of a buried P wave somewhere.

   The morphology of a T wave will usually be altered by a buried P wave (Figure 23-4). This is because the ventricular repolarization process is slow and the forces that they generate are smaller than those that occur during an actual coordinated depolarization wave. Even the relatively low forces of atrial depolarization are enough to cause an electrocardiographic fusion to occur on the strip. (Notice that this refers to a fusion on the ECG because of the timing of the waves, and not an actual fusion of the waves themselves within the heart as we talked about in the last section.)

2. *Compensatory Pause*

   The other thing that will help you to differentiate between a PAC with a buried P wave and a PJC is the type of pause involved. PACs are usually associated with noncompensatory pauses because the sinus node is usually reset by an ectopic atrial impulse. PJCs can have either compensatory or noncompensatory pauses. PJCs are associated with compensatory pauses when there is no retrograde conduction of the depolarization wave back toward the atria. PJCs are associated with noncompensatory pauses when the sinus node is reset by a retrograde P wave. Therefore, *the presence of a compensatory pause favors the diagnosis of PJC.*

3. *Inverted P Waves in Lead II, III, and aVF with Short PR Intervals*

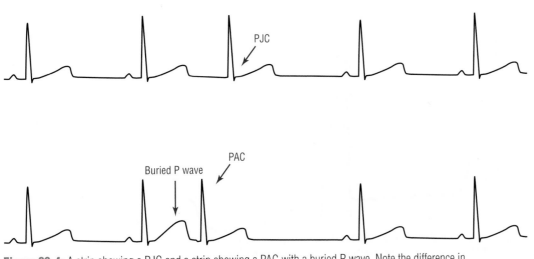

Figure 23-4: A strip showing a PJC and a strip showing a PAC with a buried P wave. Note the difference in the appearance of the T wave of the complex immediately before the PAC. The morphological difference is due to the additive effects of the ectopic P wave and the T wave.

(Continued)

Remember from Chapter 13 that ectopic atrial pacemakers may be associated with inverted P waves in leads II, III, and aVF. The P wave becomes inverted when the ectopic pacemaker is inferior and near the AV junction. By definition, therefore, a PJC will always have inverted P waves in leads II, III and aVF. In addition, the PJC's P wave can be before, after, or buried within the QRS complex. If the P wave occurs before the QRS complex in a PJC, the PR interval is almost always shorter than normal (<0.12 seconds) because it doesn't have to undergo the full physiologic block because of its site of origin.

4. *Identifying Aberrantly Conducted PJCs*
One of the toughest things in arrhythmia recognition is to correctly identify an aberrantly conducted

PJC. To accomplish this feat, you need to keep a very close eye on the "company it keeps" and to look very closely at the area right at the start of the QRS complex.

An aberrantly conducted morphology occurs when a normally transmitted depolarization wave traveling down the electrical conduction system hits an area that is refractory to impulse transmission (Figure 23-5). From that point on, the impulse has to be transmitted down to the rest of the ventricles via direct cell-to-cell transmission. Because the very early portion of the QRS complex is always transmitted down the normal electrical conduction system, that portion will always be identical to the normally conducted complexes.

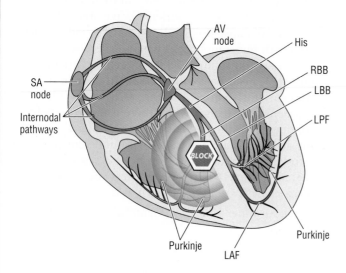

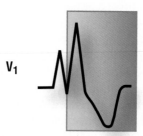

Figure 23-5: An aberrancy develops when an impulse traveling down the normal electrical conduction system hits an area of refractoriness. The cell-to-cell transmission that has to develop after that point causes the electrocardiographic aberrancy to develop.

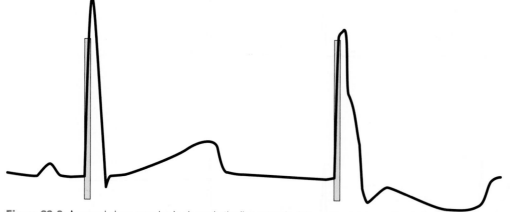

Figure 23-6: A normal sinus complex is shown in the first example, followed by an aberrantly conducted beat. Note how the initial few milliseconds of the two complexes are exactly identical. The number of milliseconds that are identically transmitted depends on the site of refractoriness that causes the aberration. If the refractory site is very close to the AV node, the amount of time will be very, very short. If the refractory site is further down the electrical conduction system, the amount of aberrancy will be longer.

ADDITIONAL **INFORMATION** *(continued)*

Always look at the first few milliseconds of the normally conducted QRS complex and compare it to the aberrantly conducted beat in question (Figure 23-6). As mentioned, this area is always identical to that of the normally conducted complexes. The number of milliseconds that are identically transmitted depends on the site of refractoriness that causes the aberration. If the refractory site is very close to the AV node, the amount of time will be very, very short. If the refractory site is further down the electrical conduction system, the amount of aberrancy will be longer.

A good clinical tip to keep in mind is that if the complexes start in the same direction, especially if it occurs in multiple leads, the wide complex is probably an aberrantly conducted complex (Figure 23-7). If they start in opposite directions *in multiple leads*, it is most assuredly ventricular ectopic complex. We will be discussing this in greater detail in Chapter 28 when we talk about PVCs.

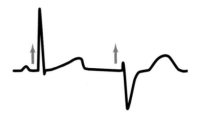

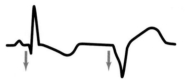

Figure 23-7: Always take a look at the direction of the start of the QRS. If the complexes are headed in the same direction, it is probably an aberrancy.

ARRHYTHMIA **RECOGNITION**

Premature Junctional Contractions

Rate:	Usually single events
Regularity:	Regular with an event
P wave:	Variable
Morphology:	Inverted
Upright in II, III, and aVF:	Inverted
P:QRS ratio:	Variable
PR interval:	Short, if present
QRS width:	Normal
Grouping:	None
Dropped beats:	None

DIFFERENTIAL **DIAGNOSIS**

Premature Junctional Contractions:

1. Idiopathic and benign
2. Anxiety
3. Fatigue
4. Drugs: nicotine, alcohol, caffeine, etc.
5. Heart disease
6. Electrolyte disorders

The list above is not all-inclusive, as the causes of PJCs are extensive. Normally, PJCs are benign and cause no hemodynamic compromise. However, hemodynamic compromise can occur rarely.

ECG Strips

ECG 23·1

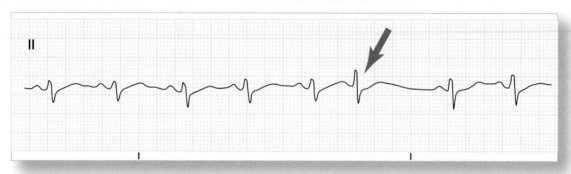

Rate:	About 80 BPM	PR intervals:	Normal, except in event
Regularity:	Regular with an event	QRS width:	Normal
P waves:	Present, except in event	Grouping:	None
Morphology:	Normal, except in event		
Axis:	Normal, except in event	Dropped beats:	Present
P:QRS ratio:	1:1, except in event	Rhythm:	**Sinus rhythm with a PJC**

Discussion:

The rhythm strip above shows a sinus rhythm. The cadence of the rhythm is interrupted by a premature complex (blue arrow) that is slightly different in morphology than the other QRS complexes. There is no real noticeable change in the T wave prior to the event, and the pause is compensatory. Both of these findings point toward a PJC. The slight irregularity is due to some aberrancy. Note that both the normal and aberrant complexes start off in the positive direction.

ECG 23·2

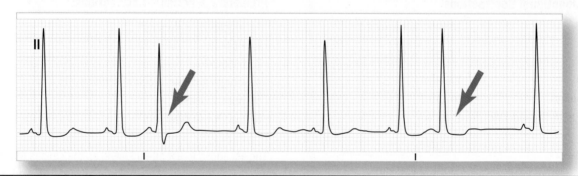

Rate:	About 72 BPM	PR intervals:	Normal, except in event
Regularity:	Regular with events	QRS width:	Normal
P waves:	Present, except in event	Grouping:	None
Morphology:	Normal, except in event		
Axis:	Normal, except in event	Dropped beats:	Present
P:QRS ratio:	1:1, except in event	Rhythm:	**Sinus rhythm with multiple PJCs**

Discussion:

This strip shows a sinus rhythm with some ST segment abnormalities, which could be due to digitalis effect (note the ladle-like or scooped-out appearance of the complexes). The two premature complexes (blue arrows) are slightly different in morphology. The first is a PJC with some aberrancy. The height is slightly shorter, but so is the fifth complex. The terminal S wave in the QRS complexes of the third complex may actually be a buried, inverted P wave. The morphology of the second PJC is exactly like the normal ones.

ECG 23-3

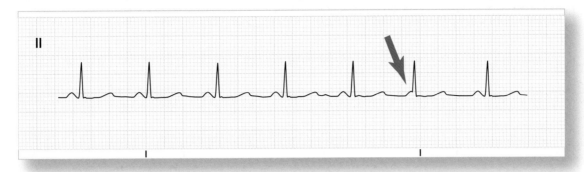

Rate:	About 80 BPM	PR intervals:	Normal, except in event
Regularity:	Regular with an event	QRS width:	Normal
P waves:	Present, except in event	Grouping:	None
Morphology:	Normal, except in event		
Axis:	Normal, except in event	Dropped beats:	Present
P:QRS ratio:	1:1, except in event	Rhythm:	**Sinus rhythm with a PJC**

Discussion:

This strip shows a nice sinus rhythm clipping along at 80 BPM. The cadence of the ventricular complexes is broken up by a premature complex that is narrow and similar in morphology to the rest of the complexes. This is obviously a PJC. The cadence of the atrial complexes, however, is not broken and persists right through the PJC making this a compensatory pause. Notice the buried upright P wave within the PJC (blue arrow). The fact the P wave is upright means that it did not come from the PJC.

ECG 23-4

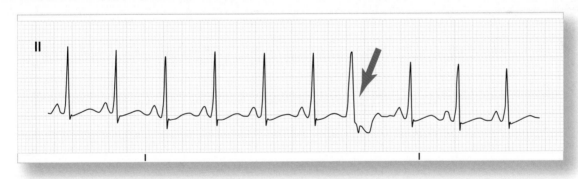

Rate:	About 110 BPM	PR intervals:	Normal, except in event
Regularity:	Regular, except in event	QRS width:	Normal
P waves:	Present, except in event	Grouping:	None
Morphology:	Normal, except in event		
Axis:	Normal, except in event	Dropped beats:	Present
P:QRS ratio:	1:1, except in event	Rhythm:	**Sinus tachycardia with a PJC**

Discussion:

This patient has an underlying sinus tachycardia and one wide, bizarre ventricular-looking complex. Is it a PVC or a PJC with aberrancy? Let's look at how they both start. They both are positive, and notice that the very early onset of both the normal beats and the aber-rant one are identical. This is an aberrantly conducted PJC. The negative deflection after the tall R wave may be an S wave and part of the complex or a buried P wave. It is difficult, if not impossible, to say which is correct from this strip.

ECG 23-5

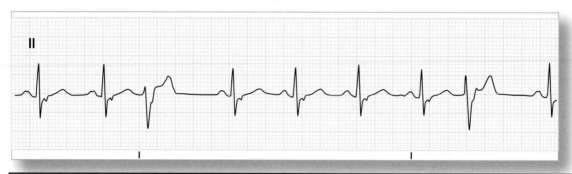

Rate:	About 86 BPM	PR intervals:	Normal, except in event
Regularity:	Regular with events	QRS width:	Normal, events are wide
P waves:	Present, except in event	Grouping:	None
Morphology:	Normal, except in event		
Axis:	Normal, except in event	Dropped beats:	Present
P:QRS ratio:	1:1, except in event	Rhythm:	**Sinus rhythm with multiple PJCs**

Discussion:

Once again, we are faced with a diagnostic challenge. Are the wide, premature complexes on the strip above of junctional or ventricular origin? How do both aberrant beats start? They start with positive waves that are identical to the start of the sinus QRS complexes. Then an aberrancy begins to develop along a slightly different location for each one, accounting for the slight differences in morphology between the two.

ECG 23-6

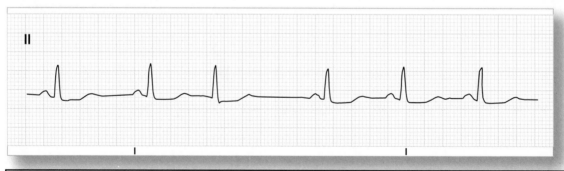

Rate:	About 58 BPM	PR intervals:	Normal, except in event
Regularity:	Regular with an event	QRS width:	Normal
P waves:	Present, except in event	Grouping:	None
Morphology:	Normal, except in event		
Axis:	Normal, except in event	Dropped beats:	Present
P:QRS ratio:	1:1, except in event	Rhythm:	**Sinus bradycardia with a PJC**

Discussion:

The strip above shows a sinus bradycardia with a PJC. The PJC causes a noncompensatory pause and the sinus rate is reset after the PJC. The ST-segment depressions found on this strip should make you think about getting a full 12-lead ECG to evaluate the possibility of ischemia. Clinical correlation would also be extremely helpful in establishing a clinical diagnosis.

ECG 23-7

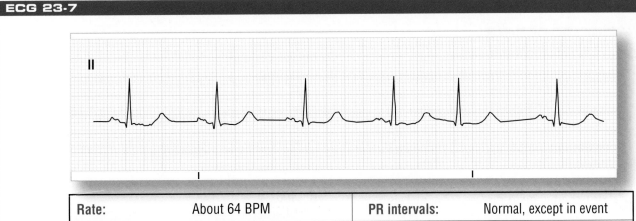

Rate:	About 64 BPM	PR intervals:	Normal, except in event
Regularity:	Regular with an event	QRS width:	Normal
P waves:	Present, except in event	Grouping:	None
Morphology:	Normal, except in event	Dropped beats:	Present
Axis:	Normal, except in event		
P:QRS ratio:	1:1, except in event	Rhythm:	**Sinus rhythm with a PJC**

Discussion:

This is another example of a PJC. The morphology of the T wave immediately prior to the PJC is a bit altered, but the PR interval would have to be exceedingly long in order for a P wave to buried in there. The QRS morphology is similar to the others and narrow, signifying a supraventricular origin.

CHAPTER **REVIEW**

1. Premature junctional contractions are _____ supraventricular complexes with QRS intervals less than _____ seconds.

2. The P waves in PJCs are either buried, absent, or _____ in leads II, III, and aVF.

3. PJCs can be associated with either compensatory or noncompensatory pauses. True or False.

4. PJCs are typically only found in patients with structural or ischemic heart disease. True or False.

5. PJCs are typically associated with:
   A. Fixed coupling intervals
   B. Variable coupling intervals
   C. Both A and B are correct.
   D. None of the above.

6. PJCs with QRS complexes wider than 0.12 seconds are found in patients with:
   A. Preexisting bundle branch block
   B. Aberrantly conducted beats
   C. Electrolyte abnormalities
   D. Fusion complexes
   E. All of the above

7. Buried P waves frequently alter the morphology of the previous ___ wave.

8. When deciding between the possibility that a complex is either a PAC or a PJC, the presence of a compensatory pause favors which type of premature complex?
   A. PJC
   B. PAC
   C. Neither

9. If the last few milliseconds of a wide-complex premature beat and the sinus beat are exactly the same, the wide-complex premature beat is probably aberrantly conducted. True or False.

10. Always take a look at the direction of the start of the QRS. If both the wide and narrow complexes are headed in the same direction, it is probably an aberrancy. True or False.

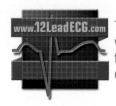

To enhance the knowledge you gain in this book, access this text's website at www.12leadECG.com! This valuable resource provides flashcards, an online glossary, web links, and more. Simply click on the Arrhythmias book cover once at the site.

Rapid Junctional Rhythms

Accelerated junctional rhythm and *junctional tachycardia* are basically the same rhythm, with rate being the only modifier separating them. The rates for accelerated junctional rhythm are between 60 and 100 BPM; those for junctional tachycardia are typically between 100 and 130 BPM (Figure 24-1). At rates between 130 and 140 BPM, the edges blur between what is considered a junctional tachycardia and what is considered an *AV nodal reentry tachycardia* (AVNRT; see Chapter 25), and either term is technically correct. At rates greater than 140 BPM, the rhythm is definitively called an AVNRT.

Accelerated junctional and junctional tachycardia are both caused by increased automaticity of the AV junction. They have the usual junctional morphology of narrow, supraventricular complexes and inverted P waves in leads II, III, and aVF that can be buried slightly before, or slightly after, the QRS complex. Junctional tachycardias are usually regular, although rarely, slight alterations in the cadence can develop. In these rare cases, the rhythm may resemble atrial fibrillation.

Junctional tachycardias with wide QRS complexes are difficult to distinguish from ventricular tachycardias. Wide-complexes can be seen in patients with pre-existing bundle branch blocks, aberrancy, or electrolyte abnormalities.

If retrograde conduction is present, the conduction ratios between the P wave and the QRS complexes remain constant. This is because the sinus node is consistently reset at a rate inherently faster than the normal sinus rate, essentially shutting off the SA node. If the retrograde conduction of the impulse is blocked, the sinus node and the atria will beat at their own pace, essentially causing two rhythms: an atrial rhythm and a ventricular rhythm, which is controlled by the junctional rate. (This is a condition known as atrioventricular dissociation. We will see this again in Chapter 35.)

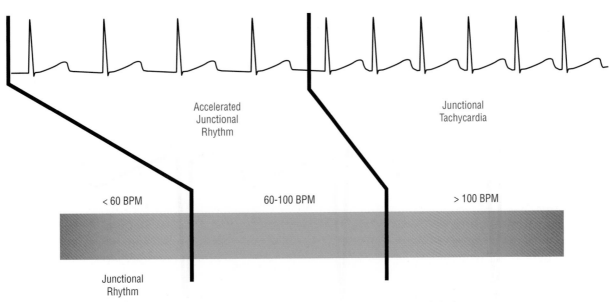

Accelerated
Junctional
Rhythm

Junctional
Tachycardia

< 60 BPM

60-100 BPM

> 100 BPM

Junctional
Rhythm

Figure 24-1: The spectrum of the junctional rhythms caused by increased intrinsic automaticity within the AV node and junctional area.

Pseudo-S and Pseudo-R' Waves

As we have seen, the P wave in the junctional rhythms can be inverted and can occur slightly after the QRS complex. In junctional tachycardias, that retrograde P wave can look just like a slurred S wave in leads II, III, and aVF and an R or R' wave in lead V_1. To differentiate these waves from "true" S and R' waves, they are known as *pseudo-S* and *pseudo-R* (or *pseudo-R'*) waves (Figures 24-2 and 24-3). The "pseudo" part is added to reflect the fact that these appear to be S waves and R waves but are not true waves; rather, they are merely an electrocardiographic reflection caused by the retrograde P waves.

These pseudo waves sometimes cause confusion when interpreting an ECG. But, they can also add a great clue to the correct arrhythmic diagnosis. Whenever you see a narrow-complex tachycardia with no obvious P waves but an s wave in the inferior leads and a small r' in lead V_1, think of an accelerated junctional rhythm, a junctional tachycardia, or AV nodal reentry tachycardia (which we will discuss in the next chapter).

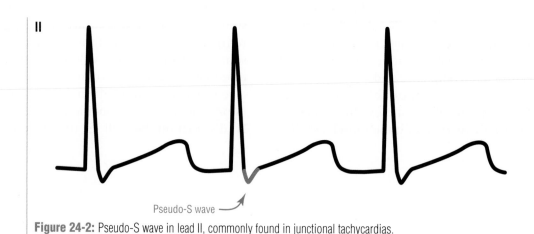

II

Pseudo-S wave

Figure 24-2: Pseudo-S wave in lead II, commonly found in junctional tachycardias.

V_1

Pseudo-R' wave

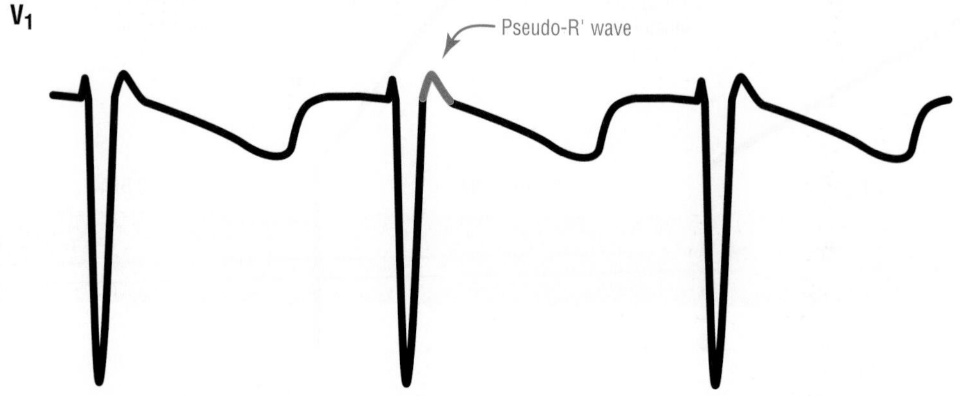

Figure 24-3: Pseudo-R' wave in lead V_1, commonly found in junctional tachycardias.

ARRHYTHMIA RECOGNITION

Accelerated Junctional Rhythm

Rate:	60 to 100 BPM
Regularity:	Regular
P wave:	Variable
Morphology:	Different, if present
Upright in II, III, and aVF:	No
P:QRS ratio:	Variable
PR interval:	Variable
QRS width:	Normal
Grouping:	None
Dropped beats:	None

ARRHYTHMIA RECOGNITION

Junctional Tachycardia

Rate:	100 to 130 BPM (may be seen up to 140 BPM)
Regularity:	Regular
P wave:	Variable
Morphology:	Different, if present
Upright in II, III, and aVF:	No
P:QRS ratio:	Variable
PR interval:	Variable
QRS width:	Normal
Grouping:	None
Dropped beats:	None

DIFFERENTIAL DIAGNOSIS

Accelerated Junctional Rhythm and Junctional Tachycardia

1. Ischemic heart disease, AMI
2. Intracardiac surgery
3. Digitalis toxicity
4. Myocarditis
5. Electrolyte disorders

The list above is not all-inclusive.

ECG Strips

ECG 24-1

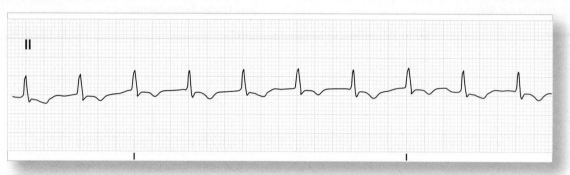

Rate:	About 98 BPM		PR intervals:	None
Regularity:	Regular		QRS width:	Normal
P waves:	None		Grouping:	None
Morphology:	None			
Axis:	None		Dropped beats:	None
P:QRS ratio:	None		Rhythm:	**Accelerated junctional**

Discussion:

This ECG shows an accelerated junctional rhythm at about 98 BPM. Since it is just under 100 BPM, we are not calling it junctional tachycardia. Note the absence of P waves, the regularity of the rhythm, and the narrow, supraventricular QRS complexes. The ST segments and symmetrically inverted T waves could easily represent ischemia or the reciprocal changes of a lateral AMI. Since accelerated junctional is associated with AMIs, clinical and electrocardiographic correlation would be a good idea.

ECG 24-2

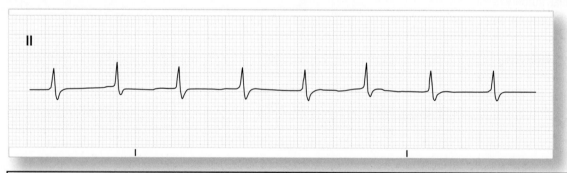

Rate:	About 85 BPM		PR intervals:	None
Regularity:	Regular		QRS width:	Wider than 0.12 sec.
P waves:	None		Grouping:	None
Morphology:	None			
Axis:	None		Dropped beats:	None
P:QRS ratio:	None		Rhythm:	**Accelerated junctional**

Discussion:

The strip above shows a wide-complex rhythm that is regular and has no apparent P waves. The width of the complex brings up a dilemma: Is this a ventricular rhythm or a junctional rhythm? Correlation with old strips and 12-lead ECGs showed a pre-existing bundle branch block with the same morphology as the ones in the strip in lead II, making this a junctional rhythm. Note that in some cases, inverted P waves may widen the QRS complex slightly, leading to a misdiagnosis of a bundle branch block.

ECG 24-3

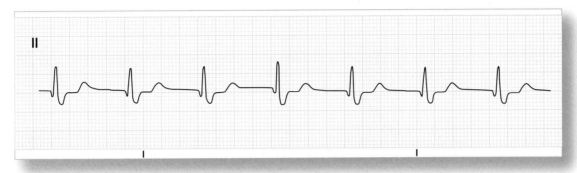

Rate:	About 78 BPM	PR intervals:	None
Regularity:	Regular	QRS width:	Wider than 0.12 sec.
P waves:	None	Grouping:	None
Morphology:	None		
Axis:	None	Dropped beats:	None
P:QRS ratio:	None	Rhythm:	**Accelerated junctional**

Discussion:

The strip above is also an example of a wide-complex accelerated junctional rhythm. This patient also had a pre-existing RBBB, which accounted for the wide complexes on the ECG. Once again, comparison with old ECGs, was crucial to determine the diagnosis and to evaluate if the small q wave and the R wave were not buried P waves. Never discount the usefulness of old ECGs, and always try to save a strip for posterity. You never know when you will need an old one to compare.

ECG 24-4

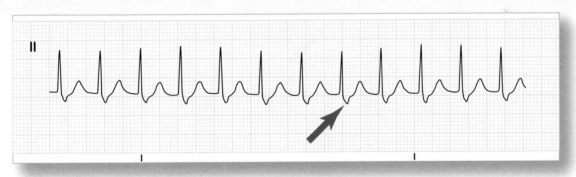

Rate:	About 135 BPM	PR intervals:	None
Regularity:	Regular	QRS width:	Normal
P waves:	Present (pseudo-S wave)	Grouping:	None
Morphology:	Pseudo-S wave		
Axis:	Abnormal	Dropped beats:	None
P:QRS ratio:	None	Rhythm:	**Junctional tachycardia**

Discussion:

This is the first example of junctional tachycardia that we have shown you. (The rate of 135 BPM is right at the borderline between junctional tachycardia and AV nodal reentry tachycardia, and either one is technically correct.) Are there any P waves on this strip? The answer is yes! The blue arrow is pointing to an inverted P wave that is occurring immediately after the QRS. This is a common finding in junctional tachycardias, known as the pseudo-S wave. It is called a pseudo-S because it is not a true S wave but is due to the inverted P wave. Comparing the morphologies with an old strip will clarify the question of S wave or pseudo-S wave.

ECG 24-5

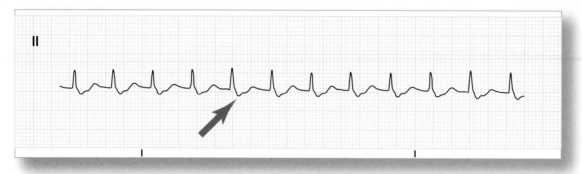

Rate:	About 135 BPM	PR intervals:	None
Regularity:	Regular	QRS width:	Normal

P waves:
  Morphology:
  Axis:
	Present (pseudo-S wave)
	Pseudo-S wave
	Abnormal
		Grouping:
		
		Dropped beats:
			None
			
			None

P:QRS ratio:	None	Rhythm:	**Junctional tachycardia**

Discussion:

The strip above shows a junctional tachycardia at about 135 BPM. (The rate of 135 BPM is right at the borderline between junctional tachycardia and AV nodal reentry tachycardia, and either one is technically correct.) The QRS complexes are narrow and obviously supraventricular in origin. There are no obvious P waves before the QRS complexes. Comparison with old strips confirmed the presence of a pseudo-S wave in lead II, which was not there on a strip with normal sinus rhythm. The pseudo-S wave was due to an inverted, retrogradely conducted P wave.

ECG 24-6

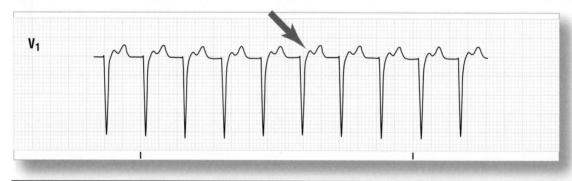

Rate:	About 135 BPM	PR intervals:	None
Regularity:	Regular	QRS width:	Normal

P waves:
  Morphology:
  Axis:
	Present (pseudo-R' wave)
	Pseudo-R' wave
	Abnormal
		Grouping:
		
		Dropped beats:
			None
			
			None

P:QRS ratio:	None	Rhythm:	**Junctional tachycardia**

Discussion:

This strip was taken on the same patient above, but the lead was switched to V_1. In this example, we see a pseudo-R' wave clearly. It is called a pseudo-R' wave because there is a small "actual" or "true" R wave present at the start of the complex. Remember, the first positive complex after an S wave is known as the R' wave.

ECG 24-7

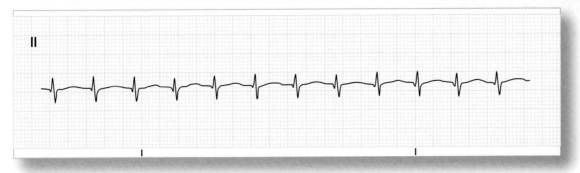

Rate:	About 135 BPM	PR intervals:	None
Regularity:	Regular	QRS width:	Normal
P waves:	None	Grouping:	None
Morphology:	None		
Axis:	None	Dropped beats:	None
P:QRS ratio:	None	Rhythm:	**Junctional tachycardia**

Discussion:

This is another example of a junctional tachycardia at about 135 BPM. (The rate of 135 BPM is right at the borderline between junctional tachycardia and AV nodal reentry tachycardia and either one is technically correct.) This strip has no obvious P waves and narrow, supraventricular QRS complexes.

ECG 24-8

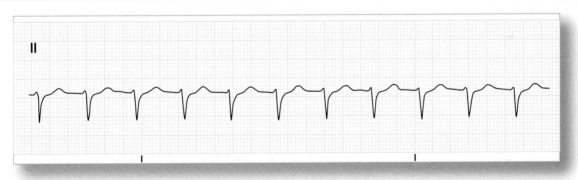

Rate:	About 112 BPM	PR intervals:	None
Regularity:	Regular	QRS width:	Normal
P waves:	None	Grouping:	None
Morphology:	None		
Axis:	None	Dropped beats:	None
P:QRS ratio:	None	Rhythm:	**Junctional tachycardia**

Discussion:

This strip is a junctional tachycardia at about 112 BPM. The QRS complexes are narrow and supraventricular in appearance. There may be a slight indentation at the end of the QRS complex, which could be indicative of a retrogradely conducted, inverted P wave, but this can-not be completely diagnosed from this strip. Comparison with an old strip will help identify the morphological appearance of the complexes and any possible buried waves.

CHAPTER REVIEW

1. Accelerated junctional rhythm and junctional tachycardia are basically the same rhythm except for the rate. True or False

2. Accelerated junctional rhythm and junctional tachycardia are due to increased automaticity of the AV junctional area. True or False.

3. Accelerated junctional rhythm is normally between ___ and ____ BPM.

4. Junctional tachycardia is typically between _____ and ____ BPM.

5. It is difficult to make the diagnosis of a junctional tachycardia at rates greater than 130 BPM on a surface ECG because it closely resembles AV nodal reentry tachycardia. True or False.

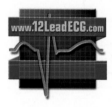

To enhance the knowledge you gain in this book, access this text's website at www.12leadECG.com! This valuable resource provides flashcards, an online glossary, web links, and more. Simply click on the Arrhythmias book cover once at the site.

CHAPTER 25

AV Nodal Reentry Tachycardia

General Overview

We are about to embark on the most complicated topic in arrhythmia recognition, AV nodal reentry tachycardia (AVNRT). Every time we have approached this topic in any lecture series (including advanced clinicians with years of experience), there is confusion as to the cause, mechanisms, and recognition of this complex but extremely common arrhythmia.

The recent changes made by the American Heart Association in their 2000 advanced cardiac life support (ACLS) guidelines have caused us to rethink the definition of what is appropriate for a beginner and what is still advanced. According to the new guidelines, every clinician should be able to differentiate between a supraventricular tachycardia with aberrancy and ventricular tachycardia. This means that every clinician—beginner or advanced—needs to know the difference between aberrantly conducted AVNRT, AVRT, and ventricular tachycardia. AVNRT and AVRT are now topics for beginners. We can no longer hide under the term "PSVT" and make the statement that they are all treated the same.

The logic behind the changes, which are appropriate, is that our pharmacological agents are becoming so sophisticated that they address the individual pathways involved in these pathological rhythms. In addition, what is indicated for the treatment of one arrhythmia can be detrimental if used in another similar-appearing arrhythmia. Wolff-Parkinson-White (WPW) greatly complicates the issue as well, because of the individual properties of the accessory pathways. Medications that slow down or block the AV node will oftentimes speed conduction through the accessory pathway, predisposing the patient to more serious arrhythmic consequences. The Chinese have a curse: May you live in interesting times! We live in a very interesting time in the field of medicine.

In this chapter, we are going to try to simplify the topic of AVNRT and make the concepts workable so that you can use them in everyday clinical life. To do this, we are going to deviate from our traditional approach and present the topic in a systematic three-step approach:

1. We are going to explain the process of reentry as it relates to AVNRT in very general, nonmedical terms.

2. We are going to take those principles and apply them to the AV junction, and to the pathology found in AVNRT in particular.

3. We are going to present the specifics of the arrhythmia clinically and electrocardiographically.

Step 1: General Concepts in AV Nodal Reentry

Normally, the AV node has only one approach or tract receiving the impulse from the atrial myocardium. As mentioned in Chapter 21, about 10% of patients have two tracts instead of one. The two tracts have their own distinct conduction properties, one conducting the current quickly, but having a much longer refractory period, and the other conducting the current much more slowly but having a shorter refractory period. Because of the differing conduction properties between the two tracts, one atrial depolarization wave could *theoretically* trigger two separate ventricular complexes. Luckily, this is not what happens in real life. Instead, the two tracts conduct the depolarization wave to the AV node in a very unique way. To help us understand how this process works, we are going to once again turn to our water model and use a simple analogy.

Suppose water were traveling down two separate channels (Figure 25-1). One of the channels is smooth and the water travels by laminar flow. The other channel is traversed with rocks and boulders, leading to the formation of turbulence. In which channel will the water travel faster?

The answer is that smooth, laminar flow is much faster than turbulent flow. Laminar flow is faster

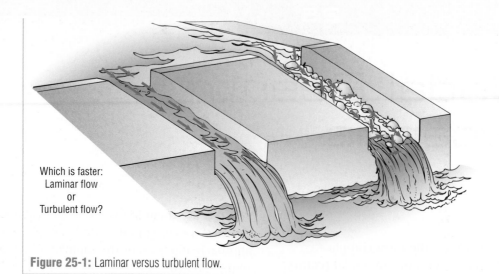

Figure 25-1: Laminar versus turbulent flow.

Which is faster:
Laminar flow
or
Turbulent flow?

because the water does not have anything holding it back or obstructing the flow (Figure 25-2). All the water is heading in the same direction and friction only occurs along the sides, where the water touches the channel walls. In turbulent flow, the water is constantly crashing into and around obstructions, which essentially slows the flow (Figure 25-3).

Now let's apply that concept to a real-life model. Suppose that you have a system of dry river channels like the one in Figure 25-4. The main channel splits into two branches that are exactly the same with the exception that one of the channels has some obstructions, which would cause turbulent flow if water were flowing through it. Can you predict the sequence of events if there were suddenly a flash flood?

First, water would travel by laminar flow until the branching point of the two channels (Figure 25-5). Then the water would proceed down the two branches. The smooth channel would continue to transport the water by direct laminar flow, and the water would travel very quickly. Let's call this one the fast channel. The obstructed channel would begin to develop turbulent flow as water winds its way slowly around the rocks (Figure 25-6). Let's call this channel the slow channel.

Now, what would happen when the water that traveled down the fast channel reaches the shallow, dry pond bed? The pond would begin to fill very quickly. Note that the pond is filling while water is still winding its way down the slow channel. What happens when the pond is completely filled?

Laminar Flow

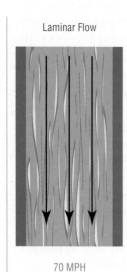

70 MPH

Figure 25-2: In laminar flow, all of the water is traveling in the same direction and the speed it accumulates is undisturbed.

Turbulent Flow

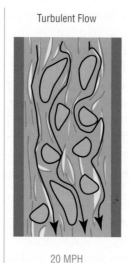

20 MPH

Figure 25-3: In turbulent flow, the water has to flow around various obstacles and is constantly crashing. Flow is much slower because the turbulence causes deceleration.

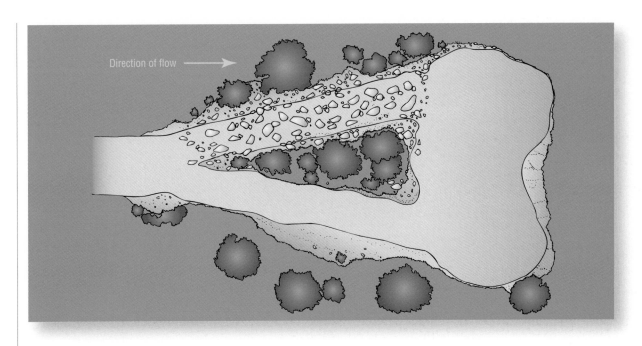

Figure 25-4: Dry riverbed.

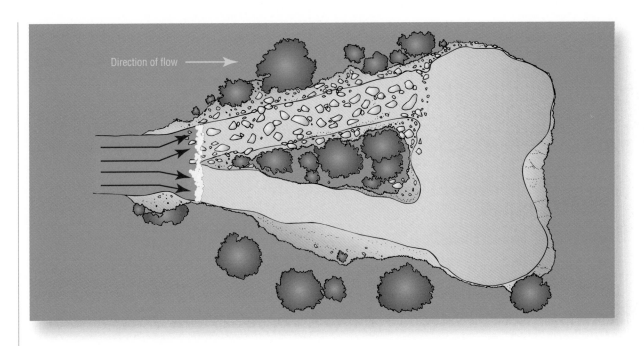

Figure 25-5: A flash flood appears.

When the pond is completely filled, the slow channel would begin to backfill with the water from the pond, which is quickly continuing to rise (Figure 25-7). The two wavefronts would travel along the slow channel until they crashed into each other (Figure 25-8). At that point, the water would stabilize and the water level would equilibrate according to the amount of water entering the system.

To recap, water entering the dry riverbed would rush downstream to the fork. There the water would spread evenly down the two channels. The flow down the smooth, fast channel would transport the water by direct

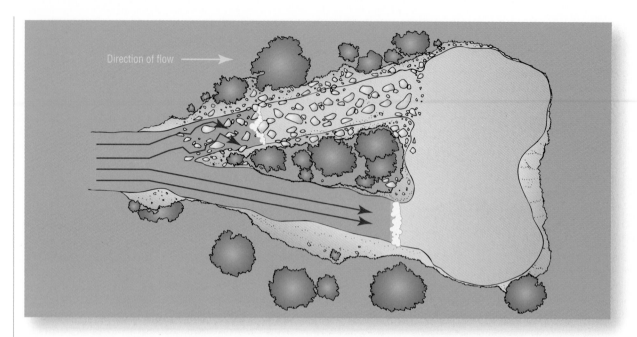

Figure 25-6: Water flows more quickly down the smooth "fast" channel than the obstructed "slow" channel.

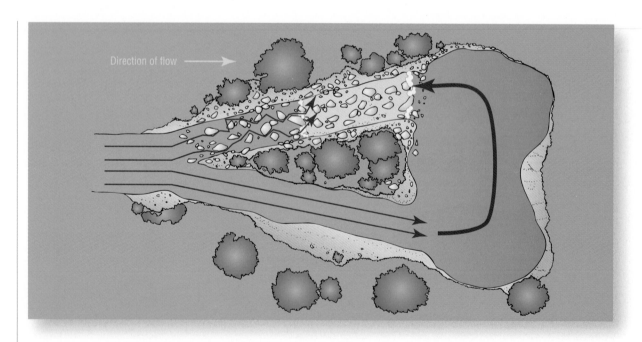

Figure 25-7: Once the pond is filled, the slow channel would begin to backfill.

laminar flow and would fill the pond first. Once the pond was filled, the water would begin to travel backward into the slow channel until the two wavefronts traveling along the slow channel met and cancelled each other out.

This sequence of events is fairly intuitive and easy to understand. As we shall see, it is also identical to what happens during a normal cycle in many patients with dual approaches to the AV node. The depolarization wave travels down the fast channel, depolarizes the AV node, and begins to return retrogradely up the slow channel. There the two currents meet, essentially canceling each other out. Note that only the depolarization wave traveling down the fast pathway depolarizes the AV node and causes only one ventricular depolarization.

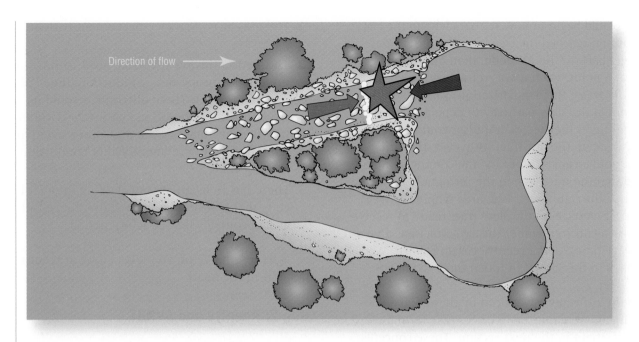

Figure 25-8: The two wavefronts traveling along the slow channel crash into each other, essentially canceling each other out.

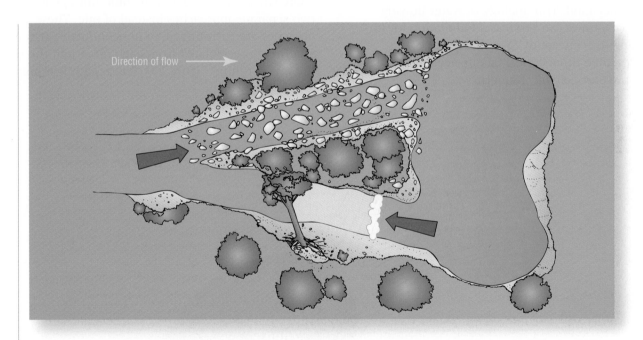

Figure 25-9: If the smooth channel is obstructed, the flow of water would be forced down the slower channel. The water would then fill the pond and flow retrogradely up the fast channel until it reached the bifurcation again.

The sequence outlined above occurs 99.99999% of the time. Now, let's move on to the other 0.00001% of the time. This very rare, but very real, scenario leads to the formation of a reentry circuit within the AV node and to the formation of AVNRT. Once again, we will turn to our water model to help simplify the process.

Suppose a tree were washed down by the rapid flow of the flash flood, and the tree propped itself right across the fast channel. What would happen to the flow of water then? Looking at Figure 25-9, we see that the flow of water would be forced down the slow channel. Eventually, the flow of water would reach the pond, fill it, and the water would begin to flow retrogradely up the fast channel until it reached the tree from the other side.

Let's get back to the AV node. If an impulse hit the fast tract at a point when it was refractory (the tree blocking the way), the depolarization wave would have to travel down the slow pathway to depolarize the AV node. From here, the electric impulse would travel retrogradely back up the fast tract. However, this time, the wave will not be canceled out by one coming simultaneously down the tract. When the retrograde impulse reaches the bifurcation area (the area where the tree would be), it would find the slow tract ready to receive the impulse again (remember the slow tract has a very fast recovery time), and a reentry circuit is born. We will get back to this circuit in much more detail later in the chapter.

Keep the concepts introduced by these two analogies in mind as we continue to discuss the formation of the reentry circuit in the next section. These concepts are key to understanding the mechanisms involved in the formation of AV nodal reentry tachycardia.

Reentry is a very foreign concept and very, very difficult to understand. This analogy of water flowing down two channels can serve as a foundation for understanding the concept of AV nodal reentry. This model presented three critical factors needed in order to establish a reentry circuit. Namely:

1. The presence of an electrical circuit with at least two pathways.

2. The two pathways involved need to have different underlying properties: conduction time, refractoriness, and so on. These differences could be due to a structural difference in the pathways, ischemia, electrolyte abnormalities, or any other event that will temporarily or permanently alter conduction and refractory time.

3. There has to be an area of slowing in one of the circuits that is just enough to allow the rest of the circuit to complete its refractory period.

Now let's move on and take a look at what really happens in the heart.

Step 2: Reentry and AVNRT

In Chapter 21 and in the previous section, we talked about the anatomy of the AV node. We saw that most people have a single area of nonspecialized tissue that approaches the AV node. But sometimes people have two separate approaches instead of one. These approaches are surrounded by nonconductive tissue and are, therefore, isolated from each other and the rest of the myocardium. Figure 25-10 is a graphic representa-

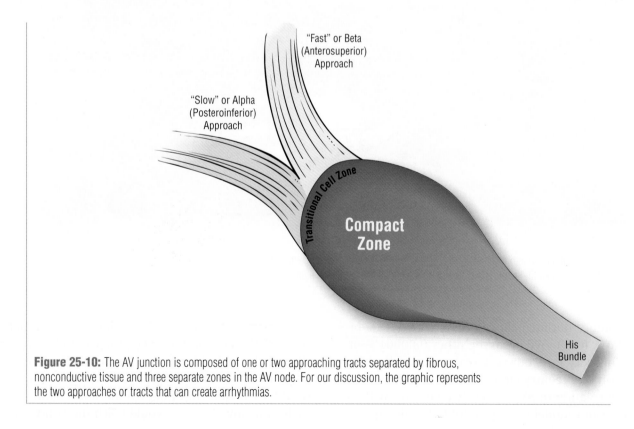

Figure 25-10: The AV junction is composed of one or two approaching tracts separated by fibrous, nonconductive tissue and three separate zones in the AV node. For our discussion, the graphic represents the two approaches or tracts that can create arrhythmias.

tion of the AV junction accentuating the two approaches or tracts leading up to the AV node.

Some people with the two tracts develop not only an anatomical separation, but a clinically relevant separation that can lead to reentry arrhythmias, specifically AVNRT. The two approaches are located at the base of the right atrium and are known as the fast or beta (anterosuperior) pathway and the slow or alpha (posteroinferior) pathway.

The pathways are functionally, as well as anatomically, different from each other, each with its own respective properties. The fast tract has very rapid conduction times but very slow refractory times. Simply, that means that the fast tract conducts impulses through the pathway very, very quickly but, once it fires, it takes a long time before it is ready to fire again. Think of a sprinter in a track race, giving his all for a short burst of speed and then needing time to recoup strength.

The slow tract has very slow conduction times but very fast refractory times. In other words, it conducts the forward impulse slowly but can conduct another one shortly afterward. This is more like a long-distance runner who can run for long distances with a short recovery time between the various bursts of speed in a race.

Now that we have covered some of the basics, can you predict what would happen when an atrial depolarization wave approaches the two tracts (Figure 25-11)? (Think back on the water model presented earlier in this chapter.)

The impulse would hit the two approaches simultaneously. The two approaches would then start transmitting the impulse at the same time, but the fast tract would transmit it faster (Figure 25-12). The result is that the fast tract stimulates the AV node and causes the depolarization wave to proceed normally down the bundle of His and on to the ventricular electrical conduction system, causing a nice tight QRS complex. The depolarization wave will also retrogradely travel back up the slow tract. Eventually, the two opposing waves (the normally conducted wave along the slow tract and the retrograde wave) would crash into each other and cancel each other out. The cancellation of the two wavefronts in the slow tract is exactly what occurs 99.99999%+ of the time during a regular sinus or atrial rhythm.

What would happen if, for any reason, the fast tract could not transmit the impulse? To understand what would happen, think about what happened when the tree blocked the fast channel in the water analogy. When the fast tract was obstructed, the water traveled down the slow tract to reach the pond. Likewise, if the fast tract were refractory for any reason, the impulse would be propagated down the slow tract. Would the two complexes look the same? The answer is that the complexes would be identical, except for the PR intervals (Figure 25-13). The PR intervals of the impulses that traveled down the slow tract would be longer than ones that used the fast tract. This is exactly what we see in many patients with a functional two-tract system. They have identical complexes with two different PR intervals present on the same strip. (Note that these two types of complexes are still both sinus complexes, as the variations in the PR intervals are not due to ectopic foci firing but rather to conduction alternating intermittently between the two different tracts.)

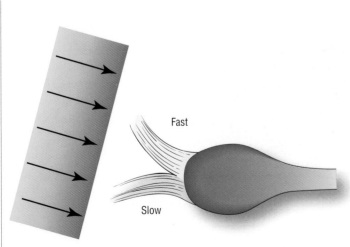

Figure 25-11: An atrial depolarization wave is approaching the AV junctional tracts. Can you predict what would happen?

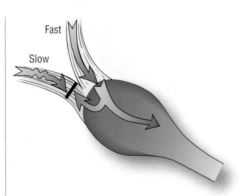

Figure 25-12: The depolarization wave travels down the fast channel faster. The result is that the AV node is depolarized by the impulse from the fast channel. The impulse then begins to spread backward from the AV node to the slow channel. Eventually, the two wavefronts traveling through the slow channel would meet and cancel each other out. Note that only one of the impulses was transmitted to the ventricles.

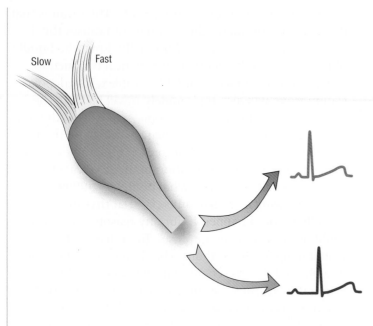

Figure 25-13: Depending on which tract transmits the impulse, the PR intervals will vary. This variation can occur beat-to-beat in many circumstances.

AVNRT is formed when a reentry loop is created along the two approaches and the AV node. Here is how the loop is created. Assume that the heart is clipping along at a nice regular pace (Figure 25-14). The impulses are being transmitted "normally" along the two pathways. Immediately after being depolarized, the two tracts would be refractory to any further impulse propagation for a short time.

Now let's suppose that an ectopic atrial focus fires prematurely, causing a PAC (see Figure 25-14). Will the fast tract be ready to handle the PAC? Will the slow tract be able to handle the PAC?

When the PAC hits the two tracts (Figure 25-15), it would find the slow tract ready to accept it because of its faster recovery time, but the fast tract would still be refractory to any new impulse due to its intrinsically slow recovery time. In other words, the PAC reached the fast tract when it was refractory and functioning exactly as the log did in our water model. Due to the obstruction to flow in the fast tract, the impulse would have to be conducted to the AV node through the only way possible—the slow tract. (Note that the PR interval

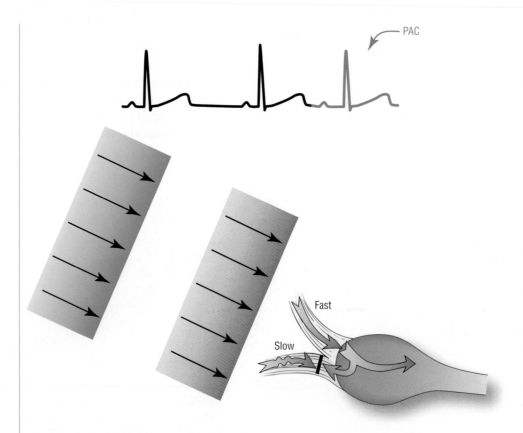

Figure 25-14: A normal sinus depolarization wave arrives at the two tracts. The fast tract transmits the impulse through as expected and as shown in the graphic. The premature impulse would then arrive, and this sequence is shown in Figure 25-15.

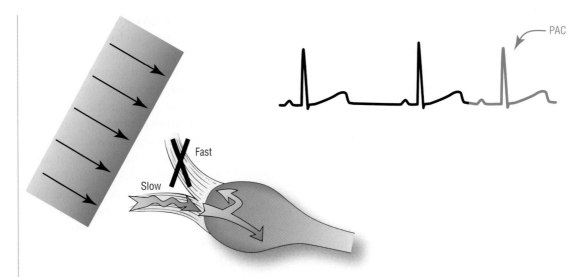

Figure 25-15: By the time the PAC arrives at the two tracts, the fast tract is refractory and the impulse must proceed through the slow tract. When the impulse reaches the AV node, it begins to fire retrogradely through the now nonrefractory fast tract.

found in this PAC would be wider than normal, reflecting the additional time needed for the impulse to be conducted through the slow tract.)

As we saw before, once the depolarization wave stimulates the AV node, it would begin to return retrogradely up the fast tract (see Figure 25-15). The reason that the fast tract would now be able to handle the new impulse is because it took additional time for the wave to travel through the slow tract. The extra time allowed the fast tract to work through its slower refractory pe-

riod, allowing it to be ready to receive the new retrograde impulse.

At this point, the retrograde wave can traverse the entire fast tract retrogradely without meeting any obstruction. When the retrogradely spread impulse reaches the other end of the fast tract, it spreads quickly over to the slow tract (Figure 25-16). Remember, electricity, like water, spreads whenever it can and wherever it can. At this point, we have completed a complete loop. What do you think happens at this point?

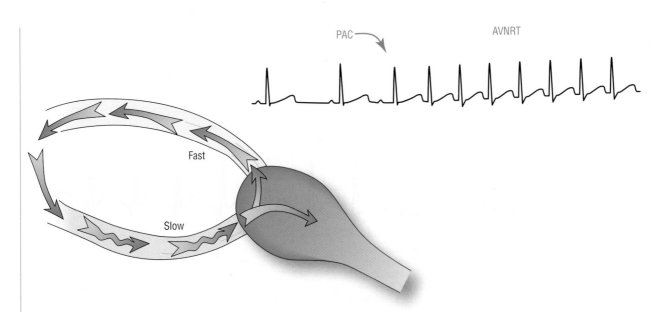

Figure 25-16: The PAC triggers a circus movement involving both tracts and the AV node. The resulting reentry circuit leads to the formation of a rhythm known as AVNRT. Note the pseudo-S pattern at the end of the AVNRT complexes representing the retrogradely conducted P wave.

The slow tract, with its short refractory period, receives the retrograde impulse and transmits it back toward the AV node, which then retrogradely spreads the impulse to the fast tract, which spreads it back to the slow tract. . .and so on, and so on (see Figure 25-16). It is now a reentry circuit or circus movement within the AV junction and the rhythm that is produced electrocardiographically is an AV nodal reentry tachycardia. The PAC was the trigger that started this.

Step 3: Identifying the Arrhythmia

A *supraventricular tachycardia* is a rough, general term for a rapid rhythm that has its origin in the atrial and junctional areas of the heart (the areas above the ventricles). The supraventricular tachycardias include sinus tachycardia, ectopic atrial tachycardia and its variations, paroxysmal atrial tachycardia, atrial flutter, atrial fibril-lation, junctional tachycardia, AV *nodal* reentry tachycardia, and AV reentry tachycardia. (The term supraventricular tachycardia is such an umbrella term that it should be avoided clinically, if possible. It is more clinically useful to determine the actual rhythm and to use the appropriate term for the arrhythmia.)

AVNRT is the most common regular paroxysmal supraventricular tachycardia found in clinical practice. Note the key words in that statement are the words "regular" and "paroxysmal." AVNRT is a regular tachycardia that is caused by a reentry loop involving the AV junctional area. It is a paroxysmal (rapid onset, rapid termination) tachycardia that, as we saw, is usually triggered by a PAC (Figure 25-17). The PAC is usually associated with a prolonged PR interval because of transmission through the slow approach to the AV node.

The most common ventricular rate is between 170 and 220 BPM, although rates can be between 140 and

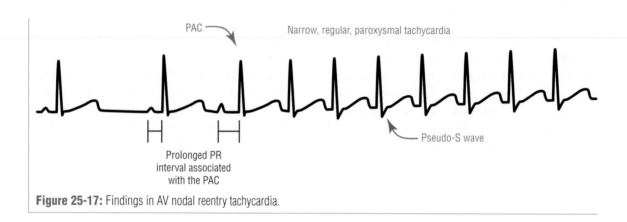

Figure 25-17: Findings in AV nodal reentry tachycardia.

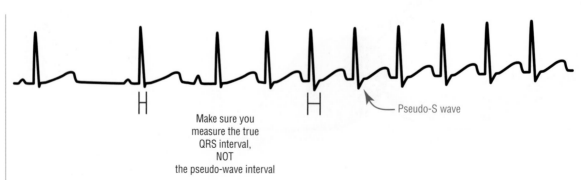

Figure 25-18: QRS interval in AVNRT. The thinner brackets are the true QRS interval. The wider brackets are the space being widened by the presence of a pseudo-S wave.

250 BPM in many circumstances. The P waves typically are buried within the QRS complex or are found immediately after the QRS complex. The P waves are rarely found in front of the QRS. The formation of pseudo-R' waves in lead V$_1$ and pseudo-S waves in lead II is a common finding in AVNRT.

The QRS complexes are typically narrow complexes with a total QRS interval width of less than 0.12 seconds. Wider complexes are found when the patient has a pre-existing bundle branch block, when the complexes are aberrantly conducted, and when there are significant electrolyte abnormalities. Care must be taken not to include the pseudo-R' or pseudo-S wave interval in the calculation of the QRS complex, as this causes a false widening of the QRS interval (Figure 25-18). Sometimes, an old strip or a section of sinus rhythm is needed to measure the true QRS interval. Other possible solutions include measuring the interval in a lead without the pseudo-waves or measuring the intervals once the rhythm is broken.

ADDITIONAL **INFORMATION**

Atypical AVNRT

We have seen that the normal reentry loop occurs when the impulse enters the slow tract and then spreads retrogradely back via the fast tract. This is the most common type of AVNRT and is known as *typical* or *common AVNRT*. In addition to this type of AVNRT, there is also an *uncommon* or *atypical* form, which occurs in 5 to 10% of the cases. Atypical AVNRT occurs when the reentry loop is backward compared to the typical form. In the atypical form, the impulse enters the fast tract and then spreads retrogradely via the slow tract.

The big difference between these two types of AVNRT is the location of the P wave. The R-P interval—the distance from the start of the QRS complex to the end of the P wave—is longer in the atypical form of AVNRT. This happens because the slow conduction time of the retrograde impulse through the slow tract, lengthens the total time to reach and spread through to the atria. In other words, slower conduction equals longer intervals (Figure 25-19).

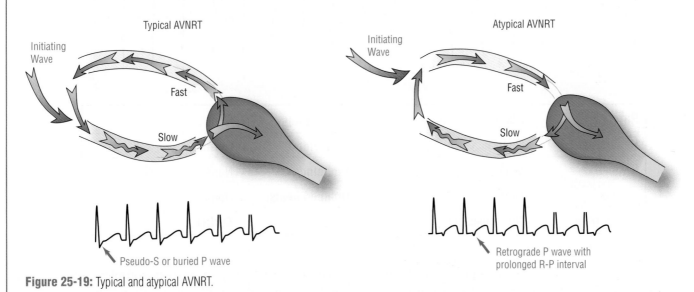

Figure 25-19: Typical and atypical AVNRT.

ARRHYTHMIA RECOGNITION

AV Nodal Reentry Tachycardia

Rate:	140 to 250 BPM (most commonly between 170 and 220 BPM)
Regularity:	Regular
P wave:	Inverted or buried
Morphology:	Inverted
Upright in II, III, and aVF:	No
P:QRS ratio:	1:1 (If P waves are present)
PR interval:	None or R-P interval
QRS width:	Normal
Grouping:	None
Dropped beats:	None

DIFFERENTIAL DIAGNOSIS

AV Nodal Reentry Tachycardia

1. Idiopathic

AVNRT is caused because of the presence of a dual pathway approaching the AV junction. It is normally found in patients without other structural heart disease.

ECG Strips

ECG 25-1

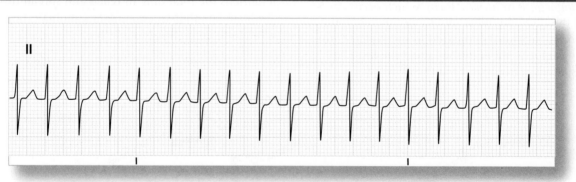

Rate:	About 180 BPM	PR intervals:	None
Regularity:	Regular	QRS width:	Normal
P waves:	None	Grouping:	None
Morphology:	None		
Axis:	None	Dropped beats:	None
P:QRS ratio:	Not applicable	Rhythm:	**AVNRT**

Discussion:

This rhythm strip shows a narrow complex tachycardia that is very regular and has no visible P waves anywhere on the strip. There is no evidence of any pseudo-S pattern on the strip. A narrow-complex tachycardia at this rate is AVNRT until proven otherwise.

ECG 25-2

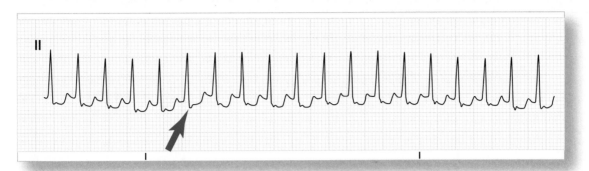

Rate:	About 200 BPM		PR intervals:	None
Regularity:	Regular		QRS width:	Normal

P waves:
  Morphology:
  Axis:
	Pseudo-S
	Inverted
	Abnormal
			Grouping:	None

			Dropped beats:	None
P:QRS ratio:	1:1		Rhythm:	**AVNRT**

Discussion:

The rhythm strip above shows a very rapid rhythm at about 200 BPM. The QRS complexes are narrow and there are no discernible P wave. There is, however, a small s wave noted at the end of the QRS complex, which was not there on old ECGs. This is a pseudo-S wave (blue arrow) and is representative of an inverted P wave. The ST segment is depressed, as is common in rapid tachycardias. This could be due to relative endocardial ischemia due to the rapid rate, but the cause is usually unclear.

ECG 25-3

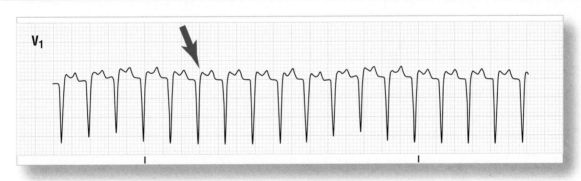

Rate:	About 200 BPM		PR intervals:	None
Regularity:	Regular		QRS width:	Normal

P waves:
  Morphology:
  Axis:
	Pseudo-R'
	Not applicable
	Not applicable
			Grouping:	None

			Dropped beats:	None
P:QRS ratio:	1:1		Rhythm:	**AVNRT**

Discussion:

This strip was obtained from the same patient as the one above, except that this is lead V_1. The extra lead was obtained in order to evaluate the patient for a pseudo-R' wave, which is present, at the end of the QS wave (blue arrow). Electrical alternans is obvious on the strip with an undulating pattern of longer and shorter QS waves. This is very common in very rapid tachycardias and does not represent any secondary pathological processes, such as pericardial effusion. Clinical correlation is indicated, however.

ECG 25·4

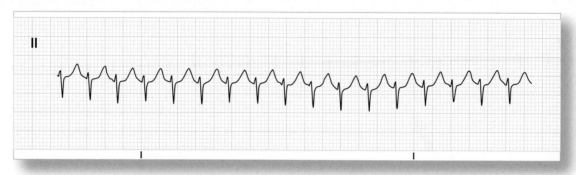

Rate:	About 195 BPM	PR intervals:	None
Regularity:	Regular	QRS width:	Normal
P waves:	None	Grouping:	None
Morphology:	None		
Axis:	None	Dropped beats:	None
P:QRS ratio:	Not applicable	Rhythm:	**AVNRT**

Discussion:

The rhythm strip above shows a rapid, narrow-complex tachycardia with negative QRS complexes in lead II. The negative complexes are composed of deep S waves, making any pseudo-s pattern difficult, if not impossible, to visualize. There is some undulation in QRS size, which is compatible with most rapid tachycardias.

ECG 25·5

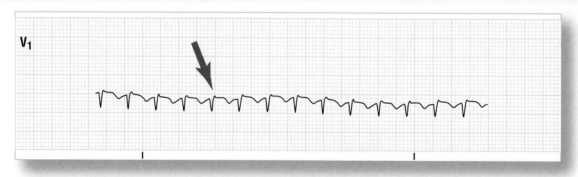

Rate:	About 195 BPM	PR intervals:	None
Regularity:	Regular	QRS width:	Normal
P waves:	Pseudo-R'	Grouping:	None
Morphology:	Not clear		
Axis:	Abnormal	Dropped beats:	None
P:QRS ratio:	1:1	Rhythm:	**AVNRT**

Discussion:

This strip is, once again, a strip of the same patient as above, but in lead V₁. Here the pseudo-R' pattern is more evident (blue arrow). This finding clinches the diagnosis of AVNRT. Please note that in all of these examples, the regularity of the rhythm is uncanny. This is due to the reentry mechanism, which causes clockwise precision in the regularity of the rhythm.

ECG 25-6

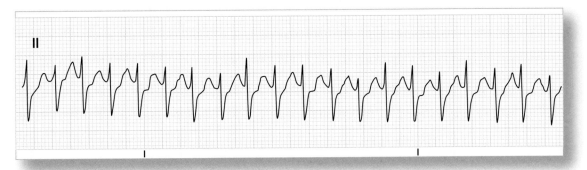

Rate:	About 200 BPM	PR intervals:	None
Regularity:	Regular	QRS width:	Normal
P waves:	None	Grouping:	None
Morphology:	None		
Axis:	None	Dropped beats:	None
P:QRS ratio:	Not applicable	Rhythm:	**AVNRT**

Discussion:

The rhythm strip above shows a narrow-complex tachycardia at about 200 BPM. The QRS complexes are negatively oriented and there appears to be a small deflection at the end of the S wave, which could indicate a pseudo-S pattern. There is some variation in the height of the R wave, which is compatible with electrical alternans seen in many rapid tachycardias. AVNRT is the diagnosis of this rhythm abnormality.

ECG 25-7

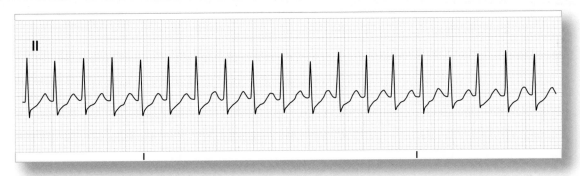

Rate:	About 190 BPM	PR intervals:	None
Regularity:	Regular	QRS width:	Normal
P waves:	See discussion below	Grouping:	None
Morphology:	See discussion below		
Axis:	See discussion below	Dropped beats:	None
P:QRS ratio:	See discussion below	Rhythm:	**AVNRT**

Discussion:

This is a rapid tachycardia at about 190 BPM with a narrow complex by initial appearance. The problem is that there is ST-segment depression and a possible pseudo-S pattern or slurred S-wave pattern (typically seen in bundle branch block). The narrowness of the initial R wave makes the diagnosis of ventricular tachycardia less likely. Comparing this strip to an old ECG or to one taken when the rhythm is broken is critical in deciding the final diagnosis. If the patient is unstable, he or she should be cardioverted or defibrillated emergently. Treatment with vagal maneuvers or adenosine initially would be appropriate if the patient were stable.

ECG 25-8

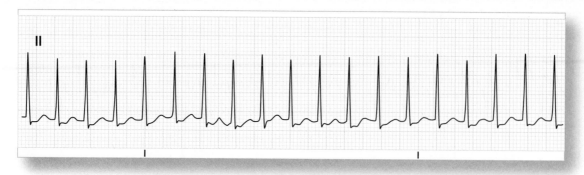

Rate:	About 185 BPM	PR intervals:	None
Regularity:	Regular	QRS width:	Normal
P waves:	See discussion below	Grouping:	None
Morphology:	See discussion below		
Axis:	See discussion below	Dropped beats:	None
P:QRS ratio:	1:1	Rhythm:	**AVNRT**

Discussion:

This strip also has ST-segment depression, which could be from the tachycardia or ischemia (relative or endocardial). Clinical correlation is indicated to evaluate this finding. There is a small s wave, which could be an actual part of the QRS complex or could be due to a pseudo-s wave pattern. Comparison with an old ECG would be helpful. The variation in QRS size is due to electrical alternans and is probably due to the tachycardia.

ECG 25-9

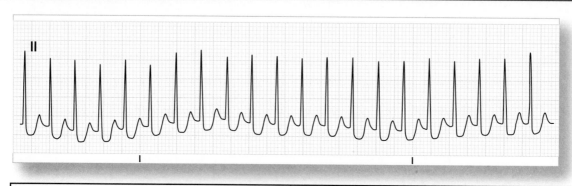

Rate:	About 210 BPM	PR intervals:	None
Regularity:	Regular	QRS width:	Normal
P waves:	None	Grouping:	None
Morphology:	None		
Axis:	None	Dropped beats:	None
P:QRS ratio:	Not applicable	Rhythm:	**AVNRT**

Discussion:

This strip shows a rapid, narrow-complex tachycardia at about 210 BPM. The QRS complexes are pretty clearly defined and the ST segments are depressed and have a scooped-out appearance. This pattern of ST depression may be due to the tachycardia, ischemia, or digitalis effect. Clinical correlation and comparison to an old ECG are critical in arriving at the final diagnosis. Remember, however, treat the tachycardia first, and then worry about the final diagnosis. AVNRT should be the first thing on your differential diagnosis list.

ECG 25·10

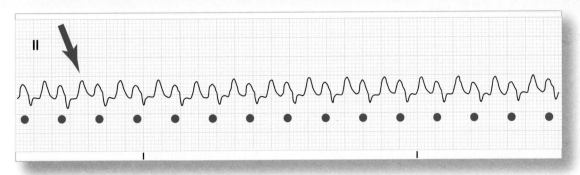

Rate:	About 145 BPM	PR intervals:	None
Regularity:	Regular	QRS width:	Normal
P waves: Morphology: Axis:	None None None	Grouping:	None
		Dropped beats:	None
P:QRS ratio:	None	Rhythm:	**AVNRT**

Discussion:

This is a real diagnostic dilemma. This is a wide-complex tachycardia that is regular and has no observable P waves. This could very easily be ventricular tachycardia and the patient should be treated for this possibility until proven otherwise. Differential diagnosis includes junctional tachycardia, AVNRT, AVRT, and ventricular tachycardia. Comparison with an old ECG showed a pre-existing bundle branch block with similar morphology, clinching the diagnosis as AVNRT. The QRS complexes are labeled with the blue dots, and the T wave is labeled with the blue arrow.

CHAPTER REVIEW

1. A reentry circuit must have:
   A. A circuit with at least two different pathways
   B. Pathways with different intrinsic properties of conduction
   C. One pathway that conducts slower than the other
   D. All of the above

2. In 10 to 35% of patients, the approach to the AV node is split into two tracts: the _____ tract and the _____ tract.

3. Under normal circumstances, the supraventricular impulse will travel down both tracts simultaneously. But, since conduction times are different, conduction through the _____ tract will be quicker.

4. When a PAC hits the two pathways, the fast tract may be refractory. The impulse may then have to travel abnormally down the slow tract. The impulse will then travel retrogradely back up the fast tract to complete the loop. True or False.

5. An indirect sign of a dual pathway system is when the patient has two different _____ but morphologically identical P waves in a normal sinus rhythm.

6. AVNRT is an example of the type of rhythm covered under the broader term paroxysmal supraventricular tachycardias. True or False.

7. The ventricular rates in AVNRT can be anywhere between:
   A. 120 and 160 BPM
   B. 140 and 180 BPM
   C. 140 and 250 BPM
   D. 170 and 250 BPM

8. The P waves in AVNRT can be found _____, _____, or _____ the QRS complex.

9. In AVNRT, the retrograde P waves can cause "pseudo" waves in various leads: pseudo-R' waves in lead II and pseudo S waves in lead V_1. True or False.

10. In addition to the typical form of AVNRT, there is an atypical form of AVNRT. The atypical form is associated with P waves that are inverted and far behind the QRS complex. In other words, the R-P interval is prolonged. True or False.

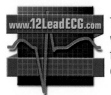

To enhance the knowledge you gain in this book, access this text's website at www.12leadECG.com! This valuable resource provides flashcards, an online glossary, web links, and more. Simply click on the Arrhythmias book cover once at the site.

AV Reentry Tachycardia

AV reentry tachycardia (AVRT) is caused by a macroreentry circuit involving the AV node and an accessory pathway. Normally, the AV node functions as the only true means of communication between the atria and the ventricles. In some people, however, a second (or multiple) tract develops elsewhere along the atrioventricular septum that allows another route of communication between the atria and the ventricles. This area is called an *accessory pathway*.

A good way to think about it is that an accessory pathway is like a backdoor into the ventricles. That backdoor does not have a guard on it like the AV node does, and so communication is unimpeded. In other words, the impulses move right through the pathway without any physiologic block or control of any kind. This lack of control can lead to some serious tachycar-

dias, which could be life threatening in many cases. AVRT is just such a rhythm disturbance.

Accessory pathways have their own rates of impulse conduction and refractory periods. These variations will be important when we begin to consider how the macroreentry circuit is formed in AVRT.

Normal Conduction Through an Accessory Pathway

Under normal circumstances, an atrial impulse will hit the AV node and the accessory pathway fairly close together, temporally speaking (Figure 26-1). The net result of this atrial depolarization wave is that the impulse begins to move through both the AV node and the accessory pathway almost simultaneously. The

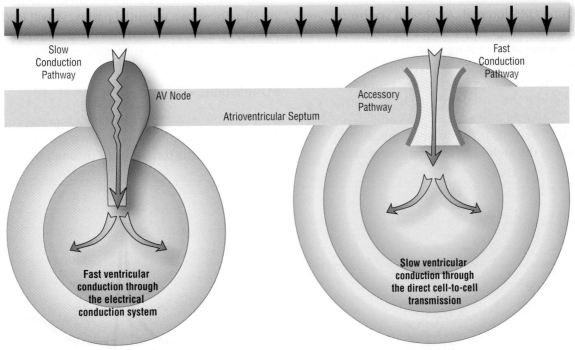

Figure 26-1: When an accessory pathway is present, the impulse has two ways of getting to the ventricles. The usual way of using the AV node is slower because of the presence of the physiologic block. The accessory pathway is not subject to the physiologic block and transmits the impulse instantaneously. Therefore, the ventricular myocardium around the accessory pathway will begin to depolarize quicker but ventricular activation will have to occur by direct cell-to-cell transmission.

AV node slows conduction briefly by applying the physiologic block. The impulse traveling through the accessory pathway, however, is unimpeded and begins to depolarize the ventricles immediately. The impulse traveling through the accessory pathway, however, moves very slowly through the ventricular myocardium because it has to travel by direct cell-to-cell transmission. Electrocardiographically, this very slow conduction through the ventricles leads to a wide, bizarre appearance at the start of the QRS complex. That wide, bizarre area of the QRS is called a *delta wave* (Figure 26-2).

Once the physiologic block is completed in the AV node, the impulse is quickly spread throughout the majority of the ventricular myocardium via the electrical conduction system. Since transmission through the normal conduction system is much faster than direct cell-to-cell transmission, the normally conducted impulse quickly overtakes and surrounds the impulse originating in the accessory pathway.

The two wavefronts eventually meet and cancel each other out. The large amount of myocardium depolarized by the normal wave causes a sharp stop to the delta wave. Electrocardiographically, this is represented as the end of the delta wave and the formation of a normal appearing mid- and terminal portion of the QRS complex. Note, however, that the QRS complex is still wide because the duration of the delta wave has to be added to the total QRS interval. As we can see from Figure 26-2, the added width of the QRS interval does come at the expense of the PR interval.

Electrocardiographically, the net result of this dual conduction is a short PR interval (because of the immediate transmission of the impulse through the accessory pathway), a delta wave, and a wide QRS complex (greater than 0.12 seconds). To round off this discussion, transmission through accessory pathways also

alters the ST segment and the T wave by altering the repolarization pattern of the ventricle. This electrocardiographic pattern is presently named after the investigators who discovered it and is known as *Wolff-Parkinson-White* (WPW) *pattern*.

An additional clinical point: If a patient with the WPW pattern also has symptoms or any clinical manifestations of rapid tachycardias, then the correct terminology for this clinical syndrome is *Wolff-Parkinson-White syndrome*. The word "syndrome" is used to focus on the pathological inclusion of life-threatening arrhythmias into the picture.

AVRT Reentry Circuits

So far, we have seen how an accessory pathway fulfills the three criteria for a reentry loop. These patients have an electrical circuit with at least two pathways, the two pathways have different underlying conduction properties, and there is an area of impulse slowing in one of the circuits (in the case of AVRT, the area of slowing is the AV node). By examining the anatomy of the two pathways, we see that the impulse from the atria can proceed in one of two ways: (1) the impulse can travel down the AV node and travel back up through the accessory pathway (Figure 26-3A); or (2) the impulse can travel down the accessory pathway and back up the AV node (Figure 26-3B). These two potential pathways will lead to the formation of the two electrocardiographic presentations of AVRT, orthodromic and antidromic AVRT.

Orthodromic AVRT

Orthodromic AVRT is created by a macroreentry circuit in which the impulse travels down through the AV node and returns retrogradely through the accessory

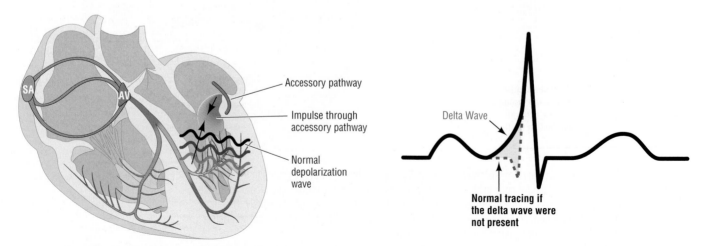

Figure 26-2: Impulse propagation through an accessory pathway and formation of the delta wave.

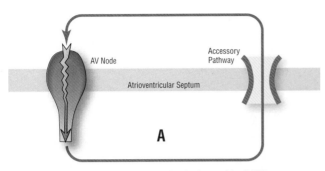
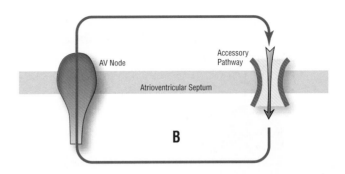
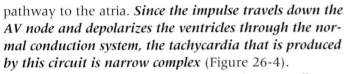

Figure 26-3: Two possible reentry circuits formed in AVRT.

pathway to the atria. *Since the impulse travels down the AV node and depolarizes the ventricles through the normal conduction system, the tachycardia that is produced by this circuit is narrow complex* (Figure 26-4).

Just as in AVNRT, the initiating impulse is usually a PAC. In AVRT, however, the initiating impulse can also be a PVC. The PVC can cause a transient block in the His-AV node area that does not allow the spread retrogradely through the AV node. However, the accessory pathway would not be blocked and would conduct the impulse retrogradely to the atria to trigger the reentry loop.

Orthodromic AVRT has one major advantage over its evil twin, antidromic AVRT—the AV node still has tremendous influence over the rates and conduction speeds. The AV node exerts its influence because it still has a functional physiologic block and responds to medications as it would under normal circumstances. This means that the rates of the tachycardia are more stable and are usually in the range of 140 to 250 BPM (although variability does occur) and are reasonably toler-

ated by most patients. The additional fact that the ventricles are contracting smoothly and synchronously because of the use of the electrical conduction system adds to the hemodynamic stability in orthodromic vs. antidromic AVRT.

The sympathetic system exerts control over the rate by altering the conduction speed through the AV node. The higher the sympathetic tone, the higher the rate. Likewise, pharmacologic agents that slow conduction through the AV node will also control or terminate the arrhythmia.

The P Wave and AVRT

A very important diagnostic clue to decide whether a rapid tachycardic rhythm is either AVNRT or AVRT is the location of the inverted P wave. As we saw in Chapter 25, the inverted P wave in AVNRT is either immediately before, during, or immediately after the QRS complex. In AVRT, the inverted P wave is usually pretty far away from the QRS complex. Can you think of why this would be?

ADDITIONAL INFORMATION

Concealed Conduction Pathways

Many times the delta wave is not formed or is so small that it is almost imperceptible. This typically occurs when the atrial depolarization wave hits the AV node before it hits the accessory pathway. The normally conducted ventricular depolarization wave will then cancel out the one traveling through the accessory pathway very quickly, before it ever becomes electrocardiographically significant. This type of conduction is, therefore, electrocardiographically silent and there is no way (short of electrophysiologic testing) to identify the presence of these silent conduction pathways. The term used to describe this silent or hidden potential conduction is *concealed conduction pathway*. This type of conduction is the most common presentation for patients with accessory pathways.

Concealed conduction pathway emphasizes the lack of electrocardiographic findings in these patients under normal circumstances. We stress the words "under normal circumstances" because the pathological process is still there and it can surface instantaneously, creating a life-threatening tachyarrhythmia by forming a reentrant circuit. Finally, some patients will intermittently move back and forth between the WPW pattern and concealed conduction on the same rhythm strip.

Clinically, patients with concealed conduction pathways are commonly encountered. A high index of suspicion is needed to correctly identify these patients and assure proper acute and definitive treatment, because their resting ECGs are completely normal. If you have any patient with a tachycardia that resembles AVRT, referral to a cardiologist or an electrophysiologist is critical.

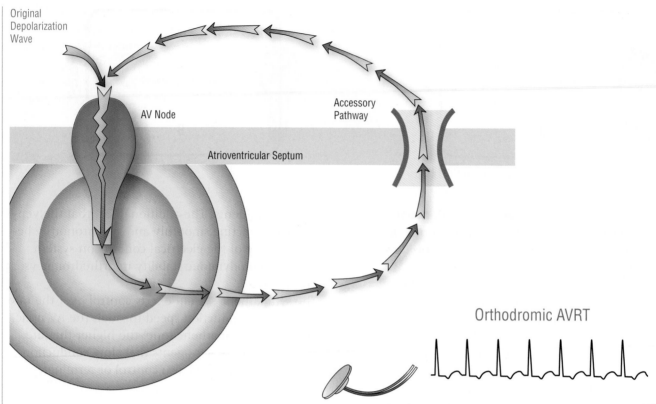

Figure 26-4: Orthodromic AVRT. In this form of AVRT, the impulse proceeds down to the ventricles via the AV node and the normal electrical conduction system. The net result is that the tachycardia is "controlled" by the AV node and the QRS complexes are narrow.

As we have seen throughout this book, if a wave has to travel farther, it will be longer. In patients with accessory pathways, the distance between the two pathways (the AV node and the accessory pathway) is relatively great in most cases. The time that the depolarization wave spends traversing those distances significantly lengthens the R-P interval.

We can use the long R-P interval found in orthodromic AVRT to help us in our differential diagnoses of narrow-complex tachycardias (Figure 26-5). In other words, if you have a narrow-complex tachycardia and you are trying to decide between AVRT and AVNRT, the location of the inverted P wave could be very helpful.

Other Important Clinical Facts

Orthodromic AVRT is the most common reentrant tachycardia found in WPW syndrome. It is found to be the mechanism involved in about 95% of the reentrant tachycardias found in WPW, and is very commonly seen in patients with concealed pathways.

Wide-complex orthodromic AVRT can sometimes be seen in cases of aberrancy, electrolyte abnormalities, or pre-existing bundle branch blocks. These cases are nearly impossible to distinguish from antidromic AVRT (as we shall see shortly) and should be treated with extreme caution, both in diagnosis and treatment strategies.

It is important to note that the delta wave is not visible during orthodromic AVRT because there is no fusion of impulse from the two pathways. Instead, the impulse travels in a sequential macroreentrant loop between the two pathways. Electrical alternans is frequently seen in these patients, just as it is in most tachycardias. ST segment depression is also commonly seen, even in young, healthy individuals.

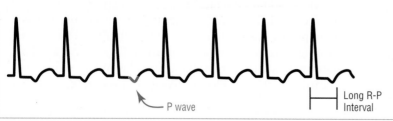

Figure 26-5: The inverted P wave is found at a longer R-P interval than that found in AVNRT. This is because the macroreentry loop has to travel longer distances between the two pathways. Longer distance means longer intervals. This fact will be very helpful in evaluating the differential diagnoses of the narrow-complex tachycardias.

Antidromic AVRT

Antidromic AVRT is created by a macroreentry circuit in which the impulse first travels down the accessory pathway to stimulate the ventricles (Figure 26-6). The impulse then moves across the ventricles by direct cell-to-cell transmission of the impulse, giving rise to a wide, bizarre QRS complex. Once the impulse reaches the area of the AV junction, it travels retrogradely through the AV node to restimulate the atria. When that impulse once again reaches the accessory pathway, the circuit will restart and continue in a looping manner giving rise to a *wide-complex tachycardia*.

The circuit can be initiated by either a PAC or a PVC and is usually associated with rates between 140 and 250 BPM (but can be as high as 360+ BPM). Note, however, that there is no AV nodal conduction control over the rate in antidromic AVRT. There is no physiologic block to help keep the rate to a ceiling of just 250 BPM. For example, what happens when the patient has an underlying atrial flutter rate at 300 BPM? What would the ventricular rate be? If you guessed 300 BPM,

you are correct. Now, can you guess what happens if the patient is in atrial fibrillation? The patient will be at very, very rapid ventricular rates and could very easily enter ventricular fibrillation. As you can imagine, antidromic AVRT is a very dangerous rhythm.

This brings us to a very important clinical discussion. Pharmacologic agents that slow conduction through the AV node but do not affect the accessory pathway are very dangerous in patients with accessory pathways. Administration of these drugs will cause the atrial impulses to travel preferentially down the accessory pathway and avoid the physiologic control exerted by the AV node. This is the main reason why certain calcium channel blockers, parasympatheticomimetic agents, beta-blockers, digitalis, vagal maneuvers, and even adenosine can be so dangerous in patients with WPW. In addition, digitalis, calcium channel blockers (especially verapamil), and adenosine can shorten the refractory period of the accessory tract and help increase conduction down the accessory pathway even further. In a patient with WPW or a concealed pathway, these agents could turn a fairly stable arrhythmia into a very highly unstable disaster.

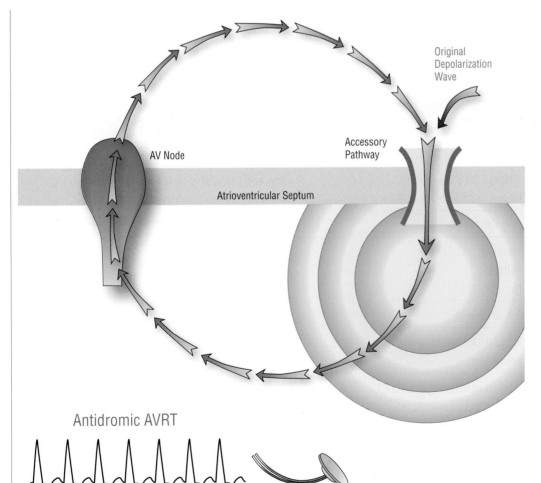

Antidromic AVRT

Figure 26-6: Antidromic AVRT. The original impulse travels down the accessory pathway. A reentry circuit is formed when the ventricular depolarization wave, being spread by direct cell-to-cell contact, reaches the AV node. It then moves retrogradely up through the AV node to restimulate the atria. The circuit is completed when the retrogradely conducted atrial impulse reaches the accessory pathway once again restarting the circuit. The resulting QRS complexes are wide and bizarre due to the slow ventricular conduction. Also note the absence of AV nodal control over the rate. The R-P interval remains long in this form of AVRT.

Remember, it is the ventricular rate and contractility that is one of the major components of the cardiac output and hemodynamic stability. A patient in atrial flutter or atrial fibrillation who is treated with the agents outlined on the previous page could easily go into a very rapid ventricular tachycardia, ventricular flutter, or ventricular fibrillation and die if he or she has a hidden accessory pathway. *Be careful of wide-complex tachycardias!* Always treat them as if they are ventricular tachycardia until proven otherwise; approach them very, very carefully and remember that they could also represent an antidromic AVRT.

ADDITIONAL INFORMATION

Wide-Complex Tachycardias

The differential diagnosis of wide-complex tachycardias includes some very dangerous rhythms, including ventricular tachycardia, ventricular flutter, torsade de pointes, and antidromic AVRT. We shall be studying these in detail in the next section. In addition, it also includes the rhythms we have seen up to this point in the book when they are associated with pre-existing bundle branch block, electrolyte abnormalities, or aberrancy. When you are approaching a patient with a wide-complex tachycardia, you should always assume the worst-case scenario. You should never assume an aberrant presentation of a more benign rhythm because the criteria that we use in surface electrocardiography are not always conclusive.

If you see an irregularly irregular rapid wide-complex tachycardia, it is going to be atrial fibrillation in a patient with WPW until proven otherwise. Ventricular tachycardia is always regular after the first few seconds of onset. Be careful of what drugs you give WPW patients! Remember, electrical cardioversion is always a possibility (especially if the patient is hemodynamically unstable). A complete discussion on the treatment of WPW is beyond the scope of this book.

Here are two major clinical pearls:

- *If the ventricular rate exceeds 200 BPM in atrial fibrillation, it is probably an atrial fibrillation in a patient with an accessory pathway or WPW syndrome.*

- *In general, as the ventricular rate exceeds 250 BPM, the possibility that you are dealing with an accessory pathway increases.*

ARRHYTHMIA RECOGNITION

AV Reentry Tachycardia

Rate:	140 to 250 BPM (can be higher in antidromic AVRT)
Regularity:	Regular
P wave:	Inverted
Morphology:	Different
Upright in II, III, and aVF:	No
P:QRS ratio:	1:1 or absent
PR interval:	None (R-P interval is prolonged)
QRS width:	Normal in orthodromic AVRT Wide in antidromic AVRT
Grouping:	None
Dropped beats:	None

DIFFERENTIAL DIAGNOSIS

AVRT

Only seen in patients with accessory pathways, either concealed conduction or WPW.

ECG Strips

ECG 26-1

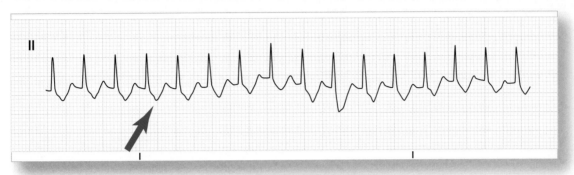

Rate:	About 180 BPM		PR intervals:	None
Regularity:	Regular		QRS width:	Normal
P waves:	Present		Grouping:	None
Morphology:	Inverted			
Axis:	None		Dropped beats:	Absent
P:QRS ratio:	1:1		Rhythm:	**AV reentry tachycardia**

Discussion:

The strip above shows a classic example of orthodromic AVRT. Note the narrow-complex tachycardia with an inverted P wave buried in the middle of the depressed ST segment. For your reference, an example of the inverted P waves is labeled with a blue arrow. The baseline of the rhythm strip is a bit wavy, adding to a variation in the QRS morphology, which is artifactual in beats 9 through 11.

ECG 26-2

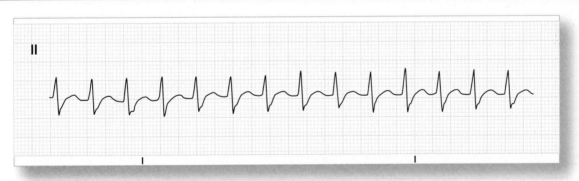

Rate:	About 150 BPM		PR intervals:	None
Regularity:	Regular		QRS width:	Wide
P waves:	None		Grouping:	None
Morphology:	None			
Axis:	None		Dropped beats:	Absent
P:QRS ratio:	None		Rhythm:	**AV reentry tachycardia**

Discussion:

This strip is not so obvious for an antidromic AVRT. All we know is that this is a wide-complex tachycardia. As such, it should be treated primarily as a ventricular tachycardia. Luckily, this patient was stable enough to obtain a full 12-lead ECG, which clearly demonstrated inverted P waves with a prolonged R-P interval consistent with an antidromic AVRT. After breaking the tachycardia, the patient demonstrated a WPW pattern on the ECG, confirming our initial suspicion that we were dealing with an antidromic AVRT.

ECG 26-3

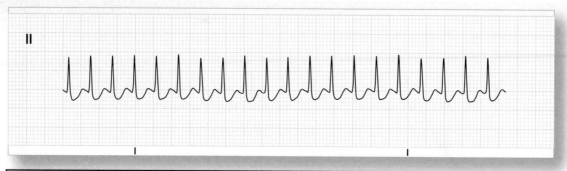

Rate:	About 230 BPM	PR intervals:	None
Regularity:	Regular	QRS width:	Normal
P waves:	None	Grouping:	None
Morphology:	None		
Axis:	None	Dropped beats:	Absent
P:QRS ratio:	None	Rhythm:	**AV reentry tachycardia**

Discussion:

This is a very rapid narrow-complex tachycardia. The differential diagnosis includes AVNRT and AVRT. It is almost impossible on this rhythm strip to determine the correct diagnosis. The only thing that makes AVRT more likely is the very rapid rate, which is slightly more con-sistent with this diagnosis. The patient was treated and responded to therapy appropriately. An ECG obtained in NSR demonstrated a WPW pattern, confirming the diagnosis of an orthodromic AVRT.

ECG 26-4

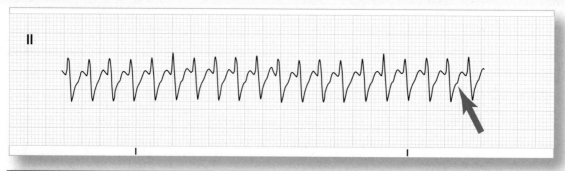

Rate:	About 235 BPM	PR intervals:	None
Regularity:	Regular	QRS width:	Wide
P waves:	See discussion below	Grouping:	None
Morphology:	See discussion below		
Axis:	See discussion below	Dropped beats:	Absent
P:QRS ratio:	See discussion below	Rhythm:	**AV reentry tachycardia**

Discussion:

This wide-complex tachycardia is very rapid and very regular. There was a consistent notching noted on the upstroke of the ST segment, which was suggestive of an inverted P wave. The very rapid rate, wide complexes, and possibly the inverted P waves all led to the diagnosis of antidromic AVRT. Ventricular tachycardias are usually not this rapid, but can occur. Luckily, the patient had a history of WPW syndrome and antidromic conduction, facilitating the diagnosis. Always remember to interpret a rhythm abnormality based on the company it keeps and the full clinical scenario.

ECG 26-5

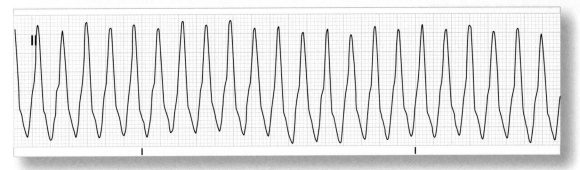

Rate:	About 215 BPM	PR intervals:	None
Regularity:	Regular	QRS width:	Normal
P waves:	None	Grouping:	None
Morphology:	None		
Axis:	None	Dropped beats:	None
P:QRS ratio:	None	Rhythm:	**AV reentry tachycardia**

Discussion:

The strip above is a really great example of a wide-complex tachycardia. Your first thought should be ventricular tachycardia. The patient should be treated as ventricular tachycardia first and foremost. Electrical cardioversion would be indicated if the patient were hemodynamically unstable. A couple of things should make you take a second look at the strip, the most important of which is the rate. This strip has an underlying rate at 215 BPM, which is very rapid for a ventricular tachycardia. After breaking the tachycardia, the patient was found to have a WPW pattern on the ECG. This is an example of antidromic AVRT.

ADDITIONAL INFORMATION

Differential Diagnosis of AVRT

The exact diagnosis is not always clear when first approaching any tachycardia, either narrow-complex or wide-complex. For that reason, we have included separate chapters on the differential diagnoses of each of these two complex subjects. We strongly suggest that you review these chapters thoroughly before completing this book.

As far as AVRT is concerned, it is not essential for you to remember the terms antidromic and orthodromic.

It is, however, vitally important that you are able to recognize the rhythm or at least to raise the possibility of these rhythms in your mind. In AVRT, thinking about the possibility is critical because of the consequences of pharmacologic therapy. This is one rhythm abnormality that could quickly deteriorate to a worse one because of the choice of an inappropriate agent.

CHAPTER **REVIEW**

1. AV reentry tachycardia is caused by a macro-reentry circuit involving the _____ and an _____ _____.

2. A good way to visualize an accessory pathway is to think of it like a "back door" to the ventricles. True or False.

3. Accessory pathways have their own intrinsic:
   A. Pacemaking rates
   B. Conduction rates
   C. Physiologic block
   D. Refractory periods
   E. Both B and D are correct.

4. The delta wave refers to the slurred onset of the QRS, which is created when the atrial depolarization wave travels unimpeded through the accessory pathway causing a slow, localized cell-to-cell ventricular depolarization wave to develop. True or False.

5. In the macroreentry circuit formed in AVRT, the slow pathway is created by:
   A. The AV node
   B. An accessory pathway
   C. Rapid ventricular depolarization
   D. Cell-to-cell ventricular depolarization

6. In the macroreentry circuit formed in AVRT, the fast pathway is created by:
   A. The AV node
   B. An accessory pathway
   C. Rapid ventricular depolarization
   D. Cell-to-cell ventricular depolarization

7. The WPW pattern consists of:
   A. A delta wave
   B. A short PR interval
   C. A QRS wider than or equal to 0.12 seconds
   D. Nonspecific ST-T wave changes
   E. All of the above

8. The WPW pattern and WPW syndrome refer to the same thing. True or False.

9. If an accessory pathway is present but it is electrocardiographically silent, it is referred to as a _____ _____ pathway.

10. A reentrant tachycardia that is formed when an impulse travels down the AV node and reenters the atria through the accessory pathway is called an _____ AVRT.

11. A reentrant tachycardia that is formed when an impulse travels down the accessory pathway and reenters the atria through the AV node is called an _____ AVRT.

12. Orthodromic AVRT is a narrow-complex tachycardia. The rate is somewhat under the control of the AV node due to the presence of the physiologic block, which is still active in these cases. True or False.

13. Antidromic AVRT is a wide-complex tachycardia. The rate is not under the control of the AV node. True or False.

14. The inverted P wave in AVRT is found immediately before, during, or immediately after the QRS complex. True or False.

15. The chance that a tachycardia involves an accessory pathway is very high if the ventricular rate exceeds 250 BPM. True or False.

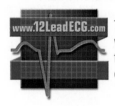

CHAPTER 27

How to Approach a Narrow-Complex Tachycardia

Narrow-complex tachycardias can create some interesting diagnostic and treatment challenges for the clinician in an acute care situation. There are two clinically important points to keep in mind when approaching a patient with a supraventricular tachycardia (SVT):

1. Isolate the exact diagnosis and cause of the tachycardia, as it will greatly assist you in providing the correct treatment.

2. In general, the hemodynamic status of the patient will usually be stable enough to allow a couple extra seconds to try to figure out the exact rhythm before having to initiate emergency treatment.

In this chapter, we will cover the thought process that you should go through when you are faced with a narrow-complex or supraventricular tachycardia.

The Hemodynamic Consequences of a Tachycardia

In a narrow-complex tachycardia, the heart rate can be anywhere from 100 BPM to over 360 BPM. Luckily, most SVTs occur in the lower to middle ranges of that rate spectrum. As you can imagine, patients can tolerate the lower end of this rate spectrum much better than they can tolerate the rates at the upper end. There are many reasons for the hemodynamic compromise that occurs in a tachycardia, but the greatest hemodynamic effect occurs because of alterations in the cardiac output.

If you remember from Chapter 1, one of the main determinants of blood pressure is the cardiac output. Cardiac output, in turn, is determined by the stroke volume and the heart rate. A rapid tachycardia will affect both the stroke volume and the heart rate negatively. In addition to its direct effects, the heart rate will also cause additional problems in ventricular filling, altering the stroke volume even further.

Heart Rate and Hemodynamics

Rapid rates affect the hemodynamic status of the heart in various ways. The most important ones include:

1. Relative ischemia due to increased myocardial oxygen demand
2. Decreasing ventricular filling times and decreasing end-diastolic volume
3. Decreasing atrial kick and ventricular overfilling

Relative Ischemia Due to Increased Myocardial Oxygen Demand   One way that an increase in heart rate causes hemodynamic compromise is by causing an increase in myocardial oxygen demand of the heart muscle itself. This increased oxygen demand, in turn, can lead to a relative myocardial ischemia. The term "relative" here refers to the fact that it is not ischemia due to atherosclerotic heart disease, but rather an imbalance of the amount of oxygen being delivered to the tissue compared to the amount of oxygen that the tissue needs. In other words, the demand for oxygen exceeds the supply of oxygen. The result is that the tissue is ischemic and does not function at its maximum (or even normal) potential.

Ischemic muscle does not contract appropriately. This decrease in the contractility of the heart leads to a decrease in the amount of blood ejected by the heart into the aorta. Remember from Chapter 1 that it is the ejection fraction of the heart (the amount of blood pumped out with each contraction) that expands the aorta. The elastic recoil of the aorta trying to return to its resting state provides enough constant pressure to push the blood forward throughout the rest of the circulatory system (Figure 27-1). As you can imagine, if the amount of blood ejected is lower, the aorta will not distend as much and the pressure exerted by the

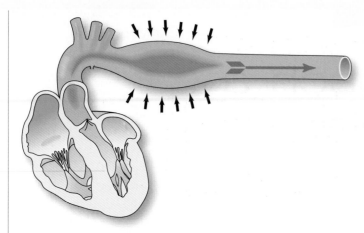

Figure 27-1: Imagine that the bolus of blood that shoots out of the heart is the red area in this figure. Notice how the aorta is distended outward by the additional bolus. As the bolus begins to mix with the rest of the blood, the built-up pressure on the arterial walls is still there and pushing the walls inward toward the lumen. This happens because the elastic walls want to return to their resting state of relaxation. This pressure causes the blood to move forward smoothly and continuously. The process is repeated over and over with each cardiac contraction.

aorta will be lessened. Less pressure equals less perfusion throughout the body tissues and leads to a shock state.

In general, the faster the tachycardia, the greater the oxygen demand of the myocardial cells. That is why patients tend to tolerate the slower rates along the SVT spectrum without much difficulty. The faster rates, however, can lead to catastrophic hemodynamic compromise and may even lead to death.

Decreasing Ventricular Filling Times and Decreasing End-diastolic Volume The heart rate also affects the cardiac output by affecting the stroke volume of the patient. Normally, the ventricles fill during the resting phase of the heart (diastole). As we saw in Chapter 1, ventricular filling occurs both passively and actively. It is in fact during the passive filling phase that most of the blood enters the heart, and passive filling occurs during diastole (Figure 27-2). The active phase of filling also occurs during diastole and is caused by atrial contraction. (Note that since most SVTs have abnormalities in the atrial rate, this atrial kick is also greatly altered in many SVTs.)

In a tachycardia, both systole and diastole are affected. The problem is that diastole is usually greatly shortened, while systole is only minimally affected. Since ventricular filling occurs during diastole, the amount of blood that actually enters the ventricles is greatly decreased. Clinically, this translates as a markedly decreased cardiac output. Therefore, the lower the end-diastolic blood volume, the lower the cardiac output. In simple terms, the faster the rate, the shorter the period of diastole. The shorter the period of diastole, the lower the ventricular filling. The lower the ventricular filling, the lower the stroke volume. The lower the stroke volume, the lower the blood pressure (Figure 27-3).

Hemodynamic stability is, therefore, strongly related to the rate of the tachycardia. At the slower end of the SVT spectrum, the amount of blood that fills the ventricles during ventricular diastole is greater than at faster

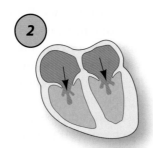

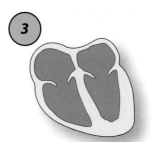

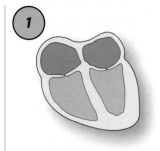

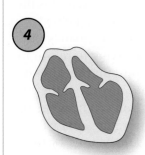

Figure 27-2: Ventricular filling.

1. This figure shows the heart in late systole. The atria are full but the ventricles are empty.

2. In early diastole, the AV valves open, allowing a large amount of blood to rush into the ventricles. This is the rapid filling phase of diastole.

3. In mid-diastole, the ventricles are full. Notice that the ventricular walls, however, are not distended in any way.

4. The atrial contraction allows an extra amount of blood to enter the ventricles causing them to stretch and overfill. The slight stretch in the ventricular muscle caused by the atrial kick will maximize stroke volume and cardiac output.

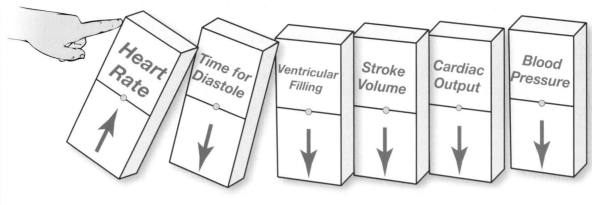

Figure 27-3: The hemodynamic consequences of high heart rates.

rates, since there is more time for the blood to enter the ventricles. The increased ventricular filling time translates to an increased ejection fraction and a stronger cardiac output. As the rates become faster, ventricular filling is decreased because, as mentioned above, the diastolic component of the cardiac cycle is shortened disproportionately. Decreased filling times leads to lower end-diastolic blood volume and lower ejection fractions, causing a weaker cardiac output. At very rapid rates, there is hardly enough time for any significant amount of blood to enter the ventricles and hardly any blood is ejected by the heart. At these rates, the blood pressure drops dramatically.

We saw above how the heart rate affects the stroke volume directly. Now let's turn our attention to how a tachycardia affects the stroke volume indirectly. The amount of blood in the ventricle at the end of diastole will greatly affect the way that the ventricle contracts. What does this mean? In general, the ventricle contracts in almost a "wringing" motion. The wringing motion is like squeezing a toothpaste tube: you start from the bottom and squeeze toward the top. The synchronized contraction allows for maximal ejection of the end-diastolic blood volume.

As mentioned earlier, synchronized depolarization leads to a synchronized and organized contraction and maximum ejection of whatever blood is present in the ventricles at that time. The synchronized "wringing" contraction can occur only because the electrical conduction system conducts the signal to depolarize, almost instantaneously, to every cell in both ventricles. As we shall see, this synchronization of the ventricular depolarization and organized contraction found in the narrow-complex tachycardias is a major factor in the inherent hemodynamic stability of the SVTs, except at extremely high heart rates.

Decreasing the Atrial Kick and Ventricular Overfilling   The atrial kick is the last important point we will look at when considering the hemodynamic effects of any tachycardia. Remember that atrial kick refers to the little extra amount of ventricular overfilling that occurs due to atrial contraction. Some patients can tolerate the loss of the atrial kick without difficulty. Unfortunately, many cannot.

The loss of the atrial kick decreases the end-diastolic ventricular blood volume by not allowing the overfilling of the ventricle. This underfilling decreases the extra "stretch" placed on the ventricular muscle that is needed to maximize contraction strength. The decreased contractility leads to a decreased stroke volume, which in turn leads to a decrease in cardiac output and blood pressure. We discussed this before in Chapter 1, where we saw that a little overstretching of the ventricular wall causes more forceful contraction of the ventricles.

Retrograde contraction of the atria, as occurs in many SVTs, does not add the atrial kick because the atrial contraction is occurring at the exact same time as ventricular contraction. The net result of a retrograde contraction is negated by contracting against closed valves. As a matter of fact, this retrograde contraction against the obstacle formed by the closed valves pushes blood *away* from the heart. (This leads to an interesting physical exam finding known as *cannon a waves*. A cannon a wave is a very large and obvious distension of the jugular vein caused by the extra blood volume from a blocked atrial ejection. The reader is referred to a book on physical diagnosis for further discussion of this very useful physical exam finding.)

As we have seen in the previous chapters in this section, some of the supraventricular tachycardias have normal, though rapid, atrial contraction and some do not have any organized atrial activity associated with them at all. In either case, the loss of the atrial kick adds further hemodynamic instability to many tachycardias.

A Few Extra Seconds. . .

The lack of synchronized ventricular activation is one of the main causes of hemodynamic instability that we see with wide-complex tachycardias. In contrast, the supraventricular tachycardias are usually well tolerated by patients in the short run unless the rates are very, very fast. The main reason behind this extra hemodynamic tolerance in the supraventricular tachycardias is that the ventricles are still contracting symmetrically and in a synchronized fashion due to the normally functioning electrical conduction system. The synchronized activation maintains the normal geometry of the ventricles and allows for maximal "wringing" action to occur in these cases. In addition, the atrial kick is often maintained in many of the SVTs.

The extra hemodynamic stability present in many of the SVTs allows us to spend a few extra seconds or minutes correctly identifying the rhythm involved. As we shall see, correctly identifying the rhythm will allow us to focus our treatment and maximize our efforts to improve patient outcome. This is a luxury that is often missing when dealing with a wide-complex tachycardia.

Please remember, the faster you treat a patient with any tachycardia, the better it is for the patient. We are not advocating taking more time before treatment. In general, however, with a supraventricular tachycardia, you could safely spend a couple of extra seconds analyzing the strip a bit more carefully, as long as the patient remains hemodynamically stable. If the patient is unstable, remember the old adage: "electricity is our friend." Electricity, in this case, refers to direct electrical cardioversion or defibrillation, whichever is needed.

Focused Treatment Requires Focused Identification

Let's suppose that your car was stolen. Which description would be more helpful to the police: (1) My car has four wheels and windows, or (2) I have a 2002 Honda Civic that is green and has a scratch on the right front bumper, with a license plate honoring arrhythmia treatment, JUICE4U? The second description will probably help them find your car a little more quickly than the first. Likewise, the term supraventricular tachycardia refers to a slew of possibilities. It is a great help to know that the arrhythmia is originating in the supraventricular area and is narrow complex. This information helps us to focus our treatment. But, knowing which one of

the supraventricular tachycardias you are dealing with can help focus treatment strategies even further.

Focused treatment to the appropriate anatomical structure or physiologic property involved leads to better results in breaking the tachycardia. In addition, certain pharmaceutical agents affect the heart rate, automaticity, conduction velocities, and refractory periods of the various components, preventing many of these tachycardias from developing in the first place. Finally, treatment that is helpful in one SVT can lead to deadly consequences in others (AVRT is an excellent example). *Focused treatment requires focused identification of the arrhythmia and a working knowledge of the mechanisms involved in each of the possibilities.*

So, how do we focus our differential diagnosis and, hopefully, arrive at the exact diagnosis? There are a few tricks and, in the rest of this chapter, we will cover them individually. Putting all of the information together in an organized manner will lead you to the right choice.

What to Look for in an SVT

As mentioned, there are certain morphological aspects of a supraventricular tachycardia that can help you arrive at a correct diagnosis. These are:

1. Rate
2. Regularity
3. The P wave
4. The P-QRS relationship
5. The company it keeps

Rate

The rate can sometimes be useful in distinguishing between the narrow-complex tachycardias (Table 27-1). However, it is usually not extremely helpful. The main reason for this lack of specificity, as you can see from the table, is that most of the rates overlap. In addition, the rates given below are the usual ranges for the tachycardia. Exceptions always occur. For example, atrial flutter usually has an atrial rate between 200 and 400 BPM. Now, with the advent of EPS studies, we have found the same macroreentry circuits can actually occur at atrial rates as low as 150 BPM.

The rate can be useful in that you can use the number of BPM to rule in or rule out some of the possibilities of your differentials list, and then use other criteria to further the analysis. In other words, do not use the rate by itself to rule in or rule out a specific supraventricular tachycardia. If you do this, you will eventually make a critical mistake.

Table 27-1: Supraventricular Tachycardias Categorized by Ventricular Response Rates

Supraventricular Tachycardia	Response Rate (BPM)
Sinus tachycardia	100 to 200
Ectopic atrial tachycardia	100 to 180
Multifocal atrial tachycardia	100 to 150
Atrial flutter	100 to 300
Atrial fibrillation	100 to 200
Junctional tachycardia	100 to 130
AVNRT	140 to 220
AVRT	140 to 250
Orthodromic	140 to 250
Antidromic	140 to 360

Table 27-2: Supraventricular Tachycardias Categorized by Regularity

Regular	Irregularly Irregular
Sinus tachycardia	Atrial fibrillation
Ectopic atrial tachycardia	Multifocal atrial tachycardia
Atrial flutter	Atrial flutter with variable block
AVNRT	
AVRT	
Junctional tachycardia	
(Atrial fibrillation when associated with a complete third-degree heart block and a junctional or ventricular escape rhythm)	

Regularity

Narrow-complex tachycardias can be divided into two main groups based on the cadence of the complexes: the regular and irregularly irregular SVTs (Table 27-2). Taking a close look at the regularity and deciding into which of these categories a particular rhythm strip fits will greatly facilitate your search for the definitive diagnosis. Let's take a look at the two groups.

The SVTs that are found under the regular category are usually extremely regular. There can be some slight variation in the regularity, but it is usually less than 0.04 seconds (a small block). An interesting phenomenon is included in parentheses in Table 27-2: When atrial fibrillation is associated with a complete third-degree heart block, the ventricular response will either be a junctional or a ventricular escape rhythm. If a junctional escape rhythm is rapid, then you can get a rapid, regular ventricular response in a patient with atrial fibrillation. Luckily, this is an extremely rare occurrence.

The most common irregularly irregular rhythm is atrial fibrillation. When you see an irregularly irregular rhythm without any visible P waves, you will usually be correct in calling this rhythm atrial fibrillation. The next most common irregularly irregular rhythm is multifocal atrial tachycardia. This is also fairly evident because of the variation in P-wave morphology. Last, but not least, you can rarely find an atrial flutter that occurs with a completely variable block, leading to a completely irregularly irregular ventricular response. Using multiple leads will facilitate being able to see the presence of the F waves in these cases.

Here is a quick clinical pearl. When the ventricular response is very rapid and uncontrolled, the amount of irregularity can be very small. *If you see a very rapid narrow-complex tachycardia with a consistent amount of irregularity (no matter how small it is) and no associated P waves, it is uncontrolled atrial fibrillation until proven otherwise! In addition, remember that a rapid irregularly irregular rhythm that is faster than 200 BPM could easily be atrial fibrillation in a patient with an accessory tract. These are very dangerous conditions and should be approached with extreme caution.*

The P Wave

The morphology of the P wave is a very useful tool when evaluating a supraventricular tachycardia. An upright P wave in leads II, III, and aVF means that the origin of the tachycardia must be in the sinus node or the atrial tissue itself (Figure 27-4). An inverted P wave is typically found in junctional or reentrant mechanisms. The presence of a pseudo-S wave or a pseudo-R′ wave is typical of AVNRT. The presence of the undulating pattern of F waves is virtually diagnostic of atrial flutter. The absence of any visible P waves can be due to either atrial fibrillation (if the ventricular response is irregularly irregular), or AVNRT or AVRT if the ventricular response is regular and the P wave is buried in the QRS complex.

If the P wave is upright, the presence of an old strip or ECG when the patient was in normal sinus rhythm is an invaluable tool. Knowledge of the P-wave morphology in NSR will greatly facilitate the diagnosis of an ectopic atrial tachycardia or a junctional tachycardia by demonstrating slight differences in morphology found in these two rhythms.

While we are on the topic, an old ECG will help identify the presence of an accessory pathway with the WPW pattern. Keep in mind, however, that most accessory pathways are electrocardiographically silent until they manifest their pathological potential by creating a tachycardia.

The P-QRS Relationship

Probably the most important tool, when it comes to identifying an exact supraventricular tachycardia, is the location of the P wave in relation to the QRS complex (Figure 27-5). This is because different SVTs have different P-R or R-P intervals associated with them, and it is this exact relationship that can help to isolate an exact SVT. In other words, it is the exact location of the P wave in relation to the QRS that we need to concentrate on when trying to establish an exact diagnosis. We not only need to look at where the P wave is situated in relation to the QRS complex (either before, buried in, or after the QRS complex), but we also need to look at the distance from the QRS complex to the P wave.

In general, any rhythm that originates in the sinus node or the atria will have either a normal or a slightly prolonged PR interval. This will quickly let you identify the rhythm as either a sinus tachycardia, a multifocal atrial tachycardia, or an ectopic atrial tachycardia. At this point, the exact morphology of the P wave will come into play. If the P wave is sinus in nature, the rhythm is sinus tachycardia. If the morphology of the P waves is changing (and there are more than three morphological types), it is multifocal atrial tachycardia (MAT). If the P wave has a normal or slightly prolonged PR interval and is slightly different from the sinus P, or they are inverted, it is ectopic atrial tachycardia (EAT).

When the P wave is found inverted and in the area immediately surrounding the QRS complex, as it is in the yellow area of Figure 27-5, the diagnosis will either be junctional tachycardia or AVNRT. In this yellow area, the morphology of the P wave is not that helpful because both possibilities have inverted P waves. A tighter relationship of the P wave to the QRS complex favors AVNRT because the reentry loop causes the P wave to fire much earlier. Pseudo-S wave in lead II or a pseudo-R′ in lead V_1 both favor AVNRT. What can be very helpful to further isolate an exact diagnosis is the rate of the tachycardia, with faster rates favoring AVNRT.

The light red area is usually reserved for AVRT associated with a concealed pathway or a WPW syndrome. This longer R-P interval is caused by the long reentry loop that occurs in many of these patients. Narrow-complex tachycardias with P wave in the light red zone should be approached as an orthodromic AVRT until proven otherwise.

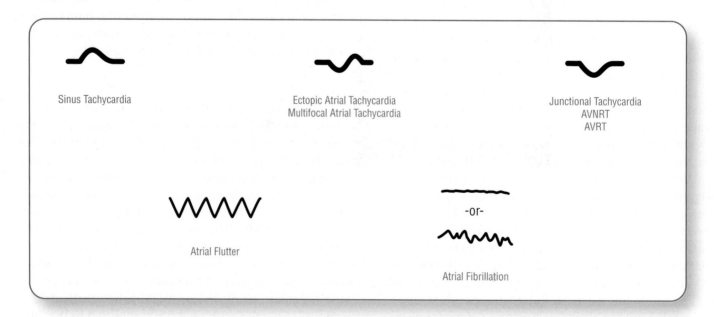

Figure 27-4: The morphology of the P wave in the various supraventricular tachycardias.

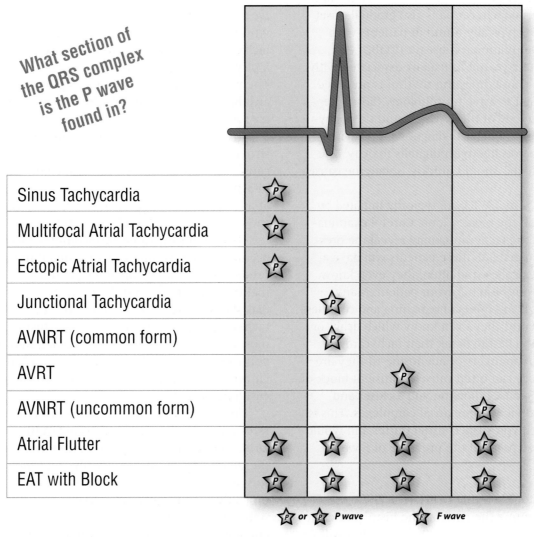

Figure 27-5: The location of the P wave in the various supraventricular tachycardias. First, isolate the exact location of the P wave on your rhythm strip and identify the corresponding colored area on the figure above. Then, look down and see which rhythms have a colored star in your particular colored area.

If the P wave is located very far away from the QRS complex, in the pink area of Figure 27-5, it is usually the uncommon or atypical form of AVNRT. Luckily, this is a very rare occurrence. Pharmaceutical agents used to treat AVNRT will work in the uncommon form as well.

Finally, atrial flutter and ectopic atrial tachycardia with block have been included in all of the sections of Figure 27-5. The reason is that these two rhythms have rapidly occurring F or ectopic P waves that recur so frequently that they are found at least twice for every typical ventricular response in most cases. These rapid atrial rates are typically associated with some accompanying AV block leading to varying conduction ratios, for example 2:1, 3:1, 4:1, and so on. Atrial flutter with 1:1

block will typically have the F waves in the green area of Figure 27-5.

The Company It Keeps

When evaluating any arrhythmia, you should pay special attention to the things that are occurring around the rhythm itself. This is what we mean by "the company it keeps." In particular, you should pay attention to the start and the end of the tachycardia. Many times this area can give you some important clues and can lead you to the correct diagnosis. The clinical scenario surrounding the arrhythmia also fits into this category.

Sinus tachycardia has a very gradual onset and termination. This is because it is typically a physiologic response to some precipitant (e.g., fever, exercise, anxiety). Multifocal atrial tachycardia is also gradual onset in most cases and is typically found in patients with chronic obstructive pulmonary disease (COPD).

Ectopic atrial tachycardia is usually associated with a rapid onset, but many times the rhythm is preceded by PACs with similar P-wave morphology. Close attention to the morphology of the PACs around the tachycardia can often help clinch the diagnosis. EAT with block is typically associated with digitalis toxicity. The history and drug levels should quickly isolate the cause in these cases.

Runs of AVNRT and AVRT are typically initiated by PACs that trigger off the reentry loop. Careful examination of the start of the tachycardia may reveal the presence of the PAC. In general, these patients will have a history of similar episodes, and often, they even know their diagnosis. Always listen to your patient. Many times they will save you hours of searching and countless headaches. Frequently, they even know which drugs or maneuvers work the best to break their tachycardias.

Finally, vagal maneuvers or adenosine (if they are not contraindicated) can often cause a transient block of the ventricular response, allowing you a closer and clearer unimpeded view of the atrial complexes. This is especially helpful if you suspect atrial flutter and would like some definitive proof of the presence of F waves.

A Final Word

In general, you should be able to arrive at the correct diagnosis by examining the patient, the history, and the arrhythmia carefully. Many times, however, you will only be able to narrow it down to a couple of possibilities. That's okay as this narrowing process will greatly help you in deciding on a clearer, more focused course of action.

If you can avoid it, do not treat sinus tachycardia! Treat the underlying cause. We have all seen trained clinicians who use drugs to try to control perfectly stable sinus tachycardia. This is a mistake because the tachycardia is a physiologic response to some underlying problem. The problem could be anemia, hypoxemia, fever, or anything else that alters the heart rate. The body will try to compensate for the physiologic abnormality with a tachycardia (remember, cardiac output = heart rate × stroke volume). Treating the tachycardia can sometimes cause significant hypotension and could introduce a pharmacologic agent that can come back to haunt you at a later time. If the patient has fever, cool her off. If she is anemic, give blood. Treat the underlying cause!

Remember that a narrow-complex tachycardia can become a wide-complex tachycardia if the patient has a pre-existing bundle branch block, an electrolyte abnormality, or aberrant conduction. Wide-complex tachycardias should always be treated as if they were ventricular tachycardia until proven otherwise. Just remember that most of the time, with careful evaluation of the rhythm, you can isolate the rhythm down to the supraventricular area, and this will allow you to provide more focused treatment.

Finally, always think of an accessory pathway if the rates are greater than or equal to 250 BPM or irregularly irregular rates greater than 200 BPM. Statistically, these very fast rates are typically associated with accessory pathways. Remember that any unstable patient probably requires electricity to convert. If the patient is stable, think of the possibility of an accessory pathway and adjust your therapy accordingly. Remember the statement, *Primum non nocere: Above all else, do no harm!*

If the rate is 150 BPM, it is atrial flutter until proven otherwise!

CHAPTER REVIEW

1. Rapid heart rates affect the hemodynamic status of the patient in various ways. Pick the one answer that is NOT correct:
   A. Relative ischemia can develop due to increased myocardial oxygen demand.
   B. The venous return is decreased.
   C. Ventricular filling times are decreased.
   D. End-diastolic volume (the amount of blood in the ventricle at the end of diastole) is decreased.
   E. The atrial kick is lost or diminished, causing less ventricular "overfilling."

2. Focused treatment requires _____ identification of the arrhythmia.

3. The rate is the most important factor in the differential diagnosis of a narrow-complex tachycardia. True or False.

4. The three irregularly irregular supraventricular tachycardia include (fill in the blank):
   A. _____ _____
   B. _____ _____ _____
   C. _____ _____ with _____ block

5. A narrow-complex tachycardia at 240 BPM that has a small variability of anywhere between 0.02 and 0.06 seconds between the QRS complexes is still considered regular. True or False.

6. If there are no P waves visible on the strip, the diagnosis that most likely fits the description of the rhythm mentioned in question 5 is _____ _____.

7. The exact location of the P wave in relation to the QRS complex is probably the most important thing to look for when establishing the differential diagnosis of a narrow-complex tachycardia. True or False.

8. The presence of a pseudo-S or pseudo-R' wave in a patient with a narrow-complex tachycardia above 140 BPM favors the diagnosis of _____.

9. The start and the end of any supraventricular tachycardia is not that critical in the evaluation of the differential diagnosis of the rhythm. True or False.

10. The following is NOT an acceptable treatment strategy for a patient in sinus tachycardia:
    A. Administer oxygen
    B. Administer fluids
    C. Administer acetaminophen
    D. Administer morphine
    E. Electrical cardioversion

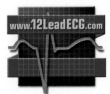

To enhance the knowledge you gain in this book, access this text's website at www.12leadECG.com! This valuable resource provides flashcards, an online glossary, web links, and more. Simply click on the Arrhythmias book cover once at the site.

Self-Test

II

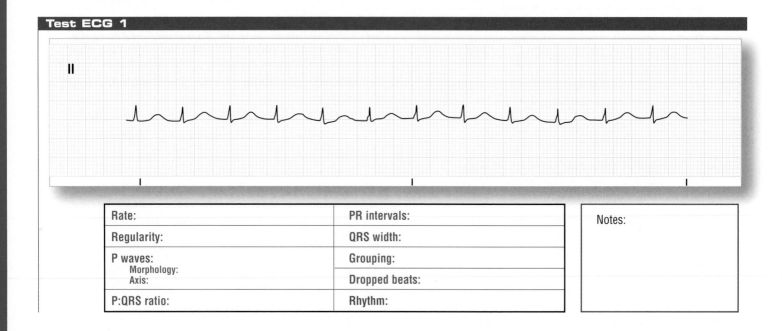

Rate:	PR intervals:	Notes:
Regularity:	QRS width:	
P waves: Morphology: Axis:	Grouping:	
	Dropped beats:	
P:QRS ratio:	Rhythm:	

II

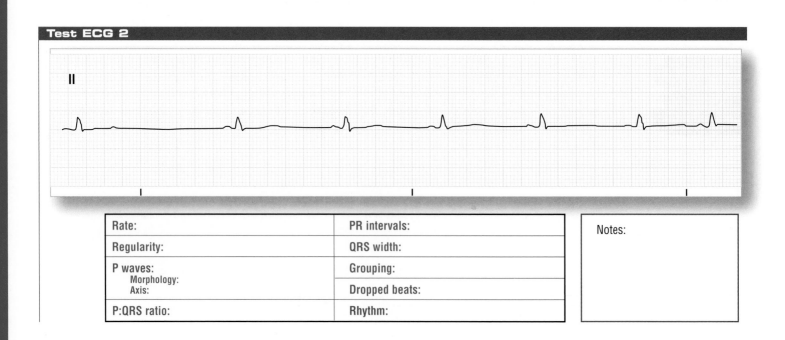

Rate:	PR intervals:	Notes:
Regularity:	QRS width:	
P waves: Morphology: Axis:	Grouping:	
	Dropped beats:	
P:QRS ratio:	Rhythm:	

Test ECG 3

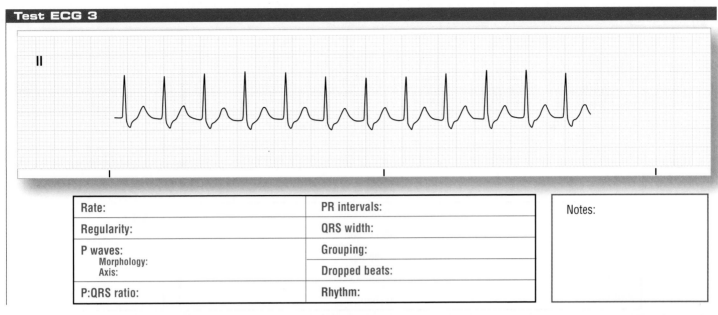

Rate:	PR intervals:	Notes:
Regularity:	QRS width:	
P waves: Morphology: Axis:	Grouping:	
	Dropped beats:	
P:QRS ratio:	Rhythm:	

Test ECG 4

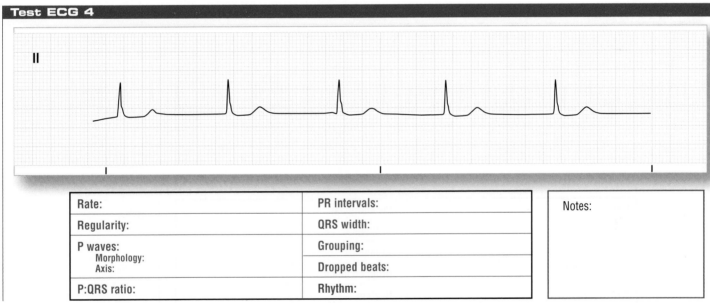

Rate:	PR intervals:	Notes:
Regularity:	QRS width:	
P waves: Morphology: Axis:	Grouping:	
	Dropped beats:	
P:QRS ratio:	Rhythm:	

Test ECG 5

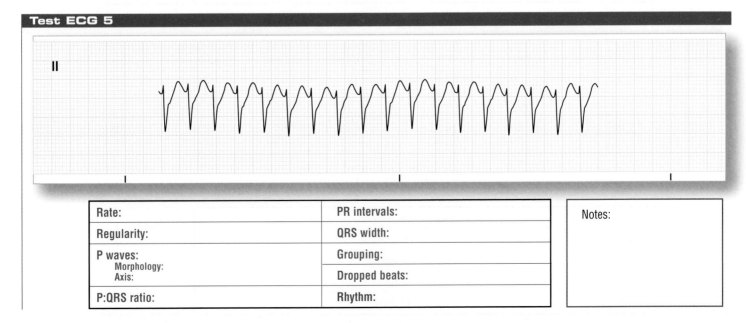

Rate:	PR intervals:	Notes:
Regularity:	QRS width:	
P waves: Morphology: Axis:	Grouping:	
	Dropped beats:	
P:QRS ratio:	Rhythm:	

Test ECG 6

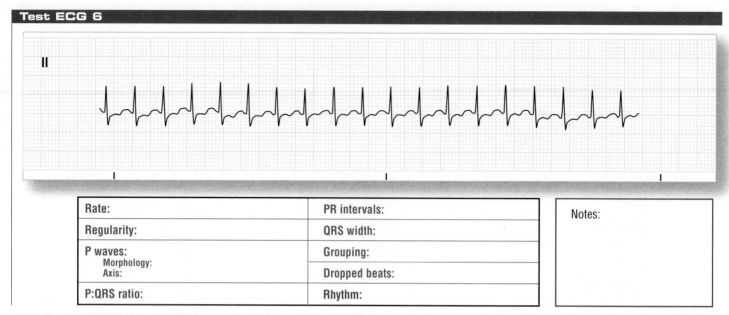

Rate:	PR intervals:	Notes:
Regularity:	QRS width:	
P waves:	Grouping:	
Morphology:		
Axis:	Dropped beats:	
P:QRS ratio:	Rhythm:	

Test ECG 7

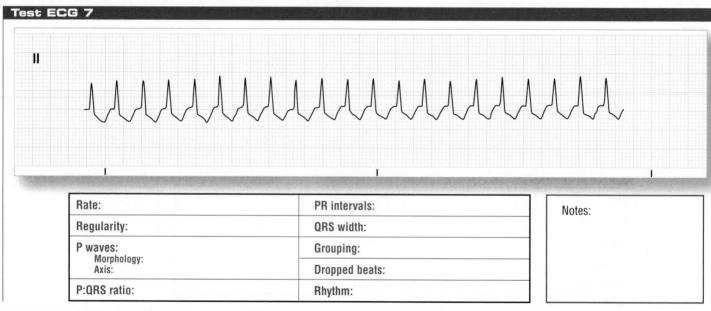

Rate:	PR intervals:	Notes:
Regularity:	QRS width:	
P waves:	Grouping:	
Morphology:		
Axis:	Dropped beats:	
P:QRS ratio:	Rhythm:	

Test ECG 8

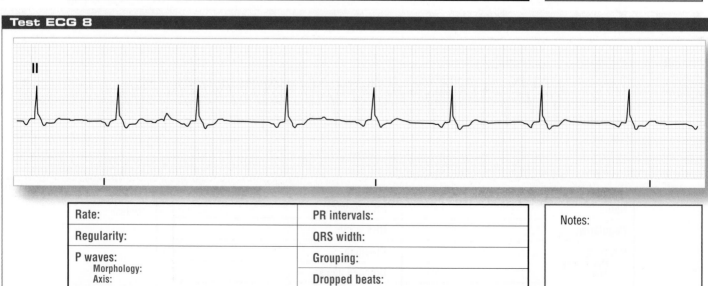

Rate:	PR intervals:	Notes:
Regularity:	QRS width:	
P waves:	Grouping:	
Morphology:		
Axis:	Dropped beats:	
P:QRS ratio:	Rhythm:	

Test ECG 9

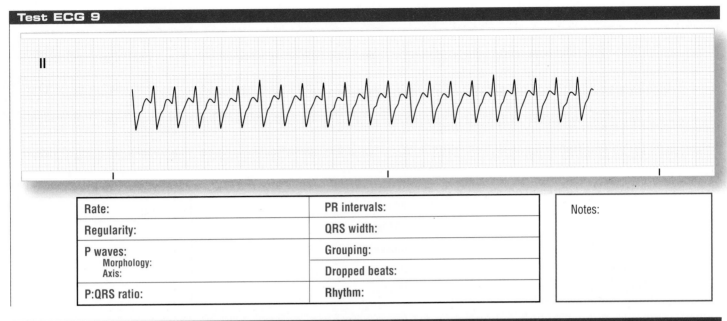

Rate:	PR intervals:	Notes:
Regularity:	QRS width:	

P waves:
    Morphology:
    Axis:
	Grouping:	

	Dropped beats:	
P:QRS ratio:	Rhythm:	

Test ECG 10

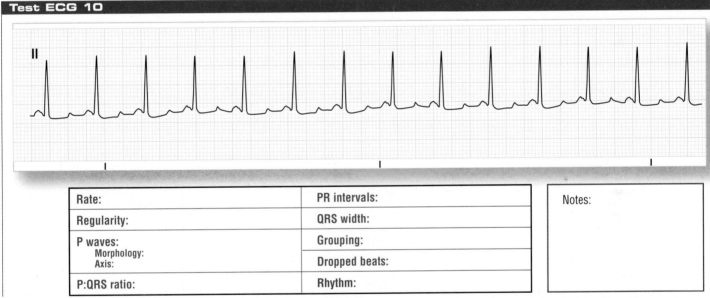

Rate:	PR intervals:	Notes:
Regularity:	QRS width:	

P waves:
    Morphology:
    Axis:
	Grouping:	

	Dropped beats:	
P:QRS ratio:	Rhythm:	

Test ECG 11

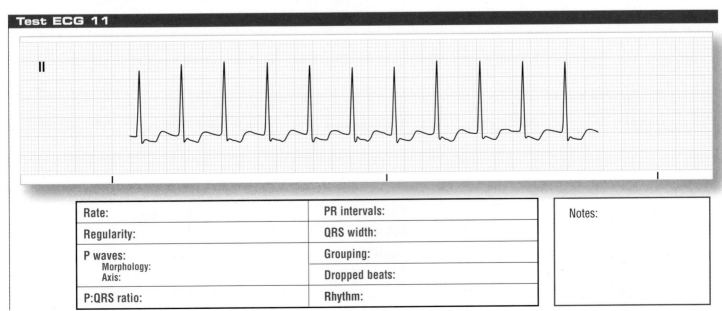

Rate:	PR intervals:	Notes:
Regularity:	QRS width:	

P waves:
    Morphology:
    Axis:
	Grouping:	

	Dropped beats:	
P:QRS ratio:	Rhythm:	

Test ECG 12

II

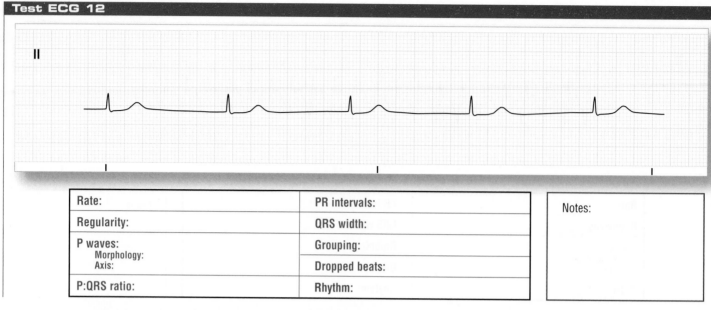

Rate:		PR intervals:	Notes:
Regularity:		QRS width:	
P waves: Morphology: Axis:		Grouping:	
		Dropped beats:	
P:QRS ratio:		Rhythm:	

Test ECG 13

II

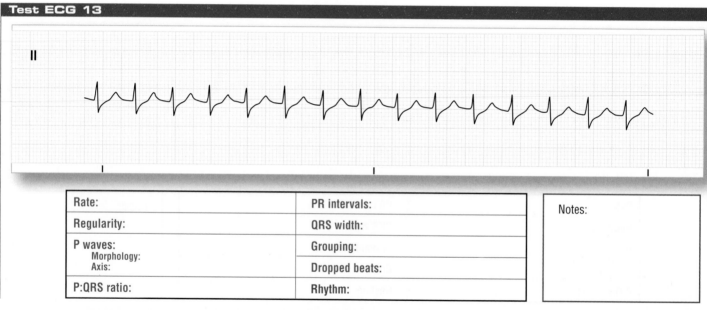

Rate:		PR intervals:	Notes:
Regularity:		QRS width:	
P waves: Morphology: Axis:		Grouping:	
		Dropped beats:	
P:QRS ratio:		Rhythm:	

Test ECG 14

V₁

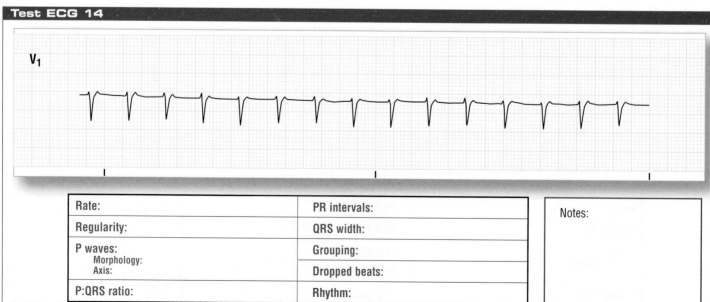

Rate:		PR intervals:	Notes:
Regularity:		QRS width:	
P waves: Morphology: Axis:		Grouping:	
		Dropped beats:	
P:QRS ratio:		Rhythm:	

Test ECG 15

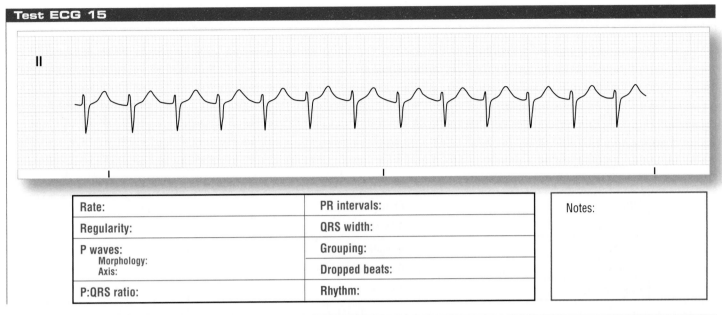

II

Rate:	PR intervals:	Notes:
Regularity:	QRS width:	

P waves:
   Morphology:
   Axis:
	Grouping:	

	Dropped beats:	
P:QRS ratio:	Rhythm:	

Test ECG 16

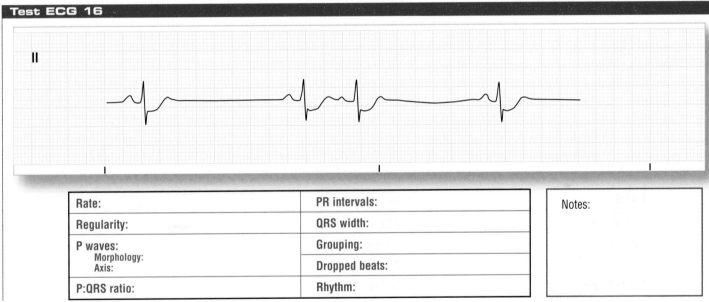

II

Rate:	PR intervals:	Notes:
Regularity:	QRS width:	

P waves:
   Morphology:
   Axis:
	Grouping:	

	Dropped beats:	
P:QRS ratio:	Rhythm:	

Test ECG 17

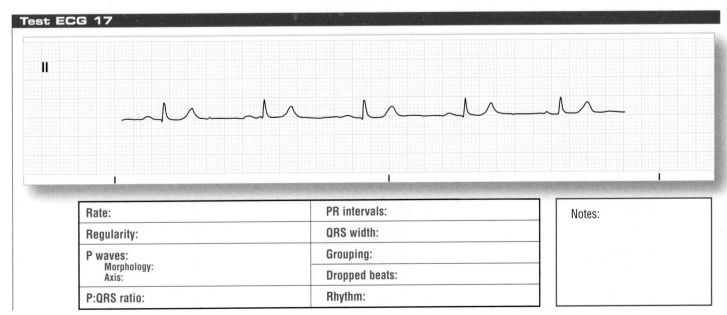

II

Rate:	PR intervals:	Notes:
Regularity:	QRS width:	

P waves:
   Morphology:
   Axis:
	Grouping:	

	Dropped beats:	
P:QRS ratio:	Rhythm:	

Test ECG 18

V₁

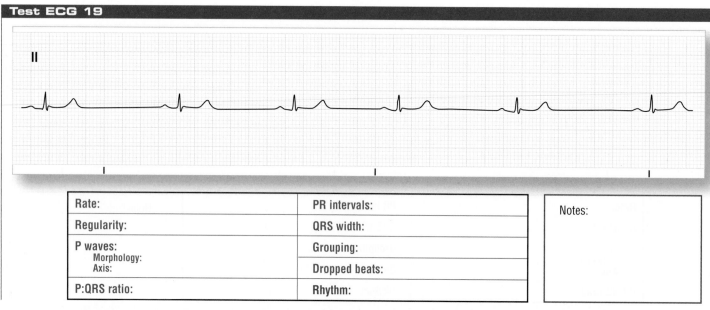

Rate:		PR intervals:	Notes:
Regularity:		QRS width:	
P waves:		Grouping:	
Morphology:			
Axis:		Dropped beats:	
P:QRS ratio:		Rhythm:	

Test ECG 19

II

Rate:		PR intervals:	Notes:
Regularity:		QRS width:	
P waves:		Grouping:	
Morphology:			
Axis:		Dropped beats:	
P:QRS ratio:		Rhythm:	

Test ECG 20

II

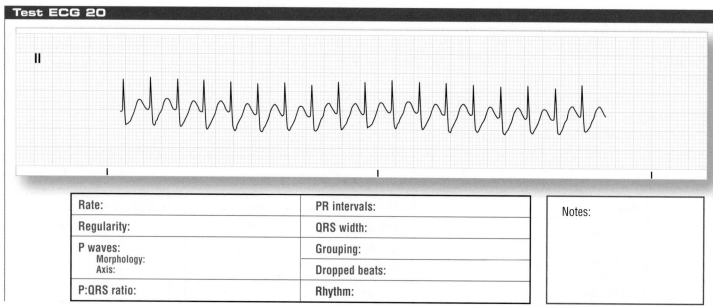

Rate:		PR intervals:	Notes:
Regularity:		QRS width:	
P waves:		Grouping:	
Morphology:			
Axis:		Dropped beats:	
P:QRS ratio:		Rhythm:	

Section 4 Self-Test Answers

Test ECG 1

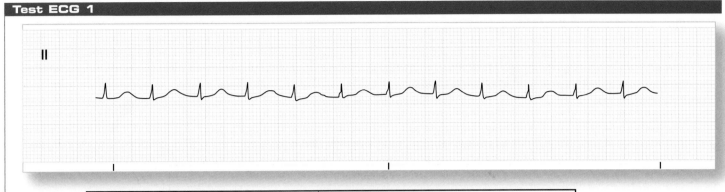

Rate:	About 115 BPM	PR intervals:	Not applicable
Regularity:	Regular	QRS width:	Normal
P waves:	None	Grouping:	None
Morphology:	None		
Axis:	None	Dropped beats:	None
P:QRS ratio:	Not applicable	Rhythm:	**Junctional tachycardia**

Discussion:

Test ECG 1 shows a rapid narrow-complex tachycardia at a rate of 115 BPM. There are no P waves noted on the strip. An argument can be made for the presence of pseudo-S waves, and this possibility can be verified or rejected by looking at the morphology of the lead II complexes in an old ECG or once the patient is back in sinus rhythm. The QT interval is prolonged on this strip, and a full 12-lead ECG should be considered to evaluate this issue further. The regular cadence, the lack of P waves, the narrow complexes, and the rate of 115 BPM all point to the diagnosis of a junctional tachycardia.

Test ECG 2

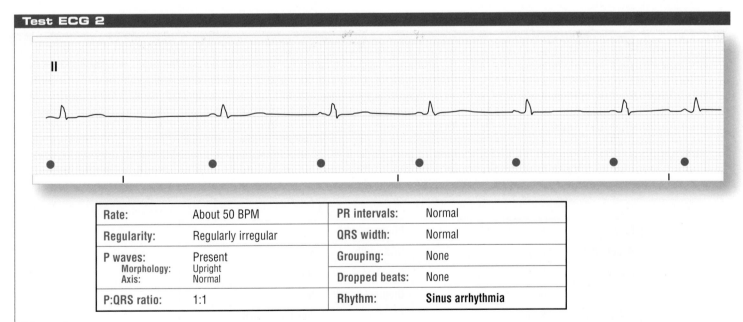

Rate:	About 50 BPM	PR intervals:	Normal
Regularity:	Regularly irregular	QRS width:	Normal
P waves:	Present	Grouping:	None
Morphology:	Upright		
Axis:	Normal	Dropped beats:	None
P:QRS ratio:	1:1	Rhythm:	**Sinus arrhythmia**

Discussion:

This strip shows an irregular rhythm with a gradual decrease in the R-R intervals. There are P waves in front of each QRS complex with nearly identical morphology. The last P wave has a different appearance on this strip but the PR interval is the same. The difference is probably due to the slight bump in the baseline. A longer strip taken on this patient verified the presence of the rhythmical slowing and speeding up, which is classic for a sinus arrhythmia.

Test ECG 3

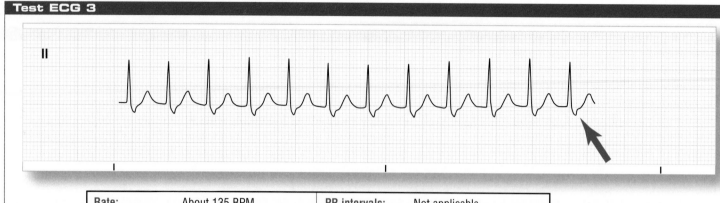

Rate:	About 135 BPM	PR intervals:	Not applicable
Regularity:	Regular	QRS width:	Normal
P waves:	Present, pseudo-S	Grouping:	None
Morphology:	Inverted		
Axis:	Abnormal	Dropped beats:	None
P:QRS ratio:	1:1	Rhythm:	**AVNRT**

Discussion:

Test ECG 3 shows a rapid, regular, narrow-complex tachycardia. There are no P waves before the QRS complexes, but there are obvious pseudo-S waves visible at the end of the QRS complexes. As mentioned, these pseudo-S waves (blue arrow) represent the retrogradely conducted, inverted P waves that are formed due to the microreentry circuit of AVNRT. There is some variation in the amplitude of the complexes due to the electrical alternans pattern, which is typically seen in very fast tachycardias.

Test ECG 4

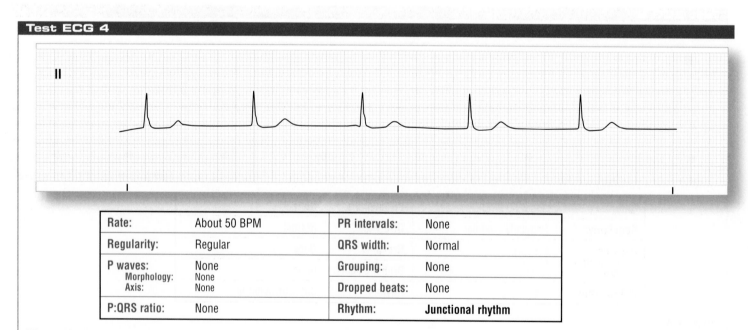

Rate:	About 50 BPM	PR intervals:	None
Regularity:	Regular	QRS width:	Normal
P waves:	None	Grouping:	None
Morphology:	None		
Axis:	None	Dropped beats:	None
P:QRS ratio:	None	Rhythm:	**Junctional rhythm**

Discussion:

Test ECG 4 shows a slow ventricular rhythm with no associated P waves. The narrow complexes are consistent with a supraventricular origin and conduction through the normal electrical conduction system. These findings and the rate of approximately 50 BPM are all consistent with a junctional rhythm. If you want to be more specific, the diagnosis is a junctional escape rhythm.

Test ECG 5

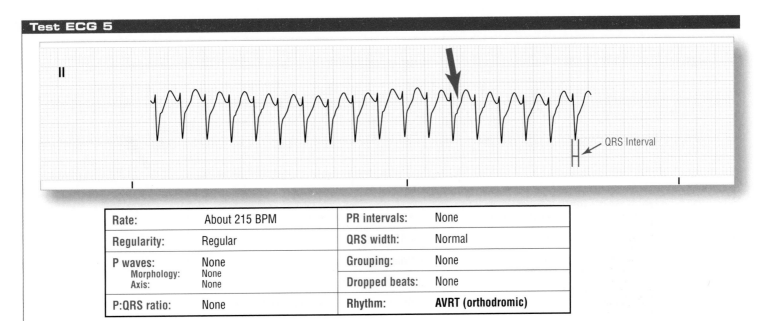

Rate:	About 215 BPM	PR intervals:	None
Regularity:	Regular	QRS width:	Normal
P waves:	None	Grouping:	None
Morphology:	None		
Axis:	None	Dropped beats:	None
P:QRS ratio:	None	Rhythm:	**AVRT (orthodromic)**

Discussion:

This strip shows a very fast narrow-complex tachycardia. There appears to be some pretty significant ST depression (blue arrow), which is probably due to the tachycardia, but could be the result of an underlying relative or actual ischemia. A case could be made for a very fast AVNRT or an AVRT. The rapid rates favor the presence of an accessory pathway. On clinical correlation, the patient did have a history of Wolff-Parkinson-White syndrome and an accessory pathway. The 12-lead ECG after the patient was converted did show the presence of a delta wave, which is typically found in WPW syndrome. If you remember, there are two kinds of conduction in AVRT: orthodromic and antidromic. This is an example of orthodromic AVRT because of the narrow complexes associated with the tachycardia.

Test ECG 6

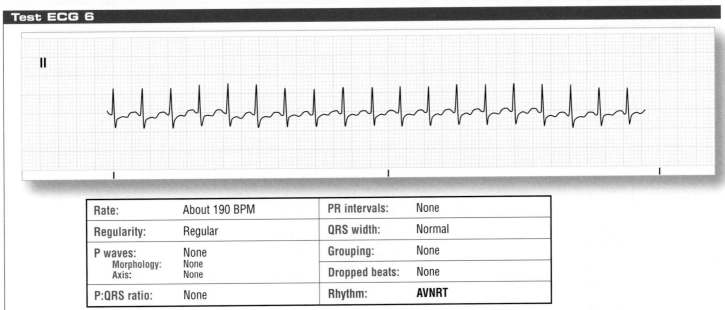

Rate:	About 190 BPM	PR intervals:	None
Regularity:	Regular	QRS width:	Normal
P waves:	None	Grouping:	None
Morphology:	None		
Axis:	None	Dropped beats:	None
P:QRS ratio:	None	Rhythm:	**AVNRT**

Discussion:

Test ECG 6 is an example of a rapid AVNRT. It shows a narrow-complex supraventricular tachycardia with associated ST depression. What makes this an example of AVNRT and Test ECG 5 an example of AVRT? The clinical scenario and the appearance of the 12-lead ECG after the rhythm is broken. Morphologically, it would be difficult to tell from the strips, and both strips could be either AVNRT or AVRT on surface examination. In Test ECG 5, the fact that the rate is over 200 BPM is the only thing that would favor AVRT, but that could also occasionally be seen in AVNRT. The reason we bring this up is that you need to have a high index of suspicion when approaching these rapid tachycardias and use all the tools you have available to effectively make your diagnosis.

Test ECG 7

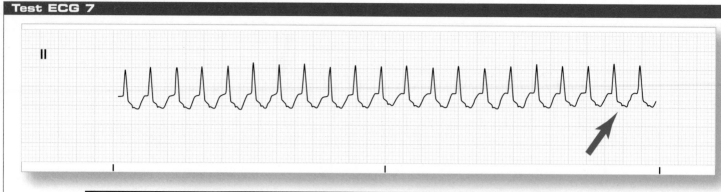

Rate:	About 210 BPM	PR intervals:	None
Regularity:	Regular	QRS width:	Normal
P waves: Morphology: Axis:	Present Inverted Abnormal	Grouping:	None
		Dropped beats:	None
P:QRS ratio:	1:1	Rhythm:	**AVRT (orthodromic)**

Discussion:

This strip is another tough diagnostic case, which could represent either AVNRT or AVRT. There is one finding, however, that helps make your decision a little easier. T waves can either be inverted, upright, or biphasic. However, they are typically smooth, gradually changing waves. Sharp changes along their lines are not typically seen in T-wave morphologies. On our strip, there appears to be a fairly sharp negative deflection on the downward slope of the T-wave (blue arrow). These sharp, negative waves are actually inverted P waves associated with very prolonged R-P intervals. Long R-P intervals are consistent with AVRT. Hence, this is an orthodromic AVRT. Clinical correlation and a 12-lead ECG verified the diagnosis.

Test ECG 8

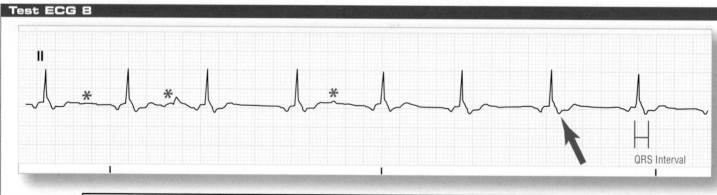

QRS Interval

Rate:	About 64 BPM	PR intervals:	Normal
Regularity:	See discussion below	QRS width:	Wide
P waves: Morphology: Axis:	Present Inverted Abnormal	Grouping:	None
		Dropped beats:	None
P:QRS ratio:	1:1	Rhythm:	**Ectopic atrial rhythm**

Discussion:

Test ECG 8 presents some interesting dilemmas. First of all, the rhythm is slightly irregular. Could the irregularity be caused by premature complexes? Not really, because all of the P waves are exactly identical and the PR intervals remain the same. Could this be a straight sinus arrhythmia? No, because the P waves are inverted, meaning that they originate in either an ectopic atrial or a junctional site. The normal PR intervals favor an ectopic rhythm. This is an ectopic atrial rhythm with some irregularity, probably due to a respiratory variation of a sinus arrhythmia. Secondly, there are some slight abnormalities noted along the baseline due to artifact (blue asterisks). Lastly, the blue arrow points to an S wave at the end of the QRS complex (verified by a 12-lead ECG), which could easily be mistaken for a blocked inverted P wave.

Test ECG 9

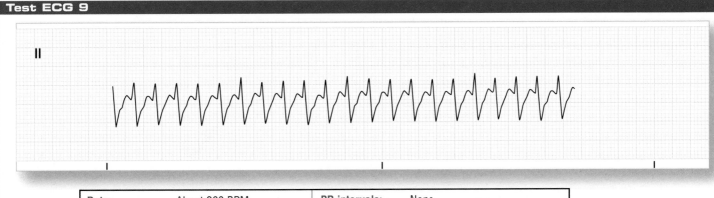

Rate:	About 260 BPM	PR intervals:	None
Regularity:	Regular	QRS width:	Wide
P waves:	None	Grouping:	None
Morphology:	None		
Axis:	None	Dropped beats:	None
P:QRS ratio:	None	Rhythm:	**AVRT (antidromic)**

Discussion:

Test ECG 9 shows a very dangerous rhythm. The rate of 260 BPM and the wide complexes noted on the tachycardia are consistent with an antidromic AVRT. Antidromic AVRTs are associated with accessory pathways and WPW syndrome. The conduction of the macroreentry electrical circuit is through the accessory pathway into the ventricles, and then retrogradely against the AV node to return to the atria. In this type of AVRT, there is no AV nodal control over the rate, hence, the danger. These very rapid rhythms can become so fast as to break down completely, sending the patient into ventricular fibrillation and cardiac arrest. Prompt, focused treatment is indicated in these patients and electrical cardioversion should be emergently performed for any hemodynamic instability.

Test ECG 10

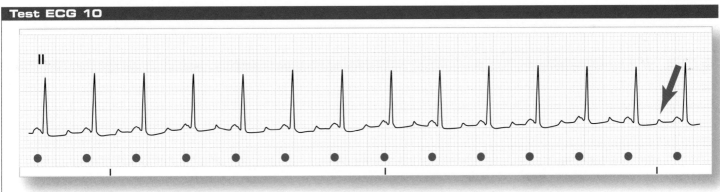

Rate:	About 110 BPM	PR intervals:	Normal
Regularity:	Regular	QRS width:	Normal
P waves:	Present	Grouping:	None
Morphology:	Upright		
Axis:	Normal	Dropped beats:	None
P:QRS ratio:	1:1	Rhythm:	**Sinus tachycardia**

Discussion:

Test ECG 10 shows a sinus rhythm with an upright P wave, a normal PR interval, and some slight ST depression. Since the rate is 110 BPM, this makes the rhythm a sinus tachycardia. The PR interval appears short, but measurement with your calipers should show you that it is 0.12 seconds and within the normal range. The QT interval appears prolonged at 0.31 seconds but, when you consider that the ventricular rate is 110 BPM, it is within the normal range. The T wave in this lead is a small, positive deflection, which could be mistaken for another P wave (blue arrow).

Test ECG 11

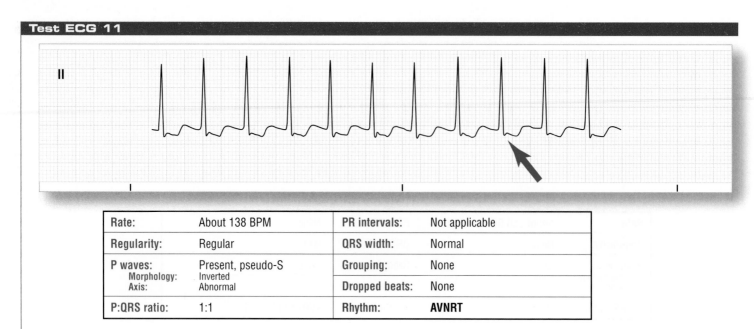

Rate:	About 138 BPM	PR intervals:	Not applicable
Regularity:	Regular	QRS width:	Normal
P waves:	Present, pseudo-S	Grouping:	None
Morphology:	Inverted		
Axis:	Abnormal	Dropped beats:	None
P:QRS ratio:	1:1	Rhythm:	**AVNRT**

Discussion:

Test ECG 11 shows a narrow-complex tachycardia at about 138 BPM. This rate is right at the upper end of the threshold between AVNRT and junctional tachycardia.

There are inverted P waves present, which cause a pseudo-S wave pattern in lead II (blue arrow). Because of the rate, we favor the diagnosis of AVNRT in this case.

Test ECG 12

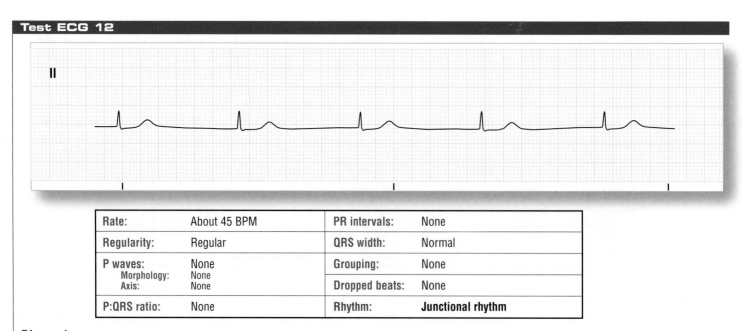

Rate:	About 45 BPM	PR intervals:	None
Regularity:	Regular	QRS width:	Normal
P waves:	None	Grouping:	None
Morphology:	None		
Axis:	None	Dropped beats:	None
P:QRS ratio:	None	Rhythm:	**Junctional rhythm**

Discussion:

Test ECG 12 shows aslow rhythm with no associated P waves noted anywhere along the strip. The QRS complexes are narrow. This strip is consistent with a junctional (escape) rhythm.

Test ECG 13

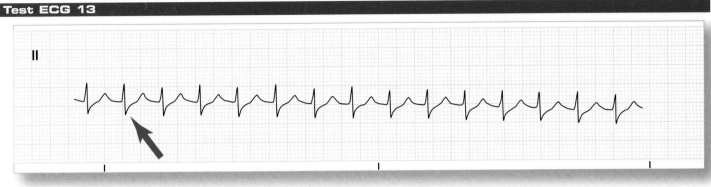

Rate:	About 145 BPM	PR intervals:	None
Regularity:	Regular	QRS width:	Normal
P waves: Morphology: Axis:	Present, pseudo-S Inverted Abnormal	Grouping: Dropped beats:	None None
P:QRS ratio:	None	Rhythm:	**AVNRT**

Discussion:

Test ECG 13 and Test ECG 14 are both from the same patient, but in different leads. Test ECG 13 shows lead II and Test ECG 14 shows lead V₁. The reason we put these next to each other is to reinforce the need to look for the pseudo-S wave in lead II (blue arrow) and pseudo-R' waves in lead V₁ of any patient in AVNRT. Multiple leads or a full 12-lead ECG are invaluable tools in seeing these two findings, which clinch the diagnosis of AVNRT as the cause of a narrow-complex tachycardia.

Test ECG 14

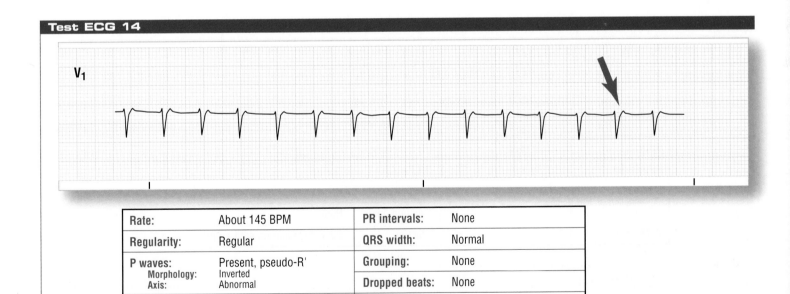

Rate:	About 145 BPM	PR intervals:	None
Regularity:	Regular	QRS width:	Normal
P waves: Morphology: Axis:	Present, pseudo-R' Inverted Abnormal	Grouping: Dropped beats:	None None
P:QRS ratio:	None	Rhythm:	**AVNRT**

Discussion:

Test ECG 14 shows a lead V₁ rhythm strip of the same patient as in Test ECG 13. Both of these strips show AVNRT. Note the presence of the pseudo-R' wave on this strip (blue arrow). Make it a habit to always check the lead that you are using to view a strip. The orientation and the appearance of the complexes will change drastically, depending on the lead that is being viewed.

Test ECG 15

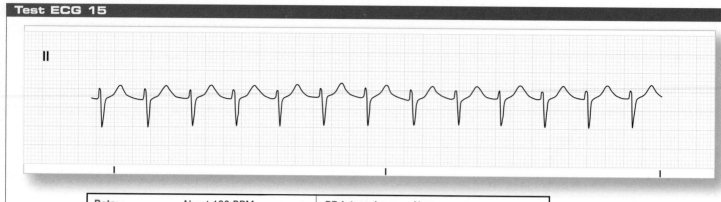

Rate:	About 120 BPM	PR intervals:	None
Regularity:	Regular	QRS width:	Normal
P waves:	None	Grouping:	None
Morphology:	None		
Axis:	None	Dropped beats:	None
P:QRS ratio:	None	Rhythm:	**Junctional tachycardia**

Discussion:

Test ECG 15 shows a rapid, regular narrow-complex tachycardia. The heart rate is 120 BPM and there are no visible P waves on the strip. These findings are consistent with a junctional tachycardia.

Test ECG 16

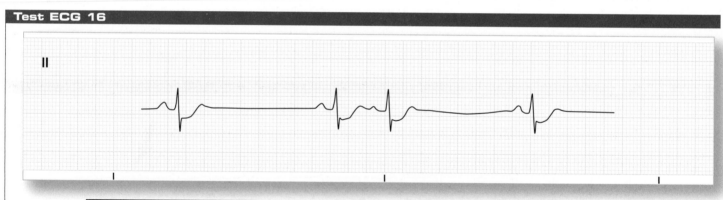

Rate:	About 34 BPM	PR intervals:	Normal, except in event
Regularity:	Regularly irregular	QRS width:	Normal
P waves:	Present	Grouping:	None
Morphology:	Upright		
Axis:	Normal	Dropped beats:	None
P:QRS ratio:	1:1	Rhythm:	**Sinus bradycardia with a PAC**

Discussion:

Test ECG 16 was taken from a patient with a very slow sinus bradycardia. The third complex arrives prematurely and has a different morphology and PR interval than the others on the strip. By definition, this makes the third complex a PAC. The PAC is probably a protective event by the heart, as it is trying to compensate for the severity of the underlying bradycardia. The patient has very significant ST depressions in lead II. The ST changes could be due to direct inferior wall ischemia or could represent reciprocal changes of an acute lateral wall MI. A full 12-lead ECG would be invaluable on this patient. Clinical correlation and evaluation for an AMI should also be emergently undertaken. Temporary pacemaker placement may be indicated if this patient is hemodynamically unstable.

Test ECG 17

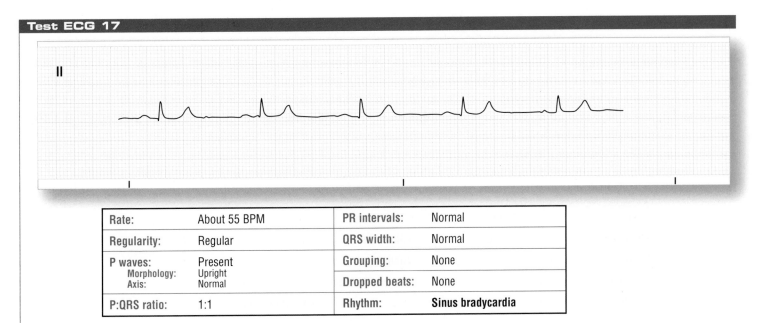

Rate:	About 55 BPM	PR intervals:	Normal
Regularity:	Regular	QRS width:	Normal

P waves:
   Morphology:
   Axis:
	Present
	Upright
	Normal
		Grouping:	None

		Dropped beats:	None
P:QRS ratio:	1:1	Rhythm:	**Sinus bradycardia**

Discussion:

Test ECG 17 shows a P wave before each QRS complex. The PR intervals are all consistent and within the normal range. The origin of the complexes is, therefore, in the sinus node. The rate of 55 BPM makes the final diagnosis sinus bradycardia.

Test ECG 18

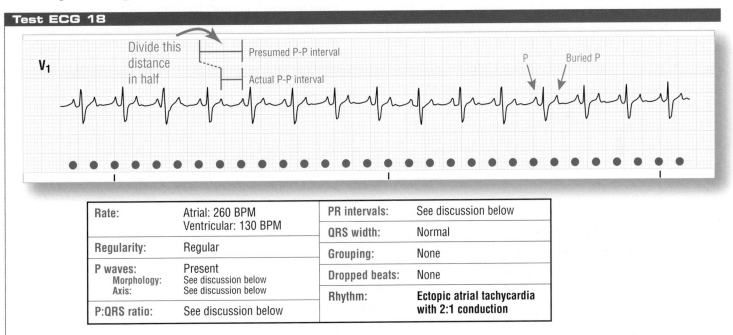

Rate:	Atrial: 260 BPM Ventricular: 130 BPM	PR intervals:	See discussion below
		QRS width:	Normal
Regularity:	Regular	Grouping:	None

P waves:
   Morphology:
   Axis:
	Present
	See discussion below
	See discussion below
		Dropped beats:	None

		Rhythm:	**Ectopic atrial tachycardia with 2:1 conduction**
P:QRS ratio:	See discussion below		

Discussion:

This strip can be quite troubling. We can all clearly see the first P wave right before the QRS complexes. However, many people miss the other P wave buried in the T wave right after the QRS complex (see purple arrows and labels), thinking that this second peak is the T wave. It isn't. Here is the proof: Use your calipers to measure the distance between the peaks that are obviously P waves. Next, divide that distance in half. Now, place your calipers over the obvious P wave and you will see that the other pin falls directly on top of the second peak—the buried P wave.

This extra P wave makes this rhythm either an ectopic atrial tachycardia with block (2:1 conduction) or an atrial flutter with 2:1 conduction. What is the deciding factor? The space between the P waves. If there is a constantly undulating saw-tooth pattern, then the rhythm is atrial flutter. If there is a return to an isoelectric baseline between the P waves, then it is an atrial tachycardia with block. A 12-lead ECG on this patient, including lead II, verified the diagnosis of ectopic atrial tachycardia with block.

Test ECG 19

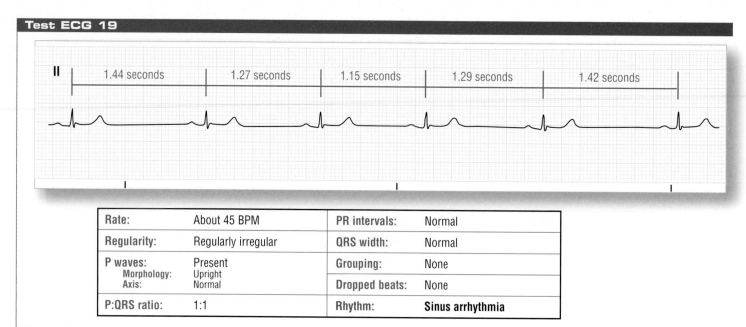

Rate:	About 45 BPM	PR intervals:	Normal
Regularity:	Regularly irregular	QRS width:	Normal
P waves:	Present	Grouping:	None
Morphology:	Upright		
Axis:	Normal	Dropped beats:	None
P:QRS ratio:	1:1	Rhythm:	**Sinus arrhythmia**

Discussion:

Test ECG 19 shows a regularly irregular rhythm with narrow QRS complexes. Each QRS complex has its own P wave, and both the P wave morphology and the PR intervals throughout the strip are identical. The rhythm strip has a regularly irregular pattern due to a gradual narrowing and widening of the P-P intervals. The differ-ence between the widest and the narrowest P-P interval is greater than 0.16 seconds, clinching the diagnosis of a sinus arrhythmia. Normally, sinus arrhythmia occurs at rates between 60 and 100 BPM, but exceptions do exist. Many times, the slower rates in these patients are due to the presence of drugs like the beta-blocking agents.

Test ECG 20

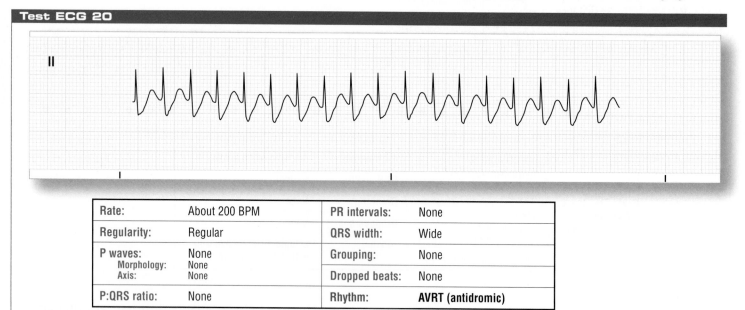

Rate:	About 200 BPM	PR intervals:	None
Regularity:	Regular	QRS width:	Wide
P waves:	None	Grouping:	None
Morphology:	None		
Axis:	None	Dropped beats:	None
P:QRS ratio:	None	Rhythm:	**AVRT (antidromic)**

Discussion:

Test ECG 20 shows a wide-complex tachycardia at 200 BPM. There are no obvious P waves noted throughout the strip. These findings are consistent with an antidromic AVRT. The presence of an accessory pathway should be evaluated further.

As a side note, could this strip represent an AVNRT in someone with a preexisting bundle branch block? The answer is yes. Always remember to obtain clinical corre-lation and to obtain multiple leads or a full 12-lead ECG to help in your decision making. An old ECG or rhythm strip will also prove invaluable in evaluating any com-plex rhythm. Finally, for completeness, just as in every wide-complex tachycardia, you need to think of and rule out the possibility of a ventricular tachycardia.

Ventricular Rhythms

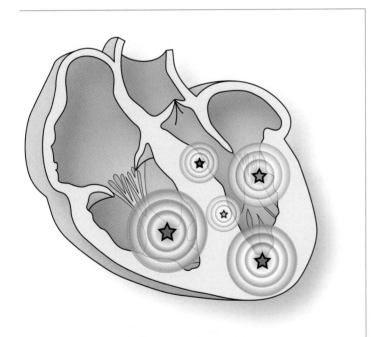

CHAPTER 28

Introduction to Ventricular Rhythms

Ventricular rhythms are the most clinically feared cardiac rhythms because of the hemodynamic instability that they cause. As we shall see, there is no such thing as a completely benign ventricular rhythm. Even PVCs, which are generally considered benign, can cause significant hemodynamic compromise in the right clinical setting.

A rhythm is considered to be of ventricular origin if the ectopic pacemaker is found distal to the bifurcation of the His bundles. The pacemaker could be found in the bundle branches, the anterior or posterior fascicle, the Purkinje system, or in the ventricular muscle. Typically, ventricular depolarization is spread through direct cell-to-cell contact. However, if the impulse originates in or near the conduction system, the impulse conduction can be conducted at least partly through the electrical conduction system. Therefore, the site of origin is critical in determining the exact electrocardiographic morphology of the complexes.

In Chapter 27, we discussed how symmetrical, synchronous contraction of the ventricles is critical to maintaining a good cardiac output. In ventricular rhythms, symmetrical and synchronous contraction of the ventricles is almost nonexistent. The typical direct cell-to-cell transmission of the impulse leads to ventricular contractions that follow very bizarre, abnormal patterns. These patterns reflect defects in mechanical contraction that significantly alter the ejection fraction of the ventricles and, therefore, the cardiac output. If you add the lack of atrial kick into the equation, the problem is compounded significantly.

In this chapter, we begin by taking a look at how the morphology of a ventricular depolarization develops, and then we will review some clinically important aspects of these rhythms. A clear understanding of the mechanisms will make discussion of the individual rhythms much easier.

Morphology

As mentioned above, the typical form of transmission of the ventricular impulse is by direct cell-to-cell contact.

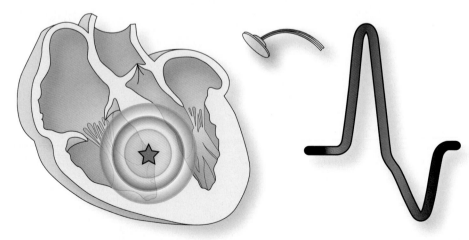

Figure 28-1: An irritable focus, represented by the red star, acts as a pacemaker and causes an impulse to occur. This gives rise to a depolarization wave that radiates outward by direct cell-to-cell transmission until all of the ventricles are depolarized. Note the color-coded sections of the depolarization wave and the complex.

As you can see in Figure 28-1, as the impulse spreads, it forms bioelectrical energy that is picked up by the ECG leads and begins to form the electrocardiographic pattern for that particular ectopic focus. The site of the ectopic focus is one of the main determinants of morphology in a ventricular complex.

Therefore, the first determinant of a ventricular depolarization is that the QRS complexes will be greater than or equal to 0.12 seconds (or three little blocks) and wide and bizarre in appearance. The "greater than" part of that statement is very critical to keep in mind because these complexes can be very, very wide. Many times ventricular complexes are even wider than 0.20 seconds. In general, ventricular depolarizations that originate in the ventricular myocardium and spread by direct cell-to-cell transmission only will tend to be in the wider end of the spectrum. Ventricular depolarizations that have some transmission through the electrical conduction system will tend to be toward the narrower end of the spectrum.

The ventricular QRS complexes are bizarre in appearance because of the delay caused by the direct cell-to-cell depolarization waves that form them and because of the atypical routes of ventricular depolarization that are taken by these waves. The vectors that are formed by these spreading waves are always abnormal; therefore, they give rise to abnormal patterns on the ECG (Figure 28-2). (It is interesting to note that one ectopic focus can lead to many different morphological presentations depending on the route taken outward from the site. For example, on one complex the route may start off spreading superiorly, while on the next complex the route may start off inferiorly. Both of those presentations will lead to remarkably different morphologies on the ECG.)

Another factor that can drastically alter the morphology of a ventricular complex is the lead in which you view it. If you remember from Chapter 3, leads are like cameras taking "pictures" of the vectors from their particular vantage point (Figure 28-3). Depending on

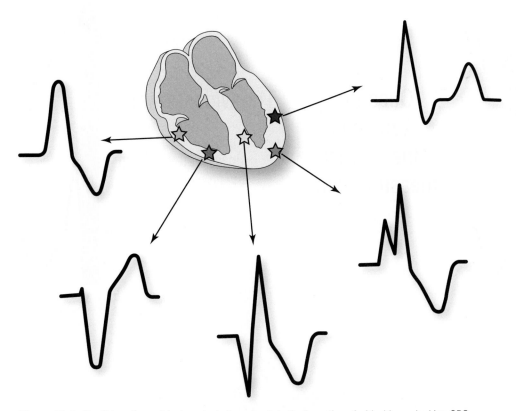

Figure 28-2: The firing of a ventricular ectopic focus leads to the formation of wide, bizarre-looking QRS complexes. The figure shows various types of possible QRS morphologies, but the actual appearance of a QRS cannot be predicted completely based on the location of the ectopic focus. In addition, the morphology will change based on the lead used to view the complexes.

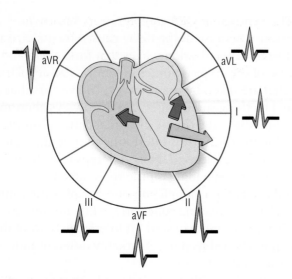

the vantage point, the same complex can appear markedly different. In addition, isoelectric segments may actually lead to errors in the correct determination of a complex's true width (Figure 28-4). Multiple leads will greatly improve the accuracy of your measurement. Always remember to use the widest complex to take your measurements (thereby avoiding the mistake of not including isoelectric segments into your measurement).

In a ventricular complex, the ST segment and T waves will always be abnormal and often may be inverted, elevated, or depressed. This occurs because of abnormal patterns of repolarization associated with these complexes. Why this occurs is a topic for a book on electrocardiography. For a further discussion of the topic, see *12-Lead ECG: The Art of Interpretation* by Garcia and Holtz.

Figure 28-3: The same complex can appear drastically different based on which lead it is viewed in.

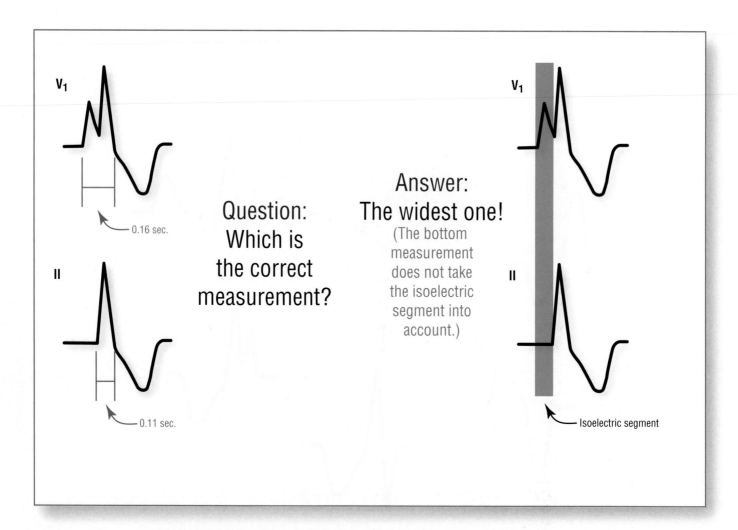

Figure 28-4: The same complex can have different widths due to isoelectric segments that can develop in certain leads. But, remember, interval widths are actually the same in every lead! Get used to always measuring the widest interval—it is the true interval without any isoelectric segments.

ADDITIONAL INFORMATION

Where is the Ectopic Focus?

Now, let's look at an interesting aspect of morphology. Since the site of origin of a ventricular depolarization is the most important factor in determining morphology, we can use the inverse of that statement to help us identify where the complex originated. In other words, we can use certain morphological types to help guide us to the most likely location of the ectopic pacemaker.

In general, ventricular complexes that originate in the left ventricle will take on a right bundle branch block pattern. Ventricular complexes that originate in the right ventricle take on a left bundle branch block pattern. These statements are generally true, but why does this occur? (For a complete review of the left and right bundle branch block patterns, please see Chapter 6.)

Take a look at Figure 28-5. In this figure, the ectopic focus is in the left ventricular myocardium. Due to its anatomical location, most of the ventricular myocardium will lie to the right of the focus. The depolarization wave has to head primarily from left to right. So, in what direction would you expect the vector formed by the depolarization wave to head? Left to right. If you think about it, this is very similar to the vector that is formed when the right bundle branch is blocked (Figure 28-6). Since the main vectors of these two complexes point in the same direction, their respective morphologies should be similar. The similar vectors are the reason why a ventricular ectopic focus on the left ventricle will give rise to a complex that is morphologically similar to one caused by a right bundle branch block. Likewise, a right ventricular ectopic focus will give rise to a main ventricular vector that heads to the left and this will resemble a left bundle branch block pattern.

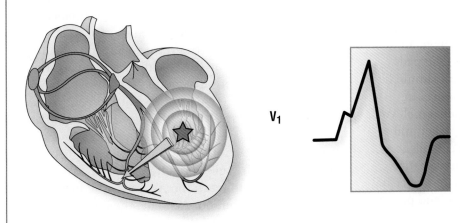

V_1

Figure 28-5: An irritable focus, represented by the purple star, acts as a pacemaker and causes an impulse to occur. This gives rise to the purple depolarization wave and the yellow vector. Electrocardiographically, this is represented by the wide slurring of the terminal portion of the QRS.

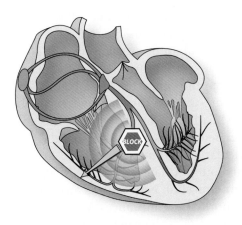

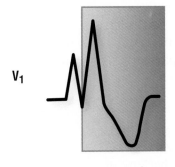

V_1

Figure 28-6: A right bundle branch block causes the depolarization wave to travel rightward to the right ventricle to depolarize the ventricle by direct cell-to-cell contact. This gives rise to the blue depolarization wave and the yellow vector and the typical RBBB pattern.

The Ventricle as a Pacemaker

The ventricular myocardium offers our last defense against asystole or the lack of any rhythm. If you remember from Chapter 1, the first and principal pacemaker is the sinus node. In cases where the sinus node fails, the atrial myocardium becomes our first line of defense. This continues down the line until you reach the ventricular pacemaker. Keep in mind, ventricular rhythms are dangerous for many reasons. One of the principal reasons is this: ***What is your failsafe if a ventricular pacemaker fails to fire? Answer: there is none!*** That is it. . .end of the line . . .the buck stops here. . .or whatever other cliché you choose to say that there is no other failsafe pacemaker after the ventricular myocardium.

The intrinsic rates of the various portions of the ventricle are as follows: The bundle branches fire at a rate of 40 to 45 BPM. The Purkinje system fires at an intrinsic rate of 35 to 40 BPM. Finally, the ventricular myocardium usually fires at an intrinsic rate of 30 to 35 BPM, but can be as low as the 20s.

Here is a little clinical pearl. Whenever you have a patient with a slow ventricular rate that is wide and bizarre, you'd better have pacemaking capabilities at hand or, better yet, on your patient. If you have an external transthoracic pacemaker available, the pads should be on the patient's chest and the unit should be accessible and ready to go at a moment's notice. In addition, if you have the capability or the personnel, you should have an internal transvenous pacemaker and wire ready, just in case the transthoracic pacer fails. Remember, there is no other intrinsic pacemaker that can save you if the ventricles fail. Your only response at that point is CPR, electricity via a pacemaker, and prayer.

The P Wave in Ventricular Rhythms

Some people never pay attention to the P waves in ventricular rhythms. That is a big mistake. The P waves are very useful in evaluating the wide-complex rhythms (and ventricular tachycardia in particular). In particular, we need to concentrate on the morphology, axis, and rate of the P waves. In addition, we need to pay particular attention to the P:QRS relationship.

P Wave Morphology in Ventricular Rhythms

Would you expect any P waves in a ventricular rhythm and, if so, what would they look like? The answer is that retrograde P waves can *occasionally* occur because of isolated ventricular firing. We say "occasionally" because the retrograde transmission of the ventricular impulse to the atria is very variable. Many times, the AV node allows the impulse to spread retrogradely to the atria. Many times, it completely blocks the retrograde transmission and the atria are totally oblivious to the occurrences in the ventricle. Other times, the atria and the ventricles are completely isolated from each other because of a third-degree AV nodal block. In these cases, the atria and ventricles are firing at their own intrinsic rates without any form of interaction.

The antegrade block or retrograde transmission of the ventricular impulse through the AV node into the atria is dependent on many variables, and it is impossible to predict when either will occur. Drugs, ischemia, intrinsic conduction system disease, electrolytes, sympathetic and parasympathetic influences, and so on, all influence the AV node in this respect.

Let's look at what happens when there is retrograde conduction through the AV node. When an ectopic ventricular pacer fires, it stimulates the ventricles by direct cell-to-cell contact. This causes a wide, bizarre-looking QRS complex to develop. When the impulse reaches the AV node, the AV node can either allow the impulse to travel retrogradely into the atria or it can block the impulse completely (Figure 28-7).

If the impulse is spread retrogradely into the atria, a P wave will be created. Since the P-wave vector is heading from inferior to superior, the P wave will be inverted on the ECG. Also, in an isolated ventricular complex, *the inverted P wave can either be buried in the QRS complex, be immediately after the QRS, or have a prolonged R-P interval.* The R-P interval can often be long because it takes time for the cell-to-cell transmission of the ventricular impulse to reach the AV node. The further the ectopic pacer is from the AV node, the longer the R-P interval (Figure 28-8).

The P:QRS Relationship in Ventricular Rhythms

Most ventricular complexes do not have a P wave associated with them. Others have an inverted P wave with a prolonged R-P interval. In this section, we are going to concentrate on the concepts involved in the dissociation of the atria from the ventricles. We are going to be spending much more time on this topic when we discuss third-degree heart block in Chapter 35. This short discussion is intended only as a quick look at the issues related to ventricular arrhythmias.

As we pointed out in Chapter 1, the AV node is the only area of communication between the atria and the ventricles under normal circumstances. We talked about the AV node functioning as the gatekeeper between the atria and the ventricles and have seen various examples

When a
ventricular impulse
reaches the AV node,
it can take one of
two routes:

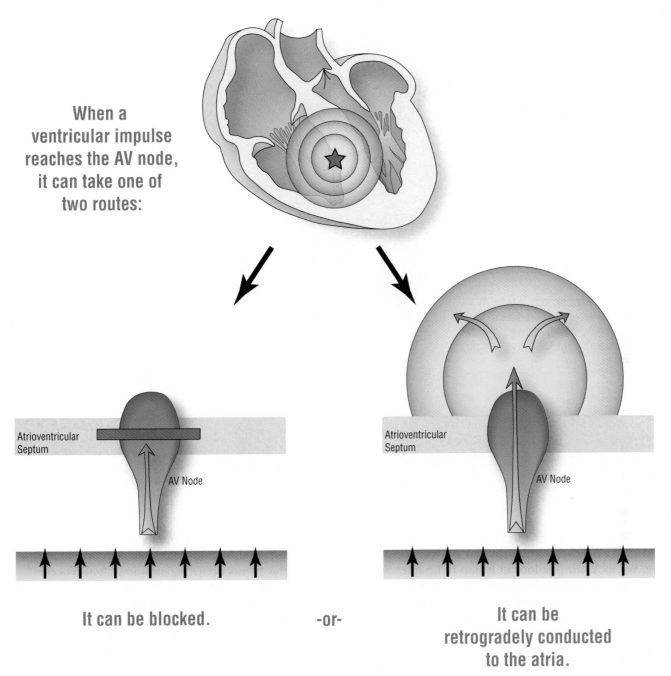

It can be blocked.   -or-   It can be
retrogradely conducted
to the atria.

Figure 28-7: Ventricular conduction through the AV node.

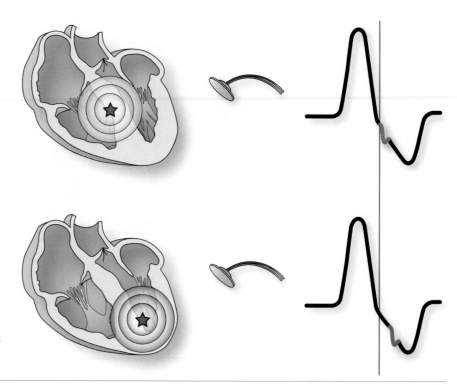

Figure 28-8: The closer the ectopic focus is to the AV node, the shorter the R-P interval. The extra distance traveled by the ventricular impulse created by the ectopic focus represented in green causes the inverted P wave to occur further along the complex.

ADDITIONAL **INFORMATION**

Fusion

Fusion of the QRS complexes and the other component waves occurs in every ventricular rhythm we will be discussing. We took our first look at fusion in Chapter 5. We will now include a short review of this topic for your convenience, but we strongly urge you to spend the time to go back and review this concept thoroughly. Fusion will greatly alter the morphology and appearance of ventricular complexes and will often lead you to misdiagnose some malignant ventricular rhythms.

Fusion refers to the merging together of two or more waves and/or vectors that are occurring at the same, or nearly the same, moment in time. The final result is that the complexes that are formed have characteristics of both of the parent waves or vectors. The complexes formed are different in morphology from the rest of the strip, as each of the parents adds its input into the final product.

In reality, fusion is actually two different electrocardiographic phenomena with one name. The first is an isolated electrocardiographic summation of waves from two different complexes. The fusion is on the ECG, but not actually in the heart. This occurs mostly during premature or fast rhythms and is fairly evident on the ECG because of the events occurring around it. It also occurs in most cases of AV block.

The second type of fusion is actual fusion of two depolarization waves occurring simultaneously. An example of this type of fusion is one in which a normally occurring ventricular depolarization begins to occur, and an ectopic pacer fires and begins to form its own depolarization wave somewhere else in the ventricle. The result is that both waves begin to form and eventually crash into one another. The complexes formed during this type of fusion are more difficult to differentiate and can be easily mistaken for complexes originating at completely different ectopic sites.

Both types of fusion occur in ventricular rhythms. We will look at fusion in the next segment of this chapter and we will look at it throughout the rest of this section. In particular, fusion complexes can be very useful in evaluating ventricular tachycardia, and we will revisit this topic in more detail when we get to that chapter.

of the arrhythmias that can develop because of malfunctions. Now, suppose that the AV node shuts down all communication completely between the atria and the ventricles. What do you think would happen?

Once again, in order to answer that question, we have to go back to our basic knowledge. If you remember, we talked about the sequential order of pacemakers in the heart, which act as a failsafe against asystole or cardiac standstill. We saw that the order went from sinus node, to atrial muscle, to AV node, to His bundles, to the bundle branches, to the Purkinje system, to the ventricular myocytes. Failure of an earlier group means that the next group would take over. So, what do you suppose would happen if the ventricles were cut off from above? The ventricular pacers would think that

the upper groups have failed and they need to begin to take over the pacing function themselves. In other words, the isolation of the ventricles causes a ventricular pacer to take over ventricular pacing (Figure 28-9).

Each respective pacemaker, one atrial and one ventricular, would beat at its own intrinsic rate and create its own rhythm (see Figure 28-9). These two rhythms are occurring simultaneously, and would appear in the electrocardiogram as a series of atrial complexes and ventricular complexes occurring completely separately. Note, however, that electrocardiographically the complexes would fuse together at certain times and possibly cause some alteration of the individual morphologies (Figure 28-10). This type of AV block is complete and is, therefore, known as a *third-degree* or *complete AV block*.

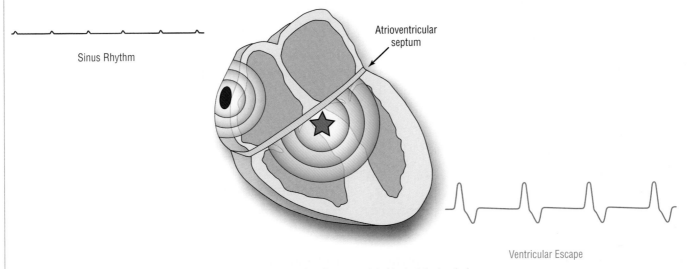

Sinus Rhythm

Atrioventricular septum

Ventricular Escape

Figure 28-9: When the AV node is not conducting, it creates, functionally, a complete block at the level of the interventricular septum. The atria and the ventricles are completely oblivious to each other, and two separate pacemakers develop. Each pacemaker will keep its own intrinsic rate and control its respective chamber.

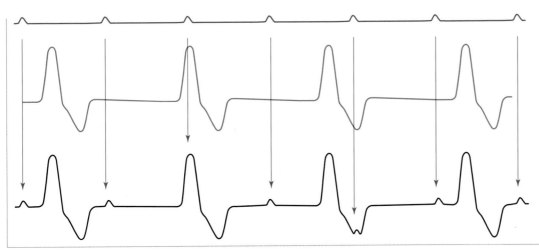

Figure 28-10: The atria and the ventricles are completely oblivious to each other and there are two separate pacemakers. Each pacemaker will keep its own intrinsic rate and control its respective chamber. The ECG fuses these two rhythms into one strip (see strip in black). This is a third-degree heart block with a ventricular escape.

Josephson's Sign

Josephson's sign refers to the presence of a notch in the downstroke of the S wave present in many complexes of ventricular origin (Figure 28-11). The presence of the notch is very useful in distinguishing a ventricular complex from an aberrantly conducted supraventricular complex or a complex with an underlying LBBB or RBBB.

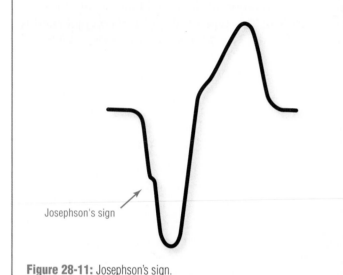

Figure 28-11: Josephson's sign.

Brugada's Sign

Brugada's sign refers to a distance of at least 0.10 seconds from the onset of the QRS complex to the very bottom (or nadir) of the S wave that is present in many complexes of ventricular origin (Figure 28-12). The presence of this distance interval is a very useful sign in distinguishing a ventricular complex from an aberrantly conducted supraventricular complex or a complex with an underlying LBBB or RBBB.

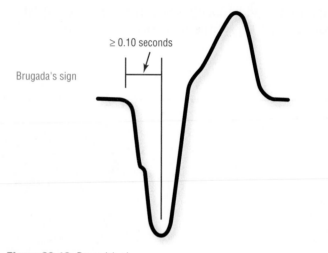

Figure 28-12: Brugada's sign.

Third-degree AV block is very common in ventricular arrhythmias. In the typical case, the AV block leads to a ventricular response that is either in the range of the normal ventricular pacemaking range (30 to 45 BPM) or increased ventricular automaticity may lead to a faster response.

Always keep the P:QRS relationship in mind when approaching any wide-complex rhythm. It is one of the most useful tools in determining whether a wide-complex tachycardia is caused by a ventricular pacemaker or if it is an aberrant form of supraventricular tachycardia due to another reason.

Ventricular Rhythms: General Overview

The ventricular rhythms occur either as a result of an escape mechanism or due to increased automaticity. Some ventricular rhythms actually occur as a result of reentry loops. In this section, we will be reviewing the most important ventricular rhythms. These include ventricular escape beats, ventricular premature depolarizations, idioventricular rhythm, accelerated idioventricular, ventricular tachycardia, ventricular flutter, and ventricular fibrillation (Figure 28-13). At the end of this section, Chapter 33 discusses the differential diagnosis of the wide-complex arrhythmias. It will be worth your while to review and thoroughly understand this particular chapter. Finally, we will take a look at the agonal rhythms and asystole (complete absence of ventricular activity).

As mentioned previously, the intrinsic rate of the ventricular pacemakers ranges from 30 to 45 BPM. The ventricular pacemakers are the last failsafe mechanism for the heart. Their failure signifies death. In addition, the hemodynamic status of the body is completely dependent on the ventricular rate and their appropriate contraction. Take every ventricular rhythm that you encounter very seriously. Wide-complex rhythms are generally dangerous and should be treated with extreme urgency and care.

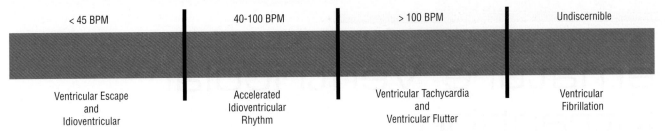

< 45 BPM	40-100 BPM	> 100 BPM	Undiscernible
Ventricular Escape and Idioventricular	Accelerated Idioventricular Rhythm	Ventricular Tachycardia and Ventricular Flutter	Ventricular Fibrillation

Figure 28-13: The spectrum of the ventricular rhythms. In addition, there are the agonal rhythms and asystole (which is considered the absence of any ventricular rhythm). Notice that in previous chapters, the bar had sections that were green, to symbolize some level of stability. In the ventricular rhythms, there is no such luxury, as any of them can be life-threatening.

CHAPTER REVIEW

1. A rhythm is considered to be of ventricular origin if the ectopic pacemaker is found below the bifurcation of the bundle of His. True or False.

2. A complex of ventricular origin may be partly spread through the normal conduction system. This can affect the width of the complex dramatically, but all of them will be over _____ seconds wide.

3. Characteristics of a ventricular complex include:
   A. Wide, bizarre-looking complexes
   B. Width greater than or equal to 0.12 seconds
   C. Inverted P waves may or may not be found
   D. ST and T wave abnormalities
   E. All of the above

4. The morphology of every complex originating from any one ectopic focus will always appear the same on the ECG. True or False.

5. In general, ectopic foci starting in the _____ventricle will have a _____ bundle branch block morphology.
   A. Left, left
   B. Left, right
   C. Right, right
   D. Right, left
   E. B and D

6. The QRS interval's direct measurement will be the same in every lead of an ECG. True or False.

7. The true QRS interval will be exactly the same in every lead of an ECG. True or False.

8. The P wave, if one occurs, in a ventricular complex has to be _____.

9. The R-P interval will vary in ventricular rhythms depending on the location of the ectopic pacemaker and the route taken by the impulse to reach the AV node. True or False.

10. Ventricular rhythms are frequently associated with _____-_____ or complete heart block.

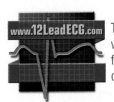

To enhance the knowledge you gain in this book, access this text's website at www.12leadECG.com! This valuable resource provides flashcards, an online glossary, web links, and more. Simply click on the Arrhythmias book cover once at the site.

Premature Ventricular Contraction

General Overview

Premature ventricular contractions (PVCs) can go by various names in the literature. They are known as ventricular premature depolarizations, ventricular premature contractions, and ventricular extrasystoles. Since there is no consensus in the literature about the correct terminology, we will stick to the tried and true nomenclature of PVCs that is very familiar to most clinicians.

A PVC is a depolarization wave that originates in a ventricular focus and that arrives prematurely when compared to the underlying rhythm. It has all of the qualities of a ventricular beat. The list of general characteristics of a PVC includes (Figure 29-1):

- Wider than 0.12 seconds
- Bizarre morphology
- ST segment and T wave abnormalities
- The complex arrives prematurely

PVCs are a very common occurrence and can occur in the normal population, as well as in patients with cardiac disease. In any one patient, the number of PVCs that occur can vary tremendously based on the time of day, medications, coffee, soda, or a hundred other variables. The PVCs usually cause no symptoms, and the patient will be completely unaware that they are occurring. Other times, the patient may just feel a slight skipping in the heart or a sense of palpitations.

In some cases, however, the unsynchronized contraction of the heart caused by a PVC may actually lead to a momentary stop in cardiac ejection. These patients may develop hemodynamic compromise if the frequency of PVCs is high enough. For example, a patient

> **NOTE**
>
> As we discussed in Chapter 5, there is a fine point in the cardiac nomenclature between a rhythm and an event. A rhythm is an intrinsic rate of the heart based on some cardiac pacemaker. An event is a single depolarization or an isolated set of depolarizations, either sinus or ectopic, that breaks up the regularity or cadence of an underlying rhythm. A PVC is an event. Two PVCs occurring sequentially, known as a couplet, is also an event. Many clinicians make the mistake of stating the couplet as the rhythm. The correct way of saying this is: The patient has a (fill in the rhythm) with a couplet.

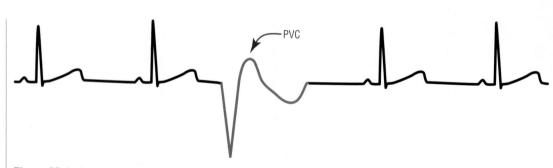

Figure 29-1: A premature ventricular contraction.

with a PVC occurring every other beat may have a monitored heart rate of 80 BPM, but the actual palpable heart rate in the peripheral arteries may be 40 BPM because every other beat is not having any form of effective contraction. As you know, a heart rate of 40 BPM may cause significant hemodynamic compromise in many patients.

A word about the treatment of PVCs: New treatment strategies and new pharmacologic agents are changing the clinical treatment spectrums of the various arrhythmias on an almost daily basis. We try to stay away from the treatment strategies of any rhythm abnormality whenever possible in order to try to keep this book current. However, there are some underlying treatment strategies related to PVCs that we feel are timeless and need to be presented here.

The drugs that we use to treat ventricular arrhythmias can be very dangerous in the wrong clinical setting. In many cases, these drugs can potentially initiate or propagate more serious, life-threatening arrhythmias

in many patients. Therefore, when treating PVCs, remember to **treat the patient and not the individual events**. If the patient is asymptomatic from the PVCs, why would you want to give him or her a drug that could potentially be more harmful?

Coupling Interval

Just like in PJCs, PVCs can have fixed or non-fixed coupling intervals. To review, the coupling interval is the distance from the previous QRS complex to the PVC. A fixed coupling interval (Figure 29-2) is a fairly common occurrence when the PVCs originate in the same ectopic focus and the depolarization wave takes the same route. Fixed coupling intervals should not be off by more than 0.08 seconds. Variable coupling distances (Figure 29-3), on the other hand, are more common in PVCs that originate from multiple ectopic pacemaker and these PVCs will each have a different morphological appearance.

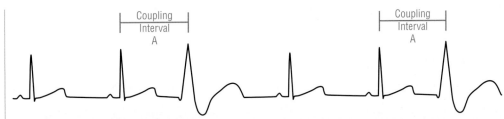

Figure 29-2: The coupling interval refers to the distance between the premature complex and the preceding normal beat found in the underlying rhythm. A fixed coupling interval is the same whenever an individual ectopic focus fires.

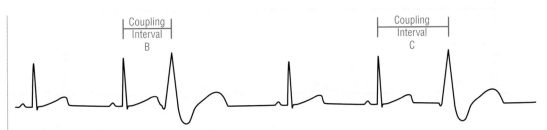

Figure 29-3: A variable coupling interval refers to a variability in the coupling distance. This can occur when the route taken by a depolarization wave is different or if the complex originated in a different ectopic focus.

ADDITIONAL INFORMATION

R-on-T Phenomenon

While we are on the topic of coupling intervals, there are a couple of special types of PVCs that we should look at more closely. These include R-on-T phenomenon and end-diastolic PVCs.

R-on-T Phenomenon

PVCs typically occur after the previous complex has finished repolarization, in other words, after the previous T wave is finished. In certain cases, however, the PVC starts during the relative refractory period of the previous complex's T wave. This is known as the *R-on-T phenomenon* (Figure 29-4). As we saw in Chapter 1, this can create the potential for some very serious reentry loops and circus movements within the ventricles. These loops can lead to serious life-threatening rhythms, including ventricular tachycardia.

There has been a lot of controversy in the literature as to the true clinical importance of the R-on-T phenomenon. For a while, the thought was that the R-on-T phenomenon was very dangerous and that these PVCs had to be treated emergently. Then the pendulum swung in the direction of completely ignoring the R-on-T phenomenon, and the thought was that these PVCs were completely benign. Recently, the pendulum is beginning to swing back in the direction of potential danger.

Here is our thought on this. If there is a potential for serious clinical consequences, you should monitor the patient closely for these serious arrhythmias. In the meantime, a clinical decision based on a sound evaluation of the risk-benefit ratio of the various pharmacologic agents and your patient can be made. Consultation with a cardiologist or electrophysiologist should be obtained quickly, if necessary.

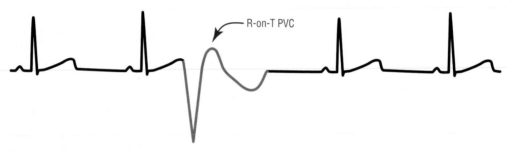

Figure 29-4: A PVC with an R-on-T phenomenon.

ADDITIONAL INFORMATION

End-diastolic PVC

Sometimes, when there is an underlying slow sinus bradycardia, a PVC can fall in such a way that it falls after the next normally occurring sinus P wave (Figure 29-5). These PVCs are known as *end-diastolic PVCs*, because they occur during the late diastolic phase of the previous complex.

End-diastolic PVCs have no additional clinical significance. They can, however, cause frequent misdiagnoses and are often mistaken for aberrantly conducted PACs and PJCs. Luckily, this type of PVC is not frequently found.

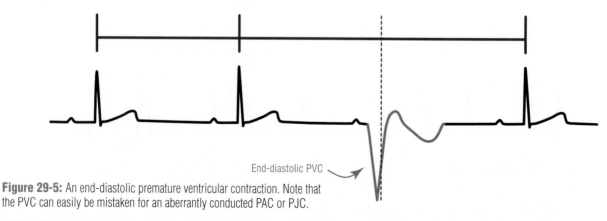

Figure 29-5: An end-diastolic premature ventricular contraction. Note that the PVC can easily be mistaken for an aberrantly conducted PAC or PJC.

Compensatory vs. Noncompensatory Pauses

PVCs can be associated with either compensatory (Figure 29-6) or noncompensatory pauses (Figure 29-7). If the ectopic ventricular depolarization wave of the PVC spreads retrogradely to the atria and resets the sinus node, the pause will be noncompensatory. If the ectopic ventricular depolarization wave is blocked from retrogradely spreading to the atria, then the pause will be fully compensatory. In general, most of the pauses associated with PVCs will be fully compensatory.

Unifocal vs. Multifocal PVCs

The morphological appearance of a PVC depends on the location of the ectopic ventricular pacer that triggered the complex and the route of depolarization. If either of those two variables is different, the appearance of the PVC will be changed.

PVCs that originate in the same ectopic pacer and depolarize via the same route through the ventricular myocardium are known as *unifocal* PVCs (Figure 29-8). These PVCs have the same coupling interval throughout the rhythm strip. They do not have to appear with a

regular timing or at a specific recurring interval during the strip, but can occur in a random pattern. Unifocal PVCs can either appear singly or in combinations.

Multifocal PVCs (Figure 29-9) originate from either different ectopic pacers or in the same ectopic pacemaker, but take different routes to depolarize the ventricles. These PVCs occur randomly throughout the rhythm strip and their coupling intervals will be completely different. Multifocal PVCs can either appear singly or in combinations.

As mentioned earlier, the number of PVCs occurring in a minute can vary in any one patient due to many reasons. The numbers of PVCs can vary because of electrolyte abnormalities, ischemia, diurnal (hormonal) changes, medications, and so on. If the number exceeds five or more per minute during an ECG strip, or 20 to 30 per hour during ambulatory or Holter monitoring, they are considered frequent.

Bigeminy, Trigeminy, and More

When a PVC occurs every second complex, it is known as ventricular *bigeminy* (Figure 29-10). When a PVC occurs every third complex, it is known as ventricular

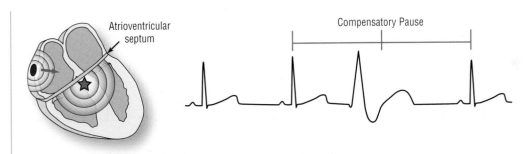

Figure 29-6: Compensatory pause. The ectopic ventricular depolarization wave does not retrogradely spread to the atria. Since the sinus node is not reset, the underlying rhythm is not disturbed.

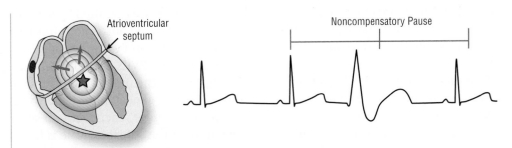

Figure 29-7: Noncompensatory pause. The ectopic ventricular depolarization wave does spread retrogradely to the atria. The sinus node is reset and the underlying rhythm or rate is changed.

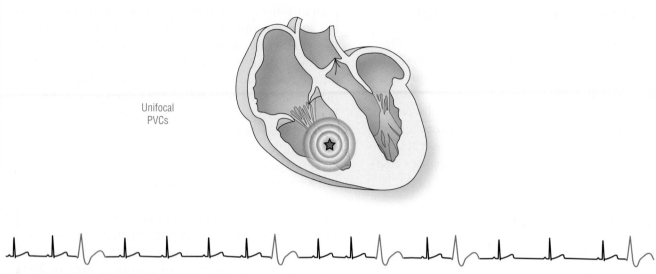

Figure 29-8: Unifocal PVCs originate in the same ectopic focus and depolarize the ventricles via the same route. The coupling interval is the same.

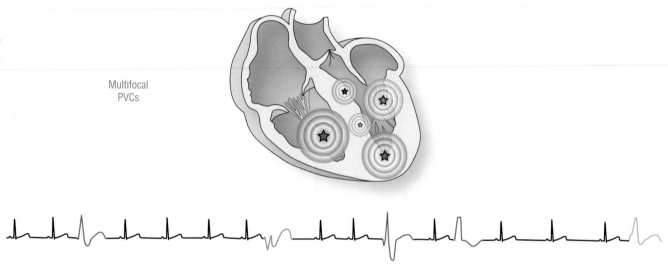

Figure 29-9: Multifocal PVCs originate in different ectopic foci or depolarize the ventricles via different routes. The coupling intervals are different.

trigeminy (Figure 29-11). Likewise, a PVC occurring every fourth complex is considered ventricular *quadrigeminy* (Figure 29-12). The word "ventricular" is present to designate the ectopic complexes as ventricular in origin (remember, you can also have supraventricular bigeminy, etc.).

Usually, the most commonly found PVCs are unifocal and have the same coupling intervals and morphological appearance. Multifocal PVCs are less commonly found, have different morphological appearances, and typically do not appear with any recurring coupling interval.

Clinically, these rhythm abnormalities are stable and are not cause for alarm. The exception to this rule, however, occurs when the PVCs do not cause an adequate mechanical contraction. In these patients, the cardiac output can be dramatically altered due to the presence of the PVCs, and clinical management and eradication of the premature complexes are indicated emergently. A good clinical habit to develop is to take the patient's pulse whenever you see a patient with bigeminy. If the palpable pulse is half of the pulse that you see on the monitor or the rhythm strip, you need to take action to eradicate the cause of the PVCs or to

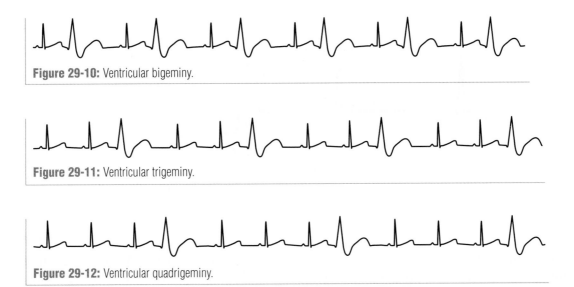

Figure 29-10: Ventricular bigeminy.

Figure 29-11: Ventricular trigeminy.

Figure 29-12: Ventricular quadrigeminy.

directly treat them. Don't forget to check the other vital signs as well!

Couplets, Triplets, and Salvos

Bigeminy, trigeminy, and the others in that group have normal complexes interspersed between single PVCs. In this section, we are going to look at what happens when PVCs occur in sequence. When two PVCs occur sequentially, they are known as a *couplet* (Figure 29-13). When three PVCs occur sequentially, they are known as a *triplet* (Figure 29-14). The term *salvo* refers to a group of three or more ectopic ventricular complexes occurring sequentially.

Fusion of the various ventricular complexes and their associated waves is a very common occurrence

> **NOTE**
>
> When there are three PVCs in a row, it starts to become difficult to tell if they are a run of PVCs or ventricular tachycardia. The term *salvo* is typically used when the clinical impression is leaning toward the presence of ventricular tachycardia. We will discuss this topic in much greater detail in Chapter 31.

when you are dealing with two or more sequential PVCs. The fusion can occur anywhere along the complexes and will affect the morphological appearance of the various complexes.

Couplets and triplets can have PVCs that are either unifocal or multifocal. The morphological appearance of

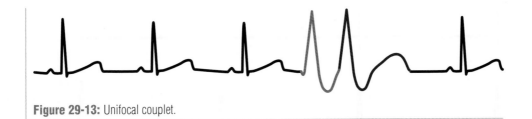

Figure 29-13: Unifocal couplet.

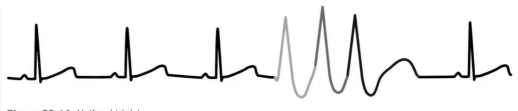

Figure 29-14: Unifocal triplet.

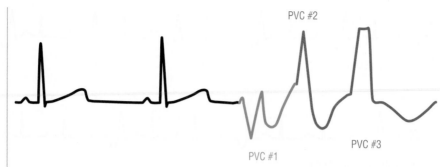

Figure 29-15: A multifocal triplet. Note the different appearance of the three ventricular beats and the varying degree of fusion between the waves.

unifocal couplets and triplets may be slightly altered because of fusion, but the general appearance of the complexes will be the same. Multifocal couplets and triplets will show a wide variation in morphological appearance and timing (Figure 29-15).

Clinically, unifocal couplets and triplets can be considered normal variants, but clinical correlation with your patient is definitely a good idea. Multifocal couplets and triplets are a bit more troubling and may be harbingers of further, more life-threatening ventricular

arrhythmias to come. Observation and treatment may be clinically indicated for these patients.

The P Wave and PVCs

Are there P waves associated with PVCs? The answer is. . .sometimes. Often, there is a retrograde P wave created as the depolarization wave travels retrogradely from the ventricle to the atria, as we saw in Chapter 28. These P waves are associated with prolonged R-P inter-

ADDITIONAL INFORMATION

Interpolated PVC

Occasionally, a PVC falls in such a time as to be completely sandwiched between two consecutive sinus complexes. As long as the PVC does not retrogradely depolarize the atria, the normal sinus rhythm and its associated ventricular

response will continue completely undisturbed. The result is a PVC placed directly between two sinus complexes. This type of PVC is known as an *interpolated* PVC (Figure 29-16). These PVCs are not associated with any additional clinical significance and are just a diagnostic oddity.

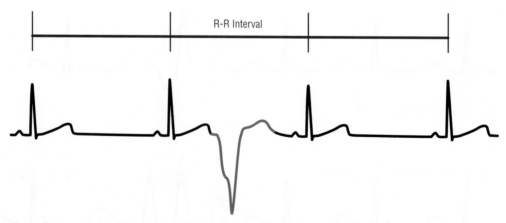

Figure 29-16: Interpolated PVC. Note that the underlying sinus rate and complexes are completely undisturbed. This can only occur if there is no ventriculo-atrial activation from the PVC.

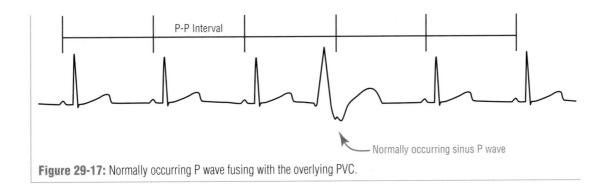

Figure 29-17: Normally occurring P wave fusing with the overlying PVC.

vals because of the long travel times needed to traverse the ventricles by direct cell-to-cell transmission. In general, the retrograde P waves associated with PVCs have an R-P interval greater than or equal to 0.20 seconds.

Can you think of a time when the P waves associated with a PVC would be upright? A P wave can only be upright if it is sinus or atrial in origin. Therefore, a retrograde P wave cannot be upright. You can, however, often see the normally occurring P wave peeking around or being fused with the PVC. This occurs when there is no ventriculo-atrial retrograde transmission of the premature depolarization wave and the underlying sinus rhythm is not interrupted (Figure 29-17). Note that these P waves, in comparison to the retrograde

ones discussed above, map out with the other ones from the underlying rhythm if you use your calipers. The pause must be fully compensatory in these cases.

Fusion Complexes

Ventricular complexes, especially when they occur in couplets, triplets, or higher, are very often morphologically altered by fusion with other waves and complexes. The fusion can occur with previous P or T waves or with other complexes of ventricular origin. The fusion of ventricular complexes is typically caused when a supraventricular complex is partially conducted at the same time that a ventricular complex is occurring. The

---

net result is that the complexes morphologically resemble the two parents (Figure 29-18) and is known as a *fusion complex*.

Fusion complexes are going to be critical to understand and diagnose in the more complex ventricular arrhythmias. They are a critical diagnostic point for accelerated idioventricular rhythms and, especially, ventricular tachycardia.

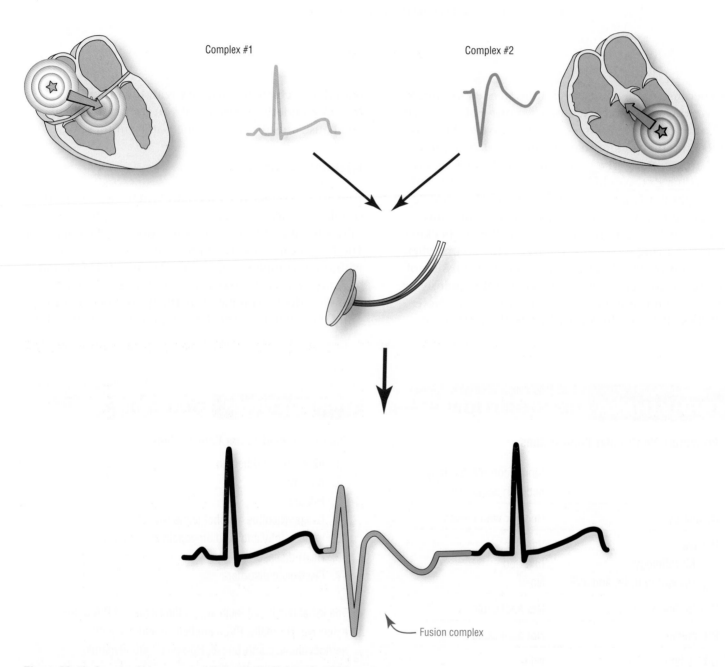

Figure 29-18: Complex #1 is a supraventricular complex being normally transmitted to the ventricles. This complex would give rise to a nice, tight QRS complex. Complex #2 originates in an ectopic ventricular focus and will give rise to an aberrant, wide QRS complex. The ECG machine translates these bits of electrical information into the fusion complex below. Note that the resulting complex resembles each parent complex slightly.

ECG Strips

ECG 29-1

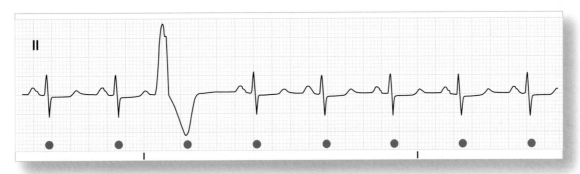

Rate:	About 78 BPM		PR intervals:	Normal, except in event
Regularity:	Regular with an event		QRS width:	Event is wide
P waves:	Present, except in event		Grouping:	None
Morphology: Axis:	Normal, except in event Normal, except in event		Dropped beats:	Present
P:QRS ratio:	1:1, except in event		Rhythm:	**Sinus rhythm with a PVC**

Discussion:

The strip above shows a sinus rhythm with a single PVC (third complex). Note that the PVC is wider than 0.12 seconds and is associated with ST and T wave abnormalities. The pause associated with the PVC is fully compensatory. Notice that the underlying cadence of the sinus rhythm is undisturbed by the PVC. The underlying sinus P wave is not visible because it is completely fused with the PVC.

ECG 29-2

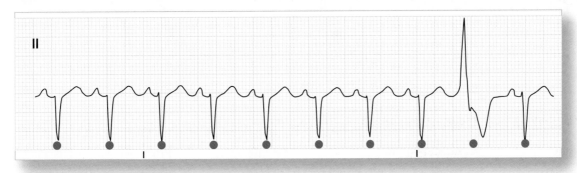

Rate:	About 104 BPM		PR intervals:	Normal, except in event
Regularity:	Regular		QRS width:	Event is wide
P waves:	Present, except in event		Grouping:	None
Morphology: Axis:	Normal, except in event Normal, except in event		Dropped beats:	Present
P:QRS ratio:	1:1, except in event		Rhythm:	**Sinus tachycardia with a PVC**

Discussion:

This strip shows your typical PVC with a wide, bizarre complex with ST and T wave abnormalities. The pause is fully compensatory. The underlying rhythm, in this case, is sinus tachycardia.

ECG 29-3

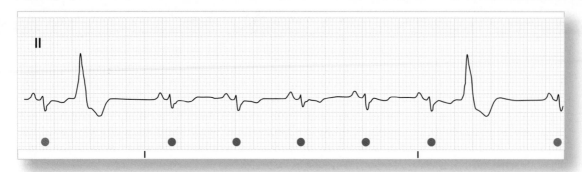

Rate:	About 82 BPM	PR intervals:	Normal, except in event
Regularity:	Regular with multiple events	QRS width:	Event is wide
P waves:	Present, except in event	Grouping:	None
Morphology:	Normal, except in event		
Axis:	Normal, except in event	Dropped beats:	Present
P:QRS ratio:	1:1, except in event	Rhythm:	**Sinus rhythm with a PVC**

Discussion:

The strip above shows a sinus rhythm at about 82 to 84 BPM. The wide complexes (complexes #2 and #8) are PVCs. Note that the pauses associated with these PVCs are noncompensatory pauses. The retrograde V-A conduction of the ectopic depolarization wave causes a resetting of the sinus node. The reset node shows varying rates after each PVC. On a longer rhythm strip, the rate was constantly being reset throughout the strip.

ECG 29-4

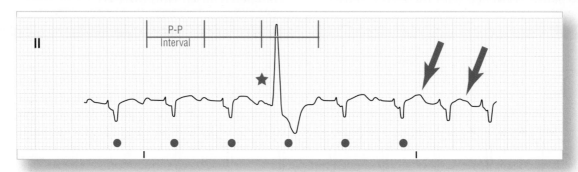

Rate:	About 94 BPM	PR intervals:	Prolonged, see discussion below
Regularity:	Regular	QRS width:	Wide
P waves:	See discussion below	Grouping:	None
Morphology:	See discussion below		
Axis:	See discussion below	Dropped beats:	Present
P:QRS ratio:	See discussion below	Rhythm:	**Sinus rhythm with a PVC**

Discussion:

This strip is much more complex than you would think at first. The underlying rhythm is sinus, but the last two complexes are premature. Note that the T waves of the complexes (labeled with the blue arrows) have a different morphology from the others. These are PACs with buried P waves. The PVC has a P wave in front of it (see blue star), but the PR interval is different. Could this be an aberrantly conducted PAC? No, it is not premature (see P-P interval brackets) and the underlying cadence is not interrupted. Finally, the pause is fully compensatory (see blue dots). This is an end-diastolic PVC.

ECG 29-5

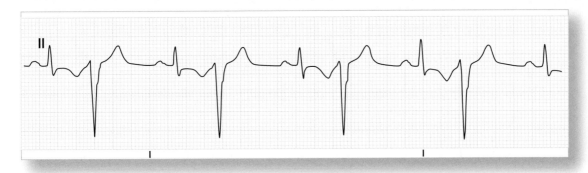

Rate:	See discussion below	PR intervals:	Normal, except in events
Regularity:	Regularly irregular	QRS width:	Events are wide

P waves:
    Morphology:
    Axis:
	Present, except in events
	Normal, except in events
	Normal, except in events
		Grouping:	Yes

		Dropped beats:	Present
P:QRS ratio:	1:1, except in event	Rhythm:	**Sinus rhythm with ventricular bigeminy**

Discussion:

The rate on the strip above is hard to state electrocardiographically. The reason is that every other beat is a PVC, making this a sinus rhythm with ventricular bigeminy. The best guess is that it is 90 BPM (9 complexes in a 6-second strip). The best thing to do is to go to the patient and actually take a manual pulse for accuracy. It is impossible in bigeminy to state if the pauses are compensatory or noncompensatory pauses because there is no clear underlying P-P interval.

ECG 29-6

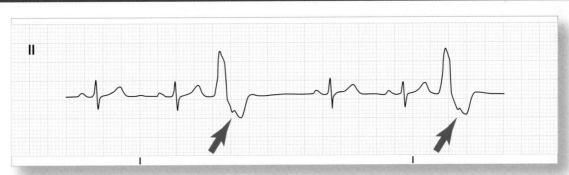

Rate:	About 70 BPM	PR intervals:	Normal, except in events
Regularity:	Regular with frequent events	QRS width:	Events are wide

P waves:
    Morphology:
    Axis:
	Present, except in events
	Normal, except in events
	Normal, except in events
		Grouping:	Yes

		Dropped beats:	Present
P:QRS ratio:	1:1, except in events	Rhythm:	**Sinus rhythm with ventricular trigeminy**

Discussion:

The rhythm strip above has a PVC for every third complex. This is an example of ventricular trigeminy. In this strip, the rate is a little over 70 BPM and slightly irregular. It would be a good idea to go and manually check the pulse on the patient to evaluate for effective mechanical contractions by the PVCs. The blue arrows are there to show the underlying P waves fusing with the PVCs.

ECG 29-7

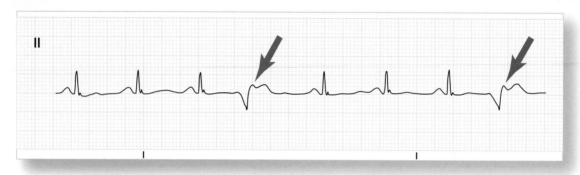

Rate:	About 88 BPM	PR intervals:	Normal, except in events
Regularity:	Regular with frequent events	QRS width:	Events are wide
P waves:	Present, except in events	Grouping:	None
Morphology:	Normal, except in events		
Axis:	Normal, except in events	Dropped beats:	Present
P:QRS ratio:	1:1, except in events	Rhythm:	**Sinus rhythm with ventricular quadrigeminy**

Discussion:

The rhythm strip above shows an underlying sinus rhythm with a PVC occurring every fourth complex. This pattern for PVCs is known as ventricular quadrigeminy. The PVCs are unifocal and the coupling intervals are identical. The pauses are fully compensatory. It is interesting to note that the hump at the end of the QRS complex of the PVCs is actually the fusion of the P wave of the underlying rhythm with the PVCs.

ECG 29-8

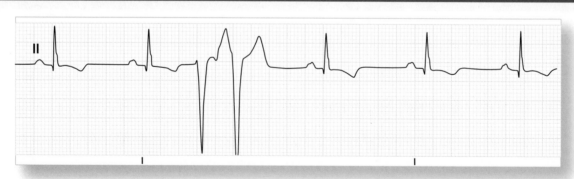

Rate:	About 57 BPM	PR intervals:	Normal, except in event
Regularity:	Regular with an event	QRS width:	Events are wide
P waves:	Present, except in event	Grouping:	None
Morphology:	Normal, except in event		
Axis:	Normal, except in event	Dropped beats:	Present
P:QRS ratio:	1:1, except in event	Rhythm:	**Sinus bradycardia with a unifocal couplet**

Discussion:

The strip above shows a sinus bradycardia with a unifocal couplet. Note the slight morphological differences between the two ventricular complexes. This morphological difference is due to fusion of the two complexes with each other or by a slight alteration in a reentry circuit.

ECG 29-9

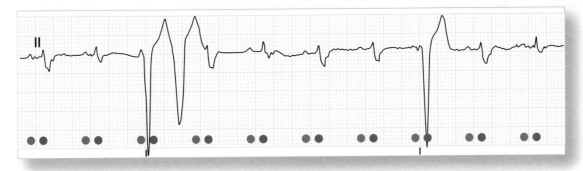

Rate:	About 98 BPM	PR intervals:	Normal, except in events
Regularity:	Regular with events	QRS width:	Wide
P waves:	Present, except in event	Grouping:	None
Morphology:	Normal, except in events		
Axis:	Normal, except in events	Dropped beats:	Present
P:QRS ratio:	1:1, except in events	Rhythm:	**Sinus rhythm with a unifocal couplet and a PVC**

Discussion:

The rhythm strip above shows an underlying sinus rhythm that is undisturbed by the extra events occurring in the ventricles (P waves timing is represented by the pink dots, QRS timing by the blue dots). Notice that the pauses are fully compensatory. The P waves show through and fuse with the morphology of the PVCs at the start of the complexes. The underlying ventricular depolarizations during the sinus complexes demonstrate a varying degree of aberrancy in ventricular conduction.

ECG 29-10

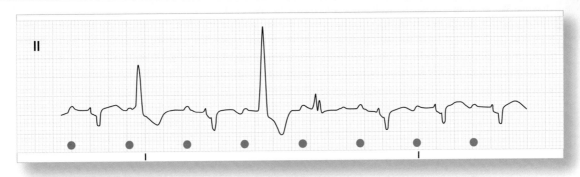

Rate:	About 94 BPM	PR intervals:	Prolonged, except in events
Regularity:	Regular with events	QRS width:	Wide in events
P waves:	Present, except in event	Grouping:	None
Morphology:	Normal, except in events		
Axis:	Normal, except in events	Dropped beats:	Present
P:QRS ratio:	1:1, except in events	Rhythm:	**Sinus rhythm with frequent multifocal PVCs**

Discussion:

This strip shows an underlying sinus rhythm with a very prolonged PR interval. There are at least 2 different morphologies to the ventricular complexes (complexes #2, #4, and #5), making them multifocal PVCs. (To be completely correct, complexes #4 and #5 should be considered a multifocal couplet.) The PVCs are also end-diastolic PVCs with the normal P waves occurring right before them. The pauses are fully compensatory.

CHAPTER REVIEW

1. Other names used for premature ventricular contractions (PVC) are:
   A. Ventricular premature contractions (VPC)
   B. Ventricular premature depolarizations (VPD)
   C. Ventricular extrasystoles
   D. All of the above

2. The general characteristics of PVCs include:
   A. Wider than 0.12 seconds
   B. Bizarre appearance
   C. ST segment and T wave abnormalities
   D. Premature arrival of the complex
   E. All of the above

3. PVCs are only found in patients with structural heart disease. True or False.

4. The R-on-T phenomenon refers to a PVC that falls within the relative refractory period of the previous complex. True or False.

5. An end-diastolic PVC is one that falls immediately after the normally occurring ___ wave.

6. PVCs are typically associated with _____ pauses, but either one can occur.

7. Multifocal PVCs commonly have identical coupling intervals because they originate in the same site. True or False.

8. When a PVC occurs every other beat, it is called a ventricular _____.

9. When two PVCs occur one after the other, it is called a _____.

10. Salvos can be:
    A. Unifocal
    B. A PVC that occurs every third beat
    C. Multifocal
    D. Trigeminal
    E. Both A and C
    F. Both B and D

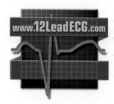

To enhance the knowledge you gain in this book, access this text's website at www.12leadECG.com! This valuable resource provides flashcards, an online glossary, web links, and more. Simply click on the Arrhythmias book cover once at the site.

CHAPTER 30

Ventricular Escape and Idioventricular Rhythms

General Overview

In this chapter we are going to cover the ventricular escape rhythms and the idioventricular rhythms. We will begin by looking at individual ventricular escape complexes. Then, we will move on to the more complicated ventricular escape rhythms. When there are three or more ventricular escape complexes in a row, we call this an *idioventricular* rhythm.

Idioventricular rhythms, however, are a bit more complicated. They can occur as an escape rhythm, or they can occur due to the increased automaticity of a single ventricular ectopic pacemaker. This increased automaticity may lead to rates that are faster than the intrinsic rate of the upper pacemakers.

When the rate is faster than the intrinsic pacemakers, the ectopic pacemaker actually takes over the pacing function of the heart, and so they are not escape rhythms in these cases. These fast ventricular rhythms are known as the *accelerated idioventricular* rhythms. At this point, the line frequently gets blurred with another lethal arrhythmia, which we will cover in the next chapter, ventricular tachycardia.

A word of caution about treatment before we begin. The ventricular escape pacemakers are the last line of defense for the heart when it comes to maintaining function and a cardiac output. *You need to be extremely careful in treating any ventricular escape or idioventricular rhythm. If you succeed in eradicating the ventricular response, you may be left without any electrical activity whatsoever.* This is not a good thing!

Ventricular Escape Complexes

When the primary supraventricular pacemakers fail for a short time, the ventricles will quickly take over and fire a ventricular escape complex. This is to make sure that a ventricular mechanical contraction occurs. As we mentioned before, it is the ventricular rate that maintains control over the cardiac output in the vast major-

NOTE

It is our opinion that when you are faced with a slow ventricular escape rhythm, you should try to speed it up by using either a transvenous or transthoracic electric pacemaker, *as long as you can place one quickly*. We make this suggestion because an external temporary cardiac pacer will let you achieve a *controlled* rate of increase, one that you can manually adjust to maximum benefit.

Pharmaceutical agents can also be used to speed up the heart and are usually faster to deliver. But, be aware that you cannot control the patient's physiologic response to them as well as you can control an external cardiac pacer. Giving a drug like atropine will typically speed up the heart, but how fast it will go is anyone's guess. In some cases, too fast a rate can be just as dangerous as too slow a rate. Pharmaceutical agents can be a great asset if you cannot get external pacemaker control quickly or if your pacer fails to capture. Please be aware that this reflects our own individual clinical practice, and there is a lot of controversy as to the best approach. For a more thorough and complete discussion, a review of the current literature is suggested.

ity of cases. In other words, the loss of the atrial kick does not compare with the loss of the ventricular "kick." The bottom line is that we need our ventricles to work if we want to stay alive.

The ventricular escape complexes have all of the characteristics of ventricular complexes, as we have seen and covered in Chapter 28. They arrive late during the cadence of the rhythm, after a supraventricular pacer fails to fire. The R-R interval, therefore, is longer than expected (Figure 30-1).

Ventricular escape complexes can occur singly or they can appear in pairs (Figure 30-2). If there are more than three sequential ventricular escape complexes, it then becomes known as an idioventricular escape rhythm.

If a P wave is present in a ventricular escape complex, it is because the supraventricular P wave failed to conduct to the ventricles or it is retrograde from the ventricular escape complex itself. Multiple ventricular escape complexes are usually associated with AV dissociation (Figure 30-3).

Idioventricular Rhythm

Idioventricular rhythm refers to an intrinsic rhythm that starts in the ventricles (Figure 30-4). It originates in the ventricular area and the depolarization wave spreads either partially through the electrical conduction system or completely via direct cell-to-cell transmission. The intrinsic rate in idioventricular rhythm is most commonly between 30 and 50 BPM, but the rhythm can be anywhere from 20 to 50 BPM. The idioventricular complexes will have the morphological characteristics of the

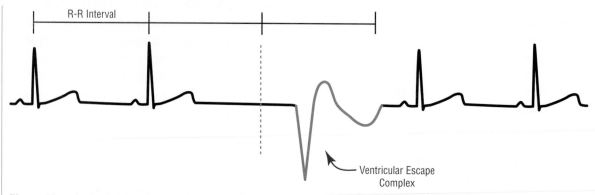

Figure 30-1: A ventricular escape complex.

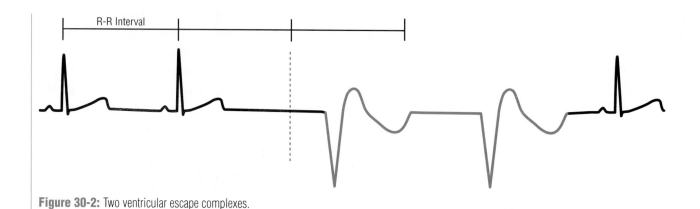

Figure 30-2: Two ventricular escape complexes.

Figure 30-3: Two ventricular escape complexes with associated AV dissociation.

ectopic ventricular complexes (wider than 0.12 seconds, bizarre appearance, ST and T wave abnormalities).

An idioventricular rhythm may develop because of increased automaticity of a ventricular escape focus. An idioventricular rhythm may also develop as an escape mechanism if the supraventricular pacemakers fail, in order to overcome a very slow supraventricular bradycardia, or if there is a block of AV conduction (Figure 30-5).

Accelerated Idioventricular Rhythm

An *accelerated idioventricular rhythm* is basically a rapid idioventricular rhythm (Figure 30-6). The rates for accelerated idioventricular rhythm are above the rates typically expected for the ventricular pacemakers and are typically between 50 and 100 BPM. The rhythm is due to increased automaticity of an ectopic ventricular

pacer. The ventricular complexes have the morphological characteristics of the intrinsic ventricular rhythms (wider than 0.12 seconds, bizarre appearance, ST and T wave abnormalities).

Accelerated idioventricular rhythm is typically very regular, but there may be some slight irregularity at the onset of the rhythm. The rhythm can usually be overcome by overdrive pacing from an external pacer or by using pharmaceutical agents that speed up the heart or suppress ventricular activity. *Once again, be careful of pharmaceutical intervention because the ventricular pacemakers are the last defense against asystole or absence of rhythm.* Overdrive pacing can be attempted as long as the patient is hemodynamically stable. But, as usual, in the case of any hemodynamic compromise, electrical cardioversion is still the treatment of choice.

Accelerated idioventricular rhythm may occur in the absence of any supraventricular rhythm, or it can occur

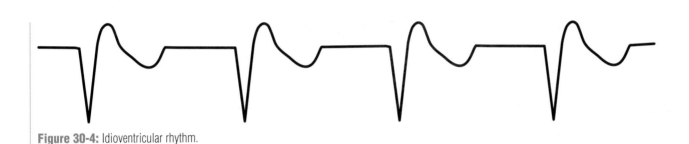

Figure 30-4: Idioventricular rhythm.

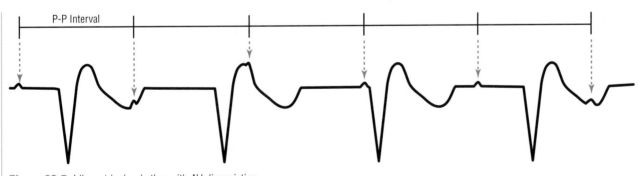

Figure 30-5: Idioventricular rhythm with AV dissociation.

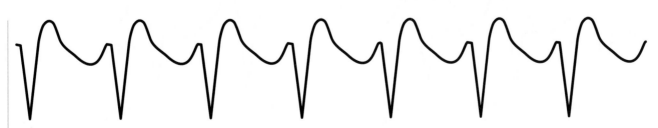

Figure 30-6: Accelerated idioventricular rhythm.

as a ventricular response to an AV dissociation or block (Figure 30-7). As you can imagine, the faster ventricular rates in accelerated idioventricular rhythms can lead to more variability in fusion complexes with the dissociated P waves and, as we shall see in the next section, with partially conducted supraventricular complexes.

Accelerated idioventricular rhythms are commonly found in patients having acute myocardial infarctions. They are also part of a set of rhythm disturbances seen commonly after reperfusion has begun during the administration of thrombolytics for an AMI. In this clinical setting, this set of arrhythmias is known as the *reperfusion arrhythmias*. The reperfusion arrhythmias are typically stable and transient in nature, although they are scary to observe on a monitor. When idioventricular or accelerated idioventricular rhythms appear as reperfusion arrhythmias, they do not require treatment unless they are causing significant hemodynamic compromise.

Capture Beats

When we use the term AV dissociation, remember that we are talking about a situation in which the atria and the ventricles are each beating to their own drummer, but there is still some occasional or limited communication between them. In other words, it is not a *complete block* of all of the transmission of information. We will be covering complete block in Chapter 35.

Since there is some limited communication between the atria and the ventricles, occasionally, the timing of a supraventricular impulse will fall in such a way as to trigger conduction through the normal conduction system in the ventricles. The normal P wave in these cases will stimulate the ventricles in such a way as to cause a QRS complex that appears normal on the strip or ECG. This normal-looking complex is known as a *capture beat* (Figure 30-8). They are called capture beats because the normal supraventricular impulse "captures" the ventricles and forces them to behave normally.

Capture beats, along with fusion complexes, are the keystone features in the diagnosis of accelerated idioventricular rhythms and ventricular tachycardia. *If you ever see a wide complex rhythm with a normal-appearing QRS complex smack in the middle of it, it is either accelerated idioventricular or ventricular tachycardia, depending on the underlying ventricular rate.*

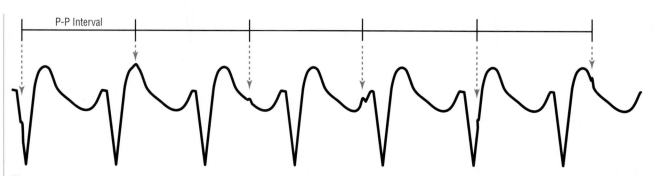

Figure 30-7: Accelerated idioventricular rhythm with AV dissociation.

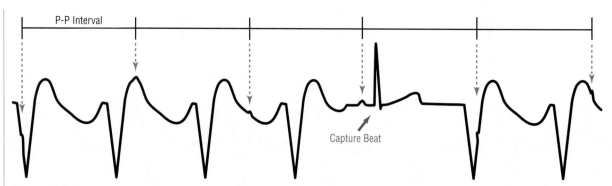

Figure 30-8: Accelerated idioventricular rhythm with AV dissociation. Note that the fourth P wave in the strip falls in such a way as to "capture" the ventricles normally. This capture gives rise to a normal, narrow QRS complex.

So, let's recap. Accelerated idioventricular rhythm is a wide complex rhythm that has complexes of ventricular morphology, is very regular, and may or may not be associated with AV dissociation, fusion complexes, and capture beats.

Here are some helpful diagnostic hints for spotting this rhythm (Figure 30-9). Use your calipers to map out any inconsistencies or "bumps" in the morphology of the complexes. Many times, these bumps turn out to be P waves and mapping them brings out the presence of AV dissociation. Look for morphological changes in the QRS complexes, and try to see if they are due to different pacemakers or to fusion. Regularity, similar cou-

pling intervals, and similarities to both parents will point in the direction of fusion. The presence of capture beats is classic for AV dissociation, which is a major determinant of accelerated idioventricular and ventricular tachycardia. As a side point, if the sinus rate and the ventricular rates are close to each other, the complexes immediately surrounding the capture beats will be fusion complexes, and you will see this pattern repeating itself on a long strip.

Now that we have given you some pointers, go ahead and analyze the complicated strip in Figure 30-9. The answer is in the Additional Information box if you would like to review it.

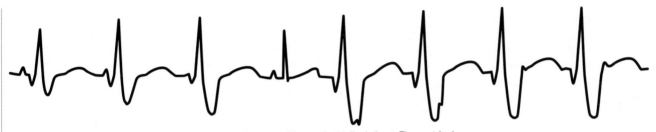

Figure 30-9: Go ahead and analyze this strip. Hint: it has everything we just talked about. The ventricular rate is 90 BPM. Don't forget to use your calipers!

ARRHYTHMIA RECOGNITION

Idioventricular Rhythm

Rate:	20 to 50 BPM
Regularity:	Regular (ventricular)
P wave:	Retrograde or AV dissociation
Morphology:	Variable
Upright in II, III, and aVF:	Sometimes
P:QRS ratio:	None or retrograde
PR interval:	None
QRS width:	Wide
Grouping:	None
Dropped beats:	None

DIFFERENTIAL DIAGNOSIS

Idioventricular Rhythm

1. Acute myocardial infarction
2. Myocardial ischemia and injury
3. Reperfusion arrhythmia
4. Cardiomyopathy
5. Drugs: Digoxin
6. Idiopathic

Idioventricular rhythm may be due to increased automaticity or it may be due to an escape mechanism, reflecting the failure of the supraventricular pacemakers. The list above is not inclusive but reflects the most common causes of the rhythm disturbance.

ADDITIONAL **INFORMATION**

Accelerated Idioventricular Rhythm

The first thing you should have done is gotten an overall feel for the rhythm. It is a wide-complex rhythm with one single event in the middle. The event is not a wide beat among narrow ones, but it is a narrow one among a bunch of wide ones. That should immediately make you think of a capture beat. The next thing is to use your calipers and map out the tips of the QRS complexes. The two areas on either side of the capture beat are perfectly regular and are composed of wide complexes. This is consistent with an idioventricular rhythm or an accelerated idioventricular. The ventricular rate is 90 BPM, so it is accelerated idioventricular.

Whenever you see a capture beat, you have AV dissociation. So, let's find the P waves. Take an overall look at the strip, starting with the P wave on the capture beat. Are there any "bumps" that are on some complexes but not others? Yes, on complex V1 there is a bump at the bottom of the S wave (see P5 on Figure 30-10). Take your calipers and put one pin on the P wave on the capture beat and the other on the bump at the bottom of V1. Now, march the calipers in both directions, placing a little mark where the pin falls. Are there other "bumps" where the pins fall? Yes! Those are your P waves marching through the strip (look at the P1–P8 markers below the strip on Figure 30-10).

Now, since we know we have a capture beat and AV dissociation, let's see if we have any fusion complexes. Do any of the ventricular complexes look different from the others? Yes, the complexes labeled F1 through F3 are definitely different from the ones on the other end of the capture beat. These complexes are a little smaller and a little narrower than the ones at the end. Notice that these complexes have P waves in front of them to varying degrees, while the ones at the end have the P waves after the QRS complexes. They have a little of the appearance of the capture beat and a little of the appearance of the full ventricular beats. F1–3 are, therefore, fusion complexes due to a *partial* capture of the supraventricular impulse from the P waves. F1 has the P wave the furthest from the QRS and is the shortest and narrowest of the three.

Let's recap. We have a wide-complex rhythm that is regular, has a ventricular rate of 90 BPM, AV dissociation, a capture beat, and some fusion beats. There is only one possibility for this combination: accelerated idioventricular!

This strip is not an easy one. It is, however, typical of what you will see in clinical practice. When you approach a strip, take a few seconds to look at it before you panic. You will see that there is a pattern that you can tease out, if you have the knowledge and the patience to see it. We hope that this analysis has helped you and that you will be able to carry away some valuable learning points as we progress through the rest of this chapter and the next. As you will see, many lessons from this chapter will carry over to your analysis of ventricular tachycardias.

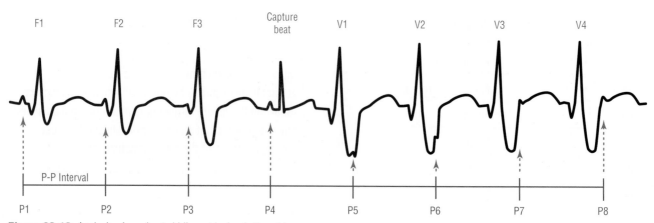

Figure 30-10: Analysis of accelerated idioventricular rhythm strip.

ARRHYTHMIA RECOGNITION

Accelerated Idioventricular Rhythm

Rate:	50 to 100 BPM
Regularity:	Regular (ventricular)
P wave:	Retrograde or AV dissociation
Morphology:	Variable
Upright in II, III, and aVF:	Sometimes
P:QRS ratio:	None or retrograde
PR interval:	None
QRS width:	Wide
Grouping:	None
Dropped beats:	None

DIFFERENTIAL DIAGNOSIS

Accelerated Idioventricular Rhythm

1. Acute myocardial infarction
2. Myocardial ischemia and injury
3. Reperfusion arrhythmia
4. Cardiomyopathy
5. Drugs: Digoxin
6. Idiopathic

The list above is not inclusive but reflects the most common causes of the rhythm disturbance.

ECG Strips

ECG 30-1

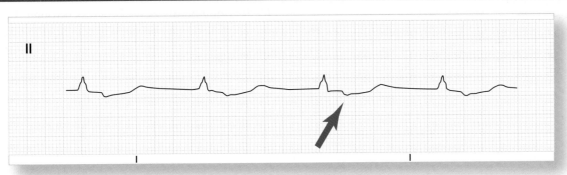

Rate:	About 45 BPM	PR intervals:	None	
Regularity:	Regular	QRS width:	Wide	
P waves:	Present	Grouping:	None	
Morphology:	Inverted and retrograde	Dropped beats:	Absent	
Axis:	Abnormal			
P:QRS ratio:	1:1	Rhythm:	**Idioventricular**	

Discussion:

This patient has an idioventricular rate at about 45 BPM. The complexes are definitely wide with very prolonged QT intervals. QT prolongation is common for ventricular rhythms because repolarization occurs on a cell-by-cell basis, which is very time consuming. However, this interval is prolonged, even for an idioventricular rhythm. CNS events, electrolyte abnormalities, and ischemia need to be ruled out. The blue arrow marks the position of the retrograde P waves. Note the long R-P interval in these complexes.

ECG 30-2

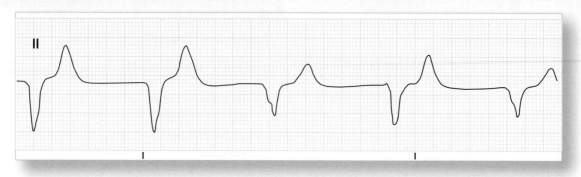

Rate:	About 45 BPM	PR intervals:	None
Regularity:	Regular	QRS width:	Wide
P waves:	None	Grouping:	None
Morphology:	None		
Axis:	None	Dropped beats:	Absent
P:QRS ratio:	None	Rhythm:	**Idioventricular**

Discussion:

The strip above shows a wide-complex, slow rhythm consistent with an idioventricular rhythm. The variation in the morphology of the complexes may be due to fusion. However, P waves are not visible on this lead. A 12-lead ECG would be very helpful in trying to spot a potential AV dissociation.

ECG 30-3

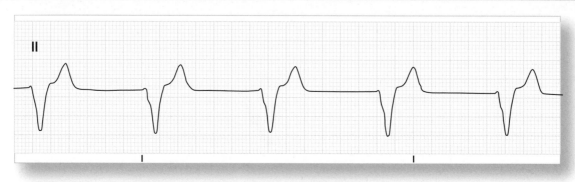

Rate:	About 47 BPM	PR intervals:	None
Regularity:	Regular	QRS width:	Wide
P waves:	None	Grouping:	None
Morphology:	None		
Axis:	None	Dropped beats:	Absent
P:QRS ratio:	None	Rhythm:	**Idioventricular**

Discussion:

This strip shows an idioventricular rhythm with a rate of about 47 BPM. The rhythm is very regular as expected in an idioventricular rhythm. The complexes are wide and bizarre in appearance with obvious ST-T wave abnormalities. Note the presence of Josephson's sign with a notching on the downstroke of the S wave. Brugada's sign is also present, with an interval of 0.10 seconds between the onset of the QRS complex and the bottom of the S wave.

ECG 30-4

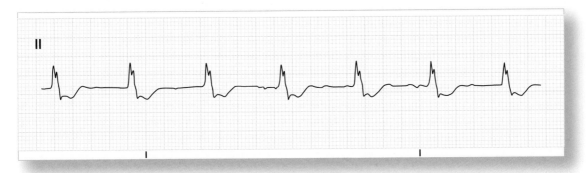

Rate:	About 72 BPM	PR intervals:	None
Regularity:	Regular	QRS width:	Wide
P waves:	None	Grouping:	None
Morphology:	None		
Axis:	None	Dropped beats:	Absent
P:QRS ratio:	None	Rhythm:	**Accelerated idioventricular**

Discussion:

This rhythm strip shows wide complex ventricular complexes with marked ST-T wave abnormalities. The ST segment depression is flat and a bit troubling because it could be evidence of ischemia. They could also be an abnormal morphology simply due to their ventricular origins. Clinical correlation and a full 12-lead ECG would be helpful.

ECG 30-5

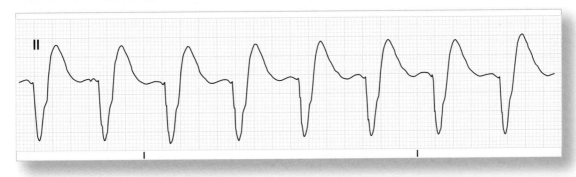

Rate:	About 82 BPM	PR intervals:	None
Regularity:	Regular	QRS width:	Wide
P waves:	None	Grouping:	None
Morphology:	None		
Axis:	None	Dropped beats:	Absent
P:QRS ratio:	None	Rhythm:	**Accelerated idioventricular**

Discussion:

This strip shows a wide-complex rhythm with an intrinsic rate of 82 BPM. There are no obvious P waves present on the ECG and there are definitely none before the QRS complexes. This is an excellent example of an accelerated idioventricular rhythm. Note the regularity of the rhythm. Also note the ST-T wave abnormalities.

The ST elevation is more obvious and taller than you would expect for ventricular complexes. The most common cause of accelerated idioventricular rhythm is AMI. This patient needs clinical correlation and a full 12-lead ECG to further evaluate this potentially life-threatening problem.

ECG 30-6

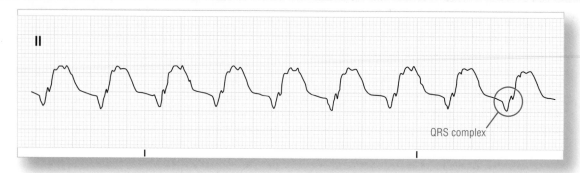

Rate:	About 82 BPM	PR intervals:	None
Regularity:	Regular	QRS width:	Wide

P waves:
    Morphology:
    Axis:
	Possibly retrograde
	Possibly inverted
	Abnormal
		Grouping:	None

		Dropped beats:	Absent
P:QRS ratio:	See discussion below	Rhythm:	**Accelerated idioventricular**

Discussion:

This strip also shows a wide-complex accelerated id- ioventricular rhythm at 82 BPM with very marked ST tombstone shape, due to an acute AMI. We have circled one of the QRS complexes for you to help you identify them, due to their small voltage. There are no obvious P waves noted, although the irregularities at the top of the ST segments could easily be a retrograde P wave.

ECG 30-7

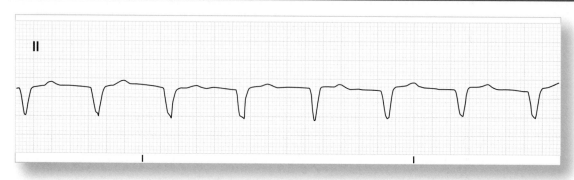

Rate:	About 75 BPM	PR intervals:	None
Regularity:	Regular	QRS width:	Wide

P waves:
    Morphology:
    Axis:
	None
	None
	None
		Grouping:	None

		Dropped beats:	Absent
P:QRS ratio:	None	Rhythm:	**Accelerated idioventricular**

Discussion:

The strip above shows a wide-complex ventricular rhythm at about a rate of 75 BPM. This is faster than the normally seen intrinsic ventricular rates of 30 to 50 BPM, making this an accelerated idioventricular rhythm. The rhythm is very regular with no obvious P waves. There could, however, be an underlying AV dissociation to explain the slight morphological differ- ence in the QRS complexes. A full 12-lead ECG would be helpful in evaluating this possibility.

ECG 30-8

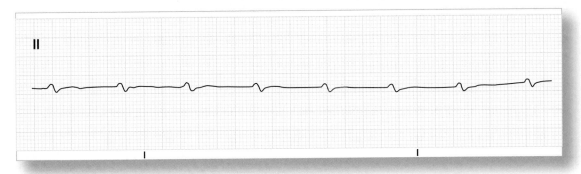

Rate:	About 80 BPM	PR intervals:	None
Regularity:	Regular	QRS width:	Wide
P waves:	None	Grouping:	None
Morphology:	None		
Axis:	None	Dropped beats:	Absent
P:QRS ratio:	None	Rhythm:	**Accelerated idioventricular**

Discussion:

No, those are not P waves. They are ventricular complexes that have a very, very small amplitude. The cause of the low amplitude is beyond the scope of this book. A full 12-lead ECG did, however, verify the ventricular origin of these complexes. The rate of 80 BPM, the wide QRS complexes, and the regularity of the rhythm make this a clear example of an accelerated idioventricular rhythm.

ECG 30-9

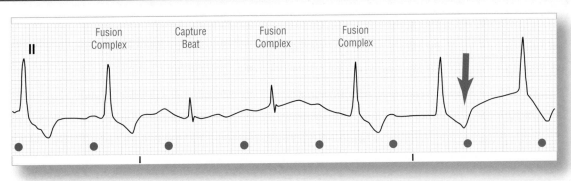

Rate:	About 66 BPM	PR intervals:	None
Regularity:	Regular	QRS width:	Wide
P waves:	Present	Grouping:	None
Morphology:	Normal		
Axis:	Upright	Dropped beats:	Absent
P:QRS ratio:	One capture beat	Rhythm:	**Accelerated idioventricular**

Discussion:

This strip shows a wide-complex rhythm quickly narrowing down to a normal-appearing complex, which is a capture beat, and then beginning to widen back out again. This is typical of an accelerated idioventricular rhythm with AV dissociation. Notice that the first and the last two complexes are the true ventricular complexes. All the rest in the middle are either fusion or the capture beat. The blue arrow points out a small deflection in the T wave, which is caused by the underlying P wave. Speaking of P waves, the P waves are upright because they are from the sinus node and are dissociated.

ECG 30-10

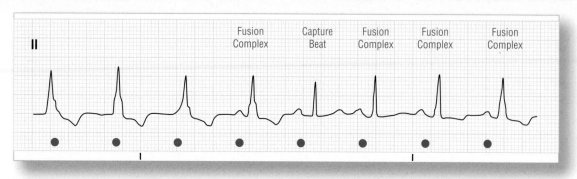

Rate:	About 80 BPM	PR intervals:	None
Regularity:	Regular	QRS width:	Wide

P waves:
  Morphology:
  Axis:
	Present
	Normal
	Upright
		Grouping:	None

		Dropped beats:	Absent
P:QRS ratio:	One capture beat	Rhythm:	**Accelerated idioventricular**

Discussion:

This strip shows very obvious AV dissociation in a patient with an accelerated idioventricular rhythm. Notice that the morphology of the first three beats changes slightly due to the fusion with the P waves. The third complex shows a slurring upward on the R wave due to the fusion. The other complexes in the strip are due to true fusion of the ventricular with a supraventricular complex. There is one capture beat with a prolonged PR interval. The true PR interval is unclear from this strip.

CHAPTER **REVIEW**

1. When there are at least _____ ventricular escape complexes in a row, we call that an idioventricular rhythm.

2. You should always give pharmaceutical agents to eradicate a ventricular escape rhythm. True or False.

3. The _____ are the last failsafe pacemaker for the heart.

4. The rates for an idioventricular rhythm are between:
   A. 10–35 BPM
   B. 20–30 BPM
   C. 20–50 BPM
   D. 30–60 BPM
   E. 50–100 BPM

5. The rates for an accelerated idioventricular rhythm are between:
   A. 10–35 BPM
   B. 20–30 BPM
   C. 20–50 BPM
   D. 30–60 BPM
   E. 50–100 BPM

6. Accelerated idioventricular rhythm is associated with:
   A. Wide, bizarre ventricular complexes
   B. Capture beats
   C. Fusion beats
   D. All of the above

7. One of the most common causes of accelerated idioventricular rhythm is _____.

8. Reperfusion arrhythmias refer to arrhythmia disturbances that occur during the reperfusion phase of thrombolytic therapy for an acute MI. Accelerated idioventricular rhythm is one such arrhythmia. True or False.

9. Reperfusion arrhythmias require immediate intervention, even if the patient is hemodynamically stable. True or False.

10. If you ever see a wide complex rhythm with a normal-looking QRS complex smack in the middle of it, it is either (name the possible rhythms) _____ _____ or _____ _____ depending on the underlying ventricular rate.

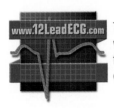

To enhance the knowledge you gain in this book, access this text's website at www.12leadECG.com! This valuable resource provides flashcards, an online glossary, web links, and more. Simply click on the Arrhythmias book cover once at the site.

Ventricular Tachycardia

General Overview

In this chapter, we are going to be reviewing one of the most deadly arrhythmias in this book: ventricular tachycardia (VTach). In reality, VTach can produce a spectrum of disease, ranging from a completely asymptomatic presentation to sudden cardiac death. It is the latter part of this spectrum that gives VTach its reputation. It is sudden and deadly. Together, VTach and ventricular fibrillation account for over 300,000 sudden cardiac deaths in the United States each year. The numbers of hemodynamically stable or mildly unstable VTach are not known but have to be much, much greater. Because of these numbers and the life-ending potential of this arrhythmia, ventricular tachycardia deserves our full attention and clinical respect.

The definition of ventricular tachycardia is simply the presence of three or more ectopic ventricular complexes in a row with a rate above 100 BPM. The rates for VTach fall between 100 and 200 BPM, but it is most commonly found running between 140 and 200 BPM. Rates above 200 BPM can occur, and when they do, the morphology of the complexes slowly begins to blur with no discernible QRS, ST, or T waves. In fact, the complexes actually become sinusoidal in morphology. When this sinusoidal pattern occurs and the rate is above 200 BPM, we call it ventricular flutter.

Morphologically, we can break down the definition of VTach a bit further. If all of the complexes have identical and uniform morphologies, the rhythm is called a *monomorphic ventricular tachycardia* (Figure 31-1). If the morphologies of the complexes change from beat-to-beat, the rhythm is called a *polymorphic VTach*. Monomorphic ventricular tachycardias are more common in clinical practice than the polymorphic variants. We will be looking at monomorphic VTach closely in this chapter and polymorphic VTach in the next chapter.

The terminology gets even more specific when we talk about the duration of the arrhythmia over time. If the arrhythmia lasts less than 30 seconds, it is labeled a *nonsustained VTach* (Figure 31-2). If the arrhythmia lasts 30 seconds or longer, or if clinical intervention is needed to prevent cardiovascular compromise (hypotension, chest pain, ischemia, severe dyspnea, etc.), the arrhythmia is labeled a *sustained VTach*. Finally, if the arrhythmia is present most of the time, it is known as *incessant VTach*.

We will begin our detailed look of monomorphic VTach, both nonsustained and sustained, by looking at the possible mechanisms that can give rise to it. We feel

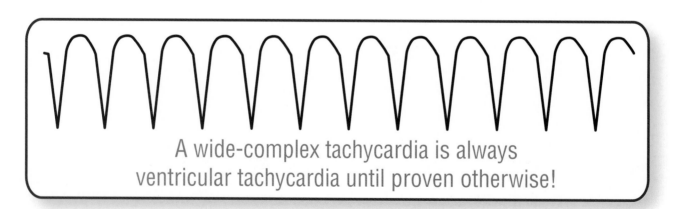

A wide-complex tachycardia is always ventricular tachycardia until proven otherwise!

Figure 31-1: Monomorphic ventricular tachycardia. Note the uniform appearance of the complexes in the strip above, and the rapid rates above 100 BPM.

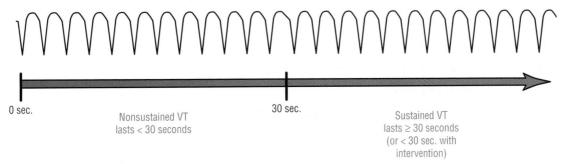

Figure 31-2: Nonsustained and sustained VTach.

that in order to understand this deadly arrhythmia and its treatment, we need to thoroughly understand how it is created. After we have looked at how it is formed, we will take a closer look at the morphology and how to diagnose it. Finally, we will look at the nonsustained and sustained forms of this rhythm disturbance separately, focusing on their differences.

Reentry and Other Possible Mechanisms

There are various mechanisms that have been proposed and could potentially be at work in any one patient for monomorphic VTach to develop. These mechanisms include intraventricular reentry mechanisms, increased automaticity (both normal and abnormal), and late and early afterdepolarizations. By far, the most common one is intraventricular reentry. In this chapter, we will review how an intraventricular reentry circuit can be formed and how it can generate monomorphic VTach. (The others are beyond the scope of this book, and the reader is referred to an advanced textbook on electrophysiology.)

We first looked at reentry in Chapter 25 when discussing AVNRT. At that time, we stated that there were some preexisting requirements needed in order to form a reentry circuit. These included:

1. The presence of an electrical circuit with at least two pathways.

2. The two pathways involved need to have different underlying properties: conduction time, refractoriness, and so on. This could be due to a structural difference in the pathways, ischemia, electrolyte abnormalities, or any other event that will temporarily or permanently alter conduction and refractory time.

3. There has to be an area of slowing in one of the circuits—just enough to allow the rest of the circuit to get over its refractory period.

Let's look at each of these requirements individually and see how they can take form to create VTach.

1. The presence of an electrical circuit with at least two pathways.

VTach is more commonly found in patients with coronary artery disease, myocardial infarctions (MIs), and congenital abnormalities. Any, and all, of these disorders can lead to the formation of various isolated areas of myocardium that can act as a pathway. For simplicity, let's look at myocardial infarctions.

Myocardial infarctions are typically caused by obstruction to flow in the larger arteries supplying blood and nutrients to the heart. Sometimes, the larger arteries communicate with each other through smaller "tributaries" and the blood will continue to flow to an area even if the main artery supplying that area is blocked. This type of cross-circulation is known as *collateral circulation*.

In addition to the type of collateral circulation we just mentioned above, there is another type that we shall call *micro-collateral circulation*. This type of collateral circulation occurs because the exact area of perfusion by any one artery is sometimes "fuzzy" along the edges of its territory, and small areas along the outskirts are covered by the adjoining arteries.

During an MI, the cells die and are eventually replaced by nonconductive fibrous scar tissue. Micro-collateral circulation will sometimes keep small islands or "bridges" of cells viable, despite the infarct that is occurring around them (see pink bridge of cells that are following the path of the collateral artery at the bottom of the gray wedge in Figure 31-3). These "bridges" of viable cells can continue to conduct the depolarization wave normally and function just like normal tissue. These "bridges," therefore, can create the pathways that are required for the formation of a ventricular reentry circuit.

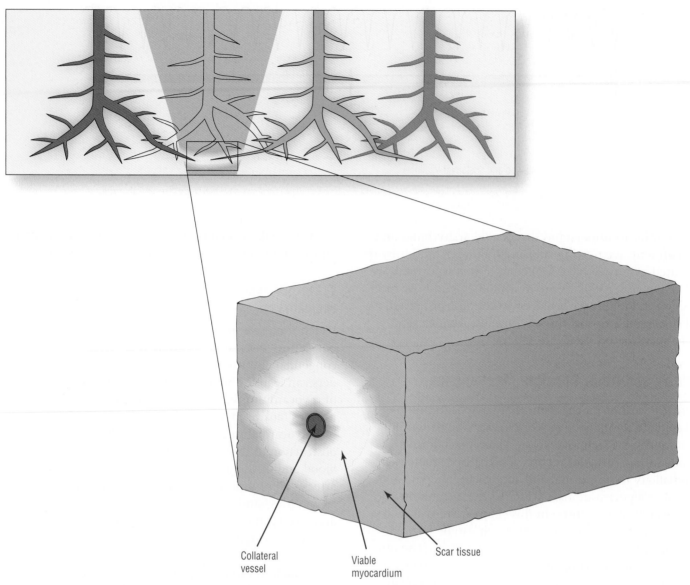

Collateral
vessel

Viable
myocardium

Scar tissue

Figure 31-3: Microscopic view of an area of infarct (gray wedge) showing circulation from three different arteries. One artery, the colorless one, is no longer perfusing an area of myocardium, giving rise to the infarct. The two surrounding arteries (the red and pink ones) have some small blood vessels penetrating the infarcted area. This redundancy of arterial supply is known as collateral circulation and is a protective mechanism for the heart. Oftentimes, the collateral circulation will keep small regions or cords of cells alive. These cords can continue to transmit the electrical depolarization wave. These pathways are completely surrounded by nonconducting scar tissue, which acts like an insulation layer.

Figure 31-4 shows how two pathways can be present around an area of infarcted tissue in the ventricle. The red pathway, labeled with the number 2, is formed when collateral circulation has caused some sparing of viable cells in the areas shown. These "tubes" can conduct the depolarization wave through the center of the dead tissue or scar tissue that is formed when an MI has healed and form the pathways for a potential reentry circuit.

2. The two pathways must have different properties.

The next condition that must be met to form a reentry circuit is that the two pathways must have different properties. How does this fit into the pathways formed above? In the normal ventricle, any one myocardial cell is surrounded by other cells. As such, there are hundreds of connection points along the membranes where communication can take place between the cells (Figure 31-5). These connection points are called *gap junctions*.

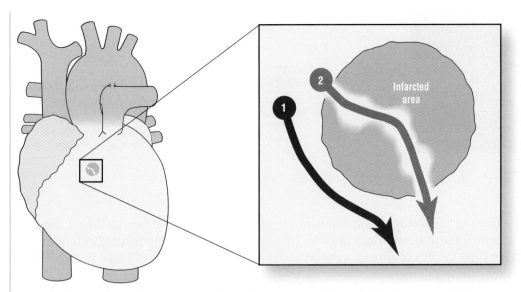

Figure 31-4: An area of infarct with some isolated islands and cords of viable cells forming an electrical pathway through the scar tissue (see red pathway #2). The blue pathway #1 is the normal route of depolarization around the infarct.

The larger the number of gap junctions present between two cells, the faster that the electrical depolarization wave is passed between them. This type of communication continues throughout the myocardium of the entire ventricle.

In general, the small viable groups and "tubes" of cells formed due to microcirculation are thin. Thinner tubes have fewer connections between cells than large three-dimensional groups of cells (Figure 31-6). In fact, these tubes can be so thin that only a few gap junctions at the end of cells may actually be in contact with each other. As you can imagine, conduction of the depolar-

ization wave along these pathways is slower than through the regular, noninfarcted ventricle. This slower cellular communication creates a difference in the individual conduction rates between the two pathways. Let's move on.

3. An area of slowing in one of the circuits—just enough to allow the rest of the circuit to get over its refractory period.

Now, let's begin to put it all together. Figure 31-7 shows an area of infarct with a viable "bridge" of myocardial cells, which acts as a second pathway. Due to the low

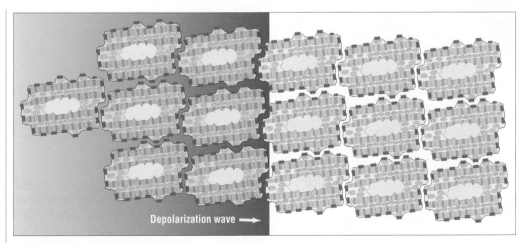

Figure 31-5: A depolarization wave as it is spread by direct cell-to-cell transmission. The transmission occurs between cells through biochemical communication at the gap junctions (red rectangles on cell membranes). Note the number of actual connections between cells.

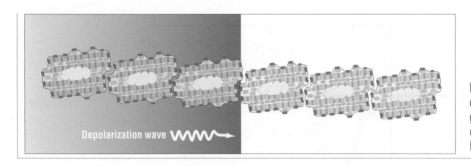

Figure 31-6: A depolarization wave as it is spread by direct cell-to-cell transmission. Note the small number of gap junctions (red rectangles) that are in contact with each other as compared with the cells in Figure 31-5. The low level of communication leads to slower conduction times.

amount of communication in the "bridge," the depolarization wave is spread much more slowly than outside the infarcted zone. This slowing allows enough time to pass so that the refractory period of the noninfarct myocardium is sufficiently repolarized to accept a new impulse. This, however, does not usually occur because the impulse enters both ends of the "bridge," essentially nullifying the two wavefronts.

Under ideal arrhythmogenic circumstances, however, a reentry circuit can easily be started by a PVC. By mechanisms very similar to the one we saw when we examined AVNRT, a PVC can arrive earlier than expected and be blocked from traveling down the refractory pathway. Since conduction will not occur

through that refractory pathway, the conduction must proceed exclusively through the other nonrefractory pathway. As we saw before in AVNRT, by the time that the impulse reaches the other end of the nonrefractory pathway, the original refractory pathway will be ready and willing to receive the impulse. This sets up the reentry circuit, which will continue to self-propagate and loop from this point on (Figure 31-8).

Note that the direction of the circuit will depend on which pathway was initially refractory. The orientation of the resulting depolarization waves as they travel through the myocardium in potentially opposite directions will give rise to vectors, which can lead to morphologically different complexes on the ECG.

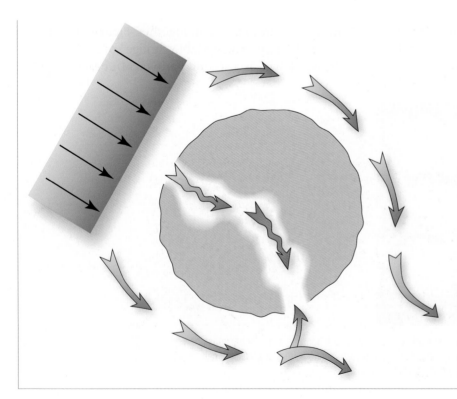

Figure 31-7: A depolarization wave (see green rectangle or wavefront) enters the intra-infarct pathway and is also normally spread around the infarct zone. The transmission through the intra-infarct "bridge" of viable tissue is conducted much slower than through the normal extra-infarct myocardium. Under normal circumstances, however, a reentry circuit is not formed because the impulses enter both ends of the bridge. The two wavefronts then meet inside the tube and cancel each other out.

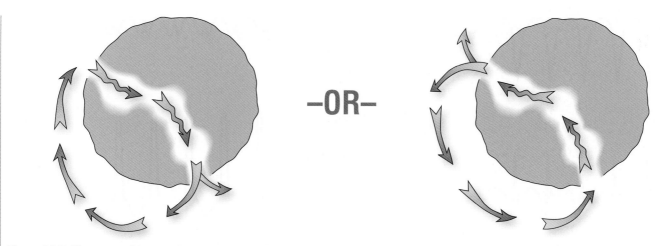

Figure 31-8: The two possible routes for a reentry using the pathway indicated.

General Characteristics of VTach

Morphology of the Complexes and Arrhythmia Recognition

If you understand the principles presented in Chapter 30, then understanding VTach will be a breeze. This is because VTach is, rhythmically speaking, just a faster, deadlier form of accelerated idioventricular rhythm. VTach is characterized by the usual ectopic ventricular appearance of wide, bizarre complexes (wider than 0.12 seconds) and ST-T wave abnormalities. Just as in any ventricular rhythm, the complexes are usually wider than you would expect to see in an uncomplicated bundle branch block, with widths of 0.16 and 0.20 seconds being common.

In addition to the general characteristics above, the presence of Josephson's sign (Figure 31-9) and Brugada's sign (Figure 31-10) are fairly commonplace in many patients with VTach, and should be actively sought because it is essential to the differential diagnosis of VTach. (As we shall see, the presence of these two morphological features will become very helpful to you in the differential diagnosis of wide-complex beats and tachycardias, as they are usually not present in supraventricular complexes with aberrant conduction or in patients with underlying bundle branch blocks.)

ST-T wave abnormalities are always present, just as in every other ventricular rhythm. The ST-T wave abnormalities are even more pronounced in VTach because of the rapid rates involved. These abnormalities can often hide an underlying P wave or a supraventricular rhythm (in the case of AV dissociation).

It is extremely important at this time to go back to the basics of electrocardiography and remember that the morphology of the complexes depends on the leads being used. A common mistake made by beginners is to

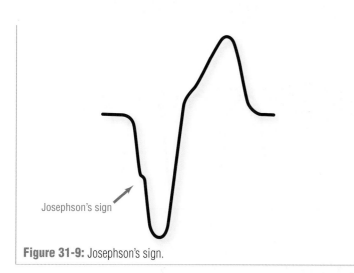

Josephson's sign

Figure 31-9: Josephson's sign.

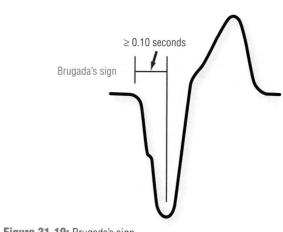

Brugada's sign

≥ 0.10 seconds

Figure 31-10: Brugada's sign.

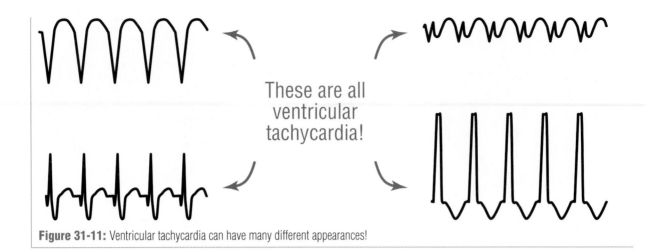

These are all ventricular tachycardia!

Figure 31-11: Ventricular tachycardia can have many different appearances!

expect to always see the same morphological appearance for VTach. Usually, it is similar to the morphology present in top left-hand strip on Figure 31-11. Often, when that expected morphological appearance is not present, the diagnosis is missed and the rhythm is mistakenly assumed to be supraventricular in nature. This can be a deadly mistake.

Remember, *if you don't think of it, you cannot diagnose it*. We need to remember that sometimes the complexes will be positive, and sometimes they will be negative. Sometimes they will be tall, and sometimes they will be short. Look for the presence of a wide-complex tachycardia first and foremost, keeping in mind that the appearance may be different depending on the lead and the direction of the ventricular vectors causing the electrocardiographic appearance.

Regularity

In general, VTach is a very regular rhythm (Figure 31-12). We say "in general" because in over 90% of the cases, it appears with clockwork precision. In the other 10%, however, there can be some slight irregularity. This irregularity causes a variation in the cadence of the complexes but by no more than 0.16 seconds (about $3\frac{1}{2}$ small boxes on the strip). These irregularities are usually found if the VTach is slow.

Patients with VTach are frequently found to have had frequent PVCs prior to onset. Tachycardia is usually triggered by a PVC; therefore the rhythm can show some irregularity at the onset (Figure 31-13). This irregularity typically lasts for a few seconds (can be up to 10 to 20 beats) but quickly corrects itself once the rate of the rhythm stabilizes.

AV Dissociation

As we saw in accelerated idioventricular rhythm, AV dissociation is very commonly found in ventricular rhythms. As we shall see, this is even more so in ventricular tachycardia. It is clearly and easily found in about 50% of the cases on close examination of the strip. (With a bit more detective work, it may actually be found in a few more cases because the P waves are frequently hidden from view by the overlying ventricular rhythm.) The diffuse ST-T wave abnormalities and the bizarre, wide morphologies of the ventricular complexes can easily obscure the relatively small underlying

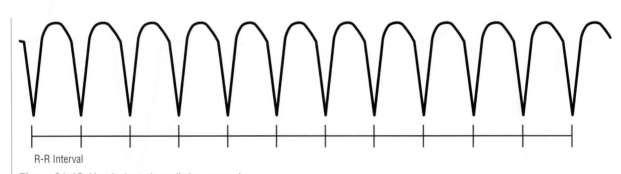

R-R Interval

Figure 31-12: Ventricular tachycardia is very regular.

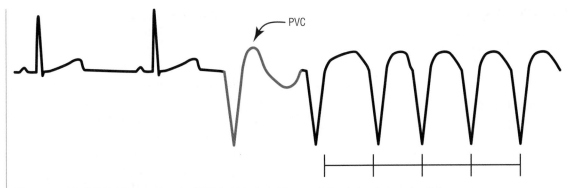

Figure 31-13: A PVC triggers off a run of VTach. Note that at the onset, the rhythm is irregular. This quickly stabilizes to the normal regular pattern typically found in VTach.

P waves. For this reason, it is extremely important to look at every little abnormality on the strip and use your calipers to map any possible connection between them.

AV dissociation is actually the most important thing you can look for when you are trying to establish ventricular tachycardia as the cause of a wide-complex tachycardia (Figure 31-14). Always look for the presence of P waves, capture beats, and fusion beats. Remember, the presence of capture beats and fusion beats is indirect evidence of an underlying AV dissociation. (AV dissociation can also occur with a junctional tachycardia with a preexisting bundle branch block or aberrancy, but as you can imagine, this combination is rarely found.)

For clinical purposes, therefore, any wide-complex tachycardia with an AV dissociation should be considered ventricular tachycardia until proven otherwise. As a matter of fact, any wide-complex tachycardia should be considered VTach until proven otherwise, PERIOD. Being conservative and playing the odds is the clinically prudent thing to do when approaching these rhythms.

That said, close clinical correlation and close examination of the strip can lead to the correct diagnosis in about 90% of the cases.

Figure 31-14 clearly shows a variation in the size of the QRS complexes. Yet, this is still an example of a monomorphic VTach. Why does this happen? The variation in the size of the complexes can be due to many reasons. Most commonly it is due to the electrical alternans that is frequently seen in most tachycardias. Other causes include: fusion with the component waves of the complexes around them, a fusion with a large underlying P wave in the case of AV dissociation, or a slight variation in the course of a reentry circuit (which could just alter the vector, and hence the morphology, slightly. Don't let the slight variations fool you into thinking that this is anything but VTach!

Similar Morphology to PVCs

Many times the complexes in monomorphic VTach will be identical to the morphology of previous PVCs associ-

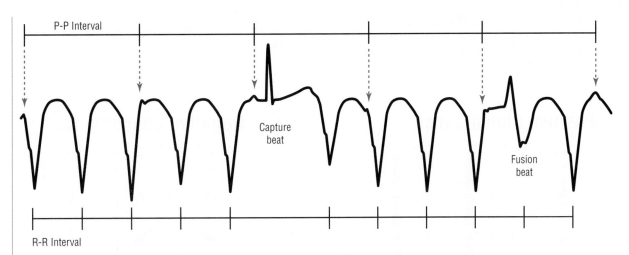

Figure 31-14: Ventricular tachycardia is quite frequently associated with AV dissociation. Always look for P waves, capture beats, and fusion beats!

ated with your patient (see Figure 31-13). The reason for this is that the reentry circuits are the same for both, but a repetitive cycle is not established with single PVCs.

Nonsustained Monomorphic Ventricular Tachycardia

Nonsustained ventricular tachycardia (NSVT), or more specifically nonsustained monomorphic VTach, is an incidental finding in some people obtaining Holter monitors for palpitations or other reasons. Electrocardiographically, it is described as the occurrence of three or more consecutive, morphologically similar, ventricular complexes occurring at an intrinsic rate of over 100 BPM. By definition, the rhythm spontaneously termi-

nates at less than 30 seconds. Clinically, it is a significant rhythm because of the symptoms with which it can present but, more importantly, it can be a harbinger for sustained VTach or ventricular fibrillation. Both of these potential rhythms are life-threatening.

Most patients typically have three to ten beat runs or salvos of NSVT. The runs are usually triggered by a PVC with the same general morphology seen on the strip (Figure 31-15). In general, patients with NSVT have a higher frequency of PVCs at baseline than patients who do not have the rhythm abnormality.

The clinical manifestations of NSVT can be anything from an asymptomatic expression to transient hemodynamic compromise, depending on the length of the run. The last part of that statement is very important, because short runs can typically be well tolerated. As a

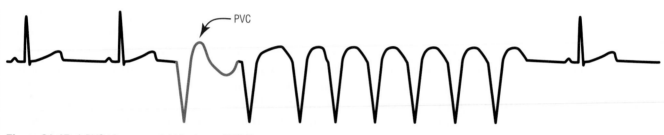

PVC

Figure 31-15: A PVC triggers an eight-beat run of NSVT.

Concordance of the Precordial Leads

A full 12-lead ECG of a patient with ventricular tachycardia will often show concordance of all of the QRS complexes in the precordial leads. What we mean by this is that *the main direction of all of the QRS complexes will be in the same direction, either all positive or all negative (Figures 31-16 and 31-17), in all of the*

chest or precordial leads (V₁ through V₆). The size of the complex is not important, just the direction and orientation of the QRS complexes.

Concordance is yet another useful tool in evaluating the differential diagnosis of a wide-complex tachycardia. It is not definitive proof of the arrhythmia, but it is highly indicative of VTach.

Positive Concordance

I	aVR	V₁ ↑	V₄ ↑
II	aVL	V₂ ↑	V₅ ↑
III	aVF	V₃ ↑	V₆ ↑

Figure 31-16: Positive concordance in VTach.

Negative Concordance

I	aVR	V₁ ↓	V₄ ↓
II	aVL	V₂ ↓	V₅ ↓
III	aVF	V₃ ↓	V₆ ↓

Figure 31-17: Negative concordance in VTach.

ADDITIONAL INFORMATION

Axis Direction and VTach

A full 12-lead ECG can also give you another useful bit of information. The axis in VTach is often found to be in the extreme right quadrant (Figure 31-18). This is not a common quadrant to find the main ventricular axis in any patient, so its presence is indicative of a vector that is originating in a bizarre ectopic site. Frequently, these sites will give rise to ventricular tachycardia. Once again, an axis in the extreme right quadrant is not definitive proof of the arrhythmia, but it is highly indicative of VTach.

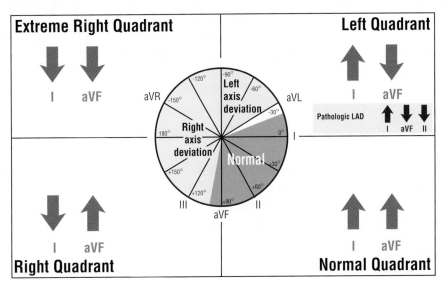

Figure 31-18: The axis in VTach is often found in the extreme right quadrant. In order to isolate the axis to that quadrant, look at the QRS complexes in leads I and AVF. If the QRS complexes are negative in both of those leads, the axis has to be in the extreme right quadrant.

matter of fact, most episodes are so short as to cause only minimal, transient symptoms.

When the run lasts longer than a few seconds, however, it can essentially cut off perfusion of the main organs, including the brain and the heart itself. A few seconds of nonperfusion to the brain could result in syncope. Other common clinical presentations include lightheadedness, near-syncope, palpitations, and visual disturbances.

Morphologically, the complexes all resemble each other. NSVT may be slightly irregular if the run is short. Longer runs will stabilize and will show a regular cadence. A quick way to decide whether a short run of irregular wide complexes is due to NSVT or intermittent atrial fibrillation with aberrancy is to compare the complexes to the PVCs that are usually found on the strip near the run in question. If the morphology is identical, or nearly identical, to the PVCs, then it is NSVT. If the run does not resemble the PVCs, it could easily be atrial fibrillation with aberrancy.

Additional things to look for include the onset of the run. If the run is triggered by a PVC, it strongly favors NSVT. Longer strips and full 12-lead ECGs are extremely helpful to look for the direct and indirect signs AV dissociation. The presence of Josephson's sign or Brugada's sign favors the diagnosis of VTach. We will look at the differential diagnosis of VTach much more closely in Chapter 33.

Sustained Monomorphic Ventricular Tachycardia

Now let's turn our attention to a very, very dangerous rhythm: Sustained monomorphic ventricular tachycardia. Electrocardiographically, sustained monomorphic VTach has all of the characteristics of NSVT. The difference lies in the length and severity of the rhythm. Sustained monomorphic VTach can either (1) last longer than 30 seconds; or (2) last shorter than 30 seconds, but requires electrical or pharmacologic intervention to terminate it because of life-threatening or severe clinical manifestations (Figure 31-19).

Runs of sustained VTach are also triggered by PVCs and are caused by reentry in over 90% of cases. The rhythm may be slightly irregular at the onset, but it quickly stabilizes into a very regular rhythm. Slight morphological changes can be present due to fusion with the beats around it, or due to capture beats and fusion beats with simultaneous supraventricular complexes. AV dissociation is very common in this rhythm abnormality and needs to be actively sought out if it is not obvious.

As you can imagine, clinical manifestations are much more serious in sustained VTach. They occur from alterations in the cardiac output produced by the rhythm due to either the length of the run, lack of ventricular filling, or lack of coordinated mechanical contraction that commonly occurs with ventricular

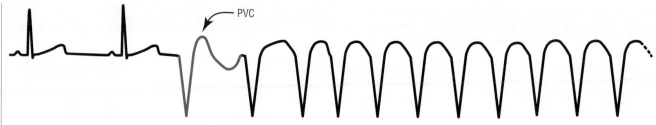

PVC

Figure 31-19: A PVC triggers a run of sustained monomorphic VTach.

complexes. The clinical manifestations include near-syncope or lightheadedness, syncope, hypotension, altered mental status, chest pain, diaphoresis, shortness of breath, myocardial infarction, stroke, pulmonary edema, cardiogenic shock, and sudden death, to name a few. Persistent stable VTach may lead to a cardiomyopathy if left untreated for an extended period of time.

In addition to the factors mentioned above, symptoms also vary with the duration of the run. The longer the run, the greater and more dangerous the clinical spectrum. Even if the patient appears to be clinically stable during a run, he or she can deteriorate quickly and unexpectedly.

A clinical word of wisdom: ***Never turn your back on a patient in VTach!*** Stable patients can turn unstable very, very quickly and you may not have enough time to get all of the equipment you need at that time. Always have the right drugs and a defibrillator by the patient's side, and make sure the patient is constantly monitored. A transcutaneous pacer is also a good idea to have on hand, as you do not know how the patient will react to therapy or to the rhythm itself if it persists. It is better to be safe than sorry in these cases and preparation is critical.

Long-term management of these patients should always include a serious discussion about placing an internal cardiac defibrillator. These could be life-saving in the case of recurrence of the rhythm in the future. ***Remember, many times the first clinical manifestation of VTach is sudden death!***

Ventricular Flutter

When an episode of ventricular tachycardia comes so fast as to obscure the morphology of the individual waves and segments (QRS, ST segment, and T wave), it is known as ventricular flutter (Figure 31-20). At this point, the rhythm resembles a very fast sinusoidal pattern.

The rates at which the morphological features become blurred vary depending on the patient and the clinical scenario. The typical rate at which the blurring occurs is usually above 200 BPM, and commonly can reach rates as high as 235 to 250 BPM. Rates above 250 BPM are uncommon, and when they occur, should raise the suspicion of an accessory pathway being involved.

Clinical manifestations are the same as for sustained VTach, but the patients are typically more unstable because of the higher rates. Once again, pharmaceutical intervention should take the possibility of accessory pathways into consideration. If the patient is hemodynamically unstable, electrical cardioversion or defibrillation is strongly recommended.

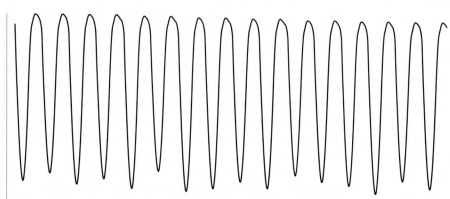

Figure 31-20: An episode of ventricular flutter. Note that the morphology of the various components of the complexes is lost and the rhythm almost becomes sinusoidal in nature.

ARRHYTHMIA RECOGNITION

Monomorphic Ventricular Tachycardia

Rate:	100 to 250 BPM
Regularity:	Regular (may be slightly irregular at onset)
P wave:	Retrograde or in AV dissociation
Morphology:	Variable
Upright in II, III, and aVF:	Variable
P:QRS ratio:	None
PR interval:	Variable, if present
QRS width:	≥ 0.12 seconds
Grouping:	None
Dropped beats:	None

DIFFERENTIAL DIAGNOSIS

Monomorphic Ventricular Tachycardia

1. Acute MI or ischemia
2. Cardiomyopathies
3. Myocarditis
4. Arrhythmogenic RV dysplasia
5. Idiopathic
6. Drugs: Cocaine, etc.
7. Electrolyte disorders

The list above is not inclusive but reflects the most common causes of the rhythm disturbance.

ECG Strips

ECG 31-1

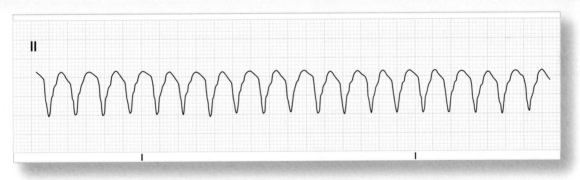

Rate:	About 200 BPM	PR intervals:	None
Regularity:	Regular	QRS width:	Wide
P waves:	None	Grouping:	None
Morphology:	None		
Axis:	None	Dropped beats:	Absent
P:QRS ratio:	None	Rhythm:	**Ventricular tachycardia**

Discussion:

The rhythm above shows a wide-complex tachycardia at about 200 BPM. The rhythm is very regular and all of the complexes are almost identical morphologically. This is an example of ventricular tachycardia. This could easily be labeled ventricular flutter, and you would not be wrong. The reason that ventricular flutter is not completely correct is that there is still some semblance of demarcation between the QRS complexes and the ST segments and T waves (although this is debatable).

ECG 31-2

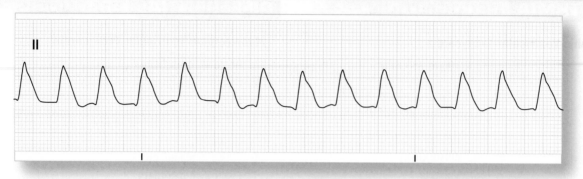

Rate:	About 135 BPM	PR intervals:	None
Regularity:	Regular	QRS width:	Wide
P waves:	None	Grouping:	None
Morphology:	None		
Axis:	None	Dropped beats:	Absent
P:QRS ratio:	None	Rhythm:	**Ventricular tachycardia**

Discussion:

This strip shows a wide-complex tachycardia clipping along at about 135 BPM. The morphology of the QRS complexes is definitely wide, even though there appears to be some fusing with the elevated ST segments.

Indeed, the patient was having a large AMI. There are no discernible P waves noted. A 12-lead ECG would be invaluable in further diagnosing the rhythm and in evaluating the AMI that appears to be present on this strip.

ECG 31-3

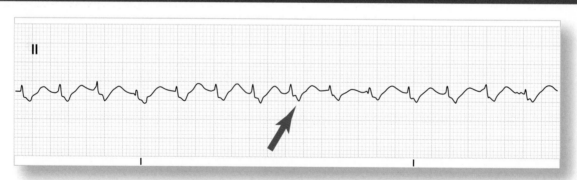

Rate:	About 140 BPM	PR intervals:	None
Regularity:	Regular	QRS width:	Wide
P waves:	None	Grouping:	None
Morphology:	None		
Axis:	None	Dropped beats:	Absent
P:QRS ratio:	None	Rhythm:	**Ventricular tachycardia**

Discussion:

The strip above shows a wide-complex tachycardia at about 140 BPM. The blue arrow is pointing toward a constant irregularity in the morphology of the S wave. This irregularity could be a retrograde inverted P wave

or it could be part of the morphological features of the S wave itself. It is unclear from this strip. Perhaps a 12-lead ECG could shed some light on this issue. There is no evidence of AV dissociation present on the strip.

ECG 31-4

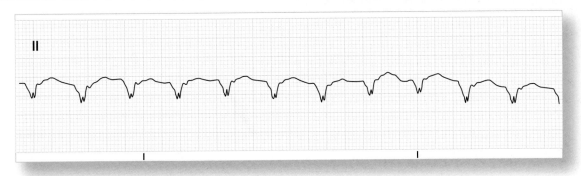

Rate:	About 112 BPM	PR intervals:	None
Regularity:	Regular	QRS width:	Wide
P waves:	None	Grouping:	None
Morphology:	None		
Axis:	None	Dropped beats:	Absent
P:QRS ratio:	None	Rhythm:	**Ventricular tachycardia**

Discussion:

This rhythm strip is also a wide-complex tachycardia. This time, the rate is around 112 BPM and there are no obvious P waves. Remember, a wide-complex tachycardia is VTach until proven otherwise! VTach is the working diagnosis. Other possibilities for the strip above include a junctional tachycardia in a patient with a pre-existing bundle branch block or in a patient with some aberrancy. An old ECG or rhythm strip while the patient was in sinus rhythm would be very helpful in establishing the definitive diagnosis.

ECG 31-5

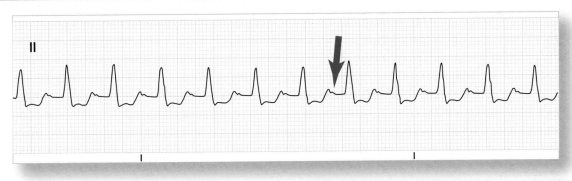

Rate:	About 115 BPM	PR intervals:	None
Regularity:	Regular	QRS width:	Wide
P waves:	None	Grouping:	None
Morphology:	None		
Axis:	None	Dropped beats:	Absent
P:QRS ratio:	None	Rhythm:	**Ventricular tachycardia**

Discussion:

Here is another example of VTach until proven otherwise. The strip above shows a wide-complex tachycardia at about 115 BPM. Take a close look at the end of the T wave. Notice that there is a slight bump (see blue arrow). Double-humped T waves are not very common and this could represent a P wave with a prolonged PR interval. But, since VTach is the diagnosis of exclusion, you should continue the treatment strategy along those lines. This was VTach. A 12-lead ECG is very helpful in these cases.

ECG 31-6

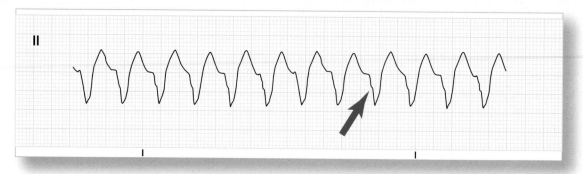

Rate:	About 150 BPM	PR intervals:	None
Regularity:	Regular	QRS width:	Wide
P waves:	None	Grouping:	None
Morphology:	None		
Axis:	None	Dropped beats:	Absent
P:QRS ratio:	None	Rhythm:	**Ventricular tachycardia**

Discussion:

This is a wide-complex tachycardia at about 150 BPM. Always think of atrial flutter when the ventricular rate is 150 BPM. There is no evidence for atrial flutter in this strip. Notice, however, that most of the complexes have a very definite hump in the downstroke of the S wave (see blue arrow). Could this be a Josephson's sign? Probably, because it is seen on almost every complex. If it only recurred on a regular pattern, such as every third or fourth complex, then it would probably be a sign of AV dissociation.

ECG 31-7

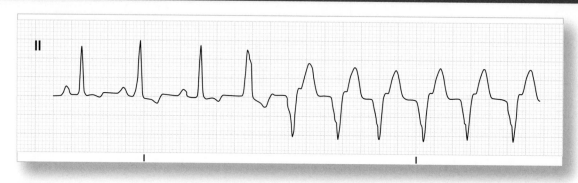

Rate:	See discussion below	PR intervals:	Normal
Regularity:	See discussion below	QRS width:	See discussion below
P waves:	Present	Grouping:	None
Morphology:	Normal		
Axis:	Upright	Dropped beats:	Absent
P:QRS ratio:	1:1 in beginning	Rhythm:	**Ventricular tachycardia**

Discussion:

This srip starts out as a normal sinus complex. The second complex shows some mild aberrancy with some slurring at the onset. The third complex appears to be sinus. The fourth complex is a PVC or an aberrantly conducted PJC. This starts a run of a wide-complex tachycardia at about 120 BPM. There are no obvious P waves or irregularities that could represent P waves with AV dissociation on this part of the strip. Each of the complexes is nearly identical in morphology. This is a monomorphic ventricular tachycardia triggered by a premature complex, either ventricular or junctional.

ECG 31-8

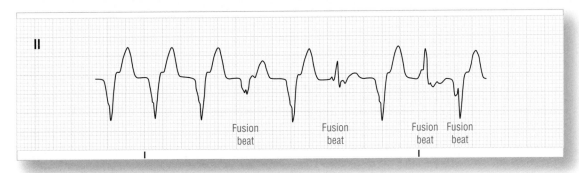

Rate:	About 115 BPM	PR intervals:	None
Regularity:	Regular	QRS width:	Wide
P waves:	None	Grouping:	None
Morphology:	None		
Axis:	None	Dropped beats:	Absent
P:QRS ratio:	None	Rhythm:	**Ventricular tachycardia**

Discussion:

This strip is a continuation of the one above. Note that there are different morphologies for the complexes in the latter two thirds of the strip. These are fusion complexes interspersed among the monomorphic complexes. This is indirect evidence of AV dissociation. We attempted to map out the P-P interval above throughout the strip, but there were no associated "bumps" in the area. However, the presence of fusion beats is clear evidence of the presence of AV dissociation.

ECG 31-9

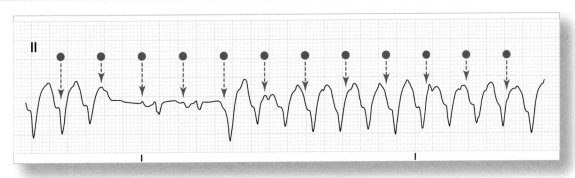

Rate:	About 190 BPM	PR intervals:	None
Regularity:	See discussion below	QRS width:	Wide
P waves:	Present	Grouping:	None
Morphology:	Normal		
Axis:	Upright	Dropped beats:	Absent
P:QRS ratio:	None	Rhythm:	**Ventricular tachycardia**

Discussion:

This strip shows a wide-complex tachycardia at about 190 BPM. There are some fusion beats present and obvious AV dissociation. Here is how you should approach the AV dissociation. Place the pins on your calipers over the two obvious P waves (third and fourth blue dots). Now, just walk your calipers in both directions, noting any irregularities in the complexes below. The presence of fusion of the P waves with the underlying complex will be apparent.

ECG 31-10

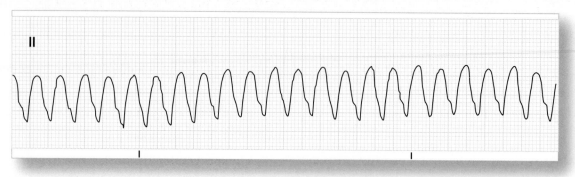

Rate:	About 215 BPM	PR intervals:	None
Regularity:	Regular	QRS width:	Wide
P waves:	None	Grouping:	None
Morphology:	None		
Axis:	None	Dropped beats:	Absent
P:QRS ratio:	None	Rhythm:	**Ventricular flutter**

Discussion:

The rhythm strip above shows a rapid, wide-complex rhythm with a sinusoidal pattern. All of the waves are nearly morphologically identical. This is a very rapid monomorphic ventricular tachycardia. The loss of the morphological identity of each of the components of the complex makes the more accurate diagnosis ventricular flutter.

CHAPTER **REVIEW**

1. Ventricular tachycardia refers to a rhythm composed of _____ or more ectopic ventricular complexes in a row with a rate above _____ BPM.

2. The typical rates for VTach are from ____ to ____ BPM.

3. If the rate is above 200 BPM and the morphology of the complexes blend to form a sinusoidal pattern, the more accurate term for this rhythm is _____ _____.

4. If all of the ventricular complexes are identical or nearly identical, the rhythm is known as a _____ ventricular tachycardia.

5. If a run of monomorphic VTach lasts less than 30 seconds, it is known as _____.

6. If a run of monomorphic VTach lasts greater than or equal to 30 seconds or if the rhythm requires an intervention in order to break it due to clinical symptoms, it is known as _____.

7. Approximately what percentage of VTachs are due to reentry?
   A. 30%
   B. 50%
   C. 70%
   D. 90%
   E. All of them are due to reentry.

8. A notch in the downstroke of the S wave in an ectopic ventricular complex is known as:
   A. Notch
   B. Johnson's sign
   C. Bruscetta's sign
   D. Josephson's sign
   E. Brugada's sign

9. A length of greater than or equal to 0.10 seconds between the onset of the QRS complex to the very bottom of the S wave is known as:
   A. Wide notch
   B. Johnson's sign
   C. Bruscetta's sign
   D. Josephson's sign
   E. Brugada's sign

10. The QRS complexes in VTach are always negative in lead II. True or False.

11. VTach can be slightly irregular at the onset of the run. However, after 20 to 30 complexes, the rhythm usually is very regular. True or False.

12. Many runs of VTach are triggered by a:
    A. Ventricular escape complex
    B. PAC
    C. PJC
    D. PVC

13. AV dissociation is a common finding in VTach. In fact, close observation yields positive evidence of AV dissociation in about ____% of the cases.

14. Indirect evidence of AV dissociation includes:
    A. Inverted P waves
    B. Capture beats and fusion beats
    C. Abnormal P wave axis
    D. A and C
    E. All of the above

15. The most common cause of sustained monomorphic VTach is an _____ _____ _____.

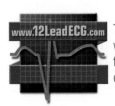

To enhance the knowledge you gain in this book, access this text's website at www.12leadECG.com! This valuable resource provides flashcards, an online glossary, web links, and more. Simply click on the Arrhythmias book cover once at the site.

Polymorphic Ventricular Tachycardia and Torsade de Pointes

General Overview

Many clinicians use the terms polymorphic ventricular tachycardia and torsade de pointes interchangeably in daily practice. In reality, these are two separate and distinct clinical syndromes presenting with an almost identical electrocardiographic presentation. There is only one morphological criterion that separates these two entities electrocardiographically: the QT interval.

Polymorphic Ventricular Tachycardia

Polymorphic ventricular tachycardia is classically described as a rhythm of ectopic ventricular origin that is characterized by an irregular cadence and a constantly changing morphological picture, amplitude, and polarity of the complexes (Figure 32-1). The complexes are wide, as you would expect for a ventricular rhythm, and typically appear to twist and turn along a central axis. The rhythm is typically triggered by a PVC that occurs along the relative refractory period of the previous complex. The QT interval is normal in polymorphic VTach.

Typically, the usual rates occur between 200 and 250 BPM. The ventricular rates, however, can be anywhere from 150 to 300 BPM (in very rare cases, there have even been cases with rates as slow as 100 BPM). The very rapid rate associated with polymorphic VTach tends to blur the distinction between the QRS waves, the ST segments, and T waves, and the complexes take on an appearance similar to ventricular flutter. Unlike ventricular flutter, however, the morphology of the complexes is constantly changing, almost on a beat-to-beat basis, due to a constant reversal of the polarity of the rhythm from positive to negative.

The changing polarity of the complexes appears to occur periodically, creating a grouped appearance in the

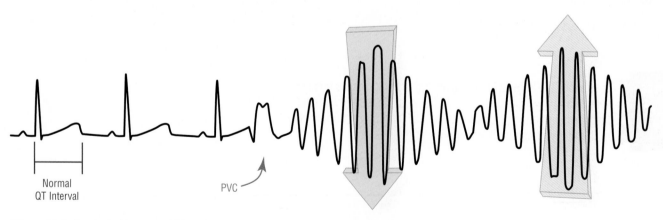

Figure 32-1: A patient with a normal QT interval has a PVC that triggers a run of polymorphic ventricular tachycardia. Note the rapid rates of the tachycardia and the lack of distinction between the components of the ventricular complexes. Finally, note that the amplitude of the complexes is constantly changing in each grouping as the polarity of the complexes changes from negative to positive (represented by the blue and pink arrows). This reversal of polarity on the same strip is virtually pathognomonic for this type of arrhythmia.

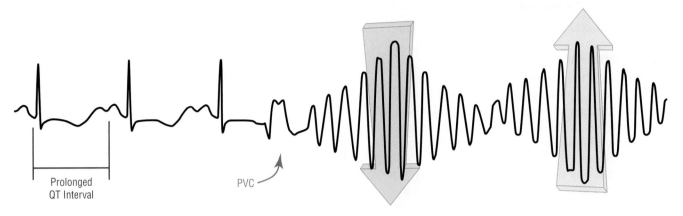

Prolonged
QT Interval

PVC

Figure 32-2: A patient with a prolonged QT interval has a PVC that triggers a run of torsade de pointes. The tachycardia has all of the morphological characteristics of polymorphic VTach, including the flipping polarity from which the rhythm derives its name (turning of the points).

rhythm. The groupings are composed of anywhere from 5 to 20 complexes on average. The number of groupings, however, depends on the duration of the arrhythmia.

Polymorphic VTach demonstrates a close relationship to the patient's underlying heart rate when the patient is not in tachycardia. Many patients develop the arrhythmia during periods of bradycardia or severe AV block. On the other hand, drugs that speed the underlying heart rate can prevent the formation of the arrhythmia.

The rhythm is typically seen in patients undergoing an acute myocardial infarction or severe ischemia. The development of this electrocardiographic arrhythmia in a patient with a normal QT interval should prompt a search for an AMI, ischemia, or silent ischemia. If ischemia or infarct is ruled out as a cause, further evaluation to isolate a cause should follow the differential diagnosis that is described in the section on torsade de pointes.

Hemodynamic instability and consequences of low cardiac output are more frequent in polymorphic VTach compared with monomorphic VTach. A large part of the reason lies in the faster rates seen with polymorphic VTach. The rhythm is usually self-limiting, but can break down into ventricular fibrillation and can cause sudden death.

Management strategies are identical to those used in monomorphic VTach. Remember, electrical cardioversion or defibrillation should be your first-line response to a significantly hemodynamically compromised patient with this arrhythmia.

Torsade de Pointes

Torsade de pointes is a variant of polymorphic ventricular tachycardia that occurs in patients with a baseline prolongation of the QT interval when measured while the

patient is in normal sinus rhythm (Figure 32-2). The prolonged QT, and the clinical scenario in which the two arrhythmias occur, are the only identifiable differences between torsade de pointes and polymorphic VTach.

The term torsade de pointes, from which the arrhythmia derives its name, means literally the "turning of the points." The "turning" is a morphological feature that is obvious on Figure 32-2. Notice how this strip is identical to Figure 32-1, except for the presence of the prolonged QT interval during the normal sinus segment of the strip.

The typical rates of torsade de pointes are between 200 and 250 BPM, although rates from 150 to 300 BPM have been documented. The complexes appear to be

CLINICAL PEARL

The causes of QT prolongation include:

1. AMI and ischemia

2. Hypocalcemia

3. Drugs: Class IA antiarrhythmics, amiodarone, phenothiazines, tricyclic antidepressants

4. CNS events

5. Hypothermia

6. Hypothyroidism

7. Congenital or idiopathic prolonged QT syndromes

Be very careful administering medications that prolong the QT to someone who has a prolonged QT!

Prolonged QT Interval and the QTc

Most of the problems that we encounter with the QT interval are related to a prolongation of the interval. Prolongation of the QT interval is different from prolongation of the PR interval. If the PR is prolonged, it is usually because of a diseased node or some pharmacologic agent. In general, a prolonged PR interval, when it occurs by itself, is not too clinically significant. QT prolongation, on the other hand, can be life threatening. Why? Because prolonged QT intervals have a tendency to break down into very bad arrhythmias, such as torsade de pointes. Take a look at the ECG strip in Figure 32-3.

The QT interval is dependent on the underlying rate of the patient. In general, the slower the heart rate, the longer the QT interval. The faster the heart rate, the shorter the QT interval. Because of these rate-related changes, a separate measure known as the QTc has been developed. The "c" stands for corrected; corrected for rate, that is. The QTc is considered prolonged if it is over 0.419 seconds, and markedly prolonged if it is over 0.440 seconds.

A good general rule of thumb is this: If the patient is not markedly tachycardic, the QT interval should not be more than half of the R-R interval. Let's look at Figure 32-3. If we place our calipers over the QT interval and then walk them over, the caliper marked B should be before the next QRS complex. If it is after the next QRS, you can bet that the QT is prolonged.

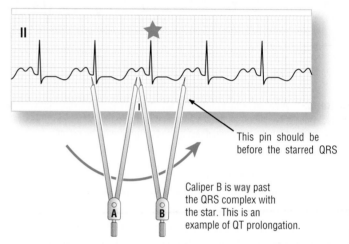

This pin should be before the starred QRS

Caliper B is **way** past the QRS complex with the star. This is an example of QT prolongation.

Figure 32-3: QT prolongation. If you place your caliper pins as marked by ECG caliper A, you are measuring the QT interval of the complex. You should be able to walk the calipers over (side B) and still have the pin fall before the next QRS complex. If the caliper pin falls after the next QRS complex, the distance is more than half of the R-R interval and the QT interval is prolonged.

"grouped" just as in polymorphic VTach, with each group being composed of anywhere between 5 and 20 complexes each. Once again, the "grouping" occurs because of a twisting of the polarity around a central baseline. The morphological appearance of each of the complexes will usually vary constantly throughout the strip.

Just as we saw in polymorphic VTach, torsade de pointes is very dependent on the underlying rate of the patient prior to the development of the tachycardia. The rate frequently develops in patients with severe bradycardia or experiencing an AV block. The arrhythmia is usually suppressed if the baseline heart rate is increased. The arrhythmia can be terminated by speeding up the tachycardia either by drugs (e.g., isoproterenol) or by overdrive pacing.

The severity of symptoms is usually associated with the duration of the tachycardia. Torsade de pointes is usually self-limiting, but it can also break down into ventricular fibrillation.

Due to the more frequent occurrence of torsade de pointes, compared with polymorphic VTach, and because they are essentially only clinical variants, torsade de pointes has literally "taken over" as the main terminology used to label this rhythm presentation. In essence, people preferentially use the term torsade de pointes to refer to either of the two rhythms and frequently use the terms interchangeably. For completeness, and because the therapeutic strategies can be different, you should be aware that they are two separate arrhythmias.

The keystone to treatment of the arrhythmia is to reverse the cause of the QT prolongation if possible. Magnesium sulfate can be very effective in terminating the arrhythmia and stabilizing cell membranes in many cases. Overdrive pacing or drugs to speed the tachycardia are also useful. If the patient is hemodynamically unstable, cardioversion or defibrillation should be attempted.

Onset of Torsade de Pointes

Torsade de pointes is also triggered by a PVC in most cases. However, due to the prolonged QT intervals present in the baseline rhythm, the chances of falling during the relative refractory period are greater in these patients (Figure 32-4). As you can imagine, if the interval is longer, the chances of having an R-on-T phenomenon are much greater than they are in a patient with a normal QT interval.

There is also a strong association between bigeminy in a patient with a prolonged QT interval and the development of torsade de pointes. Once again, the chances of an R-on-T phenomenon are greater in these patients.

The Turning of the Points

In this section, we are going to spend some time going over the actual "turning of the points" that develops in these patients due to a constant change in the polarity of the complexes. First, let's go over the actual appearance on the ECG and why we get such a strange pattern of grouping. Then, we will go into why these changes in polarity occur.

At this point in our lives, we should all be familiar with party streamers. Let's imagine that we had a party streamer with a different color on each side, and a long, uninterrupted episode of ventricular tachycardia recorded on it (Figure 32-5). How do we hang party streamers? Well, we usually twist them around to create a spiral or helical appearance. This is exactly what happens in torsade de pointes. In essence, the vectors are twisting in the heart. The ECG is just simply recording the spiral effect and this spiraling gives rise to the appearance of the "twisting of the points" and the grouping.

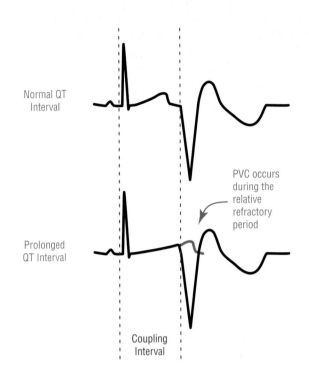

Figure 32-4: A PVC appearing at a fixed coupling interval will not fall on the relative refractory period of a patient with a normal QT interval. However, a PVC occurring with the same coupling interval would fall within the relative refractory period of a patient with a prolonged QT. This R-on-T type of phenomenon will increase the likelihood of developing torsade de pointes in these patients.

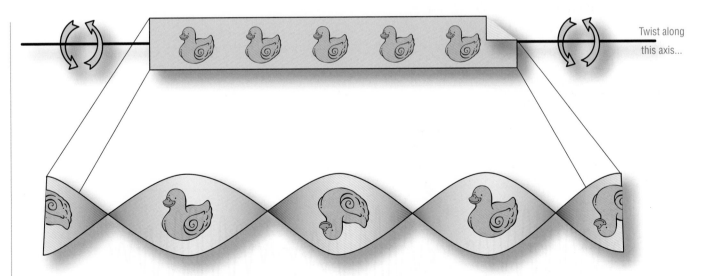

Figure 32-5: A party streamer with a different color on each side and an episode of uninterrupted VTach imprinted on it. If we were to take that streamer and twist it along a horizontal axis, we would create a spiral appearance with the two colors showing at regular intervals. In addition, the tracing would be upright in some sections and inverted in the others, depending on the length of the spiral.

This gives you a general idea of why the ECG tracings appear the way they do in patients with polymorphic VTach and torsade de pointes. Now let's turn our attention to the actual cause of the "twisting."

As you know, the ECG tracing is only a graphical representation of the vectors occurring in the heart. The mechanisms causing torsade de pointes are complex and are still being examined closely. They are beyond the scope of this book. But, we can use another analogy to help us understand the twisting a little better. Imagine you had a ventricular vector placed as the arrow of a game wheel (Figure 32-6). As you spin the vector, the electrical lead recording the vector would at first see the vector coming at it, then it would see it going away from it, then coming at it, and so forth.

A vector heading toward an electrode is recorded as a positive QRS complex. The QRS is the most positive when it is pointing directly toward the electrode. A vector heading away from an electrode is recorded as a negative QRS complex. The QRS is most negative when it is pointing directly away from the electrode. Vectors headed at a 90-degree angle from the electrode are isoelectric. Vectors falling anywhere in between these points give rise to complexes of varying sizes and polarities. ***It is this constant changing of the orientation of the electrical vector in the heart that leads to the twisting***

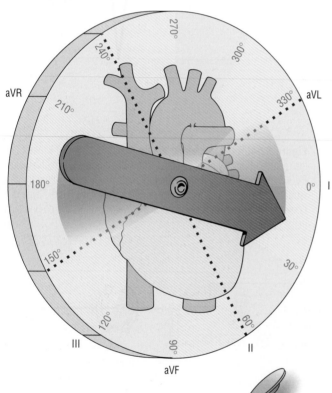

Figure 32-6: Imagine the main electrical axis of the heart (blue and pink vector) sitting on top of a big game wheel on the surface of the heart. An electrode recording the spinning motion that Vanna placed on this vector would record an undulating pattern on the paper, depending on the orientation of the vector in relation to the electrode; in this case, it is lead II. Since the orientation of the vector is constantly changing as it spins, the pattern on the ECG undulates.

When the vector points directly at the electrode, the QRS complexes will be the tallest and in a positive direction. When the vector points directly away from the electrode, the QRS complexes will be their deepest and in a negative direction. When the vectors are facing 90 degrees to the electrode, the complexes will be the smallest.

pattern found in polymorphic VTach and torsade de pointes.

Remember, the picture created on the ECG or rhythm strip by each lead is different. The helical nature of the twisting in torsade de pointes can be seen in some leads but may not be evident in others. Whenever you have a very rapid wide tachycardia, and you have the time, you should try to obtain a full 12-lead ECG to evaluate the rhythm further. An irregular wide-complex rhythm at this rate could be atrial fibrillation that is completely out of control (possibly in a patient with WPW syndrome or an accessory pathway), or it could be torsade de pointes. The 12-lead ECG is a very important tool in deciding between these two possibilities. If you cannot obtain a full 12-lead ECG because the patient is unstable, then trying several different leads may also give you the information you need to make your decision.

Causes of Torsade de Pointes

There are quite a large number of predisposing factors that can lead to torsade. In this section, we are going to list them individually and give a short description of the problem. These lists are not intended to be all-inclusive, but rather to point out the most common causes.

Slow Heart Rates   Torsade de pointes is more likely to occur in patients with severe bradycardia or in patients with severe AV blocks. There appears to be a regional repolarization abnormality found in susceptible patients who develop the arrhythmia when they are bradycardic. The bradycardia in these patients is usually associated with prolongation of the QT interval.

Direct Drug Effects   Many drugs used to treat arrhythmias prolong the QT interval and cause repolarization abnormalities. These include the class IA antiarrhythmics (quinidine, procainamide, and disopyramide), adenosine, class III drugs (sotalol, amiodarone, ibutilide). Some of the psychotropics (e.g. phenothiazines and tricyclic antidepressants), have been known to prolong the QT and lead to torsade. Intravenous haloperidol has been associated with QT prolongation. There have been many case reports for other medications and many others have an effect on the QT interval. All of those drugs should be used with caution in patients with prolonged QT intervals at baseline.

Of the drugs listed above that commonly cause torsade, quinidine appears to be the one that causes the most cases and amiodarone appears to have the least effect. The clinician needs to keep in mind the possible QT-prolonging effects of these drugs and assess and monitor patients accordingly.

Drug Combinations   In addition to direct effects, many drugs have been found to cause QT prolongation and an increased risk for torsade when used in combination with others. The major drugs that cause QT prolongation as a consequence of a drug-drug interaction include the antifungals (ketoconazole, fluconazole) and the macrolide antibiotics (erythromycin, clarithromycin). Two drugs that especially cause interactions with these are terfenadine and cispride.

These drugs should be used cautiously, if at all, in patients with prolonged QT intervals. The dangerous combinations mentioned above should not be used under any circumstances, if possible.

Electrolyte Imbalances   Hypokalemia is the biggest culprit in this bunch. Hypokalemia is frequently associated with prolongation of the QT interval and the prevalence of large U waves. These findings are due to the repolarization abnormalities that are occurring in the ventricles due to the electrolyte imbalance. The repolarization abnormalities, in turn, lead to an increased propensity for torsade de pointes.

Hypomagnesemia and hypocalcemia are also associated with an increased chance of developing torsade, although they both remain a rare cause of the arrhythmia. Both prolong the QT interval and cause repolarization abnormalities.

Congenital Long QT Syndromes   There are some genetic disorders that are related to a familial predisposition to the development of sudden cardiac death due to an underlying prolongation of the QT interval. The sudden cardiac death in these cases has been caused by either torsade de pointes or ventricular fibrillation. The genetic defects in these disorders are being isolated down to the level of the ionic channels on the cell membranes.

Prolongation of the QT interval, torsade de pointes, or sudden death, and the presence of familial deafness are the key characteristics of Jervell and Lange-Nielsen syndrome. The Romano-Ward syndrome has the same prolongation of the QT interval and an association with torsade and sudden death, but these patients have normal hearing.

Clinical presentation of individual patients is variable and there are many differences among patients in the age of onset, presenting symptoms, and severity of symptoms. Syncope is a common presenting symptom for many of these patients. We have personally treated patients with these syndromes who were misdiagnosed all their lives and considered either to have psychological issues for their syncope or thought to be simply faking their symptoms. Always check the QT interval on any patient with syncope!

Acute Myocardial Infarction   Severe ischemia and acute myocardial infarction are associated with an increased risk of both polymorphic VTach and torsade de pointes.

Metabolic Disorders   Various metabolic disorders have been associated with the development of torsade de pointes. These include hypothyroidism, "liquid protein" or fad dieting, starvation, anorexia nervosa, intracranial hemorrhages, large strokes, and encephalitis. Finally, with the increased focus on terrorism, we should men-

tion that poisoning with organophosphates can cause torsade de pointes.

A final word. . .always keep in mind the various causes of an arrhythmia. In most cases, focused treatment of the source of the problem will help terminate the arrhythmia or will be instrumental in preventing future episodes from occurring. These principles apply to torsade, just as much as they apply to every other rhythm abnormality in this book.

ADDITIONAL INFORMATION

T-wave Alternans

There is one electrocardiographic morphological abnormality that is rarely found in patients with torsade de pointes. We say rarely because it is rarely found on a plain surface rhythm strip or even a 12-lead ECG. However, digital or computerized signal averaging techniques are finding that micro-events of this nature are more common than expected in patients with proven torsade

de pointes. That electrocardiographic morphological abnormality is known as *T-wave alternans* (Figure 32-7).

The main point to keep in mind with T-wave alternans is that the patient will be at greater risk of developing torsade de pointes, especially if the underlying QT interval is prolonged. Close observation and a consultation with a cardiologist or an electrophysiologist are strongly encouraged.

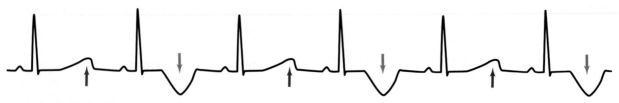

Figure 32-7: T-wave alternans.

ARRHYTHMIA RECOGNITION

Torsade de Pointes

Don't forget: Torsade de pointes is associated with a prolonged QT interval!

Rate:	150 to 300 BPM
Regularity:	Irregular
P wave:	None
Morphology:	None
Upright in II, III, and aVF:	None
P:QRS ratio:	None
PR interval:	None
QRS width:	Wide
Grouping:	5 to 20 ventricular complexes
Dropped beats:	None

DIFFERENTIAL DIAGNOSIS

Torsade de Pointes

1. Slow heart rates and AV blocks
2. Direct drug effects
   Quinidine
   Procainamide
   Disopyramide
   Sotalol
   Amiodarone
   Ibutilide
   Phenothiazines
   Tricyclic antidepressants
   IV haloperidol
   Many other drugs. . .
3. Drug combinations
   Antifungals (ketoconazole, fluconazole)
   Macrolide antibiotics (erythromycin, clarithromycin)
   Terfenadine
   Cisapride
4. Electrolyte imbalances
   Hypokalemia
   Hypomagnesemia
   Hypocalcemia
5. Congenital long QT syndrome
   Jervell and Lange-Nielsen syndrome
   Romano-Ward syndrome
6. Acute myocardial infarction and ischemia
7. Metabolic disorders
   Hypothyroidism
   Dieting
   Starvation
   Anorexia nervosa
   Intracranial hemorrhage
   Stroke
   Encephalitis
   Organophosphate poisoning

The list above is not inclusive but reflects the most common causes of the arrhythmia.

ECG Strips

ECG 32-1

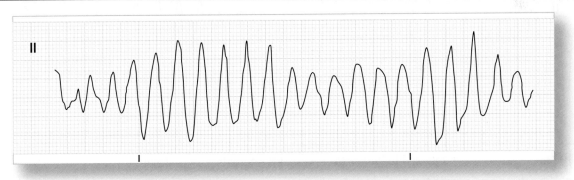

Rate:	About 250 BPM	PR intervals:	None
Regularity:	Irregular	QRS width:	Wide
P waves:	None	Grouping:	Ventricular complexes
Morphology:	None		
Axis:	None	Dropped beats:	Absent
P:QRS ratio:	None	Rhythm:	**Torsade de pointes**

Discussion:

The rhythm strip above shows the typical undulating pattern that is classic for torsade de pointes. The rate varies from beat-to-beat as expected from a completely irregular rhythm. Note the morphology differences between most of the complexes. The morphology varies not only in amplitude and polarity, but also in the actual makeup of each of the ventricular complexes.

ECG 32-2

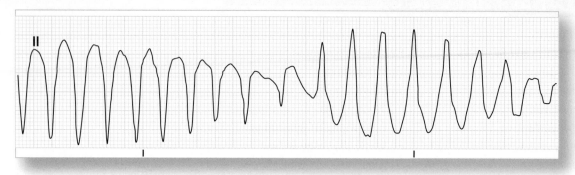

Rate:	About 170 BPM	PR intervals:	None
Regularity:	Irregular	QRS width:	Wide
P waves:	None	Grouping:	Yes
Morphology:	None		
Axis:	None	Dropped beats:	Absent
P:QRS ratio:	None	Rhythm:	**Torsade de pointes**

Discussion:

This strip also shows the same undulating pattern that is classic for torsade. In this example, the polarity of the two groups is very evident, with the group on the left showing a negative polarity (the QRS complexes are negative and point downward), while the group on the right shows a positive polarity (the QRS complexes are positive and point upward).

ECG 32-3

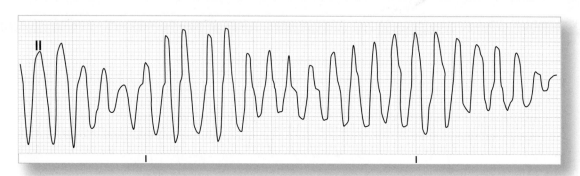

Rate:	About 260 to 280 BPM	PR intervals:	None
Regularity:	Irregular	QRS width:	Wide
P waves:	None	Grouping:	Ventricular complexes
Morphology:	None		
Axis:	None	Dropped beats:	Absent
P:QRS ratio:	None	Rhythm:	**Torsade de pointes**

Discussion:

This is another classic example of torsade de pointes. Once again, the morphological differences mentioned above are also applicable to this strip. Note that the number of complexes in each group can vary and is a normal finding in almost all strips showing torsade.

ECG 32·4

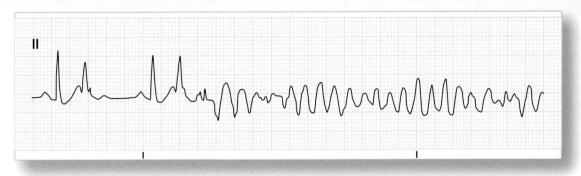

Rate:	See discussion	PR intervals:	See discussion
Regularity:	Irregular	QRS width:	Variable
P waves: Morphology: Axis:	Present at start Normal Upright	Grouping:	None
		Dropped beats:	Absent
P:QRS ratio:	See discussion	Rhythm:	**Torsade de pointes**

Discussion:

This ECG shows a patient who is having a run of bigeminy. It is unclear from this strip if the bigeminy is composed of PJCs or PVCs, because we do not see the start of the complex. The patient then begins to show a very rapid, irregular rhythm. At this point, an argument can be made as to whether this is ventricular tachycar-dia or torsade de pointes. This is because the rate is very, very fast—greater than 300 BPM in some places. Additional leads demonstrated a more traditional torsade pattern that, as mentioned, is not clearly apparent on this strip.

CHAPTER REVIEW

1. Polymorphic VTach and torsade de pointes are two separate rhythms. True or False.

2. Torsade de pointes is a variant of polymorphic VTach. True or False.

3. When the patient is in sinus rhythm, the QRS complexes in polymorphic VTach have a _____ QT interval.

4. When the patient is in sinus rhythm, the QRS complexes in torsade de pointes have a _____ QT interval.

5. Polymorphic VTach usually occurs in patients having (pick the best one):
   A. Acute myocardial infarction
   B. Hypothyroidism
   C. Ischemia
   D. Congenital syndromes
   E. Both A and C
   F. Both B and D
   G. All of the above

6. Both torsade and polymorphic VTach have groups of ventricular complexes (composed of 5 to 20 complexes) that seem to form groups. These groups are actually caused by a "twisting" of the polarity of the QRS complexes. True or False.

7. The ventricular rates in torsade and polymorphic VTach are between _____ and _____ BPM. Typically, both rhythms present around the 200 to 250 BPM range.

8. Torsade de pointes is not related to the underlying rate of the patient when he or she is not tachycardic in any way. True or False.

9. Both torsade and polymorphic VTach are usually self-limiting. They can, however, be sustained or break down into more malignant rhythms like ventricular fibrillation. True or False.

10. The following is NOT a cause of torsade de pointes:
    A. Direct drug effects
    B. Hypokalemia
    C. Intracranial hemorrhage
    D. Hypercalcemia
    E. Romano-Ward syndrome

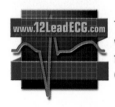

To enhance the knowledge you gain in this book, access this text's website at www.12leadECG.com! This valuable resource provides flashcards, an online glossary, web links, and more. Simply click on the Arrhythmias book cover once at the site.

How to Approach a Wide-Complex Tachycardia

General Overview

To review, a wide-complex tachycardia is a rhythm with at least three wide, ectopic ventricular complexes in a row at a rate above 100 BPM. Statistics have shown that over 80% of wide-complex tachycardias are caused by ventricular tachycardia. The rest are supraventricular tachycardias that occur in patients with pre-existing bundle branch blocks, electrolyte imbalances, accessory pathways, or are just simply aberrantly conducted in the ventricles.

In Chapter 27, we examined the differential diagnosis of narrow-complex or supraventricular tachycardias. In this chapter, we are going to address one of the most critical topics that any clinician will ever face: The differential diagnosis of the wide-complex tachycardias. The principles we are going to review in this chapter can also be used when looking at individual complexes or the slower wide-complex rhythms.

Why are we placing such importance on this one interpretive skill, especially since 80% of wide-complex tachycardias are going to be VTach anyway? There are two big reasons. The principal, most important reason is the life-threatening nature of the wide-complex tachycardias. We spent a great deal of time in Chapter 27 going over the hemodynamics involved in the narrow-complex tachycardias and discussing the need for coordinated, controlled mechanical contractions of the ventricles. Well, as you can imagine, the problems we talked about there are greatly multiplied in the wide-complex rhythms.

The second reason to accurately identify the wide-complex tachycardias, and the reason that this particular skill is becoming increasingly more important to clinicians every day, is the pharmacological advances that have recently been made for the management of arrhythmias. We now have at our disposal many drugs that specifically target the various components of the heart and the bioelectrical pathways that cause the various arrhythmias. More importantly, the future will bring even more specific and more arrhythmia-selective agents to the market every day.

Here is a typical example of how modern pharmacological options are affecting clinical decision making. No one argues that if a patient is hemodynamically unstable, emergent cardioversion is the treatment of choice for either a narrow- or wide-complex tachycardia. But that is where the similarities between the two types of tachycardias end. The American Heart Association in their *ACLS Guidelines 2000* have made it a clear point to state that any clinician treating a patient with a wide-complex tachycardia must try to distinguish between ventricular tachycardia and a supraventricular tachycardia (SVT) with aberrancy. Why?

The need to differentiate between a supraventricular tachycardia with aberrancy and a ventricular tachycardia is primarily based on the fact that the medical protocols used to treat these two rhythm disturbances vary greatly in their general approach and in the medications used to treat them. In fact, some pharmaceutical agents used to treat one arrhythmia can actually worsen another. In clear language, *an exact diagnosis leads to focused treatment and a focused cure*. Inappropriate, and unfocused, treatment of an untypable arrhythmia may lead to serious consequences, even death.

Generally speaking, a clinician should be able to distinguish between an SVT with aberrancy and a VTach with a great degree of certainty in most cases. In fact, some authors have suggested that with a little care, this level of distinction can be reached in as many as 90% of wide-complex tachycardias. All it takes is a little time and knowing what to look for.

Having a road map will usually make traveling and arriving at your destination a much smoother operation. Hopefully, after reading and understanding this chapter, you will have a road map on how to approach any wide-complex tachycardia.

That said, we cannot emphasize strongly enough that if you are faced with an untypable wide-complex tachycardia, you should treat it as if it were ventricular tachycardia. As mentioned above, statistics would be on your side, since over 80% of the wide-complex tachycardias are VTach. Missing this arrhythmia and treating it as if it were supraventricular with aberrancy could be a very costly mistake.

The Approach

When approaching a patient with a wide-complex tachycardia, it is extremely important to put together as complete a clinical picture as possible *in as little time as possible*. With a little practice, the analysis can be accomplished in seconds. The list below outlines the main things that you should look for:

1. AV dissociation
2. Capture beats
3. Fusion beats
4. Presence of P waves
5. Regular or irregular?
6. QRS morphology
   a. Multiple leads
   b. How wide are the complexes?
   c. Josephson's sign
   d. Brugada's sign
   e. Morphology of associated PVCs
   f. QRS morphology in lead V_1
   g. QRS morphology in lead V_6
7. Electrical axis in the extreme right quadrant
8. Concordance in the precordial leads
9. History
   a. Prior history of tachycardias
   b. Medications
   c. History of MI, CHF, structural heart disease
10. Physical examination
    a. Cannon A waves
    b. Response to vagal stimulation

By focusing on the main points outlined above, you should be able to develop a solid foundation to help you deal with the differential diagnosis of the wide-complex tachycardias. We have reviewed these topics at length in the previous chapters. In this chapter, we are going to revisit each one of the these points, but we will be looking at them in a different light. At the end of the chapter, we are going to pull it all together with a trial case and put our new reasoning powers to a pretty tough test.

AV Dissociation

Electrocardiographically, a complete AV block develops because of a lack of communication between the atria and the ventricles. Essentially, the AV node shuts down all communication between them. The atrioventricular septum and the nonfunctional node essentially form an electronic barrier between the atria and the ventricles (Figure 33-1). The supraventricular pacemakers are, therefore, oblivious to occurrences in the ventricles and continue to fire normally to depolarize the atria. By the

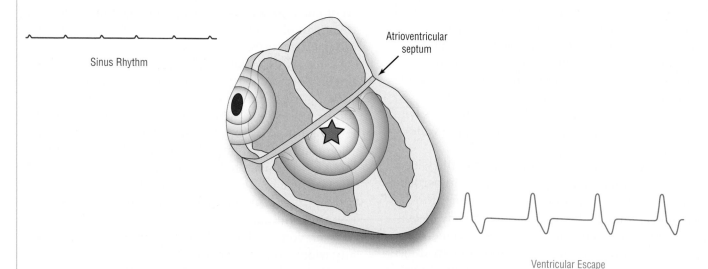

Sinus Rhythm

Atrioventricular septum

Ventricular Escape

Figure 33-1: When the AV node is not conducting, it creates, functionally, a complete block at the level of the interventricular septum. The atria and the ventricles are completely oblivious to each other, and two separate pacemakers develop. Each pacemaker will keep its own intrinsic rate and control its respective chamber.

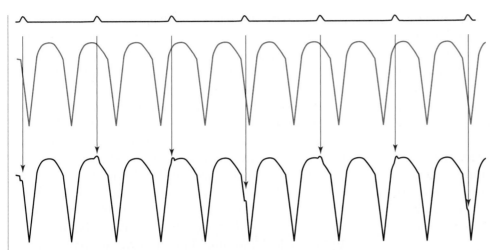

Figure 33-2: The atria and the ventricles are completely oblivious to each other and there are two separate pacemakers. Each pacemaker will keep its own intrinsic rate and control their respective chambers. The ECG fuses these two rhythms into one strip electrocardiographically (see strip in black). This is ventricular tachycardia with AV dissociation.

same token, the ventricular pacemakers, which are oblivious to occurrences in the atria, take over the pacing function for the ventricles as part of the failsafe system, essentially creating their own ventricular rhythm. The net result is two separate rhythms occurring simultaneously. One is the regular sinus or any supraventricular rhythm, and the other one is of ventricular origin.

If the ventricles and the atria were completely noncommunicable, the atrial rhythm and the ventricular rhythm would still *electrocardiographically* fuse to form a ventricular tachycardia with P waves marching through it. But, in these cases the supraventricular rhythm would not affect the ventricular rhythm in any way. This can, and does, occur in many examples of VTach (Figure 33-2).

More commonly, instead of a complete block, the constant barrage from the rapid ectopic ventricular complexes created by a ventricular reentry circuit *functionally* close down the AV node by causing it to remain in an almost constant refractory state. In other words, the AV node will almost always be refractory to the supraventricular impulses because of the constant barrage from the ventricular complexes coming at it from below. In these cases, there can still be some form of communication between the atria and the ventricles because this is really not a pathological AV node problem but a *refractory* or *functional* AV node problem.

Since the AV node is still structurally normal (in most cases), an occasional supraventricular complex will reach the AV node during just the right millisecond

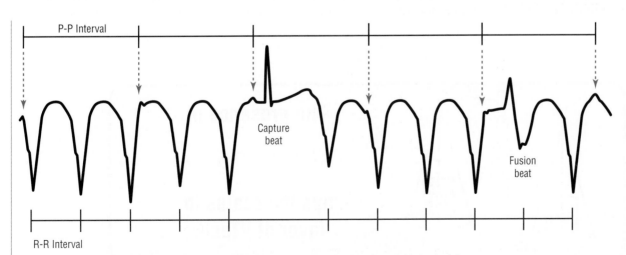

Figure 33-3: Ventricular tachycardia is quite frequently associated with AV dissociation. Always look for P waves, capture beats, and fusion beats!

and this one impulse will get through to completely capture the ventricles or cause a fusion complex (Figure 33-3). This type of partial communication between the atria and the ventricles is known as AV dissociation. The occasional transmission of a supraventricular impulse through the normal conduction system seen in AV dissociation is how capture beats and fusion complexes are formed.

With close examination, approximately 50% of wide-complex tachycardias will show some evidence of AV dissociation. That means that in approximately 50% of the wide-complex strips that you will see, you will have essentially made the diagnosis of VTach by just looking for this one finding!

Electrocardiographically, AV dissociation is the most important thing to look for in any wide-complex tachycardia. If you notice, the first three characteristics of wide-complex tachycardia that we mentioned on our original list have to do with either the direct or the indirect signs of AV dissociation. *For clinical purposes, any wide-complex tachycardia associated with AV dissociation is going to be ventricular tachycardia.* There is, however, only one rare exception. . .

Very rarely, AV dissociation can occur with a junctional tachycardia in a patient with a pre-existing bundle branch block or an accessory pathway. The rhythm and clinical conditions we are talking about are individually rare or uncommon. The fact that this can occur at the same time is so rare that, in fact, you can almost completely discount that possibility. We just mention it for completeness.

Capture Beats

As mentioned above, ventricular tachycardia is usually not associated with a complete block between the atria and the ventricles, but rather with a functional AV dissociation. This dissociation still allows for some minimal communication between the atria and the ventricles. Occasionally, the timing is just right and a supraventricular complex reaches the AV node when it is not refractory. The impulse is then normally spread to the ventricles via the electrical conduction system.

As you know, ventricular complexes are wide and bizarre in appearance. Supraventricular complexes are narrow due to the rapid conduction of the impulse through the normal electrical conduction system. What occurs in VTach is that you have a wide, bizarre, rapid ectopic ventricular tachycardia interspersed with occasional narrow complexes, which appear to be of supraventricular origin. These narrow, normally conducted complexes are known as capture beats.

Notice from the discussion of the paragraph above that you have to have perfect "timing" to get a capture beat. The timing needs to be just right and arrive at a functional, non-refractory AV node in order to get a ventricular capture by the supraventricular complex. In other words, you have to have AV dissociation in order to have a capture beat. The inverse of that corollary is also true: If you have a capture beat, there has to be an underlying AV dissociation. The presence of capture beats is, therefore, an indirect sign of AV dissociation.

Capture beats, along with fusion complexes, are keystone features in the diagnosis of accelerated idioventricular rhythms and ventricular tachycardia. *If you ever see a wide-complex tachycardia with a normal-looking QRS complex smack in the middle of it, the rhythm is ventricular tachycardia.*

Fusion Complexes

The fusion complexes seen in ventricular tachycardia are typically caused when the timing is such that a supraventricular complex is partially conducted *at the*

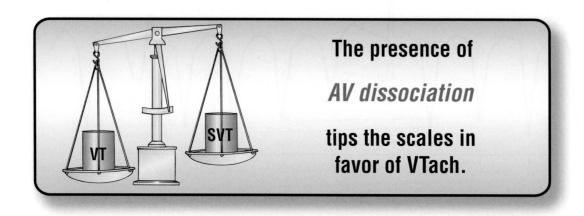

The presence of **AV dissociation** tips the scales in favor of VTach.

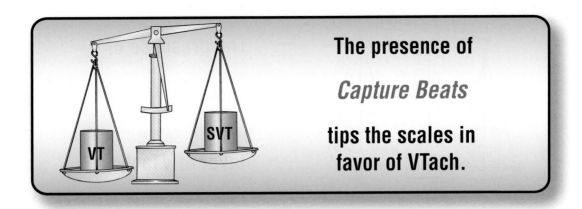

The presence of *Capture Beats* tips the scales in favor of VTach.

same time as a ventricular complex. The net result is that the fusion complex morphologically resembles the two parents (Figure 33-4). This type of fusion is an indirect sign of AV dissociation.

At the risk of being redundant, let's recap what we have said so far. *The presence of AV dissociation is the keystone feature in the diagnosis of ventricular tachycardia.* It doesn't matter whether the AV dissociation is diagnosed

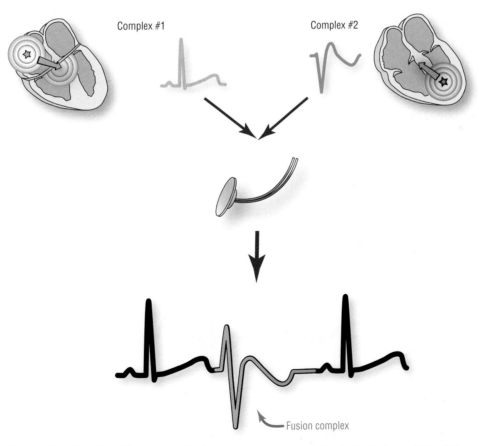

Figure 33-4: Complex #1 is a supraventricular complex being normally transmitted to the ventricles. This complex would give rise to a nice, tight QRS complex. Complex #2 originates in an ectopic ventricular focus and will give rise to an aberrant, wide QRS complex. The ECG machine translates these bits of electrical information into the fusion complex below. Note that the resulting complex resembles both parent complexes slightly.

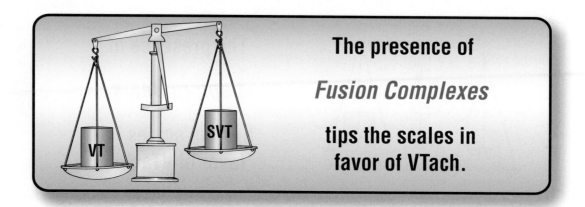

The presence of

Fusion Complexes

tips the scales in favor of VTach.

directly (by observing dissociated P waves throughout the ventricular complexes) or indirectly (by the presence of capture beats and fusion complexes).

P Waves

The presence of upright P waves on a strip from leads II, III, or aVF shows that the P waves have to originate in a supraventricular site, whether associated with a tachycardia or not. Let's take a look at why this occurs. In order for a P wave to be upright in leads II, III, or aVF, the vector causing it has to proceed from a superior direction to an inferior direction (see Chapter 8 for a full discussion). The superior-to-inferior route is the normal one taken by most supraventricular pacemakers, including the sinus node. Therefore, an upright P wave in leads II, III, and aVF has to originate in a supraventricular pacemaker.

On the other hand, P waves originating in some ectopic atrial sites, the AV node, or spread retrogradely from the ventricles, have to be inverted in leads II, III, and aVF. This occurs because their vectors proceed from an inferior to a superior direction. Therefore, inverted P waves in leads II, III, and aVF can be either supraventricular or ventricular in origin. Because of this uncertainty, you cannot use this finding to rule in or rule out either location as the origin for a wide-complex tachycardia (Figure 33-5).

Likewise, the lack of any observable P waves cannot help you either way. There are many supraventricular tachycardias in which the P waves are not visible or could be fused with the QRS complex or T wave. Ventricular tachycardia can also cause retrograde stimulation of the atria that can be lost in the wide ectopic ventricular complexes, or there could be no atrial activation whatsoever.

The presence of upright P waves in leads II, III, and aVF that are clearly dissociated from the QRS complexes in a wide-complex tachycardia are a clear sign of

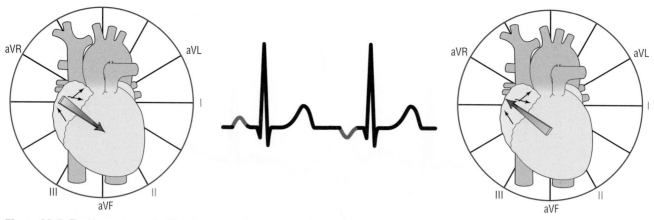

Figure 33-5: The blue vector on the left is headed inferiorly, backward, and to the left. Leads II, III, and aVF see a positive vector headed toward them, and this is represented as a positive P wave of definite supraventricular origin in those leads. The red vector on the right is headed superiorly, backward, and to the right. Leads II, III, and aVF see a positive vector headed away from them, and this is represented as a positive P wave. Inverted P waves can occur in ectopic atrial, junctional, or ventricular origin. You need to look at other variables, like the PR interval, in order to shed more light on the origin of these complexes.

NOTE

You could see dissociated and inverted P waves in a wide-complex tachycardia if the origin of the P waves was in certain lower ectopic atrial sites or if the P waves were from the AV node itself. In these cases, the rule of AV dissociation being VTach still holds true because the P waves originate in a supraventricular site. If the retrograde P waves were from a ventricular source, they would have to occur in a 1: 1 ratio with the ventricular complexes and the R:P ratio would have to remain consistent. Almost by definition, AV dissociation has to have variable and non-consistent R:P ratios. The only exception would be if the atrial and ventricular rhythms have the exact rate. This would be a rare occurrence between the rates of 100 and 300 BPM, the rate needed to call a wide-complex rhythm VTach.

a ventricular tachycardia. This is an extremely useful finding, as mentioned in the previous three sections of this chapter.

Regular or Irregular?

Wide-complex tachycardias can be either regular or irregular. The regular wide-complex tachycardias include monomorphic ventricular tachycardia and the regular SVTs with wide QRS complexes due to either a pre-existing bundle branch block, aberrancy, accessory pathways, or electrolyte disorders.

Monomorphic VTach can be slightly irregular right at the onset and in the period immediately after, but quickly becomes very regular once it gets going. Polymorphic VTach and torsade de pointes are irregular due to the morphological and polarity differences between the complexes. The undulations caused by the polarity shifts should help you identify these two possibilities.

The regular SVTs include sinus tachycardia, ectopic atrial tachycardia, junctional tachycardia, AVNRT, AVRT, and atrial flutter. AVRT can create a wide-complex tachycardia when due to one of the problems mentioned above or when the AVRT is due to an antidromic circuit. Irregular SVTs include atrial flutter and atrial fibrillation.

Rapid atrial fibrillation creates a very serious diagnostic challenge in many cases. When the atrial fibrillation is associated with wide complexes, it can easily

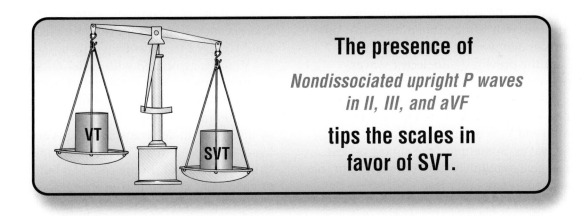

The presence of

Nondissociated upright P waves in II, III, and aVF

tips the scales in favor of SVT.

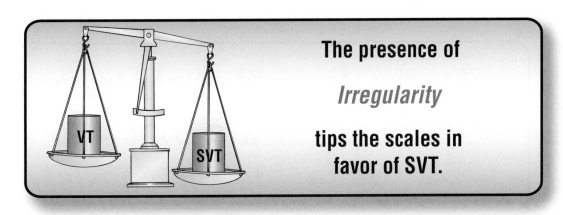

The presence of

Irregularity

tips the scales in favor of SVT.

resemble monomorphic VTach or polymorphic VTach. In general, atrial fibrillation will always have some variation in the morphology of the QRS complexes due to fusion and aberrancy. When the atrial fibrillation is above 250 BPM, you need to think very seriously about the presence of an accessory pathway.

Morphology

We will individually address the main morphological differences that can be used to differentiate between the different wide-complex tachycardias below.

Multiple Leads   The need to obtain multiple leads in evaluating any arrhythmia, let alone a wide-complex tachycardia, cannot be stressed enough. The other thing to stress about this topic is that you should obtain various leads or a full 12-lead ECG only if you have the time to obtain it safely. Remember, it doesn't matter what the arrhythmia is; if it is unstable, it needs to be shocked!

Multiple leads allow clearer identification of the morphological differences that could be critical in differentiating between the wide-complex tachycardias. Many times, isoelectric segments or small amplitude will make the QRS complexes or P waves appear to be different or even absent. By obtaining multiple leads, you will be looking at the vectors from different vantage points. The different vantage point may clear up some discrepancies about amplitude or may even clearly bring out the previously isoelectric waves.

Let's clarify one point right from the start: *lead II is not always the best lead to examine an arrhythmia.* In general, it is a good solid lead to look at, but in many cases, it isn't the best. Lead V_1 is usually the best lead to examine the P waves. Sometimes, the almost useless lead of aVR can give a uniquely different viewpoint that cannot be obtained in any other lead.

A corollary to obtaining multiple leads or, better yet, a full 12-lead ECG, is to obtain a long rhythm strip. Remember, arrhythmias usually fall along a continuum and they are constantly coming, going, and changing. Many times, you can catch little things that will help your differential greatly. One of the greatest examples of this is the period around the onset or termination of the arrhythmia. This period usually provides tons of invaluable information. A monomorphic VT, for example, will usually be triggered by a PVC of identical, or very similar, morphology to the tachycardic ventricular complexes. Another example would be a PAC triggering a run of AVNRT or AVRT. Yet another example is the variations in atrial fibrillation-flutter. Always try to obtain a long rhythm strip of at least a minute or two.

Finally, always obtain a new long rhythm strip, a new look at multiple leads, or a new full 12-lead ECG, when you see any changes in the rhythm or the patient's clinical condition. The electrocardiographic or clinical change may be due to a subtle change that could signify a hidden arrhythmia problem, like the loss of atrial kick.

How Wide Are the Complexes?   The wider the QRS complex, the greater the chance that the wide-complex tachycardia is ventricular tachycardia. If the QRS complex is greater than or equal to 0.14 seconds, it favors VTach. If the QRS complex is greater than or equal to 0.16 seconds, it makes it even more likely that the wide-complex tachycardia is VTach.

VTach is associated with wider QRS complexes because usually ***all*** of the depolarization wave spreads by direct cell-to-cell transmission through ***both*** ventricles. The transmission of the entire depolarization wave by direct cell-to-cell transmission is very time consuming and will lead to a wider QRS complex on the ECG strip (Figure 33-6). In the case of a bundle branch block or aberrancy, at least part of the QRS complex moves

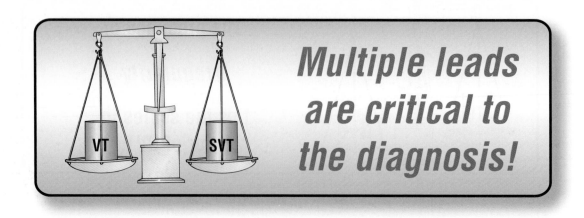

along the normal electrical conduction system (Figure 33-7). This partial transmission through the "fast" pathways significantly narrows the QRS complex. That is why the QRS complexes in bundle branch block or when associated with aberrancy are usually less than 0.14 seconds.

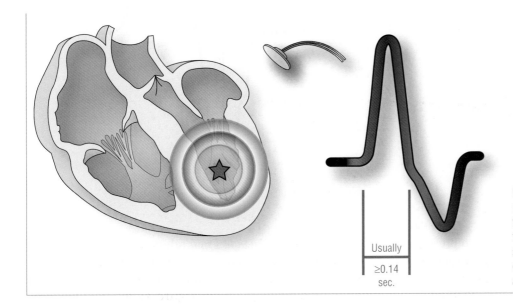

Figure 33-6: An irritable focus, represented by the red star, acts as a pacemaker and causes an impulse to occur. This gives rise to a depolarization wave that radiates outward by direct cell-to-cell transmission throughout both of the ventricles. Note the color-coded sections of the depolarization wave and the complex.

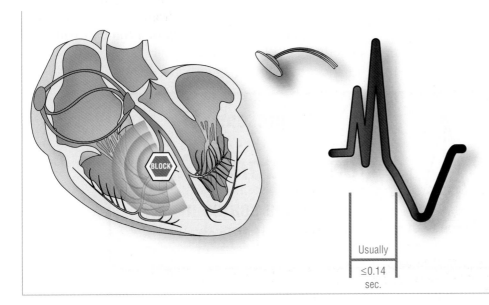

Figure 33-7: A right bundle branch block causes the depolarization wave to travel forward to the right ventricle by direct cell-to-cell contact though the right ventricle. The left ventricle was depolarized through the normal left bundle. This partial transmission through the normal left bundle branch will shorten the width of the QRS complex compared to the example above. Note: bundle branch blocks are still ≥ 0.12 seconds.

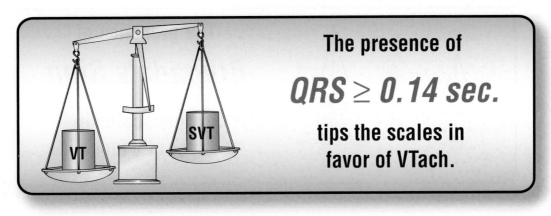

The presence of

QRS ≥ 0.14 sec.

tips the scales in favor of VTach.

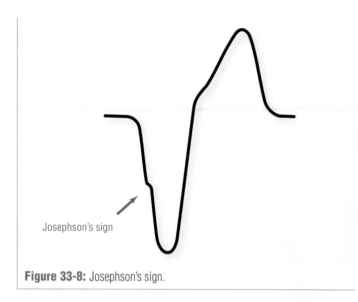

Figure 33-8: Josephson's sign.

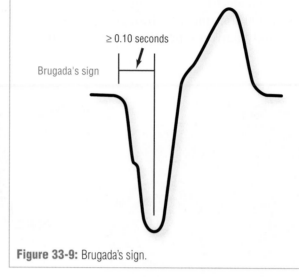

Figure 33-9: Brugada's sign.

Josephson's Sign *Josephson's sign* refers to the presence of a notch in the downstroke of the S wave present in many complexes of ventricular origin (Figure 33-8). The presence of the notch is very useful in distinguishing a ventricular complex from an aberrantly conducted supraventricular complex or a complex with an underlying LBBB or RBBB.

Brugada's Sign *Brugada's sign* refers to a distance of at least 0.10 seconds from the onset of the QRS complex to the nadir of the S wave that is present in many complexes of ventricular origin (Figure 33-9). The presence of this distance interval is a very useful sign in distinguishing a ventricular complex from an aberrantly conducted supraventricular complex or a complex with an underlying LBBB or RBBB.

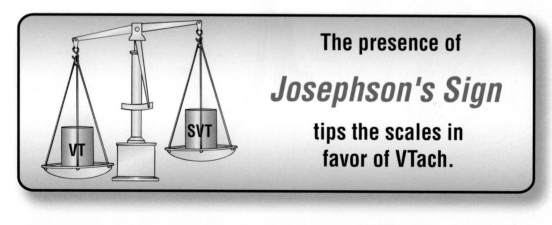

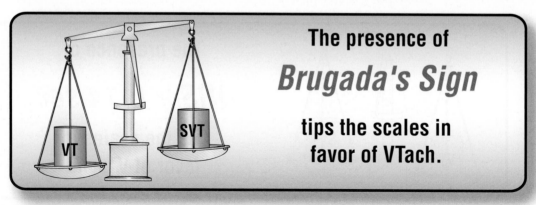

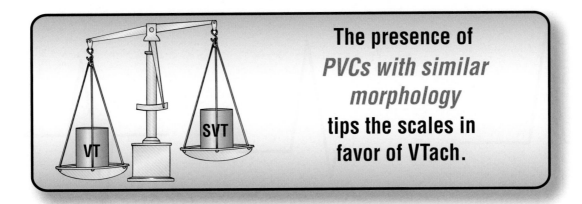

The presence of *PVCs with similar morphology* tips the scales in favor of VTach.

Morphology of the Associated PVCs   Identifiable PVCs that frequently occur during nontachycardic periods can provide a wealth of information that you can use to establish your diagnosis. If you are lucky enough to capture the onset of the arrhythmia, the morphology of any PVCs triggering the arrhythmia can really help you distinguish between your list of differentials. If the morphology of the PVC is very similar or identical to the morphology of the wide complexes, then the rhythm is probably a monomorphic VTach. Unfortunately, this rule doesn't always hold true, as any PVC can cause a reentry circuit to be formed. However, this can be used as a good indicator of VTach.

The same holds true for regularly occurring PVCs. If the morphology of unifocal PVCs found in a patient is similar or identical to that of the wide complexes in the tachycardia, the rhythm is probably monomorphic VTach.

QRS Morphology in Lead V$_1$ If the QRS complexes of the wide-complex tachycardia appear to have a right bundle branch block morphology, you have an additional clue to the possible presence of ventricular tachycardia. That additional clue is the height of the R' wave.

Normally, in a patient with supraventricular complex and a bundle branch block, the R' is taller than the R wave (Figure 33-10). This is because the vector that causes the R' is completely unopposed. Since there are no competing vectors that cancel out some of the amplitude, the R' wave is almost always taller and wider than the R wave. In an ectopic ventricular complex, there is no rule as to whether the R or the R' is taller. As a result of this discrepancy, we can state the following with some certainty: In a wide-complex tachycardia with an RBBB morphology, the presence of R greater than R' is highly suggestive of ventricular tachycardia.

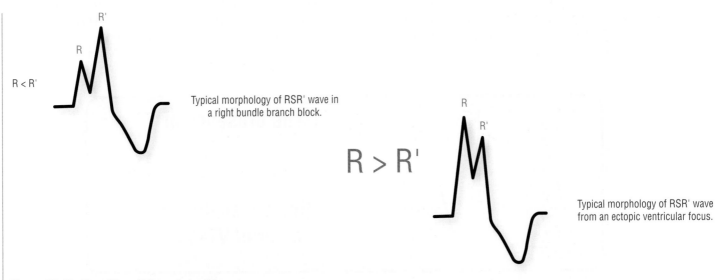

R < R'

R

R'

Typical morphology of RSR' wave in a right bundle branch block.

R > R'

R

R'

Typical morphology of RSR' wave from an ectopic ventricular focus.

Figure 33-10: Tips of the rabbit ears in lead V$_1$.

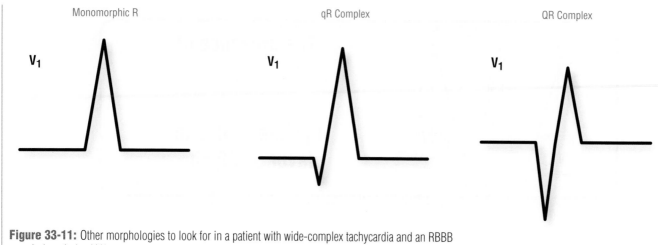

Figure 33-11: Other morphologies to look for in a patient with wide-complex tachycardia and an RBBB morphology in lead V1.

Some other things to look for include a monomorphic R, a qR, or a QR wave in lead V_1 appearing in someone with a wide-complex tachycardia with a right bundle branch block morphology. These wave patterns are graphically represented in Figure 33-11. These findings are more commonly found in ventricular tachycardia than in patients with a wide-complex supraventricular tachycardia.

QRS Morphology in Lead V_6 The criteria that can be used in lead V_6 are not as clear or as specific as those used for lead V_1. We only mention them here because of completeness. Once again, they could represent some additional findings that could help you in very difficult cases.

If the wide-complex tachycardia has a right bundle branch block morphology, the presence of an R:S ratio that is less than 1 in lead V_6 can be indicative of a ventricular tachycardia. In other words, look at lead V_6. If

NOTE

Keep in mind that these findings are more common in patients with ectopic ventricular origins for their tachycardias. However, they are not diagnostic of VTach. In other words, these findings help to point your suspicions in the direction of VTach but do not make the diagnosis a certainty. Use them as another tool in your arsenal. Remember to always interpret any arrhythmia based on all of the information and not just one or two isolated findings.

the S wave is deeper than the R wave is tall, then you have a good chance that it is VTach (Figure 33-12).

If the wide-complex tachycardia has a left bundle branch block morphology, the presence of a significant Q wave in lead V_6 can be indicative of a ventricular tachycardia (see Figure 33-12). Remember, LBBBs

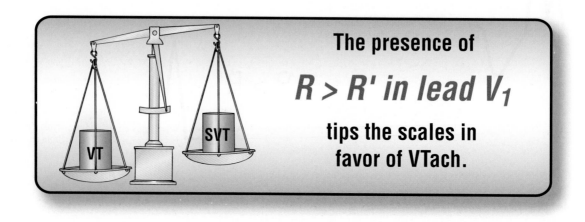

The presence of

R > R' in lead V_1

tips the scales in favor of VTach.

Examples of QRS Complexes in Lead V_6

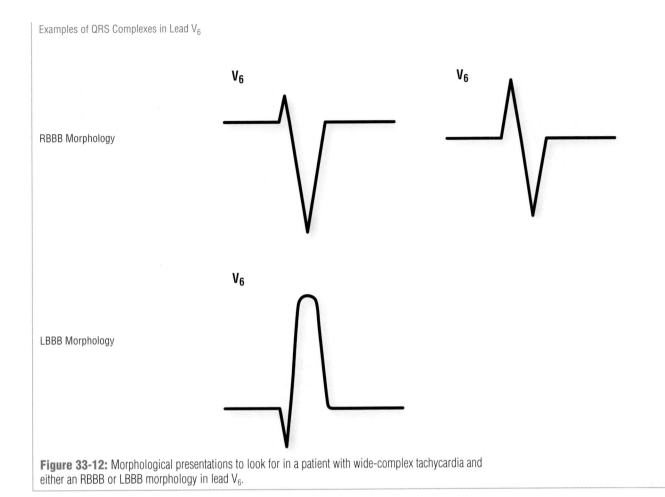

RBBB Morphology

LBBB Morphology

Figure 33-12: Morphological presentations to look for in a patient with wide-complex tachycardia and either an RBBB or LBBB morphology in lead V_6.

should not have any significant Q waves in lead V_6. They should be composed of a single monomorphic R wave. (You need to be extremely careful with these criteria, as this could also be found in a patient with LBBB and a lateral infarct. The Q wave, in these cases, would be indicative of the dead myocardium and scar formation in the ventricle.)

Electrical Axis in the Extreme Right Quadrant

We discussed the electrical axis and how to roughly calculate it in Chapter 6. As a brief review, take a look at leads I and aVF. If the complexes are negative in both leads, the axis will be in the extreme right quadrant (Figure 33-13).

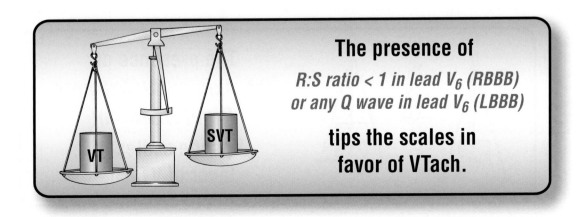

The presence of

R:S ratio < 1 in lead V_6 (RBBB)
or any Q wave in lead V_6 (LBBB)

tips the scales in
favor of VTach.

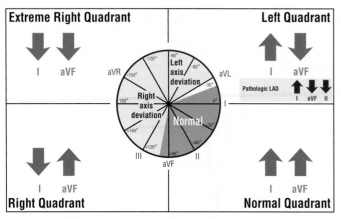

Figure 33-13: An axis is found to be in the extreme right quadrant when the QRS complexes are negative in both lead I and aVF.

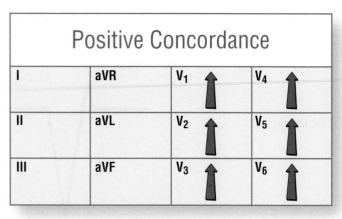

Figure 33-14: Positive concordance in VTach.

Very few things cause an axis in the extreme right quadrant. Because of this, you may sometimes hear some clinicians refer to it as having an axis in "no man's land." When you have a wide-complex tachycardia and an axis in the extreme right quadrant, the chances are great that you are dealing with ventricular tachycardia.

There are some texts that also state that an axis in the upper left quadrant also points to VTach. However, this is such a common occurrence that it is dangerous to assume that an axis in the upper left quadrant is caused by a ventricular tachycardia. Other causes include left ventricular hypertrophy, inferior and lateral myocardial infarctions, and left anterior hemiblocks.

Concordance in the Precordial Leads

A full 12-lead ECG of a patient with ventricular tachycardia will often show *concordance* of all of the QRS complexes in the precordial leads. What we mean by this is that **the main direction of all of the QRS complexes will be in the same direction, either all positive or all negative, in all of the chest or precordial leads (V_1 through V_6)**. Figures 33-14 and 33-15 show a graphical

representation of concordance of the precordial leads in a full 12-lead ECG. The size of the complex is not important, just the direction and orientation of the QRS complexes.

Concordance is yet another useful tool in evaluating the differential diagnosis of a wide-complex tachycardia. It is not definitive proof of the arrhythmia, but it is highly indicative of VTach.

History

The history is always an extremely important component of evaluating any clinical case. This is no exception in arrhythmia recognition. Many times, historical information will make the diagnosis for you. Other times, a prior history of an arrhythmia will guide you into a better strategy for the acute or long-term management of your patient. We will cover some of the relevant historical points that pertain specifically to wide-complex tachycardias in this section.

Prior History of Tachycardias   If you have the time, you should always try to obtain any relevant direct or indi-

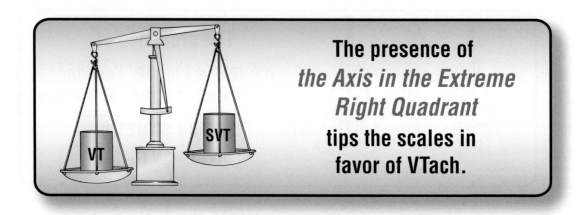

The presence of *the Axis in the Extreme Right Quadrant* tips the scales in favor of VTach.

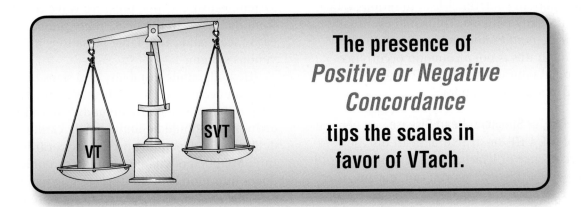

The presence of *Positive or Negative Concordance* tips the scales in favor of VTach.

Negative Concordance			
I	aVR	V₁ ⬇	V₄ ⬇
II	aVL	V₂ ⬇	V₅ ⬇
III	aVF	V₃ ⬇	V₆ ⬇

Figure 33-15: Negative concordance in VTach.

rect history of prior arrhythmias from your patient. Direct history includes any previous diagnoses of prior arrhythmias or clinical syndromes that could lead to arrhythmias. Indirect history refers to the presence of pre-syncope, syncope, palpitations, lightheadedness, or any hemodynamic compromise. Many times, the pattern and presentation of these indirect symptoms may lead you in the direction of certain arrhythmias.

A prior history of the presence of an accessory pathway or Wolff-Parkinson-White syndrome is very clinically relevant. This knowledge will certainly focus your thinking toward AV reentry tachycardia, either orthodromic or antidromic, or toward decompensated atrial flutter or fibrillation. This knowledge will also be extremely valuable in your decision regarding which pharmaceutical agents you could safely use on the patient. Accessory pathways favor SVTs as the cause of a wide-complex tachycardia.

A prior history of ventricular tachycardia, either sustained or nonsustained, will lead you in the direction of a possible recurrence. In the same way, a history of

multiple PVCs, couplets, or triplets will also steer you in the direction of a possible VTach rather than an SVT.

Ask your patients to tap out the cadence of their palpitations. Many times, patients will tap out an irregular rhythm, which will definitely be a great aid in narrowing your differential.

Medications   Always take a detailed history of medication use, prescription and nonprescription, when the clinical situation allows you the luxury of time. It is very important to remember that many medications are associated with proarrhythmic events or electrolyte abnormalities, which could lead to serious life-threatening arrhythmias.

Torsade de pointes is a great example of a proarrhythmic side effect of many medications. Any drug, prescription or nonprescription, that causes QT prolongation should be suspect. In addition to possibly causing the arrhythmia, care should be given in prescribing additional drugs that could add further fuel to the QT prolongation fire. Many times clinicians will prescribe anti-emetics without thinking about the cumulative effect that these drugs could have in extending the QT interval. Torsade de pointes or sudden death could be the result of this careless action.

Be extremely careful when dealing with any patient who could have hyperkalemia. The main group that falls into this category includes patients with renal failure. Hyperkalemia is a frequent cause of death in this patient population. Serious complications and life-threatening arrhythmias can develop within minutes in hyperkalemic patients. A full review of this topic is beyond the scope of this book, and the student is referred to the discussion on this topic in *12-Lead ECG: The Art of Interpretation* by Garcia and Holtz for further information.

Hypocalcemia can sometimes lead to serious QT prolongation in many patients. This could eventually lead to torsade de pointes and sudden death in many patients, although this is not a common occurrence. Once again, renal failure patients are frequently hypocalcemic (and hyperkalemic).

History of MI, CHF, or Structural Heart Disease   In general, any history of MI, CHF, or structural heart disease favors the occurrence of VTach over SVT. The key word in that statement is "favors." As you can imagine, there are plenty of exceptions to this statement, and both VTach and SVT will occur in these populations with great frequency. However, the statistics would be on your side if you favored VTach over SVT as the cause of a wide-complex tachycardia in these patient groups. Electrocardiographic, historical, and physical exam evidence will be needed to either corroborate or negate your suspicions of VTach in any individual patient.

MIs lead to scarring of the ventricles. Scarring can lead to the formation of pathways needed for reentry circuits. In addition, scarring frequently isolates small islands of myocardial cells, which could become irritable and lead to increased automaticity of those pacemakers.

CHF is caused, in many cases, by ventricular hypertrophy from any cause. The result of hypertrophy is to increase the irritability of the muscle cells themselves, directly or indirectly. Hypoxemia and hypoperfusion of a hypertrophied ventricle are just two of the indirect ways that arrhythmogenic foci can develop in the failing ventricle. The cardiomyopathies can lead to many different arrhythmia types, including ventricular tachycardia. Isolated hypertrophy of the atria caused by mitral or tricuspid valvular disease is more likely to cause SVTs.

Once again, structural heart disease caused by either congenital malformations or surgical manipulation can lead to some abnormal pathways which could form reentry circuits. In addition, there may be isolated islets of cells that function autonomously from the rest of the ventricle and be arrhythmogenic.

Physical Examination

AV dissociation can cause some very large venous pulsations, known as *cannon A waves*, to develop on an irregular basis. These occur because, due to the different timing of the atrial and ventricular rates found in AV dissociation, the atria sometimes contract while the heart valves leading to the ventricles are still closed. The atrial blood has to go somewhere. Since it can't go down into the ventricles, it shoots back up the venous system, causing a large pressure wave that travels away from the heart. In the neck, these pressure waves are easily seen, and cause large pulsations in the jugular venous system.

Hemodynamic instability and signs of hypoperfusion can occur in either SVTs or VTachs. The thing to keep in mind is that any hemodynamically unstable arrhythmia should be immediately cardioverted or defibrillated, depending on its electrocardiographic picture. Mild hemodynamic changes can quickly break down into serious or life-threatening hemodynamic instability in seconds. Treatment in these cases should be based on your clinical judgment, but be very, very careful with these patients.

We would be negligent if we did not talk briefly about a particular clinical event: *relative hypotension*. Blood pressure is needed by the body in order to perfuse the organs and maintain life. In general, the patient should have blood pressure within the normal range. Hypertensive patients develop thickening of their arterial walls in order to maintain the high pressures needed to perfuse their organs. These patients can usually tolerate some very high levels during their normal everyday activities.

Elevated blood pressure is needed to maintain normal perfusion in these patients because of the thickened arterial walls. Because of that arterial thickening, what is normal for the average individual and what is normal for hypertensive patients are two different things. A blood pressure of 120/80 mm Hg is smack in the middle of the normal range. But, in a hypertensive patient, this same blood pressure may not be enough to adequately perfuse the organs, leading to cell and organ death. This is what we mean by relative hypotension.

Relative hypotension is the discrepancy that can occur for any given patient between the clinical signs and symptoms of hypoperfusion while being relatively normotensive. This is why you should never treat the number, but treat the patient. If the patient appears hemodynamically unstable, despite a normal-looking BP, ask quickly about their resting BP. If they are normally hypertensive, they could be relatively hypotensive. These patients should be treated as if they were hemodynamically compromised because they *are* hemodynamically compromised. Always use your clinical judgment when treating any patient!

We hope that the preceding pages have provided you a thorough understanding of how to differentiate the various wide-complex tachycardias. Now we are going to discuss a clinical scenario that will help solidify the concepts just learned. We hope this discussion is useful and informative.

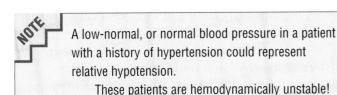

NOTE

A low-normal, or normal blood pressure in a patient with a history of hypertension could represent relative hypotension.
These patients are hemodynamically unstable!

Case Discussion

History

You are called to the side of a 52-year-old male complaining of palpitations and lightheadedness. The patient states that he had been feeling some slight indigestion after eating pizza about 2 hours earlier. The indigestion was partially relieved by antacids and didn't really worry him. However, about 15 minutes ago he began feeling lightheaded and felt some palpitations in his chest. The palpitations and lightheadedness progressed to the point that he felt he was going to pass out. This scared him and he called fire rescue.

The patient states that the palpitations have been ongoing, seem to last forever, and that he started feeling lightheaded about 15 or 20 seconds after they started. The patient describes the palpitations as a very fast, regular fluttering sensation in his chest. The episodes are associated with a subjective sensation of shortness of breath. There has been no associated diaphoresis, nausea, vomiting, or chest pain. The patient has a history of smoking (1 pack per day for 30 years) and hypertension that is controlled with some unknown medication.

Physical Examination

BP: 110/60; HR: 60 to 70 weak, thready, irregular; RR: 24 regular, unlabored; Oxygen saturation: 92%

Examination revealed occasional JVD seen in the neck. The lung fields showed some mild crackles at the bases. Cardiac exam showed a rapid, irregular rhythm but no evidence of murmurs or gallops. Abdomen was soft and nontender. Neurological exam was nonfocal. Skin was cold and clammy. Capillary refill was at 2 seconds. A rhythm strip was obtained (Figure 33-16).

1. **What do you think of this patient's history?**
2. **What do you think of this patient's exam?**
3. **What do you think of this patient's rhythm?**
4. **How can you put it all together?**

1. What do you think of the patient's history?

The patient was mainly complaining of palpitations and near-syncope. In general, palpitations and lightheadedness are very nonspecific symptoms that can be present without any observable rhythm disturbances. However, by asking some key questions, we can help make these symptoms a bit more relevant. Were the palpitations fast or slow? If so, how fast or how slow? Did the palpitations feel regular or irregular? In addition to just asking about the palpitations, you can also ask the patient to pat out the pattern of the palpitations so that you can get a feel for any possible rhythm abnormality.

The history of indigestion after ingesting pizza could be a red herring, but in light of the palpitations it could also be a symptom of cardiac ischemia or infarction. According to statistics, indigestion can be the presenting symptom for an infarct in about 20% of cases. This is especially true in women, the elderly, or anyone with any neurological problem that could alter pain perception, for example, a previous stroke.

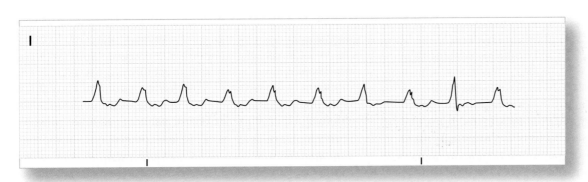

Figure 33-16: The patient's rhythm strip.

Does the history that he received some symptomatic relief with antacids make you feel more comfortable? It shouldn't. Symptomatic relief with antacids is a relatively nonspecific finding that is frequently seen in many infarct patients. The cause for this relief is unclear, but a perceived decrease in the cardiac pain is real. Please do not make the mistake of believing that relief of the pain with antacids means that the patient is having indigestion! Antacids will relieve both gastric and cardiac pain in some cases. The misconception that pain relieved with antacids or a "GI cocktail" is noncardiac can lead to the misdiagnosis of a potentially life-threatening condition.

The clinical history of the hypertension and the 30 years of smoking should elevate your suspicion about the presence of atypical cardiac ischemia or infarction. Remember, there are five main risk factors for coronary artery disease (CAD). These include hypertension, cigarette smoking, diabetes, high cholesterol level, and a family history of CAD before the age of 65.

By the way, which hypertension meds is the patient taking? The interviewer could not supply this vital piece of information. We need to keep this potential problem in mind as we go on because many drugs can actually trigger malignant arrhythmias (proarrhythmogenic). The possibility of electrolyte imbalances caused by medications will also need to be kept in mind, especially if the drugs include a diuretic or an ACE inhibitor.

With this history, your suspicion of ischemia or infarct should be high. The description of the palpitations that the patient gave as being fast and regular helps you to narrow it down to a tachycardia, but it really doesn't help much otherwise. Keep in mind, however, that any arrhythmia in a patient with ischemia or infarction can be very dangerous because it can cause an increase in the oxygen consumption of the heart or a decrease in oxygen delivery to these tissues by decreasing cardiac output.

2. What do you think of this patient's physical examination?

Let's start by looking at the vital signs. The patient's blood pressure is 110/60 mm Hg. This is a normal BP, right? It can be, as long as we keep in mind a few other factors. This patient is normally hypertensive. He is controlled on medications, but this level of control is a little too good. Hypertensive patients usually need normal or slightly elevated levels of BP in order to perfuse their organs. As mentioned on page 436 the elevated pressures in these patients is needed to overcome the anatomical consequences of hypertension. These conse-

quences include a thickening of the blood vessel walls and an increase in the vascular tone. Remember this clinical pearl: *A low or low-normal BP in a patient with a history of hypertension could represent relative hypotension due to the potentially life-threatening effects of ischemia or infarction.* Be suspicious and be careful! This patient can be having relative hypotension.

The HR is 60 to 70 BPM and irregular. The irregularity is helpful in our list of possible differentials, but the heart rate we palpate can lead to disaster. The palpable heart rate can easily mislead us into thinking that we are not dealing with a tachycardia. Lucky for us that both auscultation and, later on, the rhythm strip will let us see that we are actually dealing with a much faster rate.

Why do we get such a low palpable pulse rate? Well, sometimes the tachyarrhythmias are electrically conducted but the heart cannot mechanically contract at the same fast rate. In other words, the heart's electrical conduction system transmits the impulse that quickly, but the heart muscle itself does not contract that fast. If the heart muscle does not contract, then it also does not pump blood. It is, in essence, a missed mechanical contraction. These missed mechanical contractions can add up and lead to hypotension or relative hypotension in many cases. Sound familiar?

The oxygen saturation is decreased at 92%. This could be due to the smoking history but, with the findings of cool, clammy skin and slightly prolonged capillary refill, you have to wonder about decreased perfusion to the extremities. Once again, the concept of relative hypotension rears its ugly head.

It is unclear what the examiner meant by "occasional JVD seen in the neck." AV dissociation causes some very large venous pulsations that occur irregularly. These are the cannon A waves we talked about on page 436. Cannon A waves are a physical examination finding of the presence of some sort of AV dissociation.

At this point in your clinical reasoning, you have some strong suspicions. Sure, this could represent a vagal response causing lightheadedness in an anxious patient with indigestion after eating pizza. But, this subtle clinical scenario could be due to a more ominous problem: cardiac ischemia or an infarct. The patient appears to be having atypical chest pain and is near-syncopal. He is a smoker and is on antihypertensive medications. What about the palpitations? Are they benign or can they be representative of a life-threatening arrhythmia? You need a rhythm strip to solve this issue.

At this point, you are handed the ECG strip.

3. What do you think of this patient's rhythm?

We are dealing with a wide-complex tachycardia. As we proceed, we need to keep in mind that any structural abnormality, presence of cardiomyopathy, or presence of ischemia would favor the diagnosis of VTach over SVT with aberrancy. The patient's history and physical exam are both consistent with ischemia. In addition, statistically, you would be correct in quickly assuming that is ventricular tachycardia since over 80% of wide-complex tachycardias are VTach. But, let's look closely at the strip and make a definitive diagnosis before we move on, since the patient is at least moderately clinically stable and the clinical situation, in our judgment, allows us the luxury of a few seconds before initiating treatment.

The ECG strip shows a wide-complex tachycardia at a rate of about 125 BPM. The rhythm is regular and there appears to be some variation in the morphology of the QRS complexes throughout the strip, especially the next-to-last complex. There is a persistent hump in the ST segment of the complexes, which could represent a P wave. However, the hump is upright. Normally, retrograde P waves are inverted, so this doesn't appear to be a P wave, but just a part of the repolarization process.

What do we do now? Well, let's start by looking at the list we came up with on page 422. Remember though, we don't have to go in order. Which of the 10 things would be the most helpful in this case? How about getting multiple leads? The rhythm strip in Figure 33-17 was taken at the same time as the original strip.

As a matter of fact, the shaded area represents the strip that we showed you at the beginning. Is the rhythm a little easier to analyze now that we have multiple leads? Yes!

Obtaining multiple leads when you are stuck is a critical decision point to remember. We know that many of you are saying that we should have given you lead II because it would have been easier. You would be absolutely right in making that statement. But, you have to realize that you would be right only in this one case. For another patient, maybe lead V_1 would have been the best lead to identify the arrhythmia. In a third patient, it could have been lead III. The point is you never know which is the best lead, and you never know which lead or which part of the rhythm strip you are going to be handed. *Always obtain multiple leads or a full 12-lead ECG when you are dealing with a complex arrhythmia. Do not assume that lead II will always be the best lead to look at arrhythmias.*

As we mentioned before, a corollary to that pearl is that you should obtain long rhythm strips, if possible. This is because arrhythmias, and cardiac events in general, evolve. They are not stagnant events. The causative factors and presentation are constantly changing, moving, and evolving. Just because something is not there in this section of the strip, does not mean it will not be there in the following 10 seconds. Remember, a strip is only a static picture of the cardiac events for a few seconds (or however long your strip is). An ECG is, likewise, only 12 seconds long. Long strips help to pick up minute details that can be critical in arrhythmia inter-

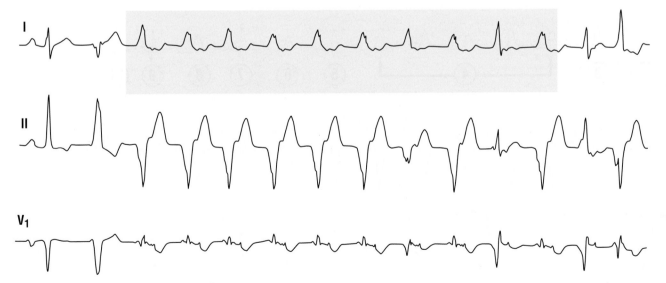

Figure 33-17: Multiple leads of a patient with wide-complex tachycardia.

pretation. For example, a long strip can be very helpful in being able to pick up the presence of capture and fusion beats, which may occur intermittently.

In this discussion, we are going to provide you with a longer three-lead strip (Figure 33-18). In addition, we have labeled the complexes from 1 through 10 to facilitate the discussion. We are going to be using the longer strip and the multiple leads to help facilitate our discussion. We could have arrived at the same diagnostic conclusion from our little strip on lead I, but it would have been a lot tougher.

The complex labeled #1 in Figure 33-18 is the patient's normal complex. Note the P wave, normal QRS complex, and inverted T wave in lead II. The PR interval is prolonged and consistent with a first-degree heart block as we shall see in Chapter 35.

Complex #2, however, is a bit different. This QRS complex is still positive, but it is wider than the normal one. It also has a different ST segment and T wave morphology. In addition, in lead V_1 we see the start of a normally occurring P wave (see the blue arrow) which is interrupted a premature complex. This premature QRS complex could be a PVC or a PJC with aberrancy. An argument can be made either way and it really doesn't matter which one it is. The important thing is that the premature complex triggers a new rhythm starting with complex #3. This new rhythm can easily be seen in all three leads.

Now let's examine this new rhythm. The morphology of the complexes is wide. They are at least 0.14 seconds wide ($3\frac{1}{2}$ small boxes, not shown). We see a small notch in the downsloping S wave that looks like a Josephson's sign (see red arrow). These two findings are both predictive of VTach. We're getting warmer, but we're not there yet.

An axis in the extreme right quadrant would be helpful. However, we can't figure out the exact electrical axis because lead aVF is not available. We can state that the axis is not in the extreme right quadrant because the complexes would have to be negative in lead I if that were the case, and they are positive on our strip. There is one thing we can tell, though, and that is that the axis of the new rhythm must point in a different direction than the normal electrical axis. We can say this because the polarity in the complexes of the new arrhythmia is pointing in the opposite direction from those of complex 1 in leads II and V_1. This is nice to know, but doesn't help us distinguish between VTach and SVT very clearly.

There is some minimal irregularity in the rhythm and some small morphological differences in complex #3 and those labeled collectively as #4. But, we know that at the onset of VTach, the rhythm can be a little irregular and the morphology can change a little bit. These changes will stabilize as the rhythm matures over time. Still could be VTach.

Complexes #5, #7, #9, and #10 provide the best diagnostic evidence for VTach on this rhythm strip. Notice that their morphologies are completely different from the others in the group. Complex #5 is a bit like complexes #3 and #4, but it is just not as deep or as wide. In addition, the T wave associated with it is different. Complex #7 is narrower and the axis is different in leads II and V_1. As a matter of fact, it is similar to the normal complex #1, isn't it? Complex #9 is somewhere between complex #5 and #7.

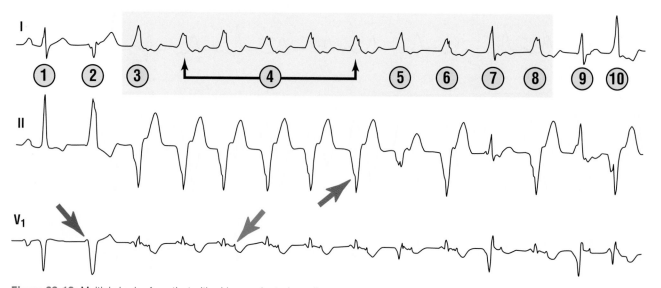

Figure 33-18: Multiple leads of a patient with wide-complex tachycardia.

Can you figure out why these complexes have these differing morphologies? The answer is that they are fusion complexes. None of them are capture beats, even though complex 7 is close, because none of them are morphologically identical to complex 1. They all have a little bit of fusion with the ventricular complexes. These morphological differences are even obvious in our lead I rhythm strip.

4. How can you put it all together?

Is there any other evidence of AV dissociation? The only hard evidence is the presence of fusion complexes. Some soft evidence is found in the fact that the T wave morphology of the complexes immediately before the fusion complexes are slightly different from the typical T waves seen prior to the ventricular beats. This happens because the P waves of the fusion complexes are buried somewhere inside those of the preceding T waves. The superimposed P and T waves alter the morphology of the resultant T wave.

Many of you are still thinking that the notches identified by the green arrow represent P waves. There are some arguments against that possibility, the main one being that the notches still occur after the QRS complexes in the fusion complexes. If they were P waves, they should occur before the QRS in the fusion complexes because there has to be some normal capture of the ventricle by definition. In other words, in order to create a fusion complex, you have to have even a minimal amount of normal capture by the P wave. A P wave occurring after the QRS complex just doesn't fit. As mentioned earlier, that notch represents a repolarization sequence found in the ventricular complexes.

In this discussion, we did most of our traditional "putting it all together" while we were analyzing the patient's rhythm. This was done purposely to facilitate discussion. We want to point out, however, that there really are no fine lines as to what should be under the answer to any of the questions. The important thing is to get to the final conclusion. The information that we have gathered from this rhythm strip does not leave much room for doubt. This rhythm is ventricular tachycardia.

We hope that you have found this review of VTach and the analysis of this very complex rhythm strip helpful. We could have made it easier but, unfortunately, you won't always get classic examples of arrhythmias in real life. This real-life strip is just one example of what you could get. Don't panic. Use your head and approach the situation with a clear head, using everything you have at your disposal to get a clear diagnosis. We feel that if you can interpret the difficult strips, the easy ones will be a cakewalk.

CHAPTER **REVIEW**

1. Approximately _____ % of wide-complex tachycardias will be VTach.

2. Generally speaking, a clinician should be able to distinguish between a supraventricular tachycardia with aberrancy and ventricular tachycardia about _____ % of the time.

3. The most important thing to look for in deciding the differential diagnosis of a wide-complex tachycardia is the presence of _____ _____.

4. Upright P waves in leads II, III, and aVF have to originate in the atria. True or False.

5. The presence of dissociated, upright P waves in lead II in a patient with a regular wide-complex tachycardia is a clear sign of _____ _____.

6. Which of the following is (are) indirect signs of AV dissociation (pick all that apply):
   A. Inverted P waves
   B. Capture beats
   C. Narrow QRS complexes with prolonged QT intervals
   D. Fusion beats

7. An irregularly irregular wide-complex tachycardia at a rate of 220 BPM is most likely ventricular tachycardia. True or False.

8. If the patient is clinically stable enough and you can obtain one quickly, you should always obtain multiple leads or a full 12-lead ECG to further evaluate any cardiac arrhythmia. True or False.

9. The presence of QRS complexes that are wider than _____ seconds tips the scales in favor of ventricular tachycardia.

10. A notch on the downstroke of the S wave in a wide-complex rhythm is known as:
    A. Joseph's sign
    B. Josephson's sign
    C. Brigadier's sign
    D. Brugada's sign

11. A distance of at least 0.10 seconds from the onset of the QRS complex to the lowest point on the S wave is known as:
    A. Joseph's sign
    B. Josephson's sign
    C. Brigadier's sign
    D. Brugada's sign

12. If the morphology of the QRS complexes in a wide-complex strip is identical to the morphology of the _____ found elsewhere on the strip, it favors the diagnosis of ventricular tachycardia.

13. Which R-R' relationship favors the diagnosis of VTach in a right bundle branch block morphology wide-complex tachycardia?
    A. R greater than R'
    B. R' greater than R
    C. An RBBB morphology in general favors VTach
    D. All of the above

14. An axis in which quadrant favors a diagnosis of VTach (pick the best choice)?
    A. Normal quadrant
    B. Left quadrant
    C. Right quadrant
    D. Extreme right quadrant

15. If you have a full 12-lead ECG with a wide-complex tachycardia, the presence of _____ of all of the QRS complexes in the precordial leads favors the diagnosis of VTach.

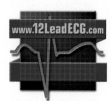

www.12LeadECG.com To enhance the knowledge you gain in this book, access this text's website at www.12leadECG.com! This valuable resource provides flashcards, an online glossary, web links, and more. Simply click on the Arrhythmias book cover once at the site.

CHAPTER 34

Ventricular Fibrillation and Asystole

Ventricular Fibrillation

Ventricular fibrillation (Vfib) is defined as a rapid, completely disorganized ventricular rhythm. The electrocardiographic characteristics of this arrhythmia are undulations of varying shapes and sizes with no pattern and no discernible P, QRS, or T waves (Figure 34-1). The undulations occur anywhere from 150 to 500 times in a minute. Notice that we did not use the word "beats" to describe the undulations. This is because in Vfib there is no organized beating of the heart in any way, shape, or form.

Some authors have commented on the presence of fine and coarse Vfib (Figure 34-2). We saw the similar fine and coarse patterns for atrial fibrillation back in Chapter 20. The actual meaning or significance of the two electrocardiographic interpretations is unclear, but we will present the two variations. Keep in mind that sometimes, fine Vfib is actually mistaken for asystole (or the absence of rhythm). In order to differentiate between the two, switching leads is extremely helpful. If you see the typical fibrillatory pattern in a different lead, then defibrillation is still indicated.

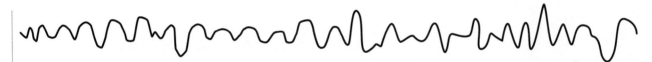

Figure 34-1: Ventricular fibrillation. Note the absence of any type of visible recurrent pattern. This is a completely chaotic electrocardiographic representation of the chaotically contracting ventricles.

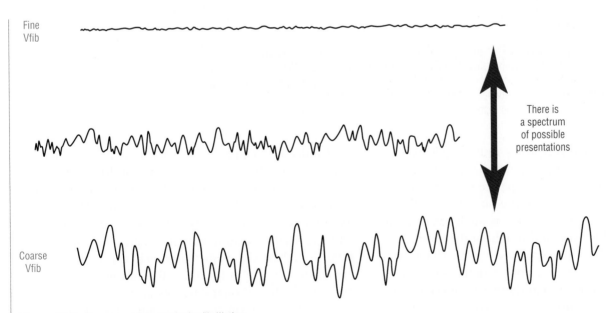

Fine Vfib

There is a spectrum of possible presentations

Coarse Vfib

Figure 34-2: Coarse and fine ventricular fibrillation.

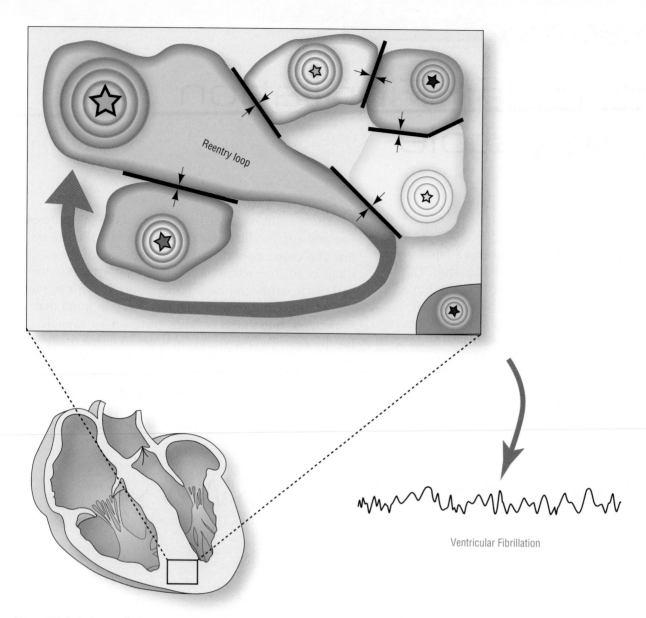

Figure 34-3: In the ventricular tissue there could be many, many individual ectopic foci acting as ectopic pacemakers at the same time. Most of these small islands of depolarization throughout the ventricles cancel each other out. These ectopic pacemakers, however, do create small vectors, which show up on the ECG strip as undulations of varying size and morphology. In addition, there are multiple reentry circuits formed and functioning at the same time. The net result is complete chaotic depolarization of the ventricles. This chaotic depolarization essentially shuts down mechanical contraction.

Ventricular fibrillation is typically caused by increased automaticity of multiple ectopic ventricular pacemakers (Figure 34-3). In addition, many separate reentry circuits are created and are functioning at the same time in the ventricles. The net result is that there is no depolarization wave of any real value formed throughout the entire ventricle. Each small section contracts, but the chaos of the regional depolarizations and contractions essentially shuts down the ventricles. When there is no mechanical contraction, there is no cardiac output. This is a condition that is not compatible with life.

Clinically, Vfib can occur spontaneously in a patient with a normal heart. It is also common for ventricular tachycardia to deteriorate into Vfib. However, the most common cause of the arrhythmia is an acute myocardial infarction. For many unfortunate patients, this lethal arrhythmia is the very first sign of an early AMI. Together with ventricular tachycardia, these two arrhythmias account for over 50% of the mortality associated with coronary artery disease.

Ventricular fibrillation is a deadly arrhythmia. Spontaneous termination of the arrhythmia does not occur.

If you get the arrhythmia, you die. The only chance of survival is immediate treatment. Within only 10 to 20 seconds of a cessation of cardiac output, life-threatening complications can begin. What is the most effective treatment for ventricular fibrillation? Immediate defibrillation. As we always say. . .*electricity is our friend!*

What exactly happens during defibrillation? *The electrical stimulus provided by emergent defibrillation causes an immediate and synchronized depolarization of all ventricular myocytes* (Figure 34-4). The heart is essentially externally stimulated, depolarized, and then left to fend for itself. Luckily, myocytes only remember as far back as the last electrical depolarization. The hope is that by shutting down the ectopic pacemakers and the reentry circuits, all during the same millisecond, the normal cardiac pacemakers will begin to take over synchronized and normal conduction of the electrical impulse throughout the heart. In essence, we stop the heart momentarily, in hopes that it will return to normal function.

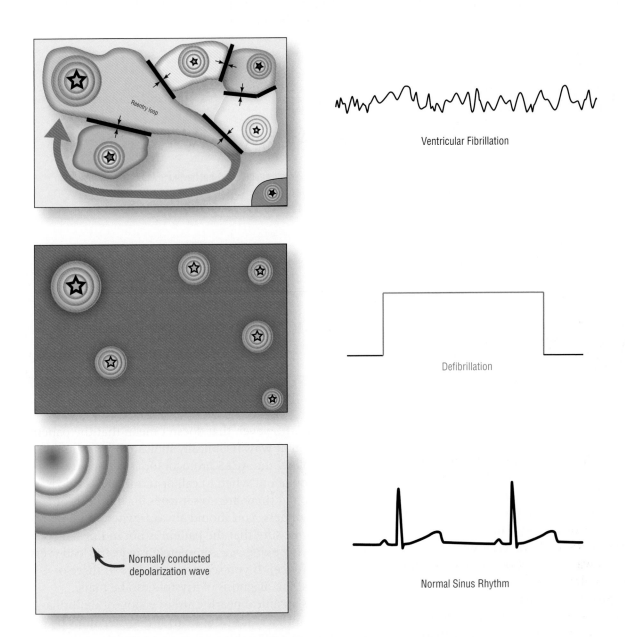

Figure 34-4: Chaotic depolarization of the ventricles leads to ventricular fibrillation. Defibrillation leads to a state where all of the myocytes of the heart are depolarized instantaneously. This essentially resets all of the myocytes. The hope is that the normal cardiac pacemakers will then be able to take over pacing function and that transmission of the depolarization wave can proceed normally through the "reset" electrical conduction system and myocardium.

ADDITIONAL **INFORMATION**

Is It Vfib or Artifact?

A clinical word of warning: Always treat the patient, not the arrhythmia! Many times, movement of the lead, the patient, or the patient's intrinsic tremors can lead to misdiagnosis of a rhythm abnormality (Figure 34-5 to 34-8). Artifact can resemble VTach, Vfib or asystole.

Take a look at your patient and use some common sense. If you see what looks like Vfib but the patient is walking to the bathroom, he is not in Vfib. On the other hand, if you see something that looks like Vfib and your patient is sleeping, shake him and wake him up. This is the first thing you are taught to do in advanced cardiac life support (ACLS), and there is a reason for this. If you can't wake him, he is in cardiac arrest. This discussion may seem like an insult to your intelligence, but we have seen seasoned clinicians begin CPR, when suddenly, the patient begins to smack him back. Treat the patient, not the monitor!

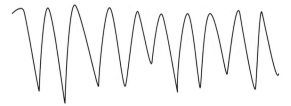

Figure 34-5: This patient was wrestling with his child. The movement of the leads caused the clinician to believe that the patient was in ventricular tachycardia. The rhythm returned to normal the second the patient stopped moving.

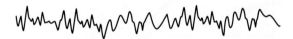

Figure 34-7: No, this patient was not having a Vfib cardiac arrest! The lead was moving on his chest as he changed his robe.

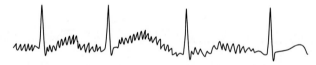

Figure 34-6: This is not atrial fibrillation—the rhythm is regular. Interference by an electrical appliance in the room was the cause of this artifact. Turning off the machine caused the baseline to return to normal.

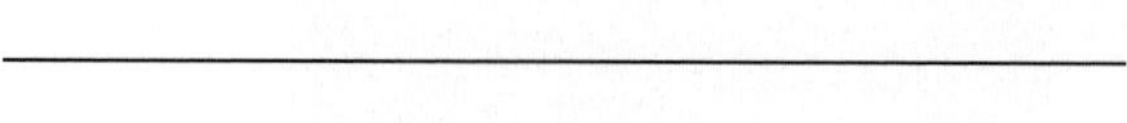

Figure 34-8: No, this patient was not in an asystolic cardiac arrest! The lead fell off his chest.

Asystole

Asystole refers to the complete absence of any electrical cardiac activity (Figure 34-9). Electrocardiographically, it is represented as a straight or almost straight line on the strip. The straight line is due to the complete lack of any depolarization waves or vectors. There is a complete absence of any P, QRS, or T waves anywhere along the strip. A good way to think of it is like this: if it looks like a straight line drawn across the ECG paper by a four year old, it is probably asystole.

As you can imagine, the patient is clinically dead at this point. There is no electrical or mechanical activity whatsoever. However, that doesn't mean that the patient has to stay that way. If clinically indicated, you should begin to follow the ACLS protocol for asystolic arrest. The decision about when to call or terminate a code is subjective, and there are no set rules for this decision. For completeness, you should always switch monitor leads to make sure that the patient is not in fine Vfib or that you are looking at a completely isoelectric lead (very rare occurrence). If you see a straight line in three or more leads, the diagnosis of asystole can be made.

Here is a clinical pearl. Cardioversion or defibrillation does not kick-start the heart but rather stops it cold. We are saying this so that you remember that

Figure 34-9: Asystole.

defibrillating or cardioverting a truly asystolic patient is contraindicated. Normally, the reason you cardiovert or defibrillate someone is to apply an electrical current to the heart in order to stop all electrical activity and allow a normal cardiac pacemaker to resume its normal role. However, in true asystole, you do not have *any* electrical activity in the first place. Applying the external current will not be effective and may actually cause damage to the myocardial tissue, further complicating your management if a spontaneous rhythm does eventually return. Use of a transvenous or transthoracic external pacing device in an asystolic arrest, on the other hand, would be an excellent idea.

Agonal

Agonal rhythm, is a variant term for asystole that is sometimes used by clinicians during daily practice (Figure 34-10). An agonal rhythm is basically asystole with an occasional P wave or QRS complex. The QRS complexes, when they occur, are very wide and very bizarre in morphological appearance. They are even bizarre by ectopic ventricular complex standards.

An agonal rhythm is a terminal event and should be treated clinically as asystole. The occasional complexes are the last efforts made by a dying heart. Remember, a ventricular rate below 20 BPM is not typically seen in an idioventricular escape rhythm.

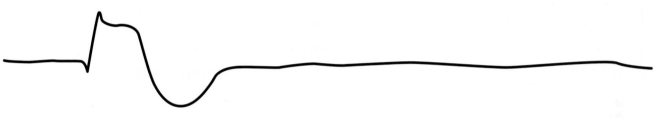

Figure 34-10: Agonal rhythm.

ECG Strips

ECG 34-1

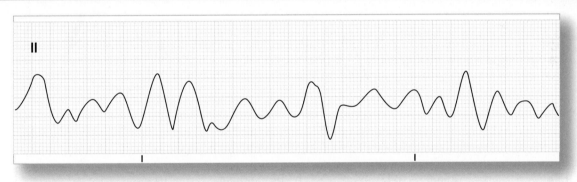

Rate:	None	PR intervals:	None
Regularity:	None	QRS width:	None
P waves:	None	Grouping:	None
Morphology:	None		
Axis:	None	Dropped beats:	Absent
P:QRS ratio:	None	Rhythm:	**Ventricular fibrillation**

Discussion:

The strip above shows a completely chaotic rhythm with no recurring regularities that could represent either P, QRS, or T waves. The undulations appear at various intervals and are of various amplitudes and pos-sible polarities. This is a typical example of ventricular fibrillation. Clinical correlation with the patient and obtaining samples from multiple leads are indicated to rule out artifact.

ECG 34-2

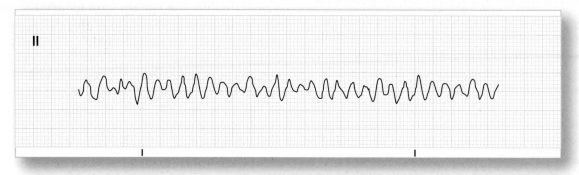

Rate:	None	PR intervals:	None
Regularity:	None	QRS width:	Normal
P waves:	None	Grouping:	None
Morphology:	None		
Axis:	None	Dropped beats:	Absent
P:QRS ratio:	None	Rhythm:	**Ventricular fibrillation**

Discussion:

The undulations in this ECG are a bit tighter than the ones in ECG 34-1, but the characteristics mentioned above can also be applied to this strip. This is an example of ventricular fibrillation. Clinical correlation with the patient and obtaining samples from multiple leads are indicated to rule out artifact.

ECG 34-3

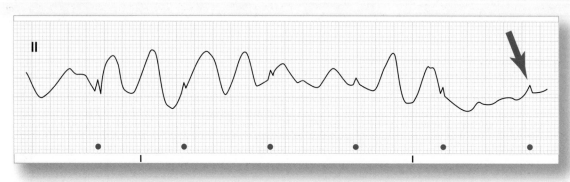

Rate:	About 65 BPM	PR intervals:	Unclear
Regularity:	Regular	QRS width:	Unclear
P waves:	Unclear	Grouping:	None
Morphology:	None		
Axis:	None	Dropped beats:	Absent
P:QRS ratio:	Unclear	Rhythm:	**See discussion below**

Discussion:

This rhythm strip is really fascinating to tease apart. First of all, take a look at the area highlighted by the blue arrow. It shows a nice, sharp peak that is different from the other undulations on the page. On closer examination, we see similar peaks occurring throughout the strip. This could represent an undulation in a patient in Vfib. Multiple leads, and clinical correlation with the patient, showed that the patient was in normal sinus rhythm and this was just artifact in lead II.

ECG 34-4

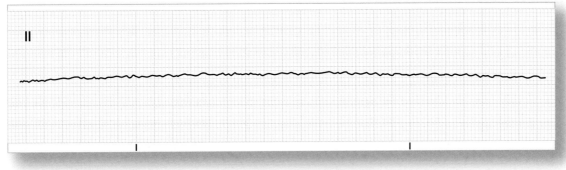

Rate:	None	PR intervals:	None
Regularity:	None	QRS width:	Normal
P waves:	None	Grouping:	None
Morphology:	None		
Axis:	None	Dropped beats:	Absent
P:QRS ratio:	None	Rhythm:	**Ventricular fibrillation**

Discussion:

This strip has the appearance of a fine line straight across the strip. This strip could represent fine Vfib or asystole. When we looked at multiple leads, it became obvious that this is fine Vfib. Always remember to obtain clinical correlation with the patient and to look at multiple leads in order to rule out artifact.

ECG 34-5

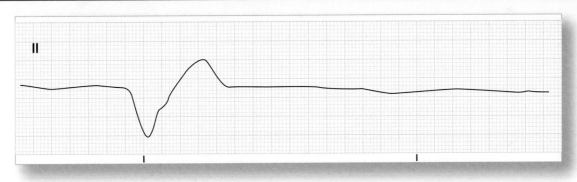

Rate:	None	PR intervals:	None
Regularity:	None	QRS width:	Normal
P waves:	None	Grouping:	None
Morphology:	None		
Axis:	None	Dropped beats:	Absent
P:QRS ratio:	None	Rhythm:	**Agonal or asystole**

Discussion:

The strip above shows a single very wide, very bizarre complex on a straight baseline. This rhythm is incompatible with life and is well below the rate expected for idioventricular escape rhythm. This is an example of an agonal rhythm.

ECG 34-6

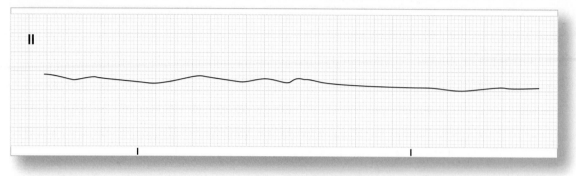

II

Rate:	None	PR Intervals:	None
Regularity:	None	QRS Width:	Normal
P Waves:	None	Grouping:	None
Morphology:	None		
Axis:	None	Dropped Beats:	Absent
P:QRS Ratio:	None	Rhythm:	**Asystole**

Discussion:

This strip just shows a straight line with some minor undulations. There is no evidence of any wave-like activity anywhere on the strip. This is an example of an asystolic strip. Clinical correlation with the patient and obtaining samples from multiple leads are indicated to rule out artifact.

CHAPTER REVIEW

1. Ventricular fibrillation is defined as a rapid, completely disorganized ventricular rhythm. True or False.

2. In Vfib, there are undulations present on the ECG anywhere from 150 to 500 BPM. True or False.

3. _____ Vfib is often mistaken for asystole.

4. The most common cause of Vfib is an _____ _____ _____.

5. The most effective treatment for Vfib is emergent _____.

6. Electrical defibrillation causes a spontaneous depolarization of every myocyte in the heart at the same exact time. The hope is that one of cardiac pacemakers will then take over pacing functions of the "silent" heart. True or False.

7. You should check at least three different leads for fibrillatory activity before calling a rhythm asystole. True or false.

8. An _____ rhythm is basically asystole with an occasional P wave or QRS complex.

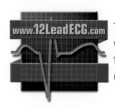

To enhance the knowledge you gain in this book, access this text's website at www.12leadECG.com! This valuable resource provides flashcards, an online glossary, web links, and more. Simply click on the Arrhythmias book cover once at the site.

Self-Test

Test ECG 1

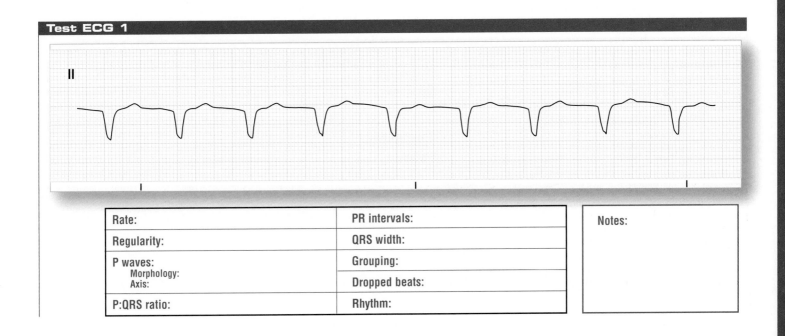

Rate:	PR intervals:
Regularity:	QRS width:
P waves:	Grouping:
Morphology:	Dropped beats:
Axis:	
P:QRS ratio:	Rhythm:

Notes:

Test ECG 2

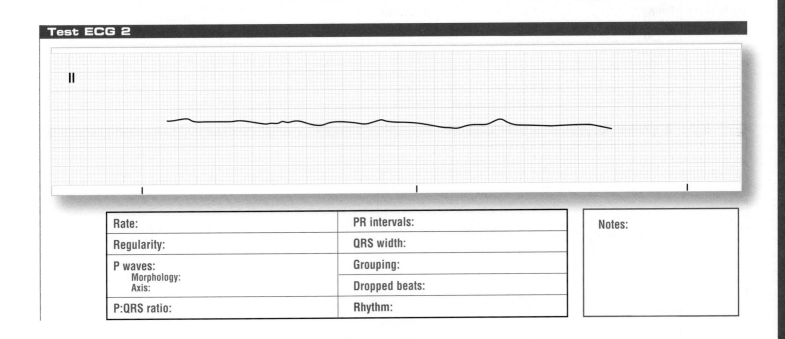

Rate:	PR intervals:
Regularity:	QRS width:
P waves:	Grouping:
Morphology:	Dropped beats:
Axis:	
P:QRS ratio:	Rhythm:

Notes:

Test ECG 3

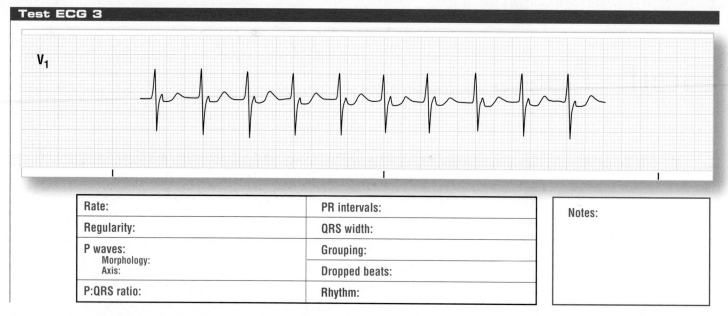

Rate:	PR intervals:	Notes:
Regularity:	QRS width:	

P waves:
   Morphology:
   Axis:
	Grouping:	

	Dropped beats:	
P:QRS ratio:	Rhythm:	

Test ECG 4

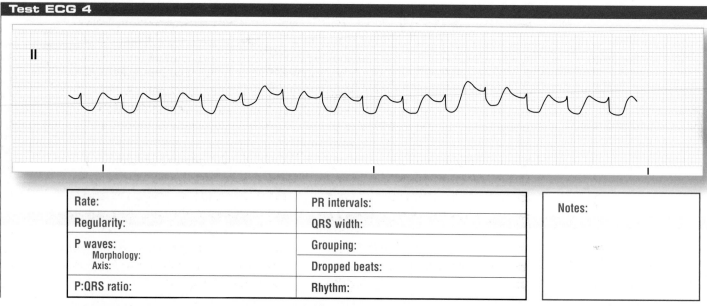

Rate:	PR intervals:	Notes:
Regularity:	QRS width:	

P waves:
   Morphology:
   Axis:
	Grouping:	

	Dropped beats:	
P:QRS ratio:	Rhythm:	

Test ECG 5

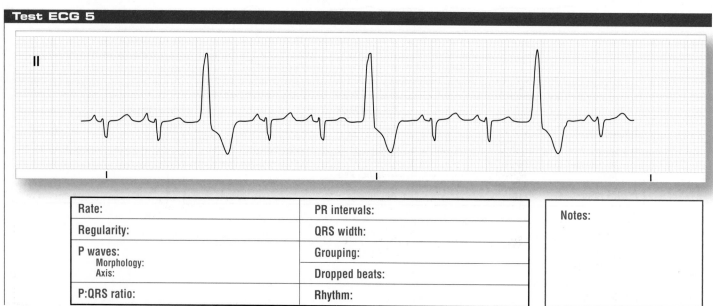

Rate:	PR intervals:	Notes:
Regularity:	QRS width:	

P waves:
   Morphology:
   Axis:
	Grouping:	

	Dropped beats:	
P:QRS ratio:	Rhythm:	

Test ECG 6

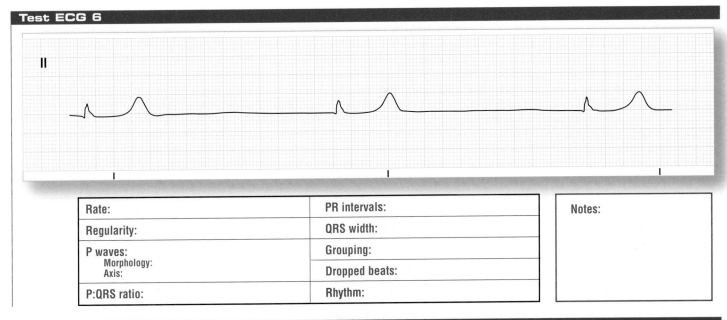

Rate:	PR intervals:	Notes:
Regularity:	QRS width:	
P waves: Morphology: Axis:	Grouping:	
	Dropped beats:	
P:QRS ratio:	Rhythm:	

Test ECG 7

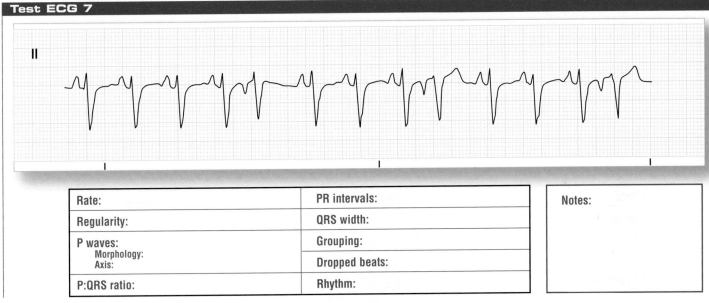

Rate:	PR intervals:	Notes:
Regularity:	QRS width:	
P waves: Morphology: Axis:	Grouping:	
	Dropped beats:	
P:QRS ratio:	Rhythm:	

Test ECG 8

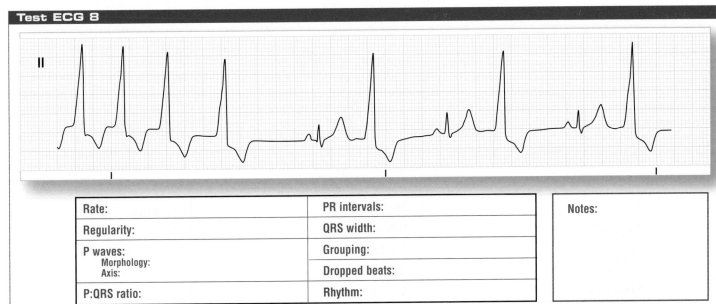

Rate:	PR intervals:	Notes:
Regularity:	QRS width:	
P waves: Morphology: Axis:	Grouping:	
	Dropped beats:	
P:QRS ratio:	Rhythm:	

Test ECG 9

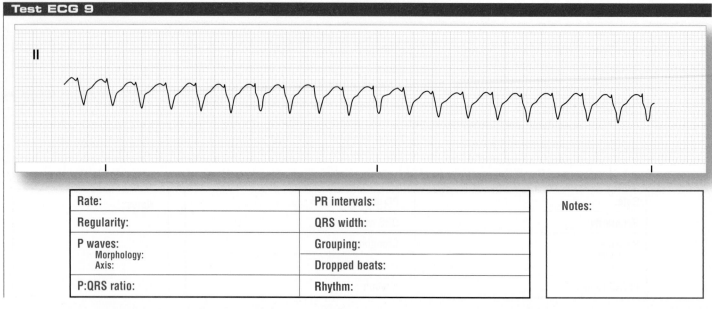

Rate:	PR intervals:		Notes:
Regularity:	QRS width:		

P waves:
    Morphology:
    Axis:
	Grouping:		

	Dropped beats:		
P:QRS ratio:	Rhythm:		

Test ECG 10

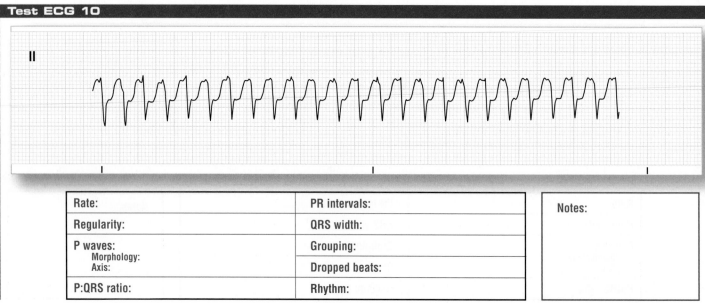

Rate:	PR intervals:		Notes:
Regularity:	QRS width:		

P waves:
    Morphology:
    Axis:
	Grouping:		

	Dropped beats:		
P:QRS ratio:	Rhythm:		

Test ECG 11

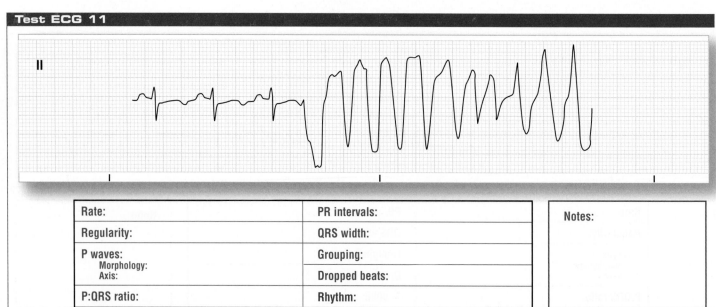

Rate:	PR intervals:		Notes:
Regularity:	QRS width:		

P waves:
    Morphology:
    Axis:
	Grouping:		

	Dropped beats:		
P:QRS ratio:	Rhythm:		

Test ECG 12

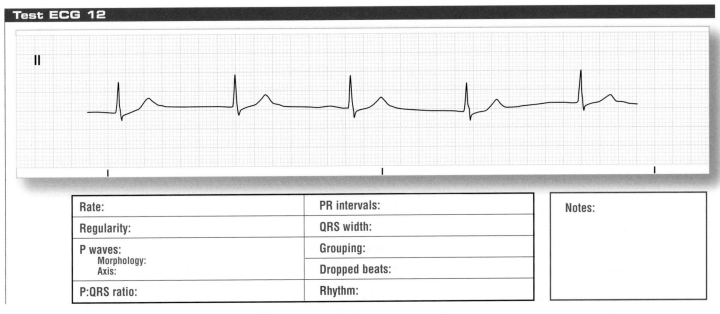

Rate:		PR intervals:	Notes:
Regularity:		QRS width:	
P waves: Morphology: Axis:		Grouping:	
		Dropped beats:	
P:QRS ratio:		Rhythm:	

Test ECG 13

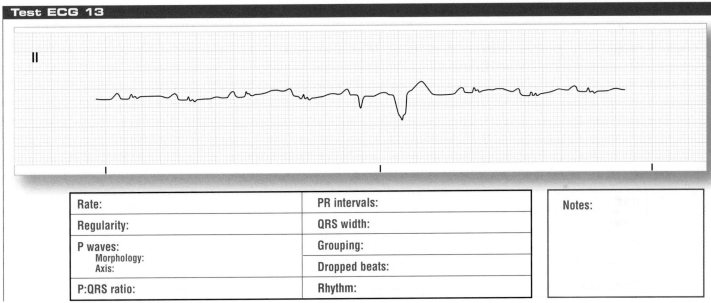

Rate:		PR intervals:	Notes:
Regularity:		QRS width:	
P waves: Morphology: Axis:		Grouping:	
		Dropped beats:	
P:QRS ratio:		Rhythm:	

Test ECG 14

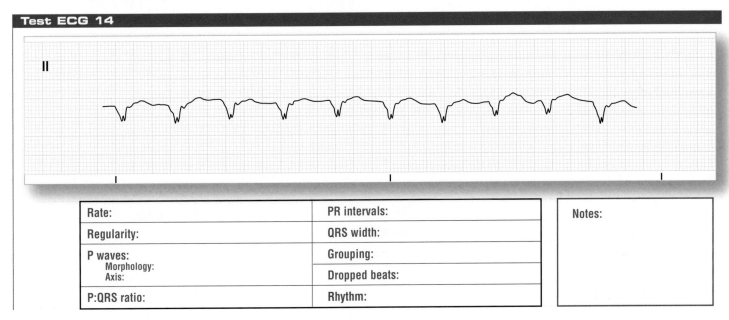

Rate:		PR intervals:	Notes:
Regularity:		QRS width:	
P waves: Morphology: Axis:		Grouping:	
		Dropped beats:	
P:QRS ratio:		Rhythm:	

Test ECG 15

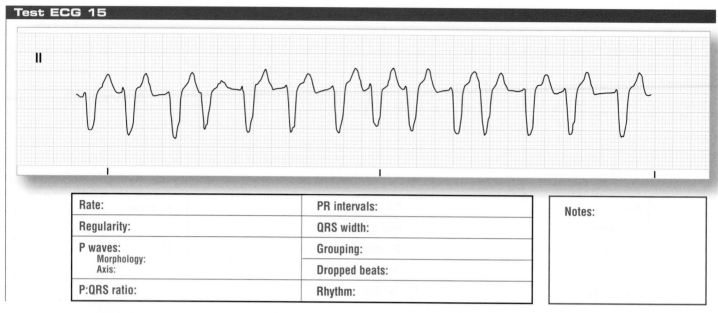

Rate:	PR intervals:	Notes:
Regularity:	QRS width:	
P waves: Morphology: Axis:	Grouping:	
	Dropped beats:	
P:QRS ratio:	Rhythm:	

Test ECG 16

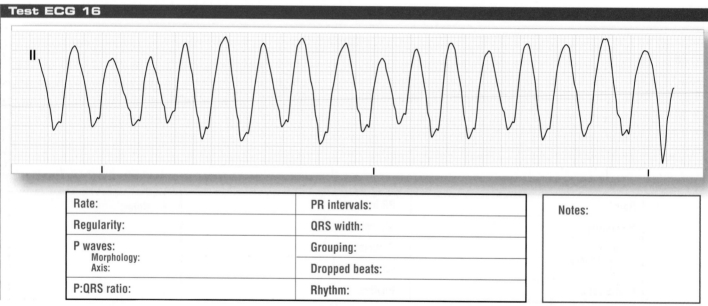

Rate:	PR intervals:	Notes:
Regularity:	QRS width:	
P waves: Morphology: Axis:	Grouping:	
	Dropped beats:	
P:QRS ratio:	Rhythm:	

Test ECG 17

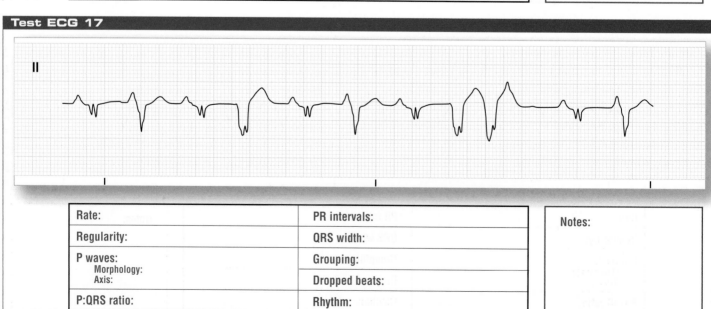

Rate:	PR intervals:	Notes:
Regularity:	QRS width:	
P waves: Morphology: Axis:	Grouping:	
	Dropped beats:	
P:QRS ratio:	Rhythm:	

Test ECG 18

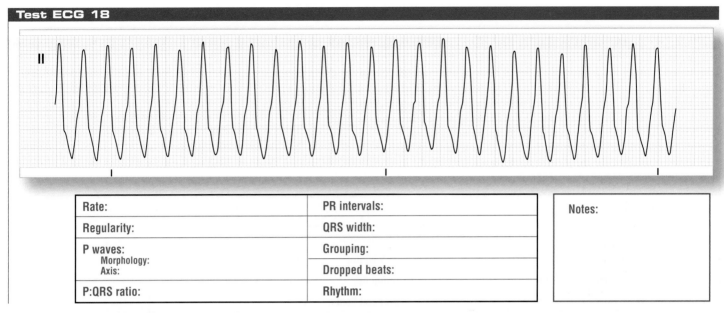

Rate:		PR intervals:	Notes:
Regularity:		QRS width:	

P waves:
    Morphology:
    Axis:
		Grouping:	

		Dropped beats:	
P:QRS ratio:		Rhythm:	

Test ECG 19

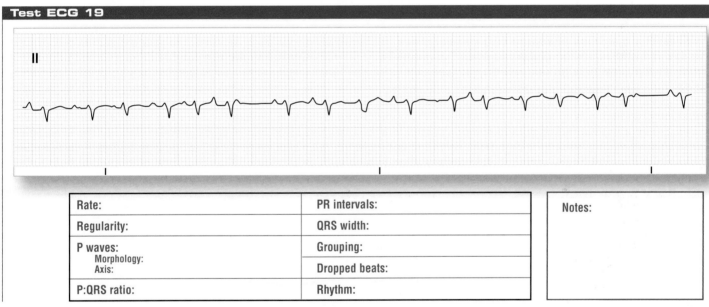

Rate:		PR intervals:	Notes:
Regularity:		QRS width:	

P waves:
    Morphology:
    Axis:
		Grouping:	

		Dropped beats:	
P:QRS ratio:		Rhythm:	

Test ECG 20

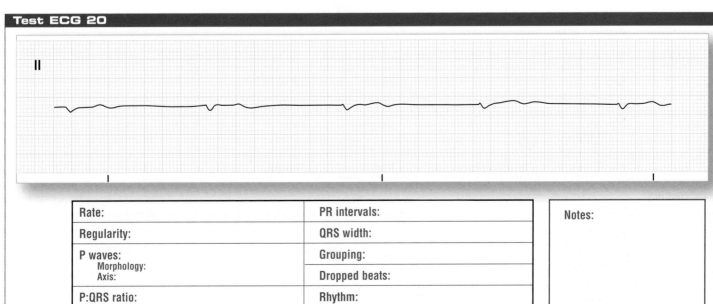

Rate:		PR intervals:	Notes:
Regularity:		QRS width:	

P waves:
    Morphology:
    Axis:
		Grouping:	

		Dropped beats:	
P:QRS ratio:		Rhythm:	

Section 5 Self-Test Answers

Test ECG 1

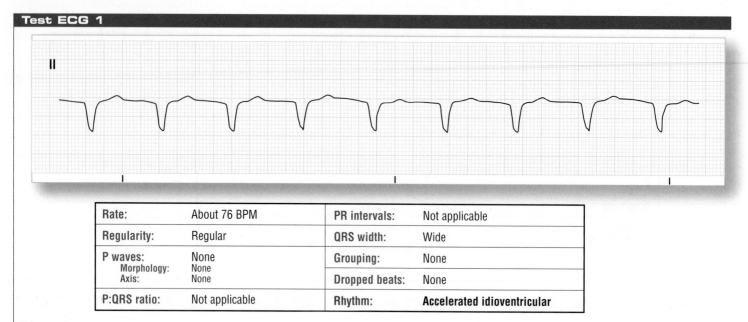

Rate:	About 76 BPM		PR intervals:	Not applicable
Regularity:	Regular		QRS width:	Wide
P waves:	None		Grouping:	None
Morphology:	None			
Axis:	None		Dropped beats:	None
P:QRS ratio:	Not applicable		Rhythm:	**Accelerated idioventricular**

Discussion:

Test ECG 1 shows a wide-complex rhythm at about 76 BPM. The rhythm has no obvious P waves anywhere along the strip. The rate and the ventricular origin for this rhythm make the diagnosis accelerated idioventricular rhythm.

Test ECG 2

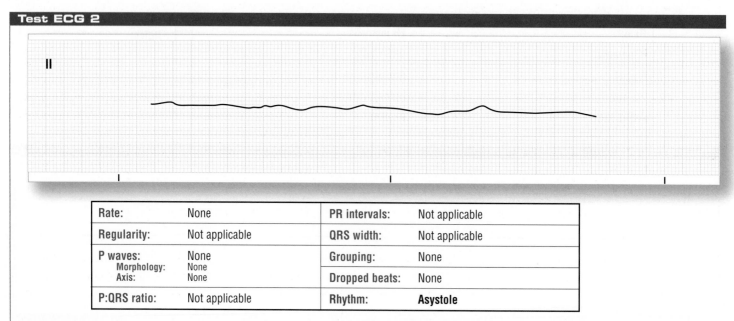

Rate:	None		PR intervals:	Not applicable
Regularity:	Not applicable		QRS width:	Not applicable
P waves:	None		Grouping:	None
Morphology:	None			
Axis:	None		Dropped beats:	None
P:QRS ratio:	Not applicable		Rhythm:	**Asystole**

Discussion:

There are no obvious waves anywhere along this strip. This is an example of asystole. For completeness, remember to try various leads to make sure that you are dealing with asystole and not artifact or a completely isoelectric lead. Remember to always try to interpret any rhythm strip based on information gained from the clinical correlation with the patient.

Test ECG 3

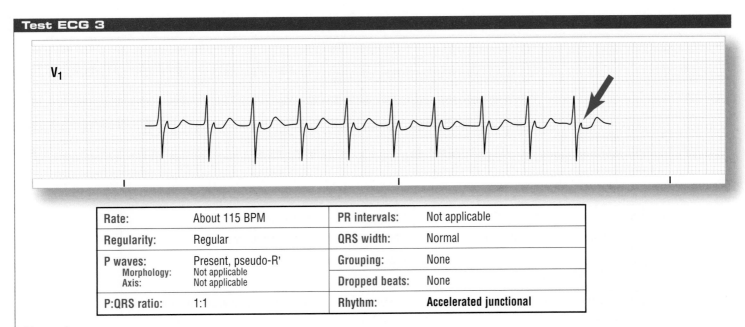

Rate:	About 115 BPM	PR intervals:	Not applicable
Regularity:	Regular	QRS width:	Normal
P waves:	Present, pseudo-R'	Grouping:	None
Morphology: Axis:	Not applicable Not applicable	Dropped beats:	None
P:QRS ratio:	1:1	Rhythm:	**Accelerated junctional**

Discussion:

Test ECG 3 shows a narrow-complex tachycardia at a rate of about 115 BPM. There are no P waves noted before the QRS complexes. The R', however, is consistent with the presence of a pseudo-R' wave (see blue arrow).

Remember, the pseudo-R' is caused by an upright P wave buried within the QRS complex in lead V_1 that simulates the presence of an R' or r' peak. They occur in either junctional, accelerated junctional, or AVNRT rhythms.

Test ECG 4

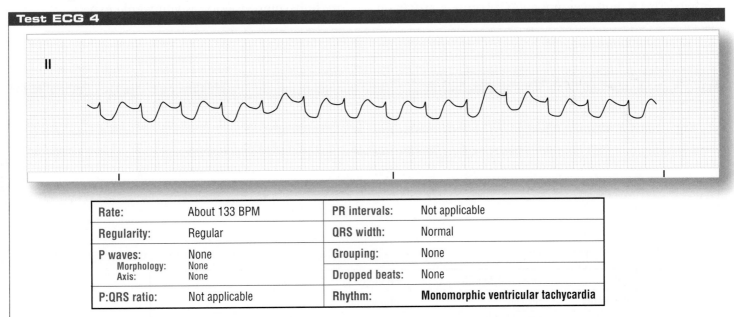

Rate:	About 133 BPM	PR intervals:	Not applicable
Regularity:	Regular	QRS width:	Normal
P waves:	None	Grouping:	None
Morphology: Axis:	None None	Dropped beats:	None
P:QRS ratio:	Not applicable	Rhythm:	**Monomorphic ventricular tachycardia**

Discussion:

This ECG brings up a typical problem seen when analyzing many patients with ventricular tachycardia: the small voltage of lead II. We are all used to seeing examples of VTach with large QRS complexes that are unmistakably ventricular in nature. The problem comes in when the VTach has a right bundle branch morphology. Typically, lead II shows small voltage, which could be either positive or negative. RBBB is a common morphological presentation for VTach, so you will see this pre-

sentation very frequently. Because it appears benign, clinicians tend to downplay its importance. Be careful! A wide-complex tachycardia with or without AV dissociation should always be considered for VTach. A 12-lead ECG on this patient verified the presence of both VTach and an acute anteroseptal MI with lateral extension. The ST segment depression present on this ECG was due to the reciprocal changes of the MI.

Test ECG 5

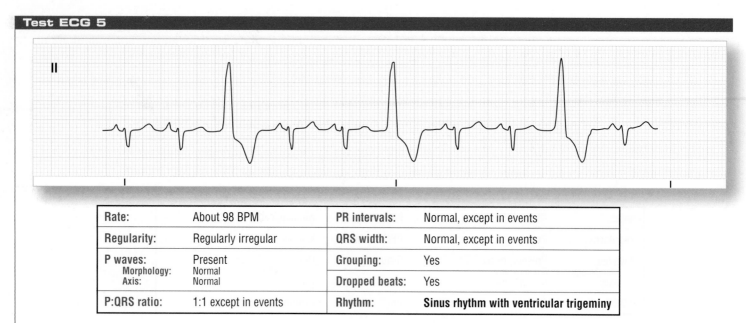

Rate:	About 98 BPM	PR intervals:	Normal, except in events
Regularity:	Regularly irregular	QRS width:	Normal, except in events
P waves:	Present	Grouping:	Yes
Morphology:	Normal		
Axis:	Normal	Dropped beats:	Yes
P:QRS ratio:	1:1 except in events	Rhythm:	**Sinus rhythm with ventricular trigeminy**

Discussion:

This strip shows a sinus rhythm with a monomorphic PVC recurring every third beat. This is an example of a ventricular trigeminy. Note on the strip that the second P wave is a slightly different morphology than the others. This is, however, not a PAC because it arrives on schedule and has the same PR intervals as the others. This could be due to the firing of a different pacemaker within the sinus node itself or due to some slight artifactual difference. The pauses associated with the PVCs are fully compensatory, as you would expect.

Test ECG 6

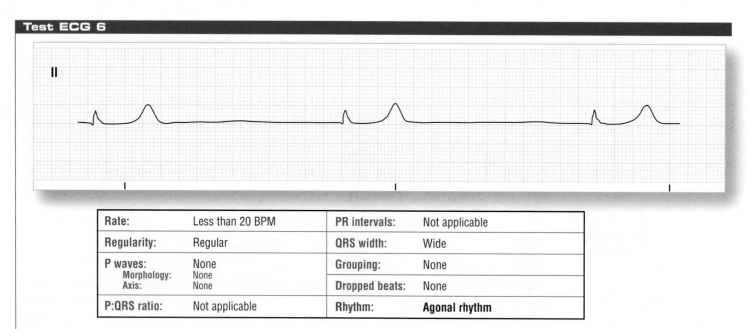

Rate:	Less than 20 BPM	PR intervals:	Not applicable
Regularity:	Regular	QRS width:	Wide
P waves:	None	Grouping:	None
Morphology:	None		
Axis:	None	Dropped beats:	None
P:QRS ratio:	Not applicable	Rhythm:	**Agonal rhythm**

Discussion:

Test ECG 6 shows ventricular complexes that are occurring at a very slow rate. It is slower than the lower limit typically seen in idioventricular rhythms. This is an example of an agonal rhythm. Remember, this is usually a terminal rhythm. If your patient has this rhythm, he or she doesn't have much time. External or transvenous pacing, as well as drugs like atropine, are emergently indicated to try to speed up the rate and maintain a viable cardiac output. Epinephrine may also be helpful in these cases, but its use needs to be considered carefully.

Test ECG 7

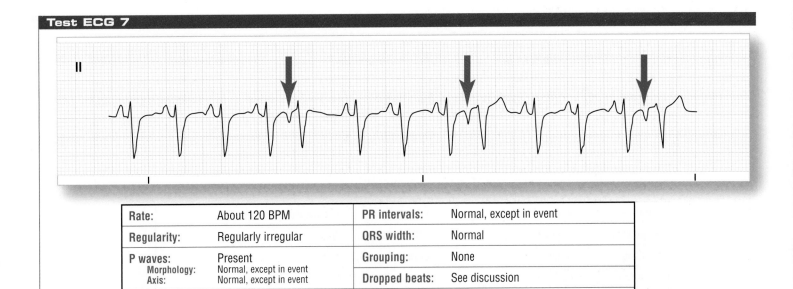

Rate:	About 120 BPM	PR intervals:	Normal, except in event
Regularity:	Regularly irregular	QRS width:	Normal
P waves: 　Morphology: 　Axis:	Present Normal, except in event Normal, except in event	Grouping:	None
		Dropped beats:	See discussion
P:QRS ratio:	1:1	Rhythm:	**Sinus tachycardia with frequent PACs**

Discussion:

This strip shows an underlying sinus tachycardia at a rate of about 120 BPM. The sinus tachycardia is broken up by occasional PACs (see blue arrows). Notice that these complexes are triggered by inverted P waves with normal PR intervals. These findings indicate that the premature complexes originate in an ectopic atrial site and not in the junctional area. However, the pauses are fully compensatory, which is less typically found in PACs.

Test ECG 8

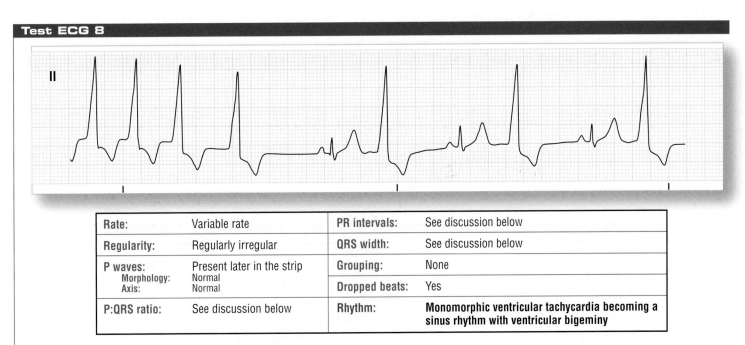

Rate:	Variable rate	PR intervals:	See discussion below
Regularity:	Regularly irregular	QRS width:	See discussion below
P waves: 　Morphology: 　Axis:	Present later in the strip Normal Normal	Grouping:	None
		Dropped beats:	Yes
P:QRS ratio:	See discussion below	Rhythm:	**Monomorphic ventricular tachycardia becoming a sinus rhythm with ventricular bigeminy**

Discussion:

Test ECG 8 is an example of the events that occur at the termination of a run of VTach. Notice that at the onset of the strip, there is a monomorphic VTach at a rate of about 125 BPM. Then there is some slight irregularity in the rhythm, which is commonly seen in VTach at the start and the end of runs. The patient then has a sinus rhythm with ventricular bigeminy. Notice that the PVCs have the exact morphology as the complexes in the run of monomorphic VTach. Clinical correlation and a full 12-lead ECG should be considered to further evaluate this patient.

Test ECG 9

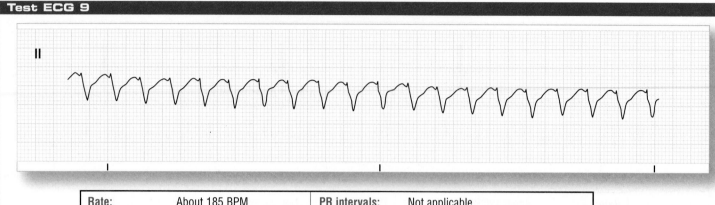

Rate:	About 185 BPM	PR intervals:	Not applicable
Regularity:	Regular	QRS width:	Wide
P waves:	None	Grouping:	None
Morphology:	None		
Axis:	None	Dropped beats:	None
P:QRS ratio:	Not applicable	Rhythm:	**Monomorphic ventricular tachycardia**

Discussion:

This is a tough strip! It is tough because there are a few things that this could be: AVNRT, AVRT, or ventricular tachycardia. There are no P waves and no evidence of AV dissociation present. The only thing that we know for sure is that this is a regular wide-complex tachycardia. So, what do we do now? Well, we treat it as a presumed VTach. A full 12-lead ECG verified the presence of ven-

tricular tachycardia on this patient. Once again, remember that a VTach with a right bundle branch block morphology may have very small QRS complexes in lead II. Just like the patient from Test ECG 4, this patient was also having an acute myocardial infarction. As we have seen over and over again, clinical correlation and a full 12-lead ECG made the diagnosis clearer.

Test ECG 10

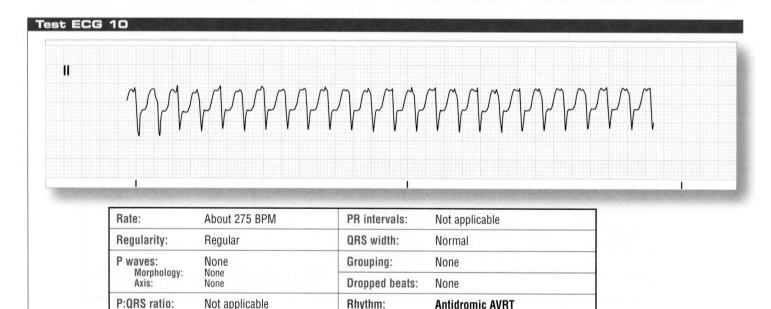

Rate:	About 275 BPM	PR intervals:	Not applicable
Regularity:	Regular	QRS width:	Normal
P waves:	None	Grouping:	None
Morphology:	None		
Axis:	None	Dropped beats:	None
P:QRS ratio:	Not applicable	Rhythm:	**Antidromic AVRT**

Discussion:

Is this another example of small QRS complexes in a patient in VTach? The answer is no. The important diagnostic feature of this strip is the very rapid rate. A rate of about 275 BPM is simply too fast for a ventricular tachycardia. Ventricular flutter at this rate would have to have, by definition, an almost sinusoidal pattern with no

discernible QRS or T waves. This strip shows clearly evident and discrete QRS complexes and T waves. Remember, when the rate exceeds 250 BPM, start thinking about rhythms caused by conduction through an accessory pathway. In this case, the wide QRS complexes make this an example of an antidromic AVRT.

Test ECG 11

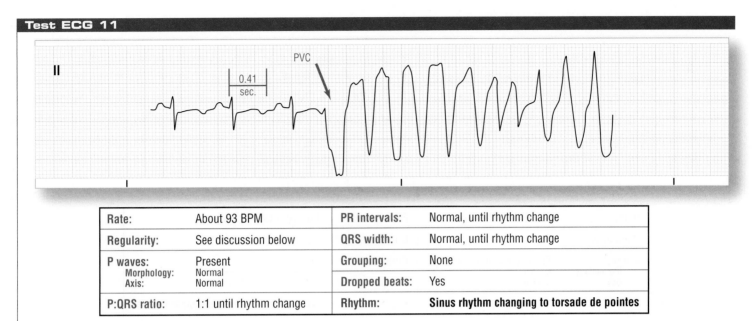

Rate:	About 93 BPM	PR intervals:	Normal, until rhythm change
Regularity:	See discussion below	QRS width:	Normal, until rhythm change
P waves: Morphology: Axis:	Present Normal Normal	Grouping:	None
		Dropped beats:	Yes
P:QRS ratio:	1:1 until rhythm change	Rhythm:	**Sinus rhythm changing to torsade de pointes**

Discussion:

Test ECG 11 shows a patient who is in sinus rhythm at a rate of 93 BPM. The patient's complexes, however, show an obvious QT prolongation, with a QT interval of 0.40 seconds. The QTc is 0.51 (QTc = QT/square root of R-R interval in seconds), which is markedly prolonged. Remember that the QTc is a value that takes into consideration the physiologic changes that occur in the QT interval due to rate. The patient has a PVC that falls on the T wave of the previous complex (R-on-T phenomenon) and triggers an episode of an undulating, irregular, wide-complex rhythm associated with polarity changes. This new rhythm is torsade de pointes.

Test ECG 12

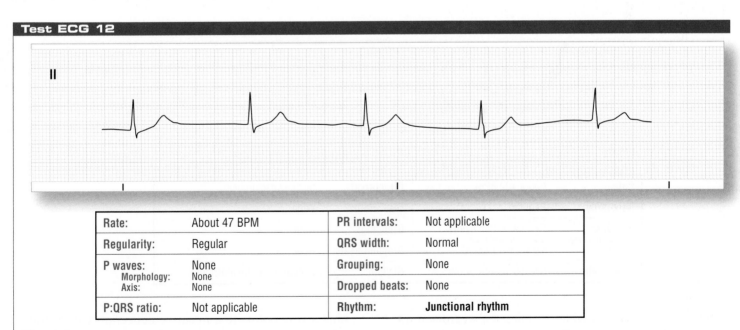

Rate:	About 47 BPM	PR intervals:	Not applicable
Regularity:	Regular	QRS width:	Normal
P waves: Morphology: Axis:	None None None	Grouping:	None
		Dropped beats:	None
P:QRS ratio:	Not applicable	Rhythm:	**Junctional rhythm**

Discussion:

Test ECG 12 shows a slow narrow-complex rhythm that is regular. There are no obvious P waves anywhere along the strip. This is an example of a junctional rhythm.

Test ECG 13

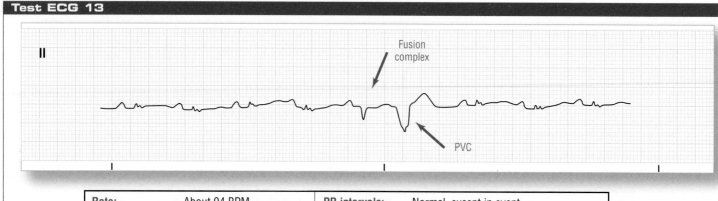

Rate:	About 94 BPM	PR intervals:	Normal, except in event
Regularity:	Regularly irregular	QRS width:	Normal, except in event
P waves: Morphology: Axis:	Present, except in event Normal Normal	Grouping:	None
		Dropped beats:	Yes
P:QRS ratio:	1:1, except in event	Rhythm:	**Sinus rhythm with a ventricular couplet**

Discussion:

Test ECG 13 shows a patient with very small voltage on the QRS complexes. The patient has an underlying sinus rhythm. After the fifth P wave, two different QRS complexes are noted. The second of these complexes is a clear PVC. The first of these two complexes, however, is completely different from either the normal QRS

complex or the PVC. The PR interval of this complex is different, but the P wave is the same and the cadence is unchanged throughout the strip. This QRS complex is most probably a fusion complex involving the normally conducted supraventricular impulse and the PVC.

Test ECG 14

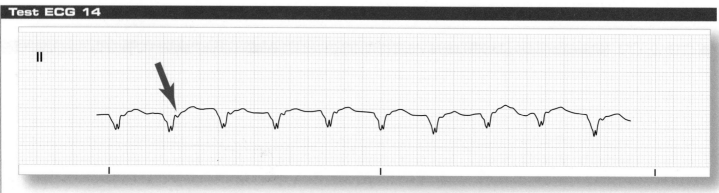

Rate:	About 102 BPM	PR intervals:	See discussion below
Regularity:	Regular	QRS width:	Wide
P waves: Morphology: Axis:	See discussion below See discussion below See discussion below	Grouping:	None
		Dropped beats:	None
P:QRS ratio:	See discussion below	Rhythm:	**Accelerated idioventricular**

Discussion:

Test ECG 14 shows a wide-complex tachycardia at a rate of about 102 BPM. The rhythm is regular and monomorphic in appearance. This is an example of an accelerated idioventricular rhythm. As a side point, the

blue arrow points to a negative deflection within the ST segment. This is an inverted P wave due to the retrograde conduction of the ventricular impulse into the atria.

Test ECG 15

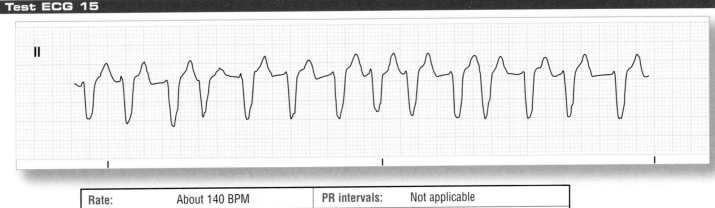

Rate:	About 140 BPM	PR intervals:	Not applicable
Regularity:	Irregularly irregular	QRS width:	Wide
P waves:	None	Grouping:	None
Morphology:	None		
Axis:	None	Dropped beats:	None
P:QRS ratio:	Not applicable	Rhythm:	**Atrial fibrillation**

Discussion:

Test ECG 15 brings up a common clinical scenario that often causes patients to be misdiagnosed—the presence of an preexisting condition which causes wide QRS complexes. To start, the rate on this strip is rapid at about 140 BPM. Is this rhythm regular, regularly irregular, or irregularly irregular? The rhythm is irregularly irregular. The three main irregularly irregular rhythms are atrial fibrillation, WAP, and MAT. Are there any P waves anywhere on the strip? Since there are no visible P waves any-

where on this strip, the most probable diagnosis is atrial fibrillation. Why are the complexes wider than 0.12 seconds? The reason for the wide complexes in this patient is that there was a preexisting left bundle branch block. This is an example of an uncontrolled atrial fibrillation in a patient with a preexisting LBBB. The key to making the diagnosis in this patient was to answer the question about the chaotic timing of the complexes and not the presence of the wide complexes themselves.

Test ECG 16

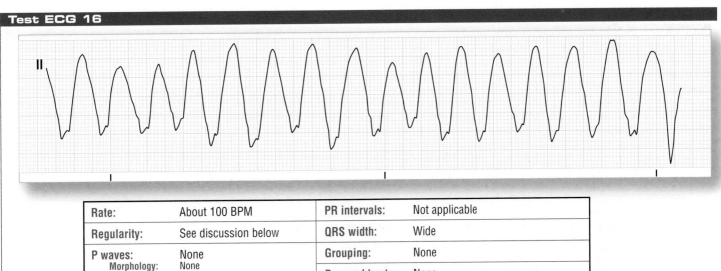

Rate:	About 100 BPM	PR intervals:	Not applicable
Regularity:	See discussion below	QRS width:	Wide
P waves:	None	Grouping:	None
Morphology:	None		
Axis:	None	Dropped beats:	None
P:QRS ratio:	Not applicable	Rhythm:	**Polymorphic ventricular tachycardia**

Discussion:

This rhythm is also very irregular. But, compare it to Test ECG 15. You will see that there are no obvious QRS complexes and T waves on this strip. There is also a wave-like undulation in the size of the QRS complexes throughout the strip. In addition, the undula-

tions involve multiple complexes forming small groups. This is an example of a very slow polymorphic ventricular tachycardia. Clinical correlation was consistent with an acute MI in this patient.

Test ECG 17

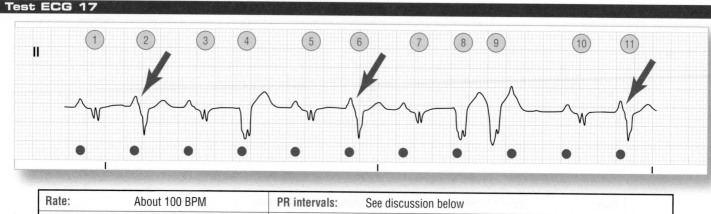

Rate:	About 100 BPM	PR intervals:	See discussion below
Regularity:	Regularly irregular	QRS width:	Normal, except in events
P waves: Morphology: Axis:	Present, except in events Normal Normal	Grouping:	None
		Dropped beats:	Yes
P:QRS ratio:	See discussion below	Rhythm:	**Sinus tachycardia with frequent PVCs and a ventricular couplet**

Discussion:

We figured that you were ready for a challenge by now. We have labeled the ventricular complexes for easier identification and are using the blue circle to signify the atrial complexes. The morphology of the QRS complex labeled #1 is representative of the normally conducted complex. The baseline rhythm on this strip is a sinus tachycardia. Complexes #2, 6, and 11 are fusion complexes formed by the normally transmitted supraventric-ular complexes and PVCs. Complexes #4, 8, and 9 are PVCs. Note that the supraventricular rhythm marches throughout the strip essentially unchanged and causing a fusion between the P waves and the underlying PVCs and fusion complexes. Finally, the P waves in complex #2, 6, and 11 are themselves fused with the onset of their respective ventricular fusion complexes (see blue arrows). All in all, a very confusing rhythm strip.

Test ECG 18

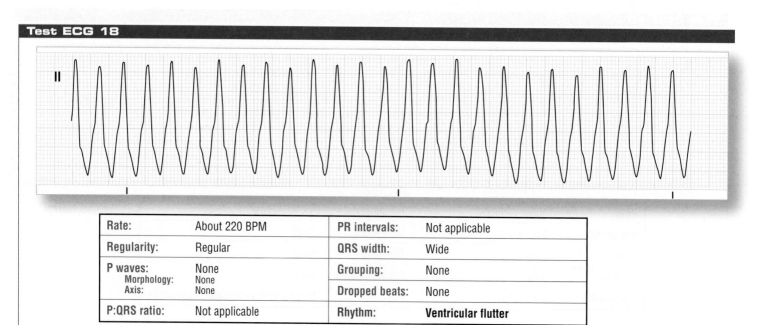

Rate:	About 220 BPM	PR intervals:	Not applicable
Regularity:	Regular	QRS width:	Wide
P waves: Morphology: Axis:	None None None	Grouping:	None
		Dropped beats:	None
P:QRS ratio:	Not applicable	Rhythm:	**Ventricular flutter**

Discussion:

This strip shows a wide-complex tachycardia with an almost constant sinusoidal pattern of the QRS complexes and the T waves. This is an example of ventricu-lar flutter. Note that the polarity of the complexes does not change in this type of rhythm, compared to poly-morphic ventricular tachycardia.

Test ECG 19

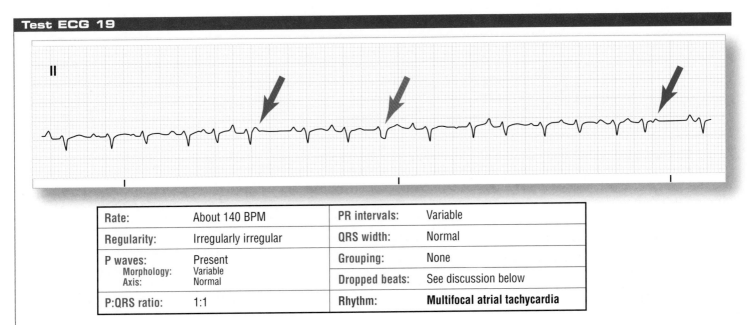

Rate:	About 140 BPM	PR intervals:	Variable
Regularity:	Irregularly irregular	QRS width:	Normal
P waves: Morphology: Axis:	Present Variable Normal	Grouping:	None
		Dropped beats:	See discussion below
P:QRS ratio:	1:1	Rhythm:	**Multifocal atrial tachycardia**

Discussion:

Once again, there are three main irregularly irregular rhythms: atrial fibrillation, WAP and MAT. Are there any P waves noted on this ECG? Yes. This means that the rhythm, with rare exceptions, is going to be either WAP or MAT. The tachycardia makes MAT the most likely candidate. Now we need to prove our presumptive diagnosis. Do we have at least three different P wave morphologies? Yes. Are they associated with different PR intervals? Yes. The diagnosis is now definitely MAT.

There are many buried P waves throughout the strip, as would be expected in a rapid MAT. In addition, there are two blocked P waves (see blue arrows). Finally, there is one complex labeled by the red arrow that most likely represents either a PJC with aberrancy or a PAC with aberrancy in a complex with an isoelectric P wave.

Test ECG 20

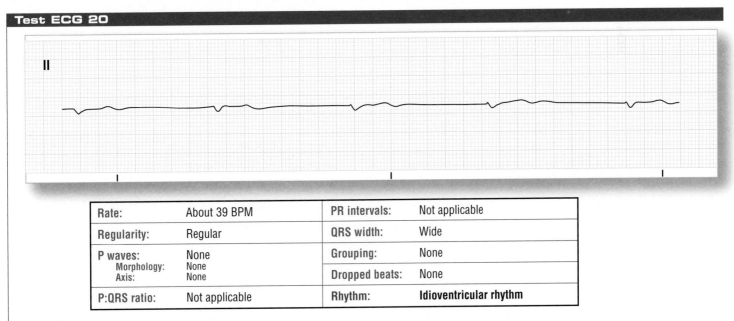

Rate:	About 39 BPM	PR intervals:	Not applicable
Regularity:	Regular	QRS width:	Wide
P waves: Morphology: Axis:	None None None	Grouping:	None
		Dropped beats:	None
P:QRS ratio:	Not applicable	Rhythm:	**Idioventricular rhythm**

Discussion:

This strip shows a series of wide complexes at a rate of 39 BPM. There are no visible P waves anywhere along the strip. This strip could be due to a junctional rhythm with aberrancy, a preexisting condition leading to wide QRS complexes, or an idioventricular rhythm, the most probable option being an idioventricular rhythm. A full 12-lead ECG and clinical correlation would be needed in this patient to be completely sure of the diagnosis.

Additional Rhythms and Information

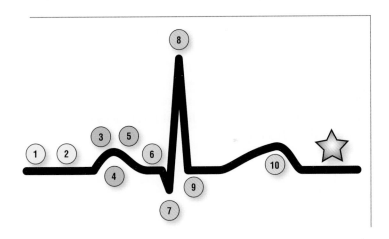

Atrioventricular Block

General Overview

Many of you may be wondering why the AV blocks (AVBs) are being placed in the miscellaneous arrhythmias section of this book instead of in the section on junctional rhythms. The main reason is that the AVBs are not really arrhythmias in and of themselves; instead, they are obstruction to conduction through the electrical conduction system. As such, they may not necessarily be the primary arrhythmia, but rather represent a secondary or a protective process. For example, we typically say a rhythm is a sinus tachycardia with a ____-degree AV block.

In very simple terms, an AV block is formed when conduction of the supraventricular impulses, through the AV node or the ventricular portion of the electrical conduction system, is either partially or completely blocked from reaching the ventricles (Figure 35-1). When the impulses are simply delayed, it is called a *first-degree AV block*. These ECGs typically show a prolonged PR interval of greater than 0.20 seconds. When the impulses are intermittently blocked from reaching the ventricles completely, causing some QRS complexes

to be dropped, it is called a *second-degree AV block*. There are two main types of second-degree AV block: *Mobitz I* and *Mobitz II*. There are also two minor variations of second-degree AVB: *2:1* (or *untypable*) and *high-grade* (or *advanced*). Lastly, when there is no actual communication at all between the atria and the ventricles, we call it a *complete* or *third-degree AV block*.

In this chapter, we are going to cover the diagnostic criteria used to identify each one of these AV blocks and provide various strips of each type for your review. His bundle electrocardiography has broadened our understanding of the AV blocks and their sites of origin. However, the concepts involved in these findings are often complex and fall well above the scope of a book on arrhythmia recognition. As such, we will be concentrating on identifying the various blocks from actual rhythm strips and will provide electrophysiological information only when appropriate. Figure 35-2 shows an easy way to remember how to identify blocks by using P waves. If readers are interested in further information on this topic, see the list of references provided at the end of this book.

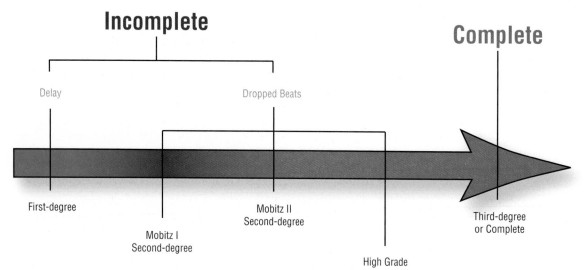

Figure 35-1: The atrioventricular blocks. The red part of the arrow signifies the potentially lethal nature of these types of AV blocks.

When **None** of the P waves are blocked,
it is a
First-degree AVB

When Some of the P waves are blocked,
it is a
Second-degree AVB

When All of the P waves are blocked,
it is a
Third-degree AVB

Figure 35-2: An easy way to remember the blocked P waves and AVBs.

ADDITIONAL **INFORMATION**

The "Blocks"

Very often, beginners have some difficulty identifying and understanding the AV blocks. This is partly because the word "block" is used to describe many different processes.

As mentioned, the AV blocks are typically caused by a conduction problem and typically show characteristic ECG patterns that involve either a prolongation of the PR interval, dropped QRS complexes, or a complete pathological lack of communication between the atria and the ventricles. The conduction defect in the AV blocks can actually take place at any level of the ventricular portion of the electrical conduction system, but the more common ones involve mainly the AV node and the bundle of His or the bundle branches themselves, and can be either functional or pathological.

The bundle branch blocks, on the other hand, are caused by true pathologic and anatomic blockade at the level of the left or right bundle branches of the electrical conduction system. The block causes an obstruction to the propagation of the impulse in either one ventricle or the other. In order to depolarize the ventricle in question, the depolarization wave must proceed by direct cell-to-cell contact. The slow transmission of the impulse creates wide QRS complexes that will have one of two morphological presentations, either a right bundle branch block pattern or a left bundle branch block pattern.

Likewise, the hemiblocks are caused by localized pathologic "blocks" to impulse conduction in either the left anterior or the left posterior fascicles. The hemiblocks mainly alter the direction of the main ventricular axis on the ECG.

First-Degree AV Block

Before we look at the specifics of first-degree heart block, we should begin by looking at the various components that make up of the PR interval itself (see Figure 35-3). Electrocardiographically, conduction of the electrical impulse from the sinus node through the ventricles takes place during the PR interval through the electrical conduction system.

The depolarization of the actual sinus node takes place very shortly before the onset of the P wave. From there, the electrical impulse itself does not have to travel through the atria by direct cell-to-cell transmission in order to reach the AV node. Instead, the impulse is conducted very quickly through a specialized tract of cells known as the internodal pathways. This rapid system allows the impulse to reach the AV node while the slow process of the depolarization of the atrial myocytes takes place. The P wave itself is formed by the depolarization of the actual atrial myocyte themselves. These simultaneously occurring processes are graphically represented in Figure 35-3 by the blue dashed line seen under the P wave.

After conduction of the impulse through the atria and the AV node, the impulse then moves through the His bundles, the bundle branches, and the Purkinje system. These events are still all occurring during the PR interval. Notice that the PR interval represents conduction throughout the entire electrical conduction system. The PR interval is measured as the distance from the beginning of the P wave to the beginning of the QRS complex.

A first-degree AV block is defined as a delay in the conduction of the supraventricular impulse to the ventricles, serious enough to prolong the PR interval above 0.20 seconds (the upper limit of normal). The delay most commonly occurs at the level of the AV node or the bundle of His. (Rarely, the delay can occur distal to the bundle of His.) Note that first-degree AV block is a delay or an incomplete block and every P wave will conduct to the ventricles. It may be late. . .but it will conduct every time.

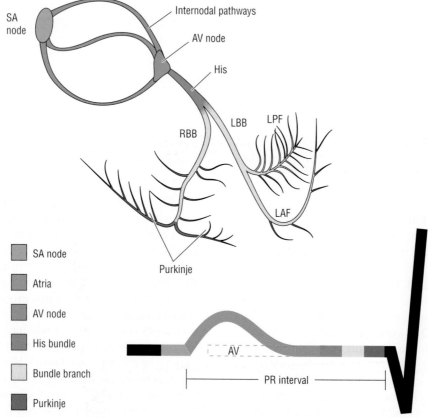

Figure 35-3: The electrical conduction system transmits the electrical impulse from the sinus node to the level of the ventricular myocytes. The portion of the complex shown breaks down the PR interval to show the various components that make up the entire interval.

So, how does a delay in conduction cause a PR prolongation? As we saw in Figure 35-3, transmission of the impulse through the electrical conduction system takes place during the PR interval. As we can further deduce from Figure 35-3, and clearly see in Figure 35-4, the prolongation of any one of the components of the PR interval will prolong the entire interval. Therefore, a serious delay in conduction through the AV node or the bundle of His will lead to a serious prolongation of that section of the PR interval, and hence, the whole thing.

As stated above, a first-degree AV block is electrocardiographically represented by a PR interval that is greater than 0.20 seconds, or one big block on the ECG paper. In general, a first-degree AV block will have a PR interval in the 0.21 to 0.40 range. The width of the PR interval, however, can be quite impressive, reaching levels of 0.60 or even 1 second wide. Figure 35-5 shows various examples of PR prolongation with various widths. Note that sometimes the P wave may actually fuse with the previous T wave. In very rare instances, the P wave of one complex may actually be before the previous QRS. Talk about a confusing presentation!

In first-degree AV block, the width of the QRS complexes should be normal, except in the case of a preexisting bundle branch block or the presence of aberrancy. Remember, ventricular depolarization is represented on the ECG by the QRS complex. The QRS complexes are normal width in first-degree AV block because ventricular depolarization is not directly affected, the onset merely occurs a little later, time-wise. In other words, the delay in conduction occurs only at the level of the electrical conduction system (represented by the PR interval) and not at the level of ventricular depolarization (represented by the QRS complex).

Figure 35-5 highlights one additional, critical fact about first-degree AV blocks: *Each P wave has its own QRS complex.* In other words, the conduction ratio is 1:1 (one P wave for every QRS complex). This is because first-degree AVBs are not really true blocks but merely reflect delays in conduction. As we shall see, the rest of the AV blocks are associated with dropped QRS complexes or complete blocks, with separate atrial and ventricular rhythms, and their conduction ratios will not be 1:1.

Finally, the width of the PR prolongation in any one patient with first-degree AV block may change slightly from time to time. This variation in PR interval may be

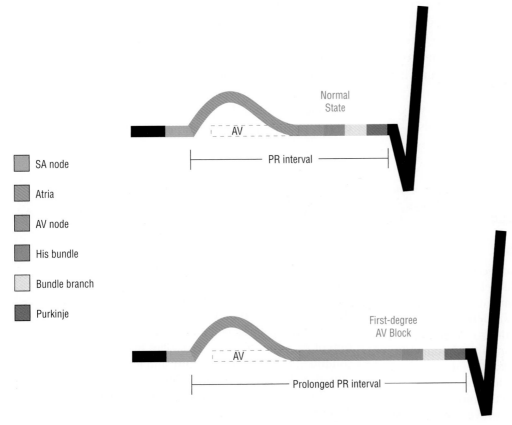

SA node

Atria

AV node

His bundle

Bundle branch

Purkinje

Normal State

AV

PR interval

First-degree AV Block

AV

Prolonged PR interval

Figure 35-4: A prolongation or delay in any one component will cause a prolongation of the entire PR interval. In this case, the prolongation occurred at the level of the AV node.

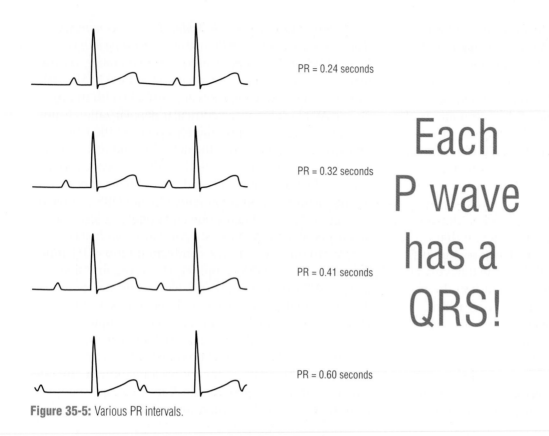

PR = 0.24 seconds

PR = 0.32 seconds

PR = 0.41 seconds

PR = 0.60 seconds

Each P wave has a QRS!

Figure 35-5: Various PR intervals.

due to various factors. For example, the heart rate itself will affect the PR interval, with bradycardias having longer intervals and tachycardias having shorter intervals. The vagal tone of the patient can also influence the PR interval, with vagal stimulation lengthening it. The presence of dual-AV nodal pathways, as we mentioned in Chapter 25, may be associated with varying PR intervals, depending on which tract the impulse takes to reach the AV node.

In this chapter, we are going to depart from our traditional method of showing the actual patient rhythm strips until the end of the chapter. This will help you become familiar with each type one at a time. At the end of the chapter, we will include a few extra rhythm strips in which all of the types will be represented for comparison. We hope that this presentation will help you form a clearer picture of this sometimes confusing topic.

Wide QRS Complexes and AV Blocks

In general, any of the AV blocks can occur in the AV node proper or in the bundle of His before the bifurcation. These complexes will have narrow QRS complex associated with them (provided that there is no preexisting bundle branch block or aberrancy). Any AV block that originates below the bifurcation of the bundle of His typically has wide QRS complexes. Remember, blocks don't always have to have wide complexes.

As we shall see when we get to the more serious kinds of AV blocks, narrow complexes typically occur if the block is above the bifurcation of the bundle of His.

This is because, in the cases when there is conduction, all of the ventricular depolarization will proceed along the normal electrical conduction system. Wide QRS complexes, on the other hand, are caused by infra-Hisian (below the bundle of His) blocks. This occurs because these blocks will always have some transmission of the impulse in the ventricles by direct cell-to-cell conduction. This process is slow and leads to the formation of wide complexes on the ECG.

This discussion is not very pertinent to first-degree AV blocks, but will become more important with the more advanced blocks to follow.

ECG 35-1

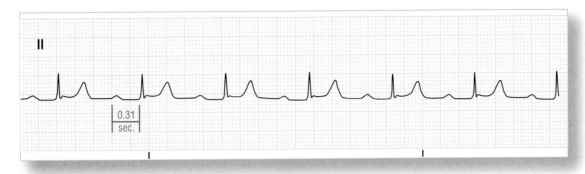

Rate:	About 65 BPM	PR intervals:	Prolonged
Regularity:	Regular	QRS width:	Normal

P waves:
   Morphology:
   Axis:
	Normal
	Normal
	Normal
		Grouping:	None

		Dropped beats:	Absent
P:QRS ratio:	1:1	Rhythm:	**Sinus rhythm with first-degree AVB**

Discussion:

The rhythm strip above shows a regular rhythm with upright P waves in lead II. This is consistent with a sinus rhythm. The PR interval is prolonged at 0.31 seconds, which is way above the upper limit of normal at 0.20 seconds. The P:QRS ratio is 1:1 with each P wave conducting to form one QRS complex. All of these findings are consistent with a sinus rhythm with a first-degree AV block.

ECG 35-2

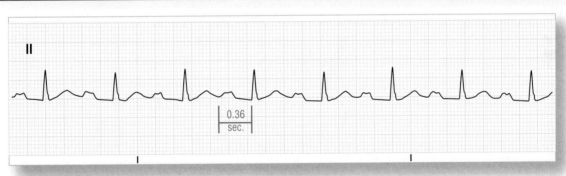

Rate:	About 77 BPM	PR intervals:	Prolonged
Regularity:	Regular	QRS width:	Normal

P waves:
   Morphology:
   Axis:
	Normal
	Normal
	Normal
		Grouping:	None

		Dropped beats:	Absent
P:QRS ratio:	1:1	Rhythm:	**Sinus rhythm with first-degree AVB**

Discussion:

This strip shows upright P waves in lead II and normal-looking QRS complexes appearing at a rate of about 77 BPM. The P: QRS ratio is 1:1 with each P wave conducting to one QRS complex. The PR intervals are approximately 0.36 seconds and are, therefore, prolonged. This strip is consistent with a sinus rhythm with a first-degree AV block.

ECG 35-3

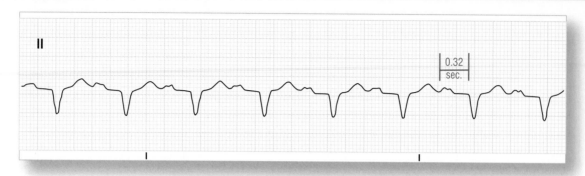

Rate:	About 77 BPM	PR intervals:	Prolonged
Regularity:	Regular	QRS width:	Wide
P waves:	Normal	Grouping:	None
Morphology:	Normal		
Axis:	Normal	Dropped beats:	Absent
P:QRS ratio:	1:1	Rhythm:	**Sinus rhythm with first-degree AVB**

Discussion:

No, this is not the same patient as in ECG 35-2. The P waves and the rates are similar, but that is where the similarities end. This patient shows upright P waves in lead II that are also humped, but the PR interval is prolonged at 0.32 seconds. Also note that these QRS complexes are exactly 0.12 seconds due to a preexisting left bundle branch block. The final diagnosis is a sinus rhythm with a first-degree AV block in a patient with a preexisting left bundle branch block.

ECG 35-4

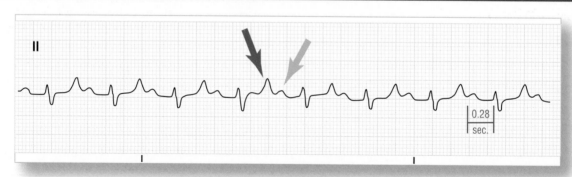

Rate:	About 85 BPM	PR intervals:	Prolonged
Regularity:	Regular	QRS width:	Normal
P waves:	Normal	Grouping:	None
Morphology:	Normal		
Axis:	Normal	Dropped beats:	Absent
P:QRS ratio:	1:1	Rhythm:	**Sinus rhythm with first-degree AVB**

Discussion:

The strip above shows prolonged PR intervals at about 0.28 seconds. The QRS complexes are small and relatively isoelectric, whereas the T waves are very prominent. The blue arrow is pointing at the T waves, and the pink arrow is pointing at the P waves. Note that the true PR interval may be slightly longer than 0.28 seconds because the P waves are partly buried in the previous T wave. This means that the early onset of the P waves, and the additional width of the PR interval, cannot be seen clearly.

ECG 35-5

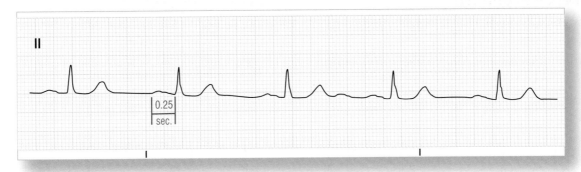

Rate:	About 52 BPM	PR intervals:	Prolonged
Regularity:	Regular	QRS width:	Normal
P waves: Morphology: Axis:	Normal Normal Normal	Grouping:	None
		Dropped beats:	Absent
P:QRS ratio:	1:1	Rhythm:	**Sinus bradycardia with first-degree AVB**

Discussion:

This ECG shows a sinus bradycardia with narrow ventricular complexes. The P waves are upright in lead II, which is a normal P wave axis. The PR intervals are prolonged at 0.25 seconds, giving this patient a first-degree AV block. Notice that in this case, the PR interval is mostly made up of a very wide P wave (P-mitrale due to left atrial enlargement). Remember, it doesn't matter what component of the PR interval is prolonged to make the call of a first-degree AV block—it just has to be prolonged.

Second-Degree AV Block

The second-degree AV blocks are characterized by both the presence of P waves and intermittently dropped QRS complexes. Usually, there is only one dropped QRS complex for each grouping, but multiple dropped complexes can occasionally occur (especially in Mobitz II second-degree block). The nonconducted P waves occur because second-degree AVBs work by an all-or-none kind of process. The conduction of the depolarization wave to the ventricles will either happen or it won't. This is in sharp contrast to the simple delay that we saw when we looked at the first-degree AVBs.

The dropped QRS complex in all types of second-degree AV blocks typically provides a natural barrier for the eye that gives the complexes the appearance of being grouped (Figure 35-6). In other words, the regular empty space created on the rhythm strip by the dropped QRS complex provides a natural break in the rhythm, which is very obvious to the naked eye. Since the dropped beats typically occur fairly frequently, the empty spaces make it look like the complexes come in groups. *The presence of grouping is one of the major things that you need to look for when considering the possibility of a second-degree AV block.*

There are two main types of second-degree AV block and two minor variations. The main types are known as Mobitz I second-degree AVB (also known as Wenckebach) and Mobitz II second-degree AVB. The differences between these two are related to the appearance of their PR intervals associated with the complexes and their most common sites of origin. The minor variations mentioned above are the high-grade or advanced AVBs and the 2:1 or untypable AVB, and we will discuss these separately.

Mobitz I Second-Degree AV Block or Wenckebach

Mobitz I second-degree AVB or Wenckebach is a very common rhythm abnormality that is usually clinically benign. It is characterized by the presence of P waves that appear with a progressive lengthening of their PR intervals until one of them fails to conduct. The process then typically begins all over again, with progressive lengthening of the PR interval until another QRS complex is dropped. The main criteria for the presence of a Mobitz I second-degree AVB are:

1. PR interval progressively lengthens until a P wave is eventually blocked.

a. The shortest PR interval is the one immediately following the dropped beat.

b. The longest PR interval is the one immediately before the dropped beat.

c. The largest incremental change in the PR interval occurs between the first and second PR intervals in a sequence.

2. The R-R intervals progressively shorten until a QRS complex is dropped.

3. The interval including the dropped P wave is less than the sum of two P-P intervals.

The site where the block most commonly occurs is at the level of the AV node. However, in about a quarter

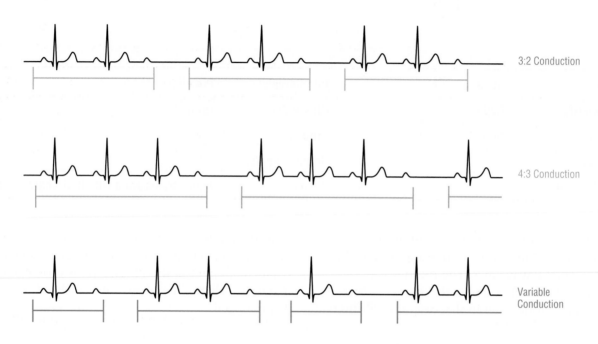

3:2 Conduction

4:3 Conduction

Variable Conduction

Grouping is one of the major diagnostic features of second-degree AVBs!

Figure 35-6: Different types of conduction in a patient with Mobitz II second-degree AVB.

The Terminology of Conduction

When referring to the conduction ratios or sequences of the various groups in second-degree AVBs, clinicians frequently use the words "conduction" and "block" interchangeably. This can lead to more confusion related to the word "block," and can lead to some serious errors.

When we use the word *conduction* in discussing the conduction ratios in AVBs, we refer to the ratio of P waves that conduct to the ventricles. For example, a 3:2 conduction means that in a grouping, there are three P waves, and two of those P waves conduct normally to create two QRS complexes. In other words, only one P wave has been blocked.

When we use the word *block* in reference to conduction ratios in groupings, we are comparing the number of P waves in the group and the number of P waves that have been blocked. For example, a 3:2 block means that for every three P waves, two get blocked and only one gets through to create a single QRS complex.

In order to avoid further problems with nomenclature, we suggest that you get used to using either "conduction" or "block" when referring to conduction ratios. We feel that "conduction" provides the maximal amount of information that is needed in clinical practice. In this book, the word "conduction" will be the terminology used exclusively.

of the cases, the block can occur below the AV nodes. The QRS complexes in Wenckebach are usually normal width unless there is a preexisting bundle branch block or there is aberrancy. An infra-Hisian site for the block may also be associated with a widening of the QRS complexes, although this is a rare occurrence.

1. PR interval progressively lengthens until a P wave is eventually blocked.
The Wenckebach phenomenon can occur with P waves that originate in either the sinus node, the ectopic atrial tissue, or the AV junction itself. In general, the P-P interval in Wenckebach is consistent, reflecting the cadence set by either the sinus node or the ectopic pacemaker.

In order for any second-degree AV block to develop, there needs to be a site of delay and eventually obstruction to the conduction of the supraventricular impulse to the ventricles. The delay and eventual obstruction occur as a result of any process that lengthens the refractory period and conduction rates of the obstructing site. For Wenckebach, this site is typically the AV node, but it can be anywhere along the electrical conduction system. For simplicity, we are going to limit this discussion to the AV node.

As the supraventricular impulses reach the AV node, the first complex after the pause finds the node normally or near normally ready to receive it (Figure 35-7). That first supraventricular impulse is conducted without difficulty because the node is set to receive it. As that first complex goes through, however, it leaves the node a little more refractory and a little less ready to receive the next impulse. This is reflected as a delay in transmitting the second impulse to the ventricles

(Figure 35-8). In other words, the PR interval temporarily lengthens for this second complex.

Now, as that second impulse goes through the node, it will in turn cause further refractoriness that will make the delay even longer for the third supraventricular impulse. This prolongs the PR interval even further during the third complex. This process of delay leading to further delay continues until, eventually, the refractoriness and delay in the AV node reaches such a point that conduction completely fails (Figure 35-9). This will be represented on the ECG strip as a P wave with a dropped QRS complex. The time supplied by the blocked impulse allows the AV node to reset, and so the next P wave will begin the whole process all over again.

This repeating cycle of delay and eventual block is what gives Wenckebach its grouped appearance. The groupings can occur at many different conduction ratios. The groupings are, however, always found in a ratio of $N:(N-1)$. In other words, there will always be one less QRS complex than there are P waves. Examples of possible conduction ratios include 2:1, 3:2, 4:3, 5:4, . . .10:9, . . . 17:16 . . . and so forth. The conduction ratios can also be variable within the same patient. Figure 35-10 shows some typical Mobitz II second-degree AV block conduction ratios.

a. The shortest PR interval is the one immediately following the dropped beat.   As you saw from the discussion above, the AV node is best able to receive a new impulse immediately after the dropped beat. This is because during the pause, the AV node had time to lose its refractoriness and to build up enough steam to conduct normally. Basically, the AV node can conduct this

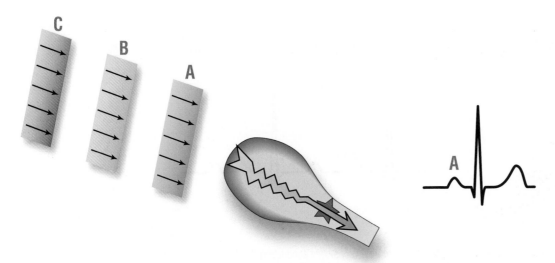

Figure 35-7: This figure represents three sinus waves that are approaching a slowly conducting or diseased AV node. In this figure, the wave labeled A reaches a rested, nonrefractory AV node. It easily makes it to the trigger zone (red star) and fires a ventricular depolarization wave.

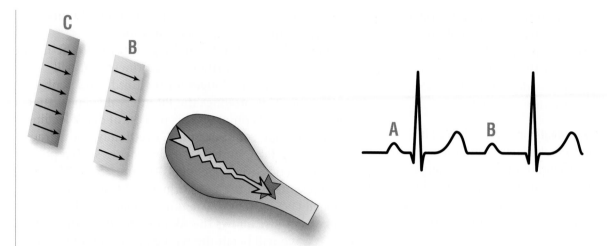

Figure 35-8: This figure represents the second wave, labeled B, reaching a slower, more refractory AV node. Conduction is delayed and the PR interval appears to be prolonged. In this figure, the wave labeled B doesn't penetrate the AV node as easily. It does, however, make it to the trigger zone and fires a ventricular depolarization wave.

first P wave with minimal, if any, variation in the PR interval. Therefore, the first PR interval in any one group (the one that occurs immediately after the dropped beat) is always the shortest (Figure 35-11).

b. The longest PR interval is the one immediately before the dropped beat. As we mentioned before, conduction through the electrical conduction system is an all-or-none phenomenon. Conduction will either occur or be blocked. Going back to our discussion on how the PR intervals become prolonged, we see that with every passing P wave, the PR interval lengthens as the AV node becomes more and more unable to trans-

mit the impulse. Eventually, the delay becomes so great that the impulse fails to conduct to the ventricles. That last, nonconducted P wave does not have a PR interval at all. Therefore, the longest PR interval has to belong to the last P wave that was conducted and has a QRS wave. That lucky P wave reached the AV node before it completely gave out. It is the one with the maximal amount of delay but still conducted. That P wave gives rise to the last PR interval in a group (Figure 35-12).

So far, we have seen that Wenckebach or Mobitz I second-degree AV block is associated with a progressive prolongation of the PR interval until a P wave gets completely blocked. We have seen that the shortest PR

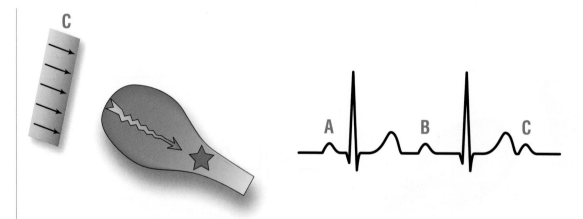

Figure 35-9: This figure represents the third wave, labeled C, approaching the now very slowly conducting or heavily refractory AV node. In this figure, the wave labeled C hardly penetrates the AV node at all. It does not reach the trigger zone and does not fire a ventricular depolarization wave.

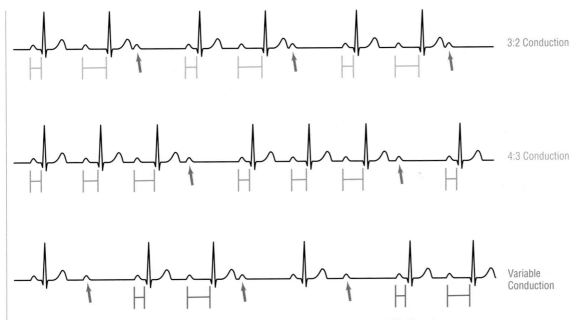

3:2 Conduction

4:3 Conduction

Variable
Conduction

Figure 35-10: Different types of conduction in a patient with Mobitz I second-degree AVB. Note the progressive prolongation of the PR interval until one P wave fails to conduct (red arrows).

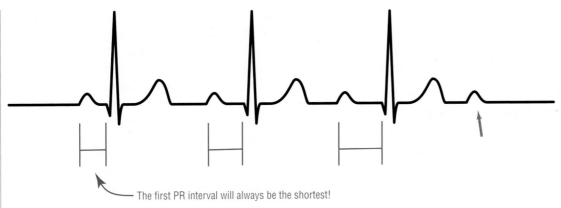

The first PR interval will always be the shortest!

Figure 35-11: The shortest PR interval is always the first one after the dropped beat.

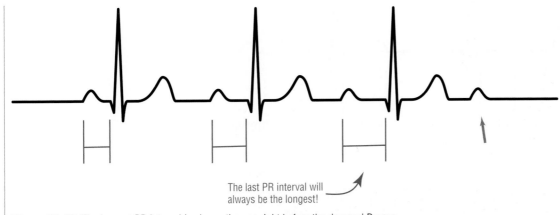

The last PR interval will always be the longest!

Figure 35-12: The longest PR interval is always the one right before the dropped P wave.

interval is the first one in the grouping, and that the longest PR interval is the last one in a grouping. Now, we need to take a closer look at what happens in between the first and last PR intervals.

c. The largest incremental change in the PR interval occurs between the first and second PR intervals.

We know that the first PR interval in a grouping is always the shortest. The next big diagnostic criterion that we are going to examine is that *the largest incremental change in the PR interval occurs between the first and the second PR intervals* (Figure 35-13).

Going back to our original progressive PR interval discussion, we see that right before the first P wave reaches the AV node, it is at its maximal amount of conductive potential. When the first P wave is conducted, the AV node remains somewhat refractory. This refractoriness leads to a delay in the conduction of the second P wave. The difference between maximal conductivity of the first P wave and the subsequent delay in the conduction of the second P wave signifies the largest amount of total change in conductivity in any one group.

The amount of additional delay that is added to each successive PR interval in a group is small in comparison to the delay between the first and second complexes. As you can see from Figure 35-13, the amount of prolongation seen between the subsequent PR intervals is smaller than between the first two.

2. The R-R intervals progressively shorten until a QRS complex is dropped.

In Wenckebach, the R-R interval shortens progressively between each QRS complex. This is because the incremental change in the delay caused by the progressing PR interval becomes shorter.

The previous comments are counterintuitive until you really break it down by looking at a strip. Take a look at Figure 35-15. In this figure, you see that the P-P interval is a value of X seconds. Under normal circumstances, the P-P intervals and the R-R interval should be the same value. But, in Wenckebach we need to add the amount of incremental change caused by the PR interval getting longer (the delay) to the normal P-P interval of X in order to get the measurement of that R-R interval. In the case of the first two complexes, the value of the true R-R interval as X + 0.08 seconds. Using the same logic, the next R-R interval would now be X + 0.04 seconds. Notice that this is shorter than the first one. As you can see, as the incremental change between the PR intervals gets shorter, the R-R intervals have got to get shorter as well. This continues to occur until the dropped P wave, then the cycle begins all over again in the next group.

Don't spend a lot of time trying to understand the math and why this occurs. Instead, just remember that the R-R intervals shorten between each complex in a group. This fact comes in handy in some tough diagnostic cases.

3. The interval including the dropped P wave is less than the sum of two P-P intervals.

The interval that includes the pause has got to be shorter than the sum of two P-P intervals (Figure 35-16). This makes sense if you think about the fact that the PR interval immediately after the pause is the shortest one in the group. Also, the blocked P contains essentially no delay at all because it was completely blocked. Therefore, the sum of any two complexes in the group would have to include at least two delays that would be longer than the nonconducted P wave and that first, short PR interval.

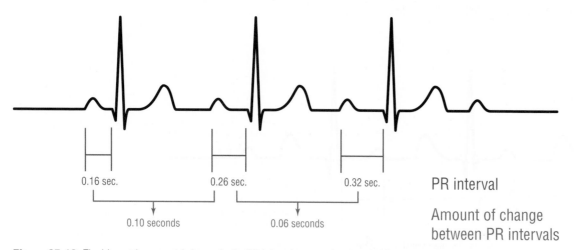

0.16 sec.　　0.26 sec.　　0.32 sec.　　PR interval

0.10 seconds　　0.06 seconds　　Amount of change between PR intervals

Figure 35-13: The biggest incremental change in the PR intervals occurs between the first and second PR intervals. In this example, the difference between the first and second PR intervals is 0.10 seconds. The difference between the second and third PR intervals is 0.06 seconds.

ADDITIONAL INFORMATION

Atypical Wenckebach or Mobitz I Second-degree AV Block

What happens if you have a really long conduction group with Wenckebach, say 10:9? Does the progressive prolongation of the PR intervals and the amount of change between them continue throughout the strip? The answer is no. Eventually, the amount of change in the PR intervals becomes zero, if the strip is long enough before the dropped beat. What probably happens is that, after a while, the amount of delay continues to increase but at electrocardiographically unmeasureable amounts until the all-or-none phenomenon fails to conduct a P wave. This type of conduction defect is known as *atypical* Wenckebach or *atypical* Mobitz I second-degree AV block (Figure 35-14).

In atypical Wenckebach, the first PR interval is still the shortest. The longest PR interval is still the last one. Finally, the largest amount of incremental change between the PR intervals is still between the first and second ones. The only difference is that the PR intervals do not continue to widen indefinitely. This can sometimes make the diagnosis of the AVB difficult. *Always look closely at the interval with the dropped beat.* If the PR interval before the dropped P wave is longer than the one immediately after the pause, you are probably dealing with an atypical Wenckebach.

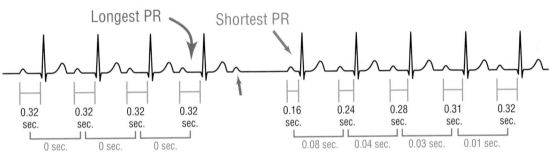

Figure 35-14: Atypical Wenckebach.

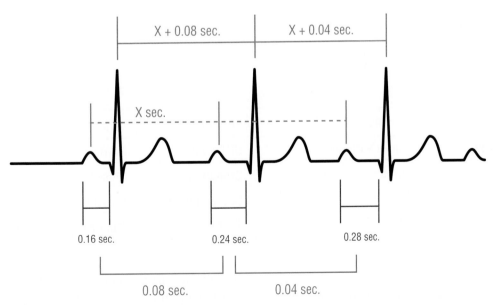

Figure 35-15: Decreasing R-R interval.

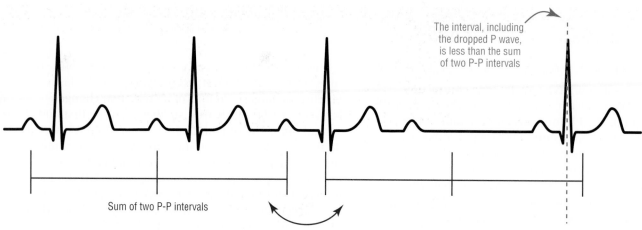

The interval, including the dropped P wave, is less than the sum of two P-P intervals

Sum of two P-P intervals

Figure 35-16: The distance of the pause.

Mobitz I Second-Degree AV Block: A Final Word

Diagnosing Wenckebach or Mobitz I second-degree AVB is simple when the conduction ratios are 3:2 or 4:3. However, the longer conduction ratios make diagnosis more difficult. Atypical presentations abound that could easily throw you off track. The key is to note the progressive PR prolongation and the eventual dropped beat. A strip that only shows you progressive prolongation of the PR interval should steer you in the right direction, and you should think about getting a longer strip. The longer strip may show the dropped P wave and the typical changes seen around the pause.

The pause is the area of any strip where the changes of Wenckebach will be the most obvious. There you will see the longest PR interval in the beat before the dropped P. There you will see that the shortest PR interval will be the first PR interval in a group. There you will see that the largest incremental change in the PR intervals occurs between the first and second conducted complexes. Above all, remember that if you don't think about the possibility, you will never make the diagnosis.

ECG 35-6

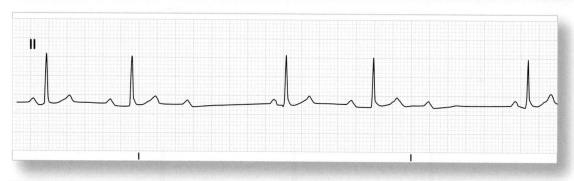

II

Rate:	About 40 to 50 BPM	PR intervals:	Variable
Regularity:	Regularly irregular	QRS width:	Normal
P waves:	Normal	Grouping:	Present
Morphology:	Normal		
Axis:	Normal	Dropped beats:	Present
P:QRS ratio:	3:2	Rhythm:	**Mobitz I second-degree AVB**

Discussion:

The rhythm strip above shows a grouped rhythm with a conduction ratio of 3:2. There is progressive widening of the PR interval between the first and second complexes and then there is a dropped P wave. The cycle then begins all over again in a recurrent pattern. This has all the earmarks of a Mobitz I second-degree AV block. Note that you cannot make a comment about shortening R-R intervals in this case because there is only one R-R interval per group.

ECG 35·7

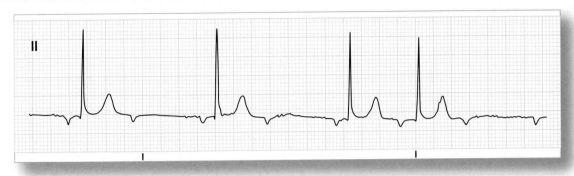

Rate:	About 40 to 50 BPM	PR intervals:	Variable
Regularity:	Regularly irregular	QRS width:	Normal
P waves: Morphology: Axis:	Present Inverted Abnormal	Grouping:	Present
		Dropped beats:	Present
P:QRS ratio:	2:1 and 3:2	Rhythm:	**Mobitz I second-degree AVB**

Discussion:

This patient starts off with two groupings that are conducted at a ratio of 2:1. After these two groupings, we see a grouping that is made up of three P waves and two QRS complexes with progressive PR interval widening and then a dropped P wave. This is consistent with a Wenckebach or Mobitz I second-degree AV block. Note that the P waves are ectopic in nature as indicated by their inverted morphology in lead II. The QRS complexes are narrow and obviously supraventricular.

ECG 35·8

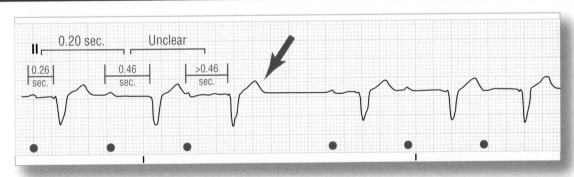

Rate:	About 50 BPM	PR intervals:	Variable
Regularity:	Regularly irregular	QRS width:	Wide
P waves: Morphology: Axis:	Normal Normal Normal	Grouping:	Present
		Dropped beats:	Present
P:QRS ratio:	4:3	Rhythm:	**Mobitz I second-degree AVB**

Discussion:

We definitely see grouping, which would be clearer if we had a longer strip. The PR intervals progressively lengthen until there is a pause. The blocked P is not visible because it is buried in the T wave of the last complex (see blue arrow). The incremental amount of the delay is definitely shorter between the second and third complexes than between the first and second complexes. However, since the third P is partially buried, the true measurement cannot be determined accurately.

ECG 35-9

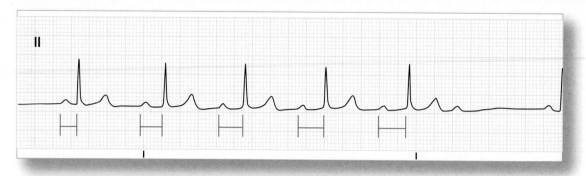

Rate:	About 60 BPM	PR intervals:	Variable
Regularity:	Regularly irregular	QRS width:	Normal
P waves:	Normal	Grouping:	Present
Morphology:	Normal		
Axis:	Normal	Dropped beats:	Present
P:QRS ratio:	6:5	Rhythm:	**Mobitz I second-degree AVB**

Discussion:

This strip is classic for Wenckebach or Mobitz I second-degree AV block. We see a pause at the start and then a normal PR interval. The PR then begins to lengthen progressively throughout the rest of the group. Finally, the group terminates with a blocked P wave. The R-R interval shortens at the beginning of the group and then the shortening levels out, which is a bit atypical. The pause is less than the sum of two P-P intervals.

ECG 35-10

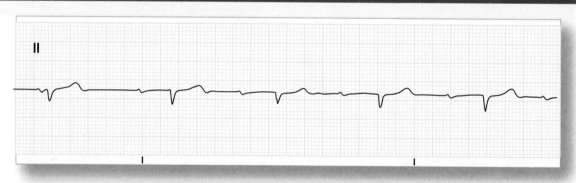

Rate:	About 50 BPM	PR intervals:	Variable
Regularity:	Regularly irregular	QRS width:	Normal
P waves:	Normal	Grouping:	Present
Morphology:	Biphasic		
Axis:	Normal	Dropped beats:	Present
P:QRS ratio:	6:5	Rhythm:	**Mobitz I second-degree AVB**

Discussion:

The strip above shows one entire grouping of a very long rhythm strip. The rhythm strip shows recurrent groupings that were identical to the strip above. This strip has all the earmarks of Mobitz I second-degree AV block, except they are a bit exaggerated. The PR pro- gressively widens throughout the group. The incremental change in PR intervals is quite dramatic between the first one and the second one in the group. By the way, the pause was less than the sum of two P-P intervals.

ECG 35-11

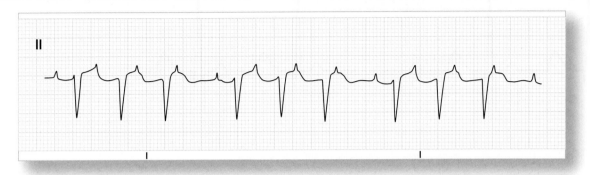

Rate:	About 90 BPM	PR intervals:	Variable
Regularity:	Regularly irregular	QRS width:	Normal
P waves:	Normal	Grouping:	Present
Morphology:	Normal		
Axis:	Normal	Dropped beats:	Present
P:QRS ratio:	4:3	Rhythm:	**Mobitz I second-degree AVB**

Discussion:

This strip also shows the classic changes for a Wenckebach or Mobitz I second-degree AVB. The PR interval starts off a bit prolonged and then continues to progressively increase throughout the strip. The groups end with a nonconducted P wave. Notice that the R-R intervals do not shorten on this strip, which is an atypical finding. The incremental change in the PR intervals is the largest between the first and second complex, as you would expect.

Mobitz II Second-Degree AV Block

Mobitz II second-degree AV block is a very simple rhythm to understand and identify compared with Mobitz I or Wenckebach. However, don't let its simplicity fool you. The mechanisms behind a Mobitz II block are much more life-threatening, and misdiagnosis can be lethal.

Simply stated, Mobitz II second-degree AVB is diagnosed when you have either a single or multiple nonconducted P waves in the face of a rhythm with constant PR intervals (Figure 35-17). The PR interval can be either normal or prolonged, just as long as it is constant before the pause and constant after the pause. The P-P intervals are constant throughout the strip and the pause is exactly equal to two.

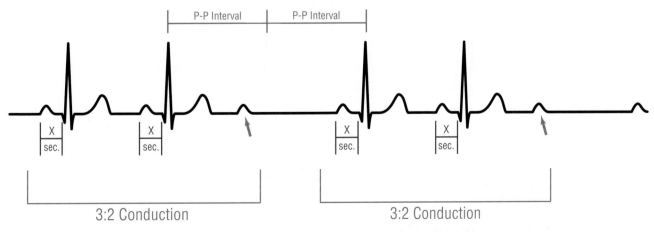

Figure 35-17: Mobitz II second-degree AVB.

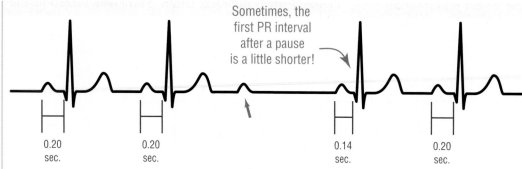

Sometimes, the
first PR interval
after a pause
is a little shorter!

0.20
sec.

0.20
sec.

0.14
sec.

0.20
sec.

Figure 35-18: The first PR interval after a pause in Mobitz II second-degree AVB may be shorter.

If you think about it, Mobitz II is the epitome of the all-or-none response. Almost all of the P waves will conduct normally. There is no delay associated with the P waves that are conducted. Occasionally, however, a P wave will simply fail to conduct.

In order to diagnose Mobitz II, you need to have at least two consecutive conducted P waves. This is important to be able to establish the consistency of the PR intervals. That said, the PR interval immediately after the pause may show some narrowing compared to the others (Figure 35-18). This can sometimes happen because of increased conduction through a well-rested conduction system. (This can sometimes lead to confusion and misdiagnosing the strip as a Mobitz I or Wenckebach.)

The conduction ratios of the Ps and QRSs can also vary in Mobitz II, just as they did in Mobitz I. Figure 35-19 is a graphical representation of various conduc-

tion ratios. The conduction ratios can also vary within the same patient at any one time.

Notice in the strips that we have shown you so far of Mobitz II, all of the QRS complexes have been narrow. *In Mobitz II, the QRS complexes can either be narrow or wide, depending on the location of the conduction block.* If the block is in the AV node or in the bundle of His, the QRS complexes will be narrow. If the conduction block occurs below the bifurcation of the bundle of His, the QRS complexes will be wide.

The most common site for the conduction block in Mobitz II second-degree AV block is in the bundle branches. It is found there about 80% of the time. In the remaining 20% of the cases, the block occurs in the bundle of His. Mobitz II rarely occurs in the AV node. From these statistics we can say that, typically, the QRS complexes in Mobitz II will be wide.

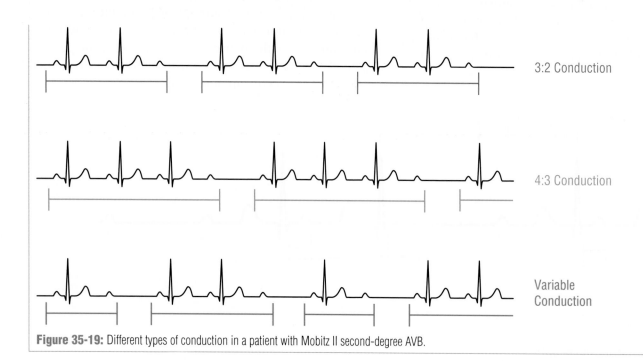

3:2 Conduction

4:3 Conduction

Variable
Conduction

Figure 35-19: Different types of conduction in a patient with Mobitz II second-degree AVB.

The location of the conduction defect is also what makes these blocks so uncommon and so dangerous. Mobitz II is much less commonly found than Mobitz I. When it is found, it is indicative of fairly advanced conduction system disease. As a matter of fact, many of these patients have concomitant bundle branch blocks.

Clinically, Mobitz II is a *permanent* conduction defect and shows a great tendency to progress to higher degrees of block. Often it progresses to complete block.

Basically, that's it. Diagnosing Mobitz II is fairly easy, and there are no variations except for an occasional narrowing of the first PR interval. When you do find it, be careful! Always have a pacemaker handy, because you are probably going to need it. This is especially true if the patient is having active ischemia or infarction.

ADDITIONAL **INFORMATION**

Mobitz II vs. Blocked PAC

There is one diagnostic problem that we would like to bring to your attention as we finish up Mobitz II second-degree AV block. Frequently, PACs are blocked from depolarizing the ventricles for whatever reason. The net result is that the P wave will be visible, but the QRS complex will not be. This resembles a Mobitz II block at first glance.

Close examination, however, will make a blocked PAC evident. First of all, a blocked PAC is still prema-ture. The prematurity of the P wave of the PAC will be in stark contrast to the metronome regularity of the Mobitz II block. Remember, the P-P interval in Mobitz II is very, very regular. If you see a prematurely occurring P wave that is blocked, it should raise the suspicion of a blocked P wave from a PAC firmly in your mind.

Secondly, the morphology of the P wave in the PAC will be different from that of the rest of the complexes in the rhythm (Figure 35-20). In Mobitz II, the morphology of *ALL* of the P waves is identical.

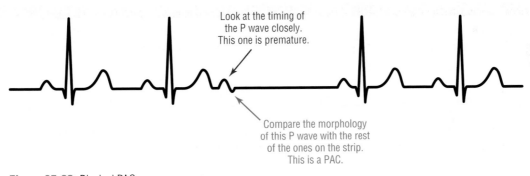

Look at the timing of the P wave closely. This one is premature.

Compare the morphology of this P wave with the rest of the ones on the strip. This is a PAC.

Figure 35-20: Blocked PAC.

ECG 35-12

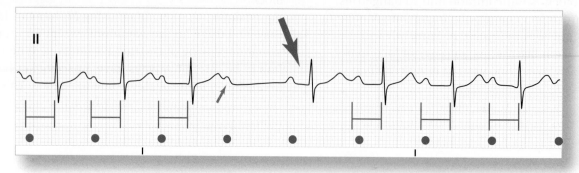

Rate:	About 70 BPM	PR intervals:	Prolonged
Regularity:	Regularly irregular	QRS width:	Narrow

P waves:
  Morphology:
  Axis:
	Normal
	Normal
	Normal
		Grouping:	Not present

		Dropped beats:	Present
P:QRS ratio:	1:1 with one dropped beat	Rhythm:	**Mobitz II second-degree AVB**

Discussion:

The strip above shows a long strip of complexes with prolonged but constant PR intervals. In the middle of the strip, there is a blocked P wave (red arrow). The blue arrow points out the first PR interval after the pause. Notice that this PR interval is a bit narrower than the others, which occurs occasionally in Mobitz II blocks. The second PR interval after the pause already is back to the constant PR interval found throughout the strip.

ECG 35-13

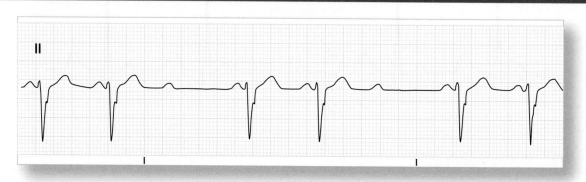

Rate:	About 50 BPM	PR intervals:	Variable
Regularity:	Regularly irregular	QRS width:	Wide

P waves:
  Morphology:
  Axis:
	Normal
	Normal
	Normal
		Grouping:	Present

		Dropped beats:	Present
P:QRS ratio:	3:2	Rhythm:	**Mobitz II second-degree AVB**

Discussion:

This strip shows a wide-complex regularly irregular rhythm with grouping. The groups are conducted in a ratio of 3:2. The important thing to note about the groups is that the PR interval remains constant throughout the strip. The P-P intervals are constant throughout, as you would expect in a Mobitz II block.

ECG 35·14

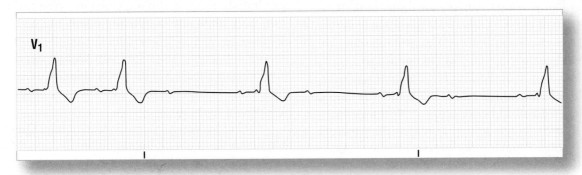

Rate:	About 75 BPM	PR intervals:	Constant
Regularity:	Regularly irregular	QRS width:	Wide
P waves:	Normal	Grouping:	Present
Morphology:	Normal		
Axis:	Normal	Dropped beats:	Present
P:QRS ratio:	3:2 and 2:1	Rhythm:	**Mobitz II second-degree AVB**

Discussion:

The strip above shows a patient who is transiently wandering between 3:2 conduction to 2:1 conduction. Whenever you have an obvious Mobitz II second-degree AVB in any section of the strip and then you have an area of 2:1 conduction, the 2:1 block is assumed to be Mobitz II second-degree as well. The QRS complexes show a wide-complex morphology that is consistent with RBBB in lead V$_1$.

ECG 35·15

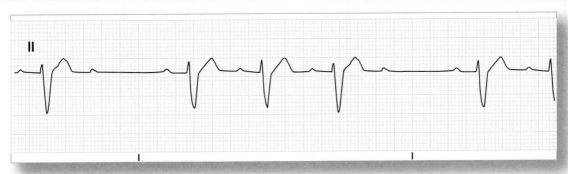

Rate:	About 75 BPM	PR intervals:	Constant
Regularity:	Regularly irregular	QRS width:	Wide
P waves:	Normal	Grouping:	Present
Morphology:	Normal		
Axis:	Normal	Dropped beats:	Present
P:QRS ratio:	4:3	Rhythm:	**Mobitz II second-degree AVB**

Discussion:

The strip above shows a regularly irregular rhythm with dropped beats. The PR intervals are constant throughout the strip, and so are the P-P intervals. This is consistent with a Mobitz II second-degree AV block. The grouping that usually occurs in any second-degree AVB would be readily apparent if you had a longer strip. The QRS complex is wide and consistent with a left bundle branch block in this patient. Bundle branch blocks are often associated with Mobitz II.

Untypable or 2:1 Second-Degree AV Block

Take a look at Figure 35-21. What rhythm is it? Well, it could be a Mobitz I second-degree AV block being conducted at a 2:1 ratio. You don't see the prolongation of the PR interval because the second P wave is the blocked P wave. But, it could also be Mobitz II second-degree AV block being conducted at a 2:1 ratio. If that were the case, you would have constant PR intervals. Once again, you could not see the constant PR intervals because the second P wave is the blocked P wave. As you can see, both possibilities could be right, and you have no way of telling.

The answer is that this strip shows a 2:1 or untypable second-degree AV block. There is definitely evidence of a second-degree AV block, but you just don't know which one. Why? Because in order to make the diagnosis of either Mobitz I or Mobitz II, you need to have at least two consecutive P waves that are conducted to the ventricles. This will allow you to establish the relationship of the PR intervals, and whether they are lengthening or staying constant. At a ratio of 2:1, you only have one conducted P wave in a group and there is no way of evaluating the relationship to the next PR interval. Since you can't make the diagnosis, the block is simply called untypable. More commonly, the term 2:1 block is used and the lack of specificity is presumed to be understood.

However, that said, if you have a long enough rhythm strip or if you happen to be lucky enough to capture the first time the block occurs, you can state the type of second-degree block with a fair degree of certainty. That is because if you see a Mobitz I pattern anywhere, you can assume the complexes that are being conducted at 2:1 are also Wenckebach (Figure 35-22). Likewise, if you see a Mobitz II pattern anywhere, you can assume the complexes that are being conducted at 2:1 are Mobitz II. Remember, always look at "the company it keeps" and you will be able to make the diagnosis.

Which is it:
Mobitz I or Mobitz II?

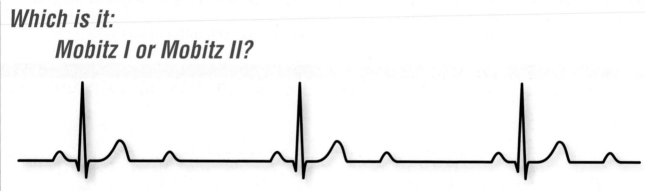

Figure 35-21: It is unclear which type of block this strip represents.

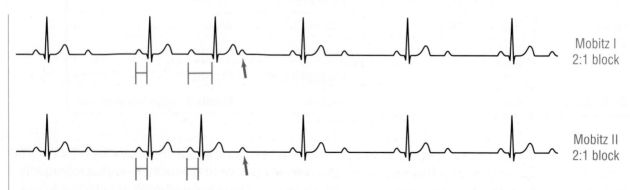

Mobitz I
2:1 block

Mobitz II
2:1 block

Figure 35-22: Mobitz I and Mobitz II 2:1 second-degree AV block.

ECG 35-16

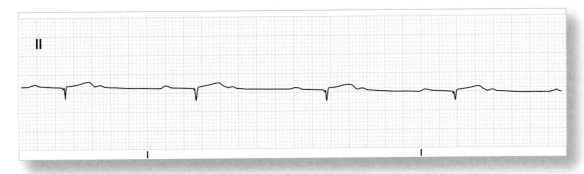

Rate:	About 42 BPM	PR intervals:	Prolonged
Regularity:	Regular	QRS width:	Narrow
P waves:	Normal	Grouping:	Present
Morphology:	Normal		
Axis:	Normal	Dropped beats:	Present
P:QRS ratio:	2:1	Rhythm:	**2:1 or untypable second-degree AVB**

Discussion:

This strip was taken from a patient with a long episode of 2:1 block. There were never any obvious segments of either Mobitz I or Mobitz II. Since you cannot tell which of them it was, the rhythm is simply labeled 2:1 or untypable second-degree AV block. The prolonged PR interval does favor the diagnosis of Mobitz II, but this is not enough to make the call.

ECG 35-17

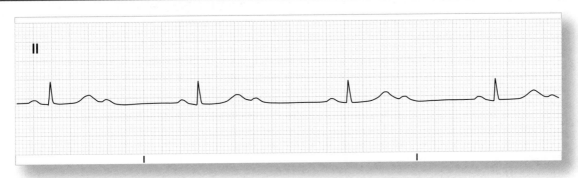

Rate:	About 35 BPM	PR intervals:	Constant
Regularity:	Regular	QRS width:	Narrow
P waves:	Normal	Grouping:	Present
Morphology:	Normal		
Axis:	Normal	Dropped beats:	Present
P:QRS ratio:	2:1	Rhythm:	**2:1 or untypable second-degree AVB**

Discussion:

This strip shows a strip with 2:1 block and a ventricular rate of 35 BPM. The PR interval is normal and consistent when it conducts. This could be compatible with either Mobitz I or Mobitz II. Based on this strip, the diagnosis can only be 2:1 AV block.

ECG 35-18

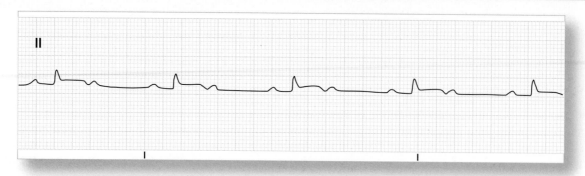

Rate:	About 45 BPM	PR intervals:	Prolonged, constant
Regularity:	Regular	QRS width:	Narrow
P waves:	Normal	Grouping:	Present
Morphology:	Normal		
Axis:	Normal	Dropped beats:	Present
P:QRS ratio:	2:1	Rhythm:	**2:1 or untypable second-degree AVB**

Discussion:

This strip shows another example of a typical 2:1 or untypable AV block. Even though you cannot officially make the call, there are a few things in this strip that favor Mobitz II. The prolonged PR interval is indicative of AV nodal dysfunction. In addition, the flat ST segment elevation could easily represent an evolving inferior wall MI. A full 12-lead ECG is indicated for evaluation of a possible MI. A longer rhythm strip may resolve the issue of this block being either a Mobitz I or II.

ECG 35-19

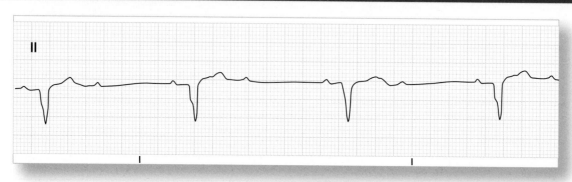

Rate:	About 33 BPM	PR intervals:	Prolonged, constant
Regularity:	Regular	QRS width:	Wide
P waves:	Normal	Grouping:	Present
Morphology:	Normal		
Axis:	Normal	Dropped beats:	Present
P:QRS ratio:	2:1	Rhythm:	**2:1 or untypable second-degree AVB**

Discussion:

Once again, you cannot make a decision on the type of second-degree AV block that this patient is experiencing based on this strip. Also once again, the presence of prolonged PR intervals and wide QRS complexes favor a Mobitz II block, but you simply cannot tell with any certainty. That is why the official diagnosis of the rhythm is 2:1 or untypable second-degree AV block.

High-Grade or Advanced AV Block

High-grade or advanced AV block is the term used to describe a conduction block that is somewhere between second-degree AVB and complete AVB. In order to meet the criteria for this type of block, *at least two consecutive P waves need to be blocked due to an underlying conduction defect*. Let's look at these criteria a bit closer.

Figure 35-23 shows a typical example of a high-grade or advanced AV block. Note that the conduction ratio is roughly 3:1 (one P wave is buried in the T wave). This means that at least two consecutive P waves were blocked before the third one finally was conducted to the ventricles. The number of P waves that have to be blocked has to be two or greater in order to meet the criteria for this type of block. This is in comparison to Mobitz I or Mobitz II, which need only one P wave to be blocked.

The second criterion is that the block has to be due to an underlying conduction defect and not simply be a normal physiologic response or block to a very rapid atrial rate. Let's take for example a rapid atrial flutter that is stimulating the atria at about 300 BPM. The constant bombardment of the AV node by such a rapid rate will often cause a physiologic block to develop due to refractoriness of the node in either a 2:1, 3:1, or higher ratio. In this case, the block is not due to an underlying conduction defect but is a normal physiologic response to a very rapid atrial rate.

The term high-grade or advanced AV block has also been used to describe certain patients whose ECGs wander between blocked P waves and complete heart block. These patients do not typically fit into the category of Mobitz II or complete heart block.

As we hinted above, this category of AV block is meant to provide clinicians with a term for blocks that don't really match any one pattern completely. As such, it is a nebulous term and there is a lot of confusion about it in the literature. In our research for this chapter, we found many different definitions and criteria for this type of block. You should be aware of the lack of consensus on this matter, and we will leave it here for now. Luckily, it is not a commonly found rhythm disturbance.

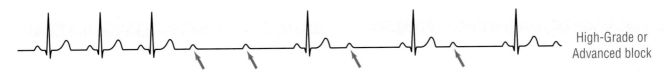

High-Grade or Advanced block

At least two consecutive
P waves are blocked

Figure 35-23: High-grade or advanced AV block.

ECG 35-20

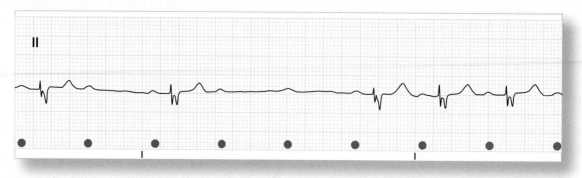

Rate:	About 81 BPM	PR intervals:	Prolonged, constant
Regularity:	Regularly irregular	QRS width:	Wide
P waves: Morphology: Axis:	Normal Normal Normal	Grouping:	None
		Dropped beats:	Present
P:QRS ratio:	Variable	Rhythm:	**High-grade or advanced AVB**

Discussion:

This rhythm strip shows a prolonged PR interval that is constant throughout the conducted beats on this strip. There is evidence of Mobitz II block at the start of the strip where one QRS complex is dropped. In the middle of the strip, there are two consecutive QRS complexes dropped. The presence of the two dropped QRS complexes is indicative of a high-grade or advanced AVB. A 12-lead ECG revealed the presence of a right bundle branch block and an acute MI in this patient.

ECG 35-21

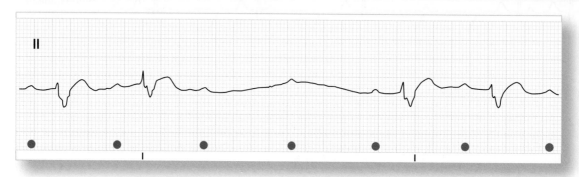

Rate:	About 62 BPM	PR intervals:	Prolonged, constant
Regularity:	Regularly irregular	QRS width:	Wide
P waves: Morphology: Axis:	Normal Normal Normal	Grouping:	None
		Dropped beats:	Present
P:QRS ratio:	Variable	Rhythm:	**High-grade or advanced AVB**

Discussion:

This patient has a strip with two consecutively blocked P waves. The PR interval is markedly prolonged, but constant throughout the conducted beats. The P-P interval remains fairly constant throughout the strip with only minimal variations that fluctuate slightly within acceptable limits, as usually happens in these patients. A 12-lead ECG was compatible with a left bundle branch block configuration in a patient having an acute MI.

Complete or Third-Degree AV Block

Complete or third-degree AV block is a fairly easy block to understand, but isn't necessarily easy to spot on a rhythm strip. Just as its name implies, complete or third-degree AV block is a *complete and total* block of conduction to the ventricles (Figure 35-24). In other words, there is a complete failure of the P waves to reach the ventricles. The conduction block can take place at the level of the AV node or lower on the electrical conduction system. This type of block is not typically caused by refractoriness of the node itself, but it is almost always due to a pathological or anatomic defect in the ventricular electrical conduction system.

In a third-degree block, almost by definition, you need to have two separate pacemakers. The supraventricular pacemaker (either sinus, ectopic atrial, or junctional), since it is a higher-order pacemaker, will usually fire spontaneously. But, a ventricular pacemaker is also mandatory in order to maintain cardiac output and, hence, life. In other words, a lower-order pacemaker from the ventricles *must* fire and set the ventricular pace in order for the patient to survive.

The morphology of the final rhythm will depend on the two individual rhythms that make it up. The two individual rhythms, in turn, depend on the ectopic site of the pacemakers involved (Figure 35-25). If the supraventricular rhythm originates in the sinus node, the morphology of the complexes will be sinus in nature. If they originate in an ectopic site, the morphological appearances of the supraventricular rhythm will depend on the location of the ectopic focus that created it and the route taken by the atrial depolarization wave to depolarize the actual atrial myocardium. Likewise, the morphological appearance of the ventricular rhythm will depend on the site of the ectopic focus that created it and the route of transmission that the ventricular depolarization wave will take through the ventricles. An ectopic focus that uses only direct cell-to-cell transmission will give rise to a very wide QRS complex. An ectopic focus that partially uses any part of the electrical conduction system will be narrower, reflecting the faster rate of transmission of the depolarization wave.

Third-degree AV block represents a failure of all of the P waves to be conducted to the ventricles. The rate of the subsidiary ventricular rhythm will depend on the ectopic site of origin for the pacemaker creating the rhythm. A junctional pacemaker will typically have narrow QRS complexes that are between 40 and 60 BPM. A ventricular pacemaker will typically have wide QRS complexes and a rate between 30 and 45 BPM. Occasionally, the ventricular rate will be very slow, sometimes occurring in the 30s or lower. That said, remember that any pacemaker can have accelerated automaticity or may trigger a reentry circuit. In those cases, the ventricular rhythm may be tachycardic.

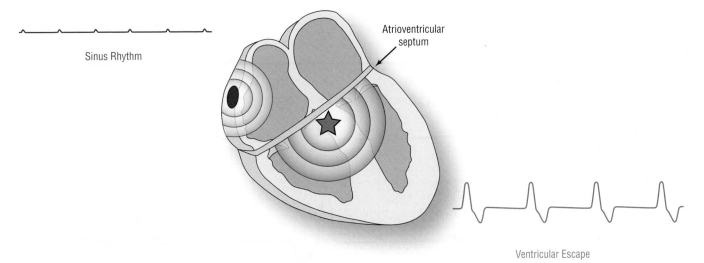

Sinus Rhythm

Atrioventricular septum

Ventricular Escape

Figure 35-24: When there is a conduction block that is complete, it basically shuts down all communication between the atria and the ventricles. For example, if the AV node is pathologically turned off, a complete block is created at the level of the interventricular septum. The atria and the ventricles are completely oblivious to each other and impulses are generated by two separate pacemakers, one supraventricular and one ventricular. Each pacemaker will keep its own intrinsic rate and control its own respective set of chambers.

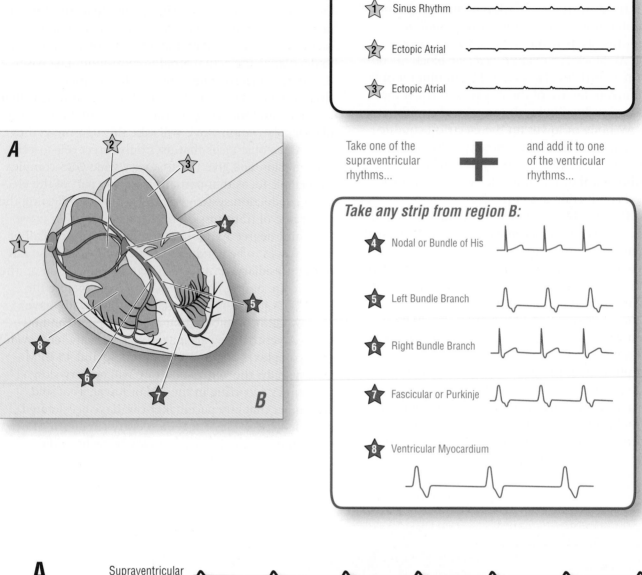

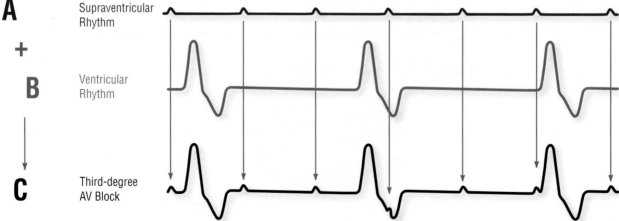

Figure 35-25: A pacemaker in the supraventricular area will create a supraventricular rhythm (blue area and blue block). A pacemaker in the ventricular area will give rise to a ventricular rhythm (red area and red block). If you take any one of the supraventricular strips and superimpose it electrocardiographically to any one of the ventricular strips, you end up with a strip showing a third-degree AV block (see figure at bottom). Note that neither the supraventricular rhythm nor the ventricular rhythm has any influence whatsoever on the other.

The width of the QRS complex can help you somewhat with the site of the block. Narrow complexes originate in either the AV node or the bundle of His in about 90%+ of the cases. Wide complexes ($\geq$ 0.12 seconds) can originate in the AV node or bundle of His if there is a preexisting bundle branch block, aberrancy, electrolyte disturbance, or some other predisposing condition. If they do not have any of these preexisting conditions, then the site of origin is usually infra-Hisian.

In third-degree AV block, the P-P intervals of the supraventricular rhythm and the R-R intervals of the ventricular rhythm will both be constant (Figure 35-26). They will, however, have no association whatsoever with each other. Each beats to its own drummer. . . or pacemaker. *The net result is that the PR interval is completely changing and never exactly repeats throughout the entire strip.* Recognizing the consistency of the individual components and the complete lack of any association between the two is the key to diagnosing a third-degree AV block.

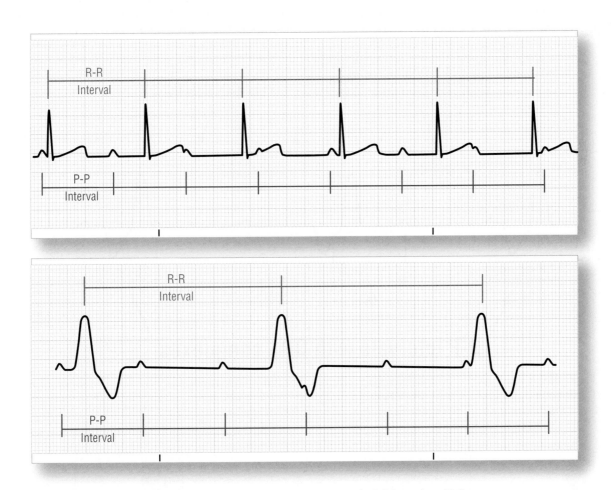

Figure 35-26: Two examples of third-degree or complete AV block. Note that the P-P intervals and R-R intervals are consistent in each strip. There is, however, no communication at all between the supraventricular and the ventricular components of each strip. This is indirectly demonstrated by the ever-changing PR intervals.

A D D I T I O N A L   **INFORMATION**

Ventriculophasic AV Dissociation

Ventriculophasic AV dissociation refers to a variation of third-degree AV block. In this variation, the R-R interval narrows slightly whenever a QRS complex falls between two P waves. The R-R intervals that do not have a QRS complex are not narrowed. The result is that the strip appears to have two different R-R intervals, one when there is a QRS involved and a different one when there is no QRS involved (Figure 35-27).

The presence of ventriculophasic AV dissociation is not clinically relevant, but it can sometimes cause a diagnostic dilemma. Awareness of this variation and close measurement of the intervals with an eye on the presence of QRS complexes will facilitate the diagnosis of the rhythm.

An easy way to remember it is that the QRS complex "pulls in" the P waves surrounding it. Another good memory aid is to think of a field goal in football (Figure 35-28). The QRS complex would be the football, which is being kicked between the two goal posts (the P waves). Making the field goal pulls the goal posts into each other. Missing the field goal doesn't do a thing.

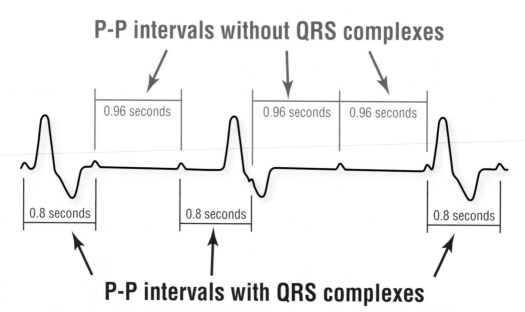

Figure 35-27: Ventriculophasic AV dissociation with the intervals that include a QRS complex at 0.8 seconds and the intervals without a QRS complex at 0.96 seconds.

Figure 35-28: Ventriculophasic AV dissociation is like a field goal. When the football makes it, the goalposts shake from the cheering and come in toward each other. When you don't make it, nothing happens.

ECG 35-22

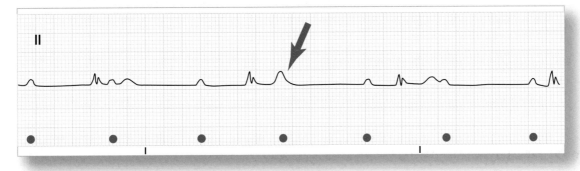

Rate:	Atrial: 65 BPM Ventricular: 35 BPM	PR intervals:	Variable
Regularity:	Regular	QRS width:	Wide
P waves:	Normal	Grouping:	None
Morphology: Axis:	Normal Normal	Dropped beats:	Present
P:QRS ratio:	Variable	Rhythm:	**Third-degree AVB**

Discussion:

This strip shows a third-degree AV block with a sinus rhythm and ventricular escape. The P waves are upright and map consistently throughout the strip. The blue arrow points out a buried P wave lying inside the T wave of the second complex. There is some slight irregularity of the P-P interval, which is ventriculophasic in nature. The P-P intervals without any QRS complexes are very consistent. The P-P intervals with QRSs inside them vary slightly in width, which is atypical.

ECG 35-23

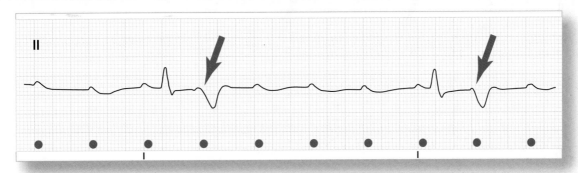

Rate:	Atrial: 100 BPM Ventricular: 20 BPM	PR intervals:	Variable
Regularity:	Regular	QRS width:	Wide
P waves:	Normal	Grouping:	None
Morphology: Axis:	Normal Normal	Dropped beats:	Present
P:QRS ratio:	Variable	Rhythm:	**Third-degree AVB**

Discussion:

This strip shows an underlying sinus tachycardia, which is completely blocked from reaching the ventricles. The ventricles are paced by a ventricular escape rhythm at about 20 BPM. Notice the wide QRS complexes with abnormal ST segments and T waves. The blue arrows point out buried P waves in the T waves of the ventricular complexes. Note the inconsistencies in the PR intervals shown, which is indicative of the complete AV block in this patient.

ECG 35-24

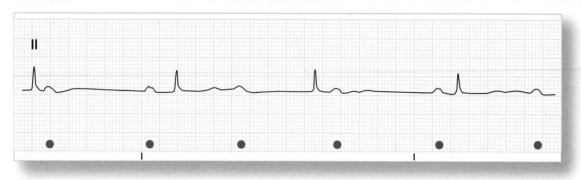

Rate:	Atrial: 57 BPM Ventricular: 39 BPM	PR intervals:	Variable
Regularity:	Regular	QRS width:	Narrow
P waves:	Normal	Grouping:	None
Morphology:	Normal		
Axis:	Normal	Dropped beats:	Present
P:QRS ratio:	Variable	Rhythm:	**Third-degree AVB**

Discussion:

This strip shows a complete or third-degree AV block with a sinus bradycardia and a junctional escape rhythm at a rate of about 39 BPM. The lack of communication between the atria and ventricles is obvious from examining the strip. Note that the PR intervals in front of the second and fourth QRS complexes are not the same.

ECG 35-25

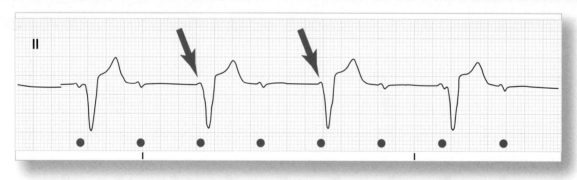

Rate:	Atrial: 90 BPM Ventricular: 45 BPM	PR intervals:	Variable
Regularity:	Regular	QRS width:	Wide
P waves:	Normal	Grouping:	None
Morphology:	Normal		
Axis:	Normal	Dropped beats:	Present
P:QRS ratio:	Variable	Rhythm:	**Third-degree AVB**

Discussion:

This strip shows a probable sinus rhythm with biphasic P waves. The ventricular rhythm is about 45 BPM, which could fall into the realm of either a junctional rhythm with a preexisting left bundle branch block or a more likely ventricular escape rhythm. An old ECG would be invaluable in confirming the final diagnosis. The presence of the third-degree AV block, however, cannot be disputed. The blue arrows point to the presence of two buried P waves.

ECG 35-26

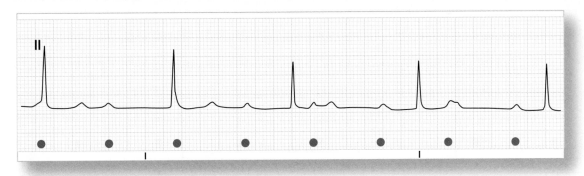

Rate:	Atrial: 79 BPM Ventricular: 44 BPM	PR intervals:	Variable
Regularity:	Regular	QRS width:	Narrow
P waves:	Normal	Grouping:	None
Morphology: Axis:	Normal Normal	Dropped beats:	Present
P:QRS ratio:	Variable	Rhythm:	**Third-degree AVB**

Discussion:

This strip shows a third-degree AV block with an underlying sinus rhythm and a junctional escape. Note how the first two QRS complexes are taller than the others. This is probably due to the fusion with the underlying P waves that just happen to fall at the same time. Using your calipers to map out a P-P interval width and then walking it back and forth across the strip is your best way to evaluate these rhythms and isolate the respective waves.

ECG 35-27

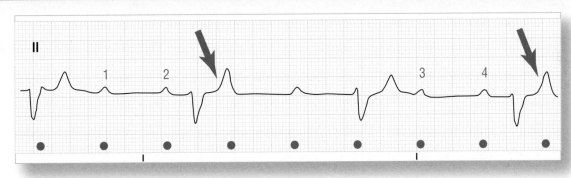

Rate:	Atrial: 88 BPM Ventricular: 33 BPM	PR intervals:	Variable
Regularity:	Regular	QRS width:	Wide
P waves:	Normal	Grouping:	None
Morphology: Axis:	Normal Normal	Dropped beats:	Present
P:QRS ratio:	Variable	Rhythm:	**Third-degree AVB**

Discussion:

This strip shows a complete heart block with an underlying sinus rhythm at about 88 BPM and a ventricular escape rhythm at 33 BPM. This ECG facilitates the diagnosis of the complete block by letting us see clearly two P waves occurring side-by-side with no QRS complexes. These P waves are labeled 1, 2, 3, and 4. Mapping out the distance between #1 and #2 and then walking the calipers over to #3 and #4 points out the consistency of the atrial rhythm. The blue arrows point to buried P waves.

ECG 35-28

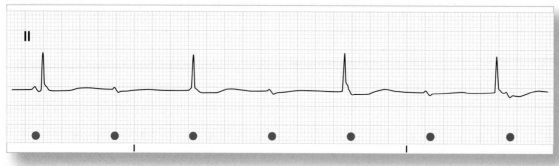

Rate:	Atrial: 70 BPM Ventricular: 36 BPM	PR intervals:	Variable
Regularity:	Regular	QRS width:	Narrow
P waves:	Normal	Grouping:	None
Morphology: Axis:	Normal Normal	Dropped beats:	Present
P:QRS ratio:	Variable	Rhythm:	**Third-degree AVB**

Discussion:

This strip shows a third-degree AV block with an underlying sinus rhythm and a junctional escape. The second and third QRS complexes have buried P waves associated with them. A clinical pearl: Whenever you have a P wave fall right in between two QRS complexes, always try to find the buried P wave. In this case, the search is simplified by the appearance of the first P wave right before the first QRS complexes. Walking this distance forward will clearly show the buried P waves.

ECG 35-29

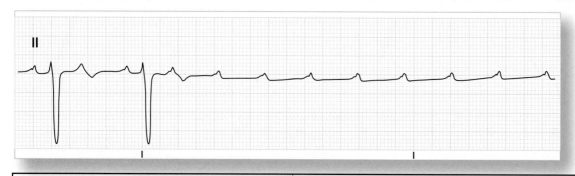

Rate:	Atrial: 60 BPM Ventricular: 115 BPM	PR intervals:	Variable
Regularity:	Regular	QRS width:	Wide
P waves:	Normal	Grouping:	None
Morphology: Axis:	Normal Normal	Dropped beats:	Present
P:QRS ratio:	Variable	Rhythm:	**Third-degree AVB**

Discussion:

This strip shows a very unfortunate patient who went from a 2:1 AV block into a complete AV block with ventricular standstill. Unfortunately for him, neither a junctional nor a ventricular pacemaker took over the pacing function for the ventricles. This patient highlights the lesson which we mentioned before, that all patients with serious AV blocks should have either a transcutaneous pacemaker or a transvenous pacemaker available at all times and ready to use. In these patients, time is critical.

ARRHYTHMIA RECOGNITION

Atrioventricular Blocks

	First-degree	Mobitz I Second-degree	Mobitz II Second-degree	2:1 or Untypable Second-degree	Third-degree or Complete
Rate	Variable	Variable	Variable	Variable	Variable
Regularity	Regular	Regular	Regularly irregular	Regular	Regular
P Wave	Present	Present	Present	Present	Present
Morphology	Normal	Normal or ectopic	Normal or ectopic	Normal or ectopic	Normal or ectopic
Upright in II, III, and aVF	Sometimes	Sometimes	Sometimes	Sometimes	Sometimes
P:QRS Ratio	1:1	X:X − 1	Variable	2:1	Variable
PR Interval	Prolonged	Variable	Normal or prolonged	Normal or prolonged	Variable
QRS Width	Normal or wide	Normal or wide	Normal or wide	Normal or wide	Normal or wide
Grouping	None	*Yes*	*Variable*	*Yes*	None
Dropped Beats	None	*Yes*	*Yes*	*Yes*	*Yes*

DIFFERENTIAL DIAGNOSIS

Atrioventricular Blocks

1. Sclerosis and fibrosis
   - Lev disease
   - Lenegre disease
   - Idiopathic
2. AMI and ischemic heart disease
3. Drugs
   - Calcium channel blockers
   - Digoxin
   - Beta blockers
   - Procainamide
   - Quinidine
   - Disopyramide
   - Propafenone
   - Amiodarone
   - Adenosine
4. Increased vagal tone: carotid sinus massage, pain, sleep, etc.
5. Surgery and trauma to the heart
6. Cardiomyopathies
7. Myocarditis
8. Infective endocarditis
9. Electrolyte disorders
10. Congenital heart disease

The list above is not inclusive but reflects the most common causes of the rhythm disturbance.

CHAPTER **REVIEW**

1. The AV blocks are caused when the conduction of the supraventricular impulses through the AV node or the ventricular portion of the electrical conduction system is either _____ or _____ blocked.

2. When the impulses are delayed but still transmitted to the ventricles, it is called a _____-degree AV block.

3. When the supraventricular impulses are intermittently blocked from reaching the ventricles causing some blocked P waves, it is called a _____-degree AV block.

4. When there is no communication at all between the atria and the ventricles, we call it a _____ or _____-degree AV block.

5. The second-degree AV blocks include various variations. These are:
    A. Mobitz I or Wenckebach
    B. 2:1
    C. Mobitz II
    D. High-grade or advanced
    E. All of the above

6. The typical finding in a first-degree AV block is a prolonged PR interval with a width greater than _____ seconds.

7. Since the block in first-degree AV block usually occurs in the AV node, the QRS complexes are usually narrow and the conduction ratio is 1:1 between the atria and the ventricles. True or False.

8. A first-degree AV block can never be wider than 0.40 seconds. True or False.

Match the following:

9. Two or more P waves blocked sequentially

10. Prolonged, constant PR intervals

11. Intermittently dropped QRS complexes in a strip with constant PR intervals

12. Noncommunicating atria and ventricles

13. Continuously prolonging PR intervals and dropped P waves

14. Two atrial complexes to one ventricular complex

A. First-degree AV block

B. Mobitz I second-degree AV block

C. Mobitz II second-degree AV block

D. High-grade or advanced AV block

E. Untypable second-degree AV block

F. Third-degree AV block

15. In some cases, second-degree AV blocks will not have any P waves at all. True or False.

16. Grouping is one of the major diagnostic features of the second-degree AV blocks. True or False.

17. The terms *conduction ratios* and *blocks* can be used interchangeably when talking about the AV blocks. True or False.

18. Which statement is incorrect about Wenckebach or Mobitz I second-degree AV block?
    A. The PR interval progressively lengthens until a P wave is eventually blocked.
    B. The longest PR interval is the one immediately after the dropped beat.
    C. The largest incremental change in the PR interval occurs between the first and second PR intervals in a sequence.
    D. The R-R intervals progressively shorten until a QRS complex is dropped.
    E. The interval including the dropped P wave is less than two times the preceding P-P interval.

19. The width of the QRS complexes in Mobitz I second-degree AV block or Wenckebach can be either _____ or _____.

20. The conduction ratio in Mobitz I second-degree AV block can be:
    A. 2:1
    B. 3:2
    C. 5:4
    D. 17:16
    E. All of the above

21. Mobitz II second-degree AV block is diagnosed when you have either a single or multiple nonconducted P waves in the face of a rhythm with a constant PR interval. If you have multiple blocked P waves, they are not sequentially blocked. True or False.

22. In Mobitz II second-degree AV block, the width of the QRS complexes can be _____ or _____.

23. A 2:1 ratio in a second-degree AV block can be either untypable, Mobitz I, or Mobitz II. However, you need to have at least *two consecutively conducted* P waves somewhere else along the strip in order to be able to diagnose Mobitz I or Mobitz II. True or False.

24. You can have capture or fusion beats in a complete or third-degree AV block. True or False.

25. The PR interval should not be constant in third-degree AV block. True or False.

Artificially Paced Rhythms

General Overview

In this chapter, we present a quick look at the specifics of the rhythms that are created artificially by either temporary or permanent artificial cardiac pacemakers. This quick look is only intended to give us the ability to recognize the presence of a paced rhythm, and not to provide an in-depth discussion of the diagnostic issues that can develop in these patients. The complexity of the problem-solving or diagnostic issues associated with pacemakers can be daunting and are well above the scope of an intermediate text on arrhythmias. In addition to the general diagnostic problems involved, there are many individual variations between the individual pacemaker manufacturers and indeed, the individual models themselves, which further complicate the issues.

An internal pacemaker typically has two components (Figure 36-1): the pulse generator and the leads. The pulse generator is basically a mini-computer that includes a power source (usually a lithium iodide battery), wave or voltage amplifiers (which include analyzing function), a transmitter system to send data to clinicians, a receiver to allow programmability or changing rates, an internal clock, and, of course, sensors. The pulse generator is the heart and soul of the pacemaker.

The leads are the electrical "wires" used to transmit the electrical data back and forth from the heart to the pulse generator. The wires can be either unipolar or bipolar in nature. Unipolar leads are composed of a single wire that transmits the impulse from the pulse generator to the heart. Since electricity has to work along circuits, the electricity must return to the pulse generator through the body tissues in order to complete the circuit. Bipolar leads have two internal wires. One of the wires terminates at the end of the lead and is used to transmit the impulse to the heart. The other wire, which usually has its end about 1 cm from the end of the lead, is meant to transmit the impulse back to the pulse generator and complete the circuit. Note that the circuit formed with bipolar leads is only about 1 cm wide. This short circuit is more than enough to cause a depolarization wave because, as we have seen, a single ectopic cell can be enough.

Pacemaker Code

Artificial pacemakers can sense, depolarize, and pace either the atria, the ventricles, or both in a sequential fashion. The pacemakers can also either automatically trigger responses at a certain specified amount of time or they can function in an inhibitory manner. The pacemaker functions in an inhibitory manner when any electrical activity sets off an internal alarm clock that will not fire a complex for a certain length of time. The artificial pacemakers can also be programmed to perform certain functions and to respond differently in the presence of a tachyarrhythmia.

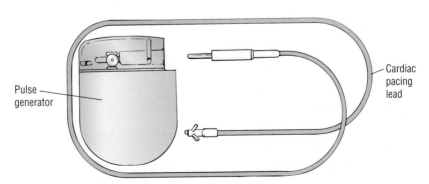

Figure 36-1: The pulse generator and lead of a typical pacemaking unit.

In order to organize all of the various functions of the artificial pacemakers into a usable system, the Intersociety Commission for Heart Disease (ICHD) came up with a system that is presently in use. This system uses a five-letter code with each letter representing a specific function (Figure 36-2).

The first letter in the code refers to the chamber that is paced—in general, pacemakers will either pace the atria (A), the ventricles (V), both (D for dual), or none (O). If the pacemaker paces both the atria and the ventricles, the pacing occurs sequentially to try to normalize the mechanical contraction of the various chambers as much as possible.

The second letter in the code refers to the chamber that is sensed—in other words, the chamber that the pulse generator will monitor for spontaneous depolarizations. The chambers that are sensed are either the atria (A), the ventricles (V), both (D for dual), or none (O).

Position I

Chamber paced

A = Atrium

V = Ventricle

D = Dual (A+V)

O = None

Position II

Chamber sensed

A = Atrium

V = Ventricle

D = Dual (A+V)

O = None

Position III

Response to sensing

T = Triggered

I = Inhibited

D = Dual (D+I)

O = None

X X X X X

Position IV

Programmability
Rate Modulation

P = Triggered

M = Inhibited

C = Dual (D+I)

R = Rate modulation

O = None

Position V

Antitachyarrhythmia
functions

P = Pacing

S = Shock

D = Dual (P+S)

O = None

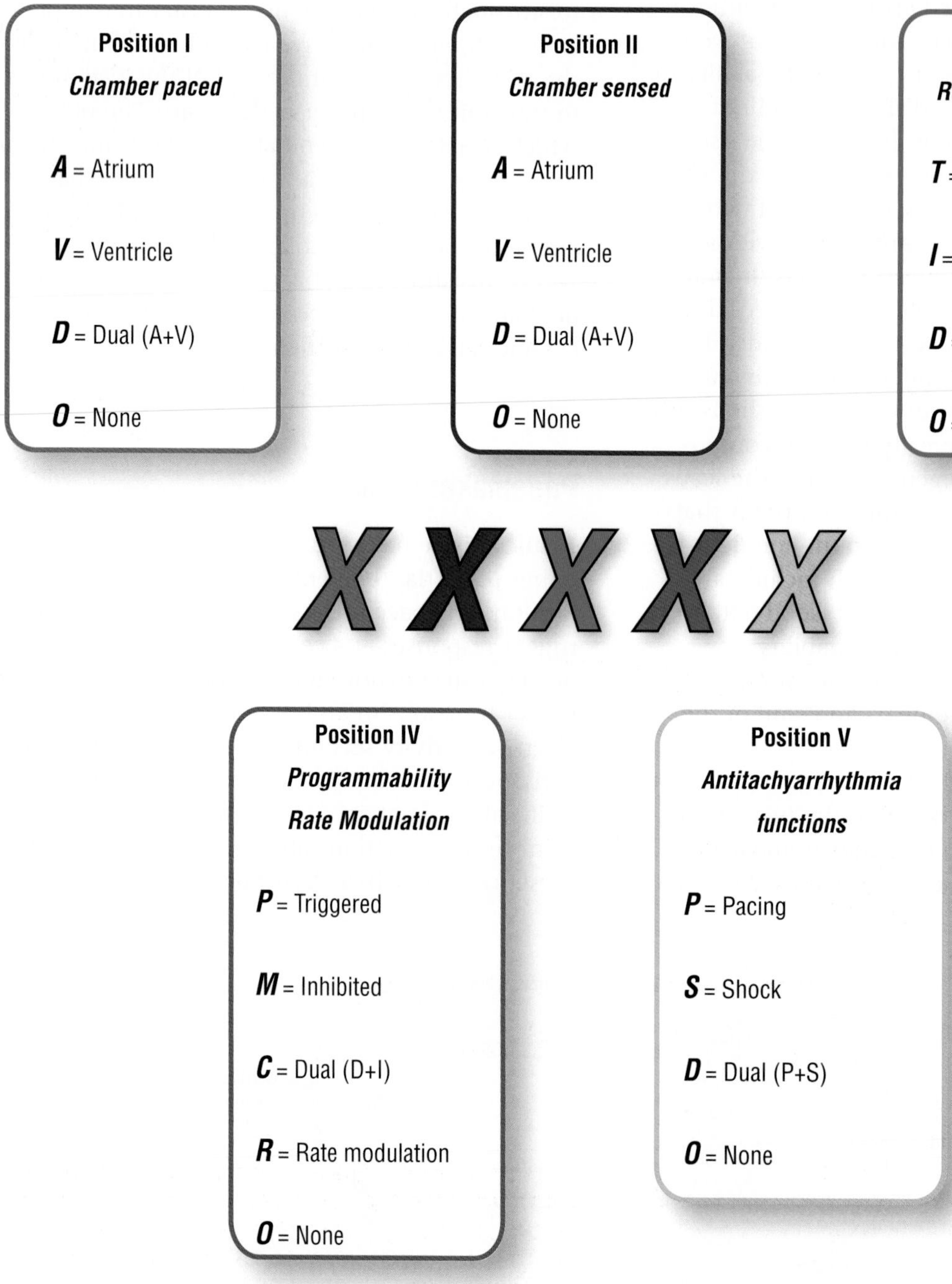

Figure 36-2: ICHD pacemaker code.

The third letter in the code refers to the response that the pacemaker will take when it senses an event. The *triggered* (T) response is when the pacemaker activates a depolarization wave to a sensed event. An example of a triggered response is when the pacemaker fires an impulse to the ventricles after it senses an atrial depolarization.

The *inhibited* (I) response is when the pacemaker responds to a sensed event by *not* firing a response for a certain amount of time. This concept appears at first glance to be counterintuitive; the pacemaker is programmed to fail in response to an event. But, it is actually a failsafe method to prevent the pacemaker from competing with an intrinsic cardiac pacemaker. Let's look a little closer at this type of response.

Let's suppose that a pacemaker senses an atrial depolarization (Figure 36-3). The pacemaker will then automatically set up a time period, known as the *ventricular escape interval* or VEI, during which it patiently waits for the ventricles to respond to the atrial impulse. The hope of the pacemaker is that the atrial impulse will proceed normally through the AV node and the electrical conduction system and eventually cause a ventricular depolarization. The VEI is usually a little bit longer than the normally occurring PR interval would be, in order to allow for normal conduction to occur

and finish through the conduction pathways. After the VEI is completed, if the ventricles failed to respond because of an AV block or whatever, or if an intrinsic ectopic ventricular pacemaker failed to fire, then and only then would the pulse generator fire an impulse.

The third possibility that can occur is the *dual* (D) response. This refers to the possibility of the pulse generator to respond in a triggered manner for some pre-programmed cases and in an inhibitory manner for other pre-programmed events.

Finally, the fourth possible response to an event is *none* (O). In this case, the pulse generator responds in neither a triggered nor an inhibitory way to an event.

The fourth and fifth letters in the pacemaker code relate to advanced functions of certain pulse generators. The review of those features is beyond the scope of this book, and the reader is encouraged to seek additional information in more advanced books on artificial pacemakers or from the individual manufacturers of specific pacemaker models.

The Pacemaker Spike

One of the most important diagnostic features to look for in any paced rhythm is the presence of the pacemaker spike or artifact. Electrocardiographically, the

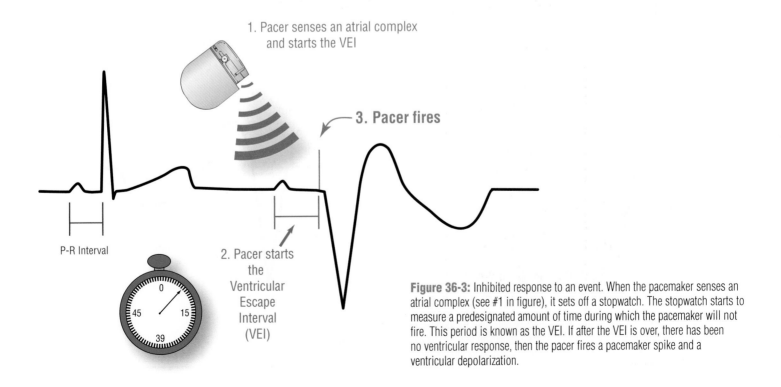

1. Pacer senses an atrial complex and starts the VEI

3. **Pacer fires**

P-R Interval

2. Pacer starts the Ventricular Escape Interval (VEI)

Figure 36-3: Inhibited response to an event. When the pacemaker senses an atrial complex (see #1 in figure), it sets off a stopwatch. The stopwatch starts to measure a predesignated amount of time during which the pacemaker will not fire. This period is known as the VEI. If after the VEI is over, there has been no ventricular response, then the pacer fires a pacemaker spike and a ventricular depolarization.

pacemaker spike is represented as a very short, very fast fluctuation from the baseline that occurs immediately before the paced complex (Figure 36-4). This spike can be either positive, negative, or biphasic, but it is always sharp and fast.

The pacemaker spike is created when the pulse generator fires a short, sharp electric burst of electricity with the intention of pacing the heart. This burst of electricity is then transmitted by the pacing wire or lead toward either the atrial or the ventricular myocardium. When the burst of electricity actually reaches the myocardium, the sudden electric jolt is picked up by the ECG lead as the classic spike pattern.

The electric pulse causes a localized depolarization of that area of the atria or the ventricles immediately in contact with the pacing wire or lead. That very localized area of depolarization immediately under the pacing wire in turn acts very similar to an ectopic pacemaker, triggering a depolarization wave that spread through the rest of the myocardium by direct cell-to-cell transmission. As we saw before, these slow, direct cell-to-cell depolarization waves give rise to wide, bizarre QRS complexes that are morphologically similar to PVCs.

It is critical to realize that the pacemaker spike may not be visible in every lead! Just as waves present differently in different leads, so too will the pacemaker spike be more prominent or be completely absent in certain leads (Figure 36-5). Once again, we are going to recommend that whenever you have a complex arrhythmia, including the ventricular rhythms, always obtain multiple leads or a full 12-lead ECG. By viewing the different leads, your chances of missing the spike will be greatly decreased.

QRS Morphology in a Paced Rhythm

As we saw in Figure 36-4, the morphology of the QRS complex in the paced rhythms is wide and bizarre. The morphology is due to the slow ventricular depolarization wave that is created by the direct cell-to-cell transmission of the impulse. As mentioned, the morphology of the QRS complexes is similar to those found in ventricular rhythms.

The morphology of the paced complexes also has something else in common with the ectopically formed ventricular rhythms—the morphology of the complexes will depend on where they started and the vectors formed as the ventricles are depolarized. Since the most common site of pacing wire insertion is in the right ventricle, many paced rhythms will have a right bundle branch block morphology. However, this is not always the case, as some paced rhythms will have a left bundle branch block morphology.

Even though this is a book on arrhythmias, we should mention that you should not make any comments on axis or chamber enlargement and hypertrophy in any paced rhythm. There are some criteria for infarct changes in paced rhythms, but great care should be taken in interpreting them unless you are very experienced in electrocardiography. Unless you are skilled in electrocardiography, we suggest using 12-lead ECGs and multiple strips to strictly evaluate only the patient's rhythm.

Popular Pacemaker Modes

Clinically, there are some commonly used pacemaker types. Each has its own strengths and weaknesses,

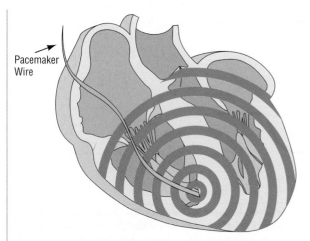

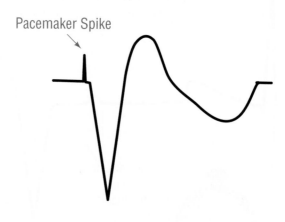

Figure 36-4: An electric burst travels from the pulse generator through the pacing wire to the ventricles. The burst is picked up on the ECG as a quick, sharp deflection from the baseline. The burst triggers a depolarization wave which is spread by direct cell-to-cell contact throughout the ventricles.

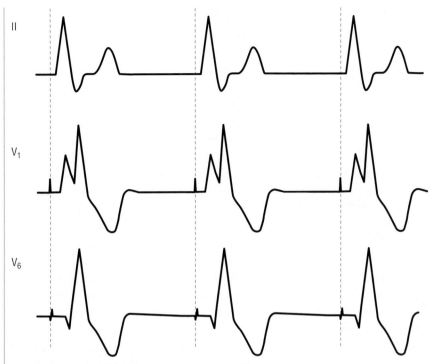

Figure 36-5: The pacemaker spike may be more visible in some leads. The leads vary between patients and there is no "best lead" in which to view them. A full 12-lead ECG or multiple leads will help in diagnosis of paced rhythms in these cases.

making them ideally suited for certain conditions. In this book, we shall review the most popular types and show you some examples of each for your review. As is customary, we will present various clinical strips at the end of the chapter.

Atrial Demand Pacemaker

When a patient has problems with bradycardia-related symptoms but has a normally functioning AV node, the atrial demand pacemaker (AAI) may be the ideal solu-

tion. The AAI pacemaker senses the atria and paces the same atria in an inhibitory fashion. Basically, the pulse generator senses the atria for spontaneous activity. If no spontaneous atrial activity is detected during a specified period (the atrial escape interval), then the pacemaker fires an atrial depolarization wave. The wave then spreads normally through the rest of the atria, the AV nodes, and the ventricles. If spontaneous atrial activity is detected, the pacemaker is inhibited from firing, allowing the normal complex to proceed unimpeded (Figure 36-6).

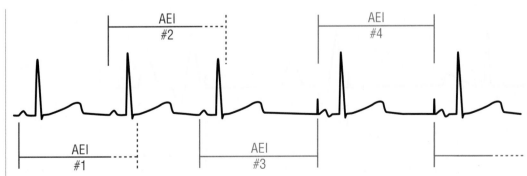

Figure 36-6: An AAI pacemaker senses an atrial complex and begins to time out an atrial escape interval (AEI #1). The interval is broken by a normally occurring P wave and the interval is reset (AEI #2). AEI #3 and #4 are not reset and so the pacemaker fires an atrial impulse.

Ventricular Demand Pacemaker

The ventricular demand pacemaker (VVI) is the ventricular counterpart of the AAI pacemaker discussed above. This type of pacemaker senses and paces only the ventricles in an inhibitory manner. The pacemaker senses the ventricles for any type of spontaneous activity. When it senses activity, the pacemaker begins to time out a specified period (the ventricular escape interval, or VEI, discussed before). If no spontaneous ventricular activity is detected during the VEI, the pacemaker fires a ventricular depolarization wave. If spontaneous ventricular activity is detected, the pacemaker is inhibited from firing, allowing the normal complex to proceed unimpeded (Figure 36-7).

Atrial activity will in no way interfere with the functioning of a VVI pacemaker. If a P wave occurs but does not conduct to the ventricles, the pacemaker will not be affected in any way and does not get reset. Only ventricular activity is sensed and only the ventricles are paced. These are the main functional characteristics of the VVI pacer.

The main functional characteristics above are also the cause of the major complications associated with this type of pacer, the so-called *pacemaker syndrome*. The lack of atrial contribution to ventricular filling and the inability of the heart rate to compensate for any form of exertion or exercise will give rise to various clinical symptoms related to decreased cardiac output and hypotension. These include fatigue, lightheadedness, syncope, dyspnea, exercise intolerance, congestive heart failure, and anginal symptoms due to myocardial ischemia.

AV Sequential

The AV sequential or DVI pacemaker was the first attempt to maintain AV synchrony. The DVI paces both the atria and the ventricle in a sequential manner when it does fire (Figure 36-8). The atria are depolarized first, and then a few milliseconds later, the ventricles are stimulated. This allows for ventricular filling and helps to maintain a more efficient and effective cardiac output. It does counter some of the events that lead to the pacemaker syndrome but is not as effective as the DDD pacemaker, which we will examine next.

The DVI pacemaker senses the ventricle for any spontaneous ventricular activity and then paces in an inhibitory manner. If spontaneous ventricular activity is sensed by the pacemaker during the VEI that is set for that particular patient, then the pacemaker holds off and does not fire. If the pacemaker does not sense any ventricular activity during the VEI, then it fires a sequence of an atrial and then a ventricular depolarization.

The DVI pacemaker does not sense atrial activity in any way. As such, a supraventricular complex will be completely disregarded by the pacer unless it triggers a ventricular complex. This is the main drawback of the DVI pacer. By disregarding supraventricular complexes, the pacer will compete with the normal heart in some cases. PVCs and PJCs are sensed and will inhibit the pacer.

Automatic Pacemaker

The automatic or DDD pacemaker is the "top-of-the-line" model of artificial pacemakers. The DDD pacer senses both the atria and the ventricles (Figure 36-9). It also

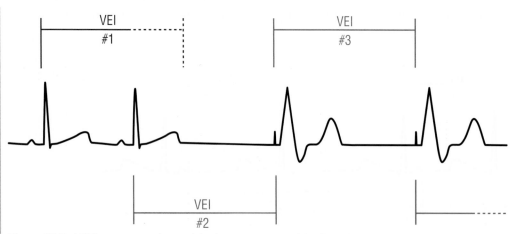

Figure 36-7: A VVI pacer senses the ventricles for spontaneous activity. If ventricular activity is sensed, no complex is fired by the pacer (see VEI #1). If ventricular activity is not sensed during the VEI (VEI #2 and #3), the pacer fires and causes a ventricular contraction.

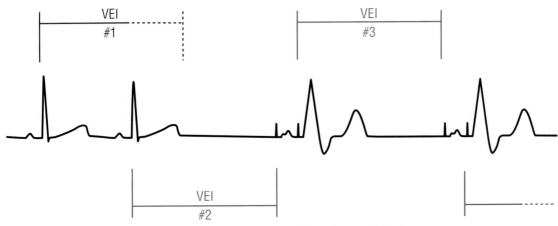

Figure 36-8: A DVI pacemaker is reset by a ventricular complex in VEI #1. During VEI #2, there is no spontaneous ventricular activity and the pacemaker fires a sequential atrial and then a ventricular complex. The same occurs in VEI #3.

has the ability to pace either the atria, the ventricles, or both in a sequential manner. The DDD pacemaker is basically a combination of the AAI, the VVI, and the DVI pacemakers due to the presence of the dual sensing/dual pacing leads.

The beauty of this pacemaker is that it will sense the heart for any atrial or supraventricular activity. If it doesn't sense any, it will trigger a supraventricular complex to stimulate the atria. The pacer will then wait an appropriate amount of time for the supraventricular complex to be normally conducted to the ventricles; if it

doesn't make it through, the ventricular lead will then pace the ventricles sequentially.

Any PAC that occurs will be sensed and will inhibit the atrial response. It will not, however, inhibit the separate ventricular sensing and pacing function. If the PAC is not conducted to the ventricles, the pacer will fire a sequentially timed ventricular complex. Likewise, PJCs and PVCs will be sensed by the pacer but these will inhibit both atrial or ventricular responses.

The exceptional capability of the DDD pacemaker to sense and respond to atrial and/or ventricular activity

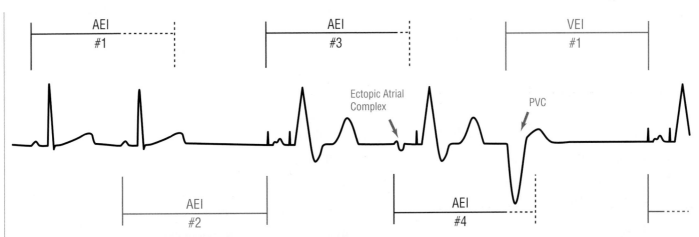

Figure 36-9: A DDD pacemaker senses spontaneous atrial and ventricular activity during AEI #1 and does not fire. During AEI #2 there is no spontaneous atrial activity and the pacemaker fires a paced atrial complex. The pacer then waits an appropriate amount of time and, when it does not sense any conduction to the ventricles, the pacer fires a sequential ventricular complex. During AEI #3, the pacemaker senses some spontaneous atrial activity and does not pace the atria. However, since conduction to the ventricles did not occur, a sequential ventricular complex was fired. Conducted PACs, PJCs, and PVCs will reset the pacer. This is what occurs during AEI #4—a PVC resets the timer. The sequence then continues as expected.

gives it a tremendous clinical edge over all of its competition. The DDD pacer will sense a sinus tachycardia that can develop due to a physiologic increase in the heart rate, as can occur when the patient is anxious, febrile, or exercising, and make sure that the ventricles match the rate in a near-normal sequential manner. This ability to respond to physiologic demand, along with the sequential nature of the atrial and ventricular depolarizations, essentially negates most complications seen in the pacemaker syndrome and allows for near-normal functioning. These advantages give the DDD pacer a preferential status as the pacemaker of choice for most patients.

We should mention that for protective measures, an upper limit to the rate of ventricular conduction of a supraventricular tachycardia is always defined in order to protect the patient from a potential disaster. For example, if the patient were in atrial flutter, a 1:1 con-

duction rate to the ventricles could result in a ventricular response of 300 BPM. As you can imagine, this rate could be life-threatening. Because of this, the upper limits of conduction can be programmed into the pulse generator by the clinician, allowing for maximal physiologic benefit for the patient under normal circumstances, while still maintaining an upper limit protection against unimpeded ventricular conduction.

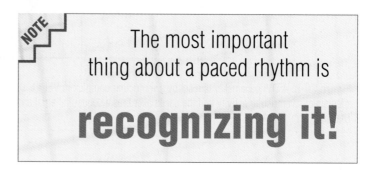

NOTE

The most important
thing about a paced rhythm is

recognizing it!

ECG Strips

ECG 36-1

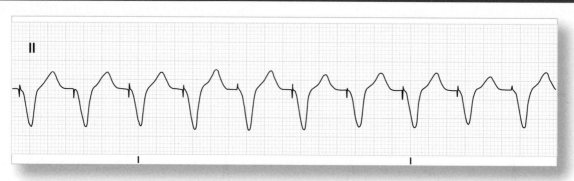

II

Rate:	About 100 BPM	PR intervals:	None
Regularity:	Regular	QRS width:	Wide
P waves:	None	Grouping:	None
Morphology:	None		
Axis:	None	Dropped beats:	None
P:QRS ratio:	None	Rhythm:	**Paced rhythm**

Discussion:

This strip shows a paced ventricular rhythm at a rate of 100 BPM. The rhythm is very regular as you would expect with an artificial pacemaker. The pacemaker spike is obvious right before the ventricular complexes.

The only troubling thing about this strip is the rate of 100 BPM, which is set very high. This could represent pacemaker malfunction. Clinical correlation is indicated.

ECG 36-2

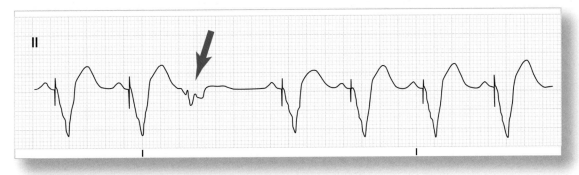

Rate:	About 72 BPM	PR intervals:	None
Regularity:	Regularly irregular	QRS width:	Wide
P waves:	None	Grouping:	None
Morphology:	None		
Axis:	None	Dropped beats:	None
P:QRS ratio:	None	Rhythm:	**Paced rhythm**

Discussion:

This strip shows a sinus rhythm at about 72 BPM. This is obvious from the constantly recurring P waves with the same morphology. The conduction of the sinus complex to the ventricles is obviously blocked because the pacemaker has to pace the ventricles sequentially in most cases. The third complex is a PVC (see blue arrow).

ECG 36-3

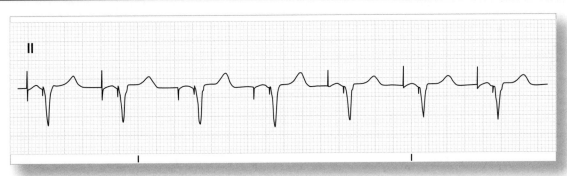

Rate:	About 72 BPM	PR intervals:	None
Regularity:	Regular	QRS width:	Wide
P waves:	None	Grouping:	None
Morphology:	None		
Axis:	None	Dropped beats:	None
P:QRS ratio:	None	Rhythm:	**Paced rhythm**

Discussion:

Unless you are very sure of your findings, get used to calling any paced rhythm just simply a paced rhythm. It usually doesn't pay to try to figure out what type of pacemaker you are dealing with. This rhythm strip shows both atrial and ventricular pacing in a sequential manner. The pacer appears to be functioning normally. Even though the ventricular complexes appear narrow, they have to be wide with isoelectric segments because they are artificially paced.

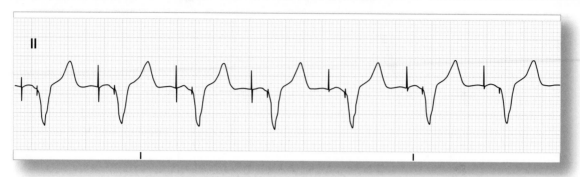

Rate:	About 70 BPM	PR intervals:	None
Regularity:	Regular	QRS width:	Wide
P waves: Morphology: Axis:	None None None	Grouping:	None
		Dropped beats:	None
P:QRS ratio:	None	Rhythm:	**Paced rhythm**

Discussion:

This strip also shows a paced rhythm with atrial and ventricular pacing in a sequential manner. The pacemaker appears to be functioning normally.

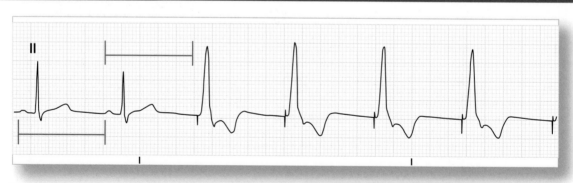

Rate:	About 62 BPM	PR intervals:	None
Regularity:	Regular	QRS width:	See discussion below
P waves: Morphology: Axis:	None None None	Grouping:	None
		Dropped beats:	None
P:QRS ratio:	None	Rhythm:	**NSR and paced rhythm**

Discussion:

This strip shows a patient in a normal sinus rhythm that suddenly stops and is replaced by a paced ventricular rhythm. Notice that if you take the first P-P interval and transfer that exact distance to that area between the second and third complexes, you will see that just an extra 0.05 seconds is all that is needed for the pacemaker to reach the end of the escape interval and fire. This pacemaker is functioning normally.

ECG 36-6

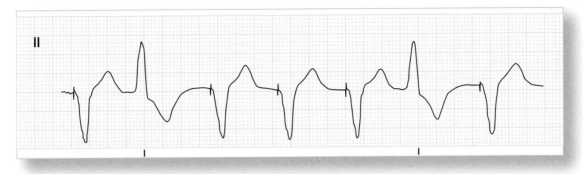

Rate:	About 80 BPM	PR intervals:	None
Regularity:	Regular	QRS width:	Wide
P waves:	None	Grouping:	None
Morphology:	None		
Axis:	None	Dropped beats:	None
P:QRS ratio:	None	Rhythm:	**Paced rhythm and PVCs**

Discussion:

This strip shows a ventricular rhythm that is obviously paced. The pacemaker spike is very obvious in this lead, making the diagnosis simple. The second and sixth complexes are PVCs. Note the different polarity of the PVCs compared with the paced rhythm. The pacemaker is obviously inhibitory in nature since the pacer was suppressed from firing by the PVCs.

ECG 36-7

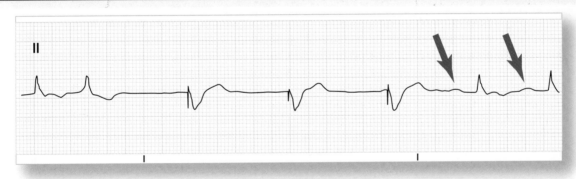

Rate:	About 55 BPM	PR intervals:	None
Regularity:	Regular	QRS width:	Wide
P waves:	None	Grouping:	None
Morphology:	None		
Axis:	None	Dropped beats:	None
P:QRS ratio:	None	Rhythm:	**Paced rhythm**

Discussion:

From this strip, it is impossible to confidently identify the first complex. The second complex, however, does not have any visible P waves and is the same morphology as the previous one and the sixth and seventh complexes in the strip. It is most probably a PJC. The third through fourth strips are obviously paced. The sixth and seventh complexes show NSR with P waves which are fairly flat in this lead (see blue arrows). Multiple leads verified the existence of those bumps as P waves.

ECG 36-8

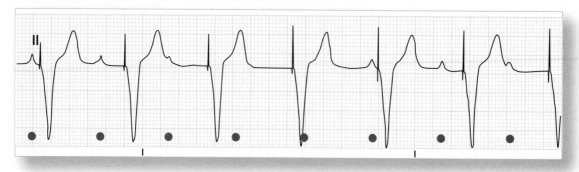

Rate:	About 65 BPM	PR intervals:	None
Regularity:	Regular	QRS width:	Wide
P waves:	None	Grouping:	None
Morphology:	None		
Axis:	None	Dropped beats:	None
P:QRS ratio:	None	Rhythm:	**Paced rhythm**

Discussion:

This strip shows the presence of a paced ventricular rhythm. The interesting thing is the presence of P waves (see blue dots) peeking out between some of the ventricular complexes. These P waves are occurring at a regular pattern and have constant P-P intervals. Obviously this pacemaker is not sensing those atrial complexes at all. On obtaining the patient's history, a VVI pacemaker was confirmed.

ECG 36-9

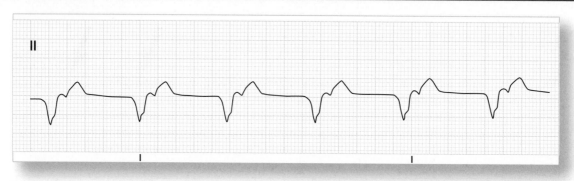

Rate:	About 62 BPM	PR intervals:	None
Regularity:	Regular	QRS width:	Wide
P waves:	None	Grouping:	None
Morphology:	None		
Axis:	None	Dropped beats:	None
P:QRS ratio:	None	Rhythm:	**See discussion below**

Discussion:

We figured that we would end this chapter with a bit of a diagnostic dilemma. Could this be a ventricular escape rhythm, for example, accelerated idioventricular? Could this be a junctional rhythm with a preexisting bundle branch block or aberrancy? Are the P waves isoelectric in this lead, and if so, could this be a sinus rhythm in somebody with a preexisting bundle branch block? These questions are difficult to answer. You need a few extra leads to make the correct diagnosis.

ECG 36-10

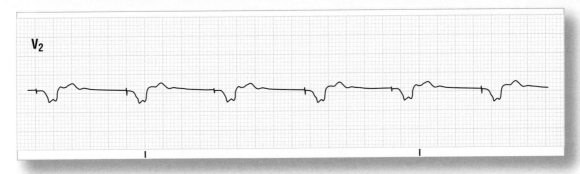

Rate:	About 62 BPM	PR Intervals:	None
Regularity:	Regular	QRS Width:	Wide
P Waves: Morphology: Axis:	None None None	Grouping:	None
		Dropped Beats:	None
P:QRS Ratio:	None	Rhythm:	**Paced rhythm**

Discussion:

This is a strip taken from the same patient in ECG 36-9 after a full 12-lead ECG showed that lead V$_2$ was the best one to see the pacer spike. Here it becomes obvious that this rhythm is a paced rhythm. It is critical to obtain multiple leads to fully evaluate any complex, or potentially complex, arrhythmia. This is just another example of a patient who would have been misdiagnosed, and probably inappropriately treated, for a rhythm abnormality he or she didn't have.

CHAPTER REVIEW

1. When examining a paced rhythm, it is more important to evaluate the presence of the actual paced complex to make the diagnosis than to try to figure out which type of pacemaker is involved. True or False.

2. Pacing wires or leads can be either:
   A. Unipolar
   B. Multiprogrammable
   C. Bipolar
   D. A and C
   E. All of the above

3. What does the first letter stand for in the code used to describe pacemaker functions and capabilities?
   A. Antitachyarrhythmia functions
   B. Chamber sensed
   C. Response to sensing
   D. Chamber paced
   E. Programmability

4. What does the second letter stand for in the code used to describe pacemaker functions and capabilities?
   A. Antitachyarrhythmia functions
   B. Chamber sensed
   C. Response to sensing
   D. Chamber paced
   E. Programmability

5. What does the third letter stand for in the code used to describe pacemaker functions and capabilities?
   A. Antitachyarrhythmia functions
   B. Chamber sensed
   C. Response to sensing
   D. Chamber paced
   E. Programmability

6. Always look for a pacemaker spike when you are looking at a wide, bizarre-looking complex or rhythm. Multiple leads or a full 12-lead ECG are very useful in these cases. True or False.

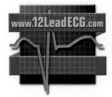

To enhance the knowledge you gain in this book, access this text's website at www.12leadECG.com! This valuable resource provides flashcards, an online glossary, web links, and more. Simply click on the Arrhythmias book cover once at the site.

CHAPTER 37

Putting It All Together

Introduction

It may seem a bit strange to put a chapter at the end of the book that shows you how to read a rhythm strip. The reason that this chapter appears at the end is because most of the advice we can give you about how to interpret strips cannot be fully appreciated until you have a strong foundation in the principles of arrhythmia recognition and the rhythms themselves.

Interpreting arrhythmias is an abstract and very individual system for each clinician. There are some principles, like obtaining the rate and looking at regularity, that are practiced routinely by everyone. However, the clinicians who are really good at interpreting rhythms practice some very subjective principles, and these change from strip to strip. As you can imagine, teaching these skills is very difficult and putting them on paper is even more of a challenge.

We are going to make every attempt to give you an overall system to look at arrhythmias. Some of the information will be very straightforward. Some will require a bit of imagination on your part. All in all, we are going to prepare you for the process of interpreting arrhythmias. How good you get at it depends on you.

We have narrowed the approach to analyzing a rhythm strip or an arrhythmia on a 12-lead ECG down to a few basic concepts. These concepts can be summed up by using the mnemonic: Always think about your *patient's IQ points* (Figure 37-1). The rest of this section is only intended as a short explanation of the concepts involved, and we will be addressing them individually later on.

The word "patient's" should always be foremost in your mind when you are approaching a rhythm strip because it is about your patient. Clinical correlation with their presenting complaints, hemodynamic status, history (present and past), physical examination, and any other pertinent information is mandatory to arrive at a correct interpretation of any rhythm strip.

"I" stands for impression. It is there to remind you to always formulate a quick impression of your strip before moving on. This does not mean, however, that this initial impression is set in stone and cannot be changed. Quite the contrary—it is basically a work in progress that needs to be either ruled in or ruled out by answering some simple questions (Figure 37-2).

Notice that in Figure 37-2, the questions relate to different parts of a typical complex. For example, the rate mostly affects the TP segment by making it shorter or longer; Questions 7, 8, and 9 are all related to the QRS complexes. We set up the questions this way so that they would be easy to remember when looking at

Always think about your...

Patient's

Impression **Q**uestions

Points!

Figure 37-1: A mnemonic to remember the approach to analyzing a rhythm strip.

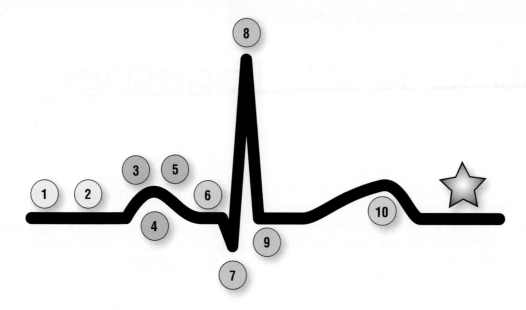

Top 10 questions:

1. Is the rhythm fast or slow?

2. Is it regular or irregular?

3. Do you see any P waves?

4. Are the P waves the same?

5. Are the P waves upright in lead II?

6. Are the PR intervals normal and consistent?

7. What is the P:QRS ratio?

8. Are the QRS complexes narrow or wide?

9. Are the complexes grouped or not grouped?

10. Have I mined for GOLD?

Then ask yourself...

 How can I put it all together?

Figure 37-2: The top ten questions to ask when analyzing a rhythm strip.

any QRS complex. You don't need to actually memorize them in any set order or to actually memorize the figure, but many people remember them a bit more easily with these visual cues to focus on.

The last part of the mnemonic (points) is a bit of a stretch. "Points" stands for getting a full 12-lead ECG and/or multiple leads and comparing them to an old ECG when needed. Why "points"? Because you want to compare the points or waves between the new strip and the patient's baseline old strip.

"Patient's"

Arrhythmias cannot be interpreted in a vacuum. We need to start off this discussion with a very simple but often overlooked fact: You need to look at, touch, and listen to your patient. When you first approach any rhythm strip, it is critical to know from whom the strip was obtained and the clinical scenario in which it was obtained. If you notice anything unusual about the rhythm, you need to physically take a look at the patient and evaluate his or her condition (or you need to inform whoever is responsible for the patient). Why? Because you can *never assume that an arrhythmia is not dangerous!*

Suppose you have been given a strip of a patient in ventricular bigeminy. Bigeminy is easy to diagnose and is fairly evident on the strip. You make the call and you are happy with yourself. The patient will be OK. . .ventricular bigeminy is usually a benign rhythm. The key word, however, is "usually." The problem is that this patient did not know that she had a benign rhythm. Instead, she had no functional mechanical contraction with the PVCs. The bigeminal episode was actually only perfusing her body at a pulse rate of 30 BPM. The patient was in cardiogenic shock and needed immediate attention in order to prevent death or, at the very least, a serious complication.

As we mentioned before, we have purposely avoided treatment strategies in this book. The reason is that we wanted the book to be useful for longer than one or two years. The principles involved in arrhythmia interpretation have remained fairly stable over the years, although treatment has not. Modern medicine is changing at such a pace that most books are outdated by the time that they are published. Emergent management of any hemodynamically unstable arrhythmia should be based on the American Heart Association's Advanced Cardiac Life Support program, or any other qualified protocols that are directed toward the management of these patients. Treatment of hemodynamically stable arrhythmias can be looked up in any book that is updated yearly, on the Internet, or on any other recently updated medium, in order to make sure that you are dealing with the latest and most up-to-date information.

If your patient is in any way hemodynamically unstable, he or she needs emergent treatment. Do not wait until matters get worse. Sometimes, the patient will show only minimal signs of instability—for example, he will be lightheaded, sweaty, his blood pressure lowered a little bit—and the next minute, he will have completely deteriorated. Early prevention and treatment (including defibrillation and cardioversion) may prevent a catastrophe. Remember that it takes time to get together all of the equipment and drugs that you will need to handle an emergency. Don't wait until the problem has completely deteriorated before you start to act.

The History

This book cannot possibly cover all of the important points about a patient's history that could shed light on your interpretation. So, we are only going to cover a few important points. The key to a good history and physical exam is to be thorough and methodical. You need to have a Sherlock Holmes-like approach to your patient's story. Nothing should be overlooked. It is usually the little things that add the most information.

To begin, for most patients, the history is the most important part of any patient evaluation. The history should include past and present information that would be pertinent to narrow your differential diagnosis. You should start by focusing your attention to the immediate incident. What was the first thing that the patient felt? In what order did the signs and symptoms present? How severe were the symptoms? How long did the symptoms last? What was the patient feeling or doing immediately before having the first symptoms? Did she pass out? Have shortness of breath? Chest pain or discomfort of any kind? Lightheadedness? Sweating? Did the pain or discomfort radiate anywhere? Did she have any palpitations? How fast were the palpitations? How regular were the palpitations? (It is a good idea to have the patient tap out the palpitations on her leg or other surface. In this way, you develop a feel for the regularity and speed of the palpitations.) Was she exposed to any toxins or allergens? Did they use any street drugs? Does she smoke? These are just a few of the questions that you should think about when you approach a patient.

Past information could include past events, for example, previous episodes of tachycardia or syncope. It should also cover predisposing conditions that could be proarrhythmic. For example, a history of a previous myocardial infarction or congestive heart failure may raise your suspicions for ventricular tachycardia as a cause of palpitations and syncope. Chronic or acute renal failure should raise the suspicion of an electrolyte abnormality that can cause some serious arrhythmias. Chronic obstructive pulmonary disease can raise your suspicion for multifocal atrial tachycardia. Leg swelling after a car trip could raise your suspicion for a pulmonary embolus and the resultant arrhythmic complications of such an event. The possibilities are endless. Every case is unique and you need to have a high index of suspicion as you approach your patient.

The family history is very important in the evaluation of many of the arrhythmias. The family history should focus on various possibilities: any family members who died suddenly at a young age; a family history of heart disease at ages less than 65 years old; a family history of frequent fainting or passing out; a family history of congenital deafness (long QT syndrome with Jervell and Lange-Nielsen syndrome); or any family history of arrhythmias or arrhythmia-related symptoms.

The medications that the patient is taking can definitely shed some light on the evaluation of an arrhythmia. Many antiarrhythmics can actually increase the occurrence of life-threatening arrhythmias. There are many medications that can prolong the QT interval, including some anti-nausea and anti-emetic medicines. Many medicines can cause gastrointestinal (GI) bleeding, renal, or hepatic complications that can, in turn, cause electrolyte abnormalities. Medications can bring to the surface certain previously undiagnosed genetic diseases or enzyme abnormalities. Finally, many medications can cause drug-drug interactions that cause untoward arrhythmic side effects.

Don't be afraid to ask questions of your patients. You are not wasting time or boring them. Trust me, they want to get to the bottom of their problem. If you cannot obtain the history from them, turn to the family members or friends who are with the patient. Many times they can provide information that your patient is embarrassed to bring up. If your patient cannot remember his medications, call the house and have someone go to the medicine cabinet. All in all, don't be afraid to use all of the resources you have available to you to come up with an answer.

Physical Examination

The first thing to look for on the physical examination is the vital signs. The pulse rate is the physical representation of the mechanical contraction caused by the underlying heart rate and rhythm. Many times, however, the pulse rate and the rate on the monitor do not match because the electrical events do not cause a mechanical contraction or an effective mechanical contraction. Always make it a habit to double-check the monitor rate and the pulse.

Besides the simple mechanical rate, the pulse can tell you whether an arrhythmia is having an effect on organ perfusion. Weak, thready pulses are usually associated with lower states of cardiac output. Cold, clammy skin is also a sign of vascular underperfusion of the skin. The *capillary refill* is obtained by pushing down on the nail until the nail bed turns white. The pressure is then released and the number of seconds it takes for the normal pink color to return is measured. Capillary refill should be less than 2 seconds in the normal patient.

The pulse rate can also tell you a lot about the regularity of the rhythm. It is easy to spot the different cadences (regular, regularly irregular, or irregularly

irregular) by taking the pulse. Events, such as premature contractions, can be picked up on the pulse. Unfortunately, it is not possible to tell the difference between PACs, PJCs, and PVCs by palpating the pulse.

The next thing to evaluate from the vital signs is the blood pressure. Most patients with significant arrhythmias, either tachyarrhythmias or bradyarrhythmias, will have some alteration in their blood pressure. The loss of atrial kick will often affect the blood pressure by altering the ejection fraction of the ventricles.

Simple gross observation of the patient can give you a quick idea about the cardiovascular status. If the patient is in extremis (looks seriously ill), it is very obvious. Patients will be diaphoretic, tachypneic, and they will usually have a look of panic or impending doom on their faces. Many times, patients will be cyanotic with a purplish discoloration to their faces. (Clinical pearl: True cyanosis, caused by low oxygen levels, will result in central cyanosis, which means that the nose and central body also appear purplish. Many rheumatological diseases can cause peripheral cyanosis, which is caused by a clamping down of the peripheral blood vessels.)

The jugular venous waves can also provide a very significant clue to an underlying arrhythmia. An interesting physical exam finding occurs when the patient is in AV dissociation. Since the atria and ventricles are contracting at their own separate pace, the atria eventually have to contract while the atrioventricular valves are still shut. In these cases, the blood being pumped by the atria has to go somewhere. That somewhere is back up through the neck veins. The sudden pressure and volume wave caused by the atrial contraction will cause a sudden, very large, venous pulsation to develop. That very large pulsation is known as a *cannon A wave*. Cannon A waves can also be seen in any other rhythm that may intrinsically have AV dissociation (idioventricular, accelerated idioventricular, and ventricular tachycardia).

The physical exam can also provide basic clues to underlying disease processes that are associated with rhythm disturbances. Congestive heart failure, cardiomyopathies, myocardial infarctions, congenital heart disease, Down syndrome, Marfan's syndrome, and the arteriovenous shunts used in chronic renal failure patients are just a few examples of these disease states.

Here is another little clinical pearl: Suppose you are asked to see a patient with unexplained syncope and a big laceration on her face which she received during the fall. Did that patient more likely lose consciousness because of a cardiac event or was it seizure? Think about it this way: An arrhythmia will cause a fast, but not instantaneous, loss of consciousness. Patients usually remember the floor coming at them as they fall and they have enough time to put their hands out to stop their faces from striking the ground. A laceration can still occur if they hit something along the way, but the chances are less likely with this type of loss of consciousness. When you have a seizure, the neurologic event is instantaneous and you lose immediate control over your body. This immediate loss of control gives you a much greater chance of hitting the ground hard with a seizure.

"Impression"

Before you start breaking down the rhythm strip, take a few seconds to formulate a general impression of what is happening and what is the main problem. Is the main problem with the strip a single event? Multiple events? Are you dealing with more than one rhythm, as occurs in AV blocks? Do you get a benign feel from the strip or is it a scary one?

Many times, what happens is that you get caught up in the minutiae of interpreting a strip and forget to formulate this overall impression. In other words, you pick up all of the little findings on the strip, but you miss the obvious diagnosis. You can't see the forest for the trees. Formulating an original impression will let you first see that there is a forest, and then you can go in and see if it is made up of pine trees, oaks, or birches.

Formulating an original impression does not mean that the thoughts are set in stone. The overall impression is basically that—an impression. An impression can change with the data that you will obtain from your more sequential analysis, or it can be verified by the same information.

First, ask yourself: Is this a patient I have to see emergently? By this point, you should have a fair idea of a dangerous rhythm versus a rhythm that is probably not so dangerous by simply glancing over the strip. Do you need to get additional leads? If you have no clue as to what the rhythm is, call for help. It pays to call for help early. If you can figure the strip out while help is arriving, so much the better. Remember, the seconds pass by very, very slowly if you wait too long before calling for help. Those seconds can seem like an eternity. Know your limitations and don't be afraid to ask for help!

Secondly, mentally compare the strip you are analyzing with a mental picture of a perfect normal sinus rhythm. Focus on the differences. If you see problems with the P waves, you need to focus on that part of the analysis and should start thinking about some supraventricular pathology. If the problem is with wide QRS complexes, you need to think about ventricular rhythms or supraventricular rhythms with preexisting conditions (such as bundle branch blocks), electrolyte abnormalities, or aberrancy (for example Ashman's phenomenon). Then you can ask some secondary questions, like: If it looks like a bundle branch block, which one is it? If you are thinking aberrancy, is it rate-related aberrancy or is there something particular about those complexes? (Right bundle branch blocks are more commonly seen in aberrancy-related blocks.)

Lastly, compare the strip mentally again, but this time to a perfect example of the arrhythmia that you are suspecting. For example, suppose you thought that the rhythm abnormality was an atrial flutter with 2: 1 conduction. Mentally compare your strip to some of the atrial flutters with 2:1 conduction that you have studied so far. What is the rate? Do they look similar? Do you see buried F waves?

Now that you have formulated your general impression, you can begin to get down to specific questions. Let's move on to them at this point.

Top 10 "Questions"

1. Is the Rhythm Fast or Slow?

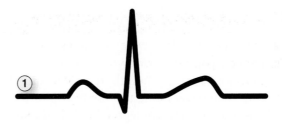

It should be simple enough for you at this point to calculate the rate and you can review this information in Chapter 4. But, just because calculating the rate is simple does not mean it is not useful or important. As we see in Table 37-1, it can quickly make a significant difference in the direction that you will head to figure out the rhythm in question.

Clinically, when you are calculating the rate, a variance of a few beats per minute will not have any significance. That is why, in this book, we have made it a point to say "about ___ BPM". Does it really matter if you calculate the rhythm to be 85 BPM and it is actually 87 BPM? No—the main thing is to focus on whether the rhythm is slow, normal, or fast. However, for completeness, you should get used to calculating the rate as closely as possible to the true number. (Author's note:

Slow	Normal	Fast	Can Be Fast, Normal, or Slow
Sinus bradycardia	Normal sinus rhythm	Sinus tachycardia	Atrial fibrillation
Junctional escape	Accelerated	Accelerated	Atrial flutter
Ventricular escape	• Junctional	• Junctional	Third-degree heart block
Idioventricular	• Idioventricular	• Idioventricular	Second-degree heart block
Wandering atrial pacemaker	Wandering atrial pacemaker	Ventricular tachycardia	First-degree heart block
		AVNRT	PACs
		AVRT	PJCs
		Multifocal atrial tachycardia	PVCs
		Aberrantly conducted supraventricular tachycardia	

Table 37-1: Differential Diagnoses by Rate

The main decision points where accuracy is very important will be around the rates of 60 BPM and 100 BPM. In these two zones, the difference of a couple of beats per minute can make a difference in whether the rhythm is called a bradycardia or normal, or whether the rhythm will be called normal or tachycardic, respectively.)

The list of potential arrhythmias causing slow, normal, or fast ventricular responses is limited in each category (see Table 37-1). This single step will narrow down the list of potential arrhythmias dramatically and will let you concentrate your attention in a more focused manner.

Remember, you can have two separate rhythms on one strip. This can occur when there is a transition from one rhythm to another along the same strip or if there is AV dissociation or a third-degree heart block. When you are approaching an AV dissociation or a third-degree heart block, it is essential that you state the rate for the atrial component and the rate for the ventricular component separately.

2. Is the Rhythm Regular or Irregular?

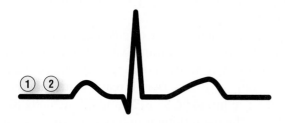

The real way that this question should be asked is as follows: Is the rhythm regular or irregular? If the rhythm is irregular, is it *regularly* irregular or *irregularly* irregular? As we have seen throughout the book, this question is essential to the interpretation of any arrhythmia. Once again, the differential diagnosis can be narrowed down greatly based on the answer to this one question (Table 37-2). Now, putting it together with the list derived from answering the previous question, your list of differentials should be getting smaller.

Regular rhythms typically have only one pacemaker setting the pace. Regularly irregular rhythms can have two or more pacemakers working simultaneously either due to escape mechanisms or due to increased automaticity or reentry. They are usually caused by events that break up the regularity of some other underlying rhythm rather than a rhythm in its own right. Irregularly irregular rhythms may have either three or more pacemakers and or pathologic transmission of the supraventricular impulses through the AV node.

Remember that there are essentially only three major irregularly irregular rhythms: Wandering atrial pacemaker, multifocal atrial tachycardia, and atrial fibrillation. If you see P waves, it is either WAP or MAT. If you do not see P waves, it is atrial fibrillation. (In atrial fibrillation, always remember to change leads to make sure that you are not dealing with an isoelectric lead for the P waves.) Can other rhythms be irregularly irregular? Yes, for example, atrial flutter with variable block, polymorphic VTach, and torsade de pointes can occasionally be irregularly irregular. But, these are uncommon rhythms. If you think of the big three, you will be right in a very, very large percentage of the cases.

Regular	Regularly Irregular	Irregularly Irregular
Normal sinus rhythm	Sinus arrhythmia	Wandering atrial pacemaker
Sinus tachycardia	Premature complexes*	Multifocal atrial tachycardia
Sinus bradycardia	• Atrial	Atrial fibrillation
Ectopic atrial rhythm	• Junctional	Atrial flutter with variable conduction
Ectopic atrial tachycardia	• Ventricular	Polymorphic VTach
Atrial flutter	Escape complexes*	Torsade de pointes
Junctional rhythm	• Atrial	
Accelerated junctional	• Junctional	
Junctional tachycardia	• Ventricular	
AVNRT	Atrial flutter with variable conduction	
AVRT	Sinus pauses*	
Idioventricular	Sinus blocks*	
Accelerated idioventricular	Sinus arrest*	
monomorphic VTach		

*These are actually events but the strips are frequently considered to be regularly irregular.

Table 37-2: Differential Diagnoses Based on the Regularity of the Ventricular Response

3. Do You See Any P Waves?
4. Are the P Waves the Same?
5. Are the P Waves Upright in Lead II?

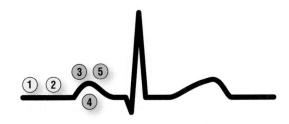

Dr. Henry J. L. Marriott asked his readers to "Cherchez Le P," which roughly translates to "look for the P wave". We like stressing the same concept, but with a bit more emphasis. We like to say: ***Beat the P's to death!*** You need to severely scrutinize each P wave for all of the information it contains. Notice that four questions out of these ten are dedicated directly to the subject of P waves (questions 3, 4, 5, and 10). Why all the fuss? Because, as we have seen so far in the book, the P waves are probably the single most important thing to look for in the evaluation of any arrhythmia.

The presence of P waves before the QRS complexes indicates a supraventricular origin for the complex. The P waves could have been formed by the sinus node, an ectopic atrial pacemaker, or an AV junctional pacemaker, but they are always formed somewhere in the supraventricular area. (The only exception is in retro-grade conduction of the impulse to the atria from an ectopic ventricular rhythms.) This bit of information will narrow down your differential diagnosis to the supraventricular rhythms (Table 37-3).

P waves that originate in the sinus node will be positive in lead II. Inverted P waves, or P waves that are negative in lead II, are found in either ectopic P waves, junctional complexes, or retrograde conduction. The site of origin in inverted P waves can be further narrowed down when we look at the PR interval (question 6). Briefly stated, normal or prolonged PR intervals are associated with ectopic atrial P waves and short PR intervals are associated with junctional complexes.

The presence of different P-wave morphologies on the same strip will also assist you in making the diagnosis. If there are irregular, premature complexes with differing P-wave morphologies, you are dealing with premature atrial contractions. If the beats in question arrive late in the cycle, you are dealing with atrial escape complexes. If you have more than three different morphologies, with differing PR intervals in an irregularly irregular rhythm, then you have either WAP or MAT depending on the underlying rate.

Sometimes it is critical to switch leads in order to obtain the most information about the P waves. In general, lead V_1 is the best lead in which to study the P waves. However, your patient is an individual; so are his P waves. Your patient's P waves may be best viewed in aVL or V_5; you never know which is the best lead. That is the reason

P Wave Is Present and Upright	P Wave Is Present but Inverted	P Wave May Be Present but Inverted
Normal sinus rhythm	Ectopic atrial rhythm*	Junctional rhythm
Sinus tachycardia	Ectopic atrial tachycardia*	Accelerated junctional
Sinus bradycardia	Wandering atrial pacemaker*	Junctional tachycardia
Sinus arrhythmia	Multifocal atrial tachycardia*	AVNRT
Ectopic atrial rhythm*		AVRT
Ectopic atrial tachycardia*		
Wandering atrial pacemaker*		
Multifocal atrial tachycardia*		
Premature atrial complexes*		
Escape atrial complexes*		

The AV blocks may be associated with either upright or inverted P waves depending on the underlying rhythm.

*P waves may be upright or inverted in these rhythms.

Table 37-3: Differential Diagnosis Based on the P Waves

why, when you have questions about the morphology or the presence of P waves, you should obtain a full 12-lead ECG. Once you know the best lead to view the P waves, then you can go back and get a longer rhythm strip from that particular lead if you need to. (Just keep in mind that inverted P waves can be normal in certain leads. In these cases, the P wave is not formed by ectopy but simply by the angle from which the lead is viewing the event.)

Look for buried P waves. We will spend much more time on this topic when we get to question #10 (Have I mined for gold?), but it is worthwhile to mention it here as well. The P waves can be buried anywhere, but usually are buried in the previous T wave.

Speaking of buried P waves, whenever the ventricular rate is 150 BPM, give or take a few beats, think about atrial flutter with 2:1 block. This association needs to become instinctual—you shouldn't even have to think about it. When you see a heart rate of 150 BPM, look at the lead with the smallest QRS complexes and try to find some buried P waves.

6. Are the PR Intervals Normal and Consistent?

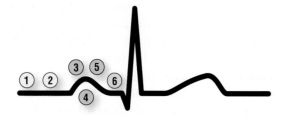

The PR interval represents conduction through the atria and the electrical conduction system, including the AV node. As such, the PR interval provides us with a win-

dow into the functional state of that system. Measuring the PR interval should be an automatic part of your analysis of any rhythm strip. As we have discussed, the PR interval is measured from the beginning of the P wave to the beginning of the QRS complex, and can be either short, normal, or prolonged (Table 37-4).

The normal PR interval is between 0.12 and 0.20 seconds. A normal PR interval is typically found in all of the sinus rhythms (normal sinus rhythm, sinus bradycardia, sinus tachycardia, and sinus arrhythmia). It can also be seen when an ectopic atrial pacemaker is at just the right distance from the AV node. The right distance is one that is neither too close nor too far from the AV node. If the ectopic pacemaker is too close to the AV node, the PR interval will be shorter because the impulse only has a short distance to travel before it reaches the AV node. If the ectopic pacemaker is too far from the AV node, the PR interval will be longer, reflecting the added distance that the impulse has to travel by direct cell-to-cell transmission in order to reach the AV node.

The PR interval is considered short if it is less than or equal to 0.11 seconds. A short PR interval can narrow down your differential into two major groups: The low ectopic atrials and the junctionals. As mentioned in the paragraph above, an ectopic atrial pacemaker that is close to the AV node will result in an impulse that only has to travel a very short distance through the atria before reaching the AV node. An AV junctional pacemaker will trigger impulses in both the atria and the ventricles simultaneously, either greatly shortening the PR interval or not forming one at all.

Now, let's start putting our PR intervals together with their P waves. You can have either upright or

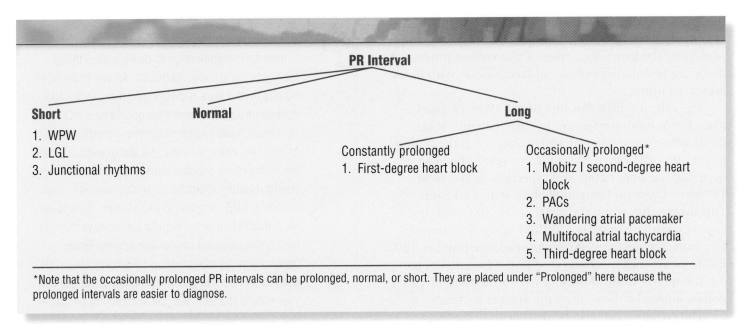

PR Interval

Short
1. WPW
2. LGL
3. Junctional rhythms

Normal

Long

Constantly prolonged
1. First-degree heart block

Occasionally prolonged*
1. Mobitz I second-degree heart block
2. PACs
3. Wandering atrial pacemaker
4. Multifocal atrial tachycardia
5. Third-degree heart block

*Note that the occasionally prolonged PR intervals can be prolonged, normal, or short. They are placed under "Prolonged" here because the prolonged intervals are easier to diagnose.

Table 37-4: Differential Diagnosis of the Various PR Interval Lengths

inverted P waves with a short PR interval. Upright P waves with short PR intervals are very rare and typically found in only two pathological states: Lown-Ganong-Levine (LGL) syndrome and WPW. LGL is a rare condition caused by having a small tract that bypasses the AV node. In essence, the bypass tract allows the impulse to avoid the physiologic block of the AV node, greatly shortening the PR interval. The QRS complexes in LGL, however, are narrow because ventricular depolarization occurred via the normal conduction pathway. WPW was covered in Chapter 26. It is associated with short PR intervals and QRS complexes that are wide due to fusion with the delta wave.

Inverted P waves with short PR intervals are associated with either very low ectopic atrial or junctional complexes. Distinguishing between these two requires invasive electrophysiological studies, which are both costly and impractical. Differentiation cannot be accomplished using a simple surface ECG recording alone. For this reason, all complexes with inverted P waves and short PR intervals are considered to be junctional complexes. Normally, there are no major clinically significant problems encountered by making this assumption and it definitely makes our lives much, much simpler.

A prolonged PR interval (greater than 0.20 seconds) is the hallmark of a first-degree AV block. As we saw in Chapter 35, first-degree AV blocks are not really blocks but delays caused by AV nodal malfunction or disease. The delay in first-degree AV blocks does not have to occur exclusively in the AV node, but can actually occur anywhere along the ventricular portion of the electrical conduction system.

In Table 37-4, the prolonged PR intervals are broken down further into those that are either constantly prolonged (all of the PR intervals in the strip are prolonged) and those that are occasionally prolonged (some of the PR intervals in the strip are prolonged and some are normal).

7. What is the P:QRS Ratio?

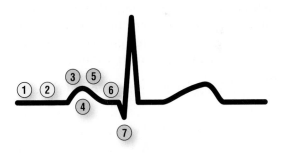

This question strikes at the heart of all the AV blocks. Normally, the P:QRS ratio is one to one because each supraventricular impulse (the P wave) causes only one ventricular depolarization (the QRS complex). When there are multiple P waves associated with only one QRS complex, you have the makings of an AV block of some sort.

The AV block can occur because of a normal physiologic response to a very fast supraventricular rate. In these cases, the supraventricular rates are so fast that, if they were conducted at a 1:1 ratio, the ventricles would be unable to function properly, causing hemodynamic compromise or maybe even cardiovascular collapse. For this reason, the AV node has a built-in safety feature that does not allow 1:1 conduction in those cases, essentially slowing down the ventricular response and protecting the heart. Examples of this type of functional block are found in ectopic atrial tachycardias with block and atrial flutter.

The rate at which this functional AV block takes place is not written in stone. In some patients, it can occur when the supraventricular rates reach the mid to lower 200 BPM range. Typically, however, the block occurs in the upper 200s and especially at 300 BPM. The most common functional block is at a 2:1 ratio. This means that when the atrial rate is 300 BPM, the typical ventricular rate is 150 BPM. Keep this number foremost in your mind. As mentioned, the number 150 BPM should trigger a visceral response that makes you ask the question: Am I dealing with atrial flutter? You will be amazed at how often the answer is "yes!"

The AV block can also be pathological, leading to either a second- or third-degree AV block. Different conduction ratios from 1:1 and grouping are the hallmarks for the second-degree AV blocks. Wenckebach or Mobitz I second-degree AV block is associated with an N:(N−1) conduction ratio. This means that there will always be one more P wave than a QRS complex in each group. Mobitz II second-degree AV block is associated with dropped QRS complexes without any widening of the PR interval.

Finally, there can be a complete absence of conduction between the atria and the ventricles. This occurs when you have a third-degree or complete AV block. In these cases, the atria and the ventricles are simply beating to the pace set by their own drummer.

Occasionally, another very rare event can occur that causes narrow complexes to develop even though the rhythm is actually ventricular. As you know, ventricular rhythms are wide because most of the conduction through the ventricles occurs by direct cell-to-cell transmission of the depolarization wave. In very rare cases, a ventricular tachycardia originating in one of the bundles transmits faster down that bundle, causing a narrow, or at least narrower than expected, QRS complex. In these cases, there is partial transmission of the depolarization wave through the normal electrical conduction system. Faster transmission equals narrower QRS complexes. This event is so rare that you will probably never see it in your clinical practice. We just want you to be aware that it can happen and that it does exist.

8. Are the QRS Complexes Narrow or Wide?

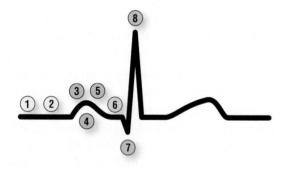

In general, supraventricular events and rhythms are narrow-complex (less than 0.12 seconds) and ventricular events and rhythms are wide-complex (greater than or equal to 0.12 seconds). There are, however, a few uncommon exceptions to this rule. To begin with, supraventricular complexes can be wide when they occur in patients with pre-existing bundle branch blocks. They can also be wide when they are aberrantly conducted in the ventricles for whatever reason. They can also be wide when there are electrolyte abnormalities causing inappropriate biochemical conduction through the atria and the ventricles.

There are a couple of other things that will affect the morphology of the complexes and possibly cause them to appear abnormally wide. One of these possibilities is fusion. Fusion with the waves from other complexes can cause abnormally wide morphology to develop in the QRS complex. Fusion is also responsible for the delta wave of WPW, giving these complexes their characteristically wide appearance (fusion of the impulse traveling through the accessory pathway and the one traveling through the regular electrical conduction system).

9. Are the Complexes Grouped or Not Grouped?

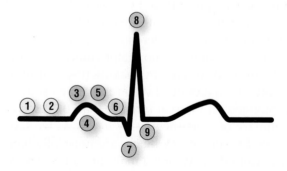

Grouped complexes are some sort of AV block until proven otherwise. Most commonly, grouping is seen with Mobitz I second-degree AV block. But, it can also be seen in Mobitz II second-degree, 2:1 second-degree AV block, advanced AV block, and sometimes even in third-degree AV block if the rates are just right.

The physiologic block that occurs at very fast supraventricular rates in atrial flutter and ectopic atrial tachycardia with block can also give the appearance of grouping. A search for the buried F or P waves in these cases will quickly lead you to the correct diagnosis.

Another common occurrence that can lead to a grouping pattern involves premature complexes. Frequent PACs, PJCs, and PVCs can give the appearance of grouping. This is especially true when the pattern involves bigeminy, trigeminy, quadrigeminy, or any other number. The rhythmic disruption of the underlying cadence of the rhythm causes the grouping appearance. In these cases, the abnormal morphology and timing of the P wave, PR interval, or the lack of P waves, will point you in the direction of premature beats rather than AV block.

10. Have I Mined for Gold?

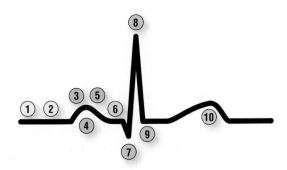

What are we getting at when we ask the question: Have I mined for gold? Well, we are asking you to examine your strip very carefully and look below the surface. Do not overlook any little irregularity, because that is where the "gold" will most likely be buried. Many times, it is these small, obscure areas of the strip that hold the key to the final diagnosis. In general, focus on

two basic principles as you answer this question: (1) Concentrate on the abnormality; and (2) Look at the "company it keeps."

Take a look at a strip you want to try to figure out. Mentally at first, and later using your calipers, compare all of the waves and intervals. Where are the differences? Is it the timing of one of the complexes that is off? Is it a wave that is a bit wider, shorter, taller, or narrower? Is the morphology different in any one wave? Are the intervals all the same? Are there any notches present that shouldn't be there? When you spot that little abnormality, do not leave it alone until you have an answer. Sometimes, the answer will be simply that it is an artifactual fluke; most of the time, however, you have found "gold."

Buried P waves are the best example that we can think of when we say "mining for gold." Typically, a buried P wave will cause the preceding T wave to be a little taller and fatter or it will cause it to lose some of its curves. This T wave will stick out like a sore thumb when compared to the others on the strip and will usually be associated with a prematurely occurring complex. If the P wave is blocked from conducting to the ventricles, however, you will only see the abnormal T wave (with the buried P) and then a long pause. These blocked, buried P waves will not conduct to the ventricles and will not have any QRS complexes or T waves associated with them.

Dr. Henry J. L. Marriott, in his book *Practical Electrocardiography,* talks about Bix's rule (named after Dr. Harold Bix). This rule basically states that if you see a P wave about halfway between two QRS complexes in a supraventricular tachycardia, you should always look for the buried P wave hidden inside the QRS complexes (Figure 37-3). This is an important principle and we can use it with many rhythms, not just the tachycardias. Practically speaking, PR intervals can be quite prolonged and intervals up to 0.60 seconds can occur, but they are extremely rare. Since they are common, you need to think of a buried P wave and an AV block

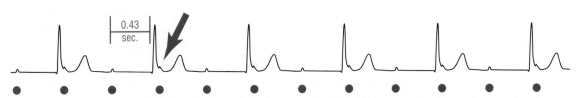

Figure 37-3: Bix's rule. Take a look at the strip above. The PR interval is 0.43 seconds. This is a markedly prolonged PR interval that only rarely occurs. The blue arrow points to a notch in the QRS complex. Is that notch a part of the QRS morphology or is it a buried P wave? It is a buried P wave and this is an example of Bix's rule. The blue dots mark the timing of the P waves along the strip.

whenever you see these markedly prolonged PR intervals. The odds will definitely be in your favor. In these cases, a little mining will clarify if you are dealing with a prolonged PR or an example of Bix's rule.

Differences in the R-R intervals also need to be addressed. Abnormal irregularity in the R-R intervals may be due to a sinus arrhythmia but, more likely, there is some other pathology involved. Premature complexes, escape complexes, blocked PACs, and AV blocks can all cause changes in the R-R interval.

Look closely at the events immediately before and after a different R-R interval or a pause. This is the area where gold is usually found. Frequently, you will see differences in the PR intervals which could represent a Wenckebach AV block. Blocked PACs can oftentimes be spotted in the T wave of the previous complex as mentioned before.

Sometimes, you may think that a notch or deflection may be a buried P wave but in reality it is part of the morphology of the QRS complex. This is especially true in looking at the pseudo-S and pseudo-R waves in AVNRT. Make sure that you check the regularity of the other P waves and see if the notch in question falls in line. If it does, it probably is a P wave; if it doesn't, it is probably not a P wave. This is exemplified in Figure 37-3. Note that the cadence of the supraventricular rhythm falls in perfect alignment with the notch on the QRS complex and that the PR interval is markedly prolonged. Why are we so sure that, in this case, we are dealing with buried P waves and not notches? Because of the company it keeps. . . .

This brings us to our other big principle in mining for gold: The company it keeps. When we say look at the "company it keeps," we are talking about a principle that we're sure your mother has told you a number of times. It could be something like "Show me your friends and I'll show you what you are." or "Birds of a feather, flock together." The company it keeps refers to the events occurring around an abnormality. In Figure 37-3, we are sure about the buried P waves not only because of the notch, but because the notch was associated with a very rare, very prolonged PR interval. In addition, the cadence of the supraventricular rhythm fits perfectly. The diagnosis was not made because of only one finding, but because of the finding and the "company" that finding "kept."

When you approach an obvious abnormality, look at everything around it in close detail. Do not leave the question unanswered. You need to be persistent when you mine for gold and if you are, eventually, you will be rewarded.

How Can I Put It All Together?

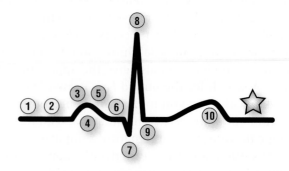

Unless you ask a question, you won't get an answer. The question we ask in this section makes perfect sense to ask oneself when approaching an arrhythmia. The problem is that most people never ask it. The result is that you will be lost in the small intricacies of the rhythm, but you will miss the diagnosis because you are not seeing the "big picture."

You need proof? When you took the end-of-section tests in this book, you probably came upon a strip that puzzled you. You saw the findings present on the strip, but couldn't put it together. When you looked up the answer, you likely saw the diagnosis very clearly and knew that it was correct. Why? Because you saw the big picture.

Chances are, you would have gotten the answer correct if it had been a multiple-choice question, because the answers themselves would have made you think of how the pieces fit together. Unfortunately, in our clinical lives, we cannot turn to the back of the book to get the answer, and the monitor does not provide multiple choices at the end of the strip. So, what should we do? We need to ask the big question: How can I put it all together?

Let's use an analogy to make our point a little differently. How do you build a jigsaw puzzle? You start out by looking at the "big picture" on the front of the box. Then, you find the corners and put them down. Then, you find the border pieces and build the outside frame. Then, you separate the rest of your pieces by color and put them down. Finally, you look at your finished work and see if it looks exactly like the "big picture." Now, suppose you had to build the puzzle without seeing the picture on the front of the box. That would be a tough way to build a puzzle. That is exactly what we are doing when we analyze a rhythm strip or an ECG—we are looking at the individual pieces with no guidance from the big picture.

To start your analysis of any strip or ECG, formulate an initial impression of the strip. This is like imagining what the puzzle picture would look like before we build it. Then look at each individual piece of the puzzle and answer the ten questions about the strip. Then step back and look at the finished picture. Does it make sense? Do all the pieces fit? Are there any pieces left over?

That last question (Are there any pieces left over?) is an important one. This is because, many times, there will be one piece of our arrhythmic puzzle that just doesn't seem to fit. It is easy to ignore that one finding because it doesn't want to fit into your diagnosis. This is a major mistake. In general, things will always fit. If it doesn't, you may be looking at the wrong picture. You have to keep looking for a solution in which all of the information fits. As we always say: If it doesn't fit, you mustn't quit.

Putting it all together includes the history and physical exam of your patient. Suppose you had a patient who was cyanotic, diaphoretic, and hypotensive—in other words, sick as a dog. You looked at the rhythm strip and the patient was in a normal sinus rhythm at 65 BPM. Does this piece of the puzzle fit? No, it doesn't; this patient should at least be tachycardic because the heart rate would increase trying to compensate for the low blood pressure. Should you just discard the physical exam and say that he is in normal sinus rhythm and the heart rate cannot be the problem, or do you quickly look around to see how this bit of information fits into the whole picture? Of course, you should look around a bit further and put it all together. In this particular case, the reason that the patient's heart rate was only at 65 BPM was that he taken a beta-blocker that was preventing his heart rate from compensating for the hypotension caused by his massive gastrointestinal bleed. Now every piece in the puzzle fits.

We believe that the one fact that separates the great clinicians from the mediocre ones is how they fit all of the pieces together. If we are meticulous and spend the time, each of us can get all of the pieces. Fitting them together is the art form. The title of this book is *Arrhythmia Recognition: The Art of Interpretation.* Putting it together is the art. We can all do it. We just need to ask the question: Why?

"Points"

The word "points" refers to the additional points from multiple leads and full 12-lead ECGs. Throughout this book, you have seen many examples of arrhythmias that would have been missed if multiple leads had not been obtained. We also talked about how the differen-

tial diagnosis was narrowed down to a couple of possibilities and the final diagnosis was made by taking a look at other leads. Remember, leads are like cameras. They shoot the same information from various angles. It is only fair to use these different vantage points to increase your odds of spotting pathology.

Should you get an ECG for every PVC you see? No, that would be overkill. But, you should get one whenever there is a question about an event, a rhythm, or a finding. It is also helpful to get one when the rhythms change, because something made that rhythm change. Getting a full 12-lead ECG may clarify what changed.

Old ECGs and strips are very helpful in arrhythmia recognition. The most important reason is that they allow us to see if the morphological features of the strip are consistent with the patient's baseline state or if they are a result of a new problem. New problems can be dangerous. It is always worthwhile to figure out why they are occurring.

Do not try to make decisions about hypertrophy, infarct, or any other pathological electrocardiographic process on a rhythm strip. Rhythm strips are notoriously bad for looking at morphology because the gain and other variables are too easily adjusted on the monitor. The result is that the complexes you see on a monitor are not a true representation of the morphology of the complexes, but an electronically manipulated facsimile of the true morphology. The ECG machine does not need to be "adjusted." When something is changed on the ECG, the machine shows the changes made on the calibration bar at the end of the strip. ECG machines are standardized and, therefore, can be used to evaluate morphology; monitors are not.

The bottom line is that if you see anything suspicious about the morphology on the rhythm strip, you should obtain a full 12-lead ECG. ST depression in lead II can be due to inferior ischemia or artifact on the monitor. It can also be due to a reciprocal change from a full-blown lateral infarct. The 12-lead ECG will help you tell the difference. Use all the tools available to you; the ECG machine is one of those tools.

One final word of wisdom: If you are serious about arrhythmia recognition, learn to use and interpret ECGs. This does not mean that you have to be an expert, but you at least have to be proficient with them. Twelve-lead ECGs and arrhythmias are all part of electrocardiography. The principles involved are the same and cross over from one to the other. Likewise, it is not realistic to think that you can study one without studying the other. You will see a major improvement in your arrhythmia recognition skills after you have studied an introductory book on 12-leads. In this book, we have tried to cross the barrier by explaining the interactions in greater depth than most other books. We hope that you have seen the connection and that you will continue to see the results of your labor over the coming years.

Let's Go Through an Example

Take a look at the strip in Figure 37-4. If you can figure out the diagnosis right away, you are doing great. Keep reading, though, because we are going to go through an exercise in the logic we have shown you in this chapter.

The first thing to look at in our "Patient's IQ Points" program is the patient. For the purposes of this discussion, we are going to say that the patient is hemodynamically stable and he is here to see you because he was experiencing some palpitations. The peripheral pulse rate is about 150 BPM. Huh? That number sounds familiar. . .

Overall Impression of the Rhythm

We can see that the rhythm is fast. The QRS complexes are small and narrow and there is a lot of undulation in the baseline. Your first impression should be that this is a narrow-complex tachycardia at about a rate of 150 BPM. The rate of 150 BPM should make you think of atrial flutter. Are we right? Let's go on. . .

Question 1: Is the Rhythm Fast or Slow?

Answer: The obvious answer is fast. The ventricular rate is about 150 BPM. Take a look at Figure 37-5. From the answer to this one question, we have already dramatically narrowed down our list of differentials to the ones in the pink blocks. The number of possibilities has gone from 21 to 11.

Question 2: Is the Rhythm Regular or Irregular?

Answer: The ventricular response is regular. We have just narrowed the pink list down again, this time to the rhythms represented by the seven blue rectangles.

Question 3: Do You See Any P Waves?

Answer: This is a tougher question to answer. What are those negative waves right before the QRS complexes: Are they inverted P waves or are they the T waves from the previous complexes? Well, if they were the T waves from the prior complexes, the QT intervals would be terribly prolonged. This can happen, but it's not too common to have that long of a QT interval with such a fast ventricular rate. Could the inverted waves be F waves? There's atrial flutter again. Let's move on. . .

Question 4: Are All of the P Waves the Same?

Answer: The inverted waves right before the QRS complexes are all the same. Are they inverted P or F waves? Still not sure. Let's move on. . .

Question 5: Are the P Waves Upright in Lead II?

Answer: No, if those are P waves, they would have to be inverted. F waves would most likely be inverted in lead II. We cannot state it with certainty, but it could be either an inverted P wave or an F wave. That narrows down our differential diagnosis to four rhythms represented by the purple boxes.

Question 6: Are the PR Intervals Normal and Consistent?

Answer: The intervals are definitely consistent. We still don't know if they are P waves, though.

Question 7: What is the P:QRS Ratio?

Answer: This raises a very important point. We are now at the major branching point for this arrhythmia. If we

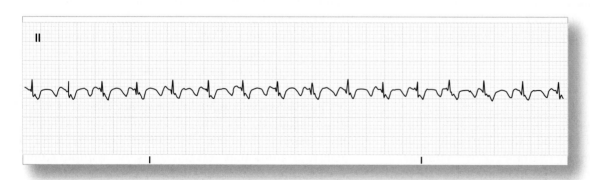

Figure 37-4: What is the rhythm?

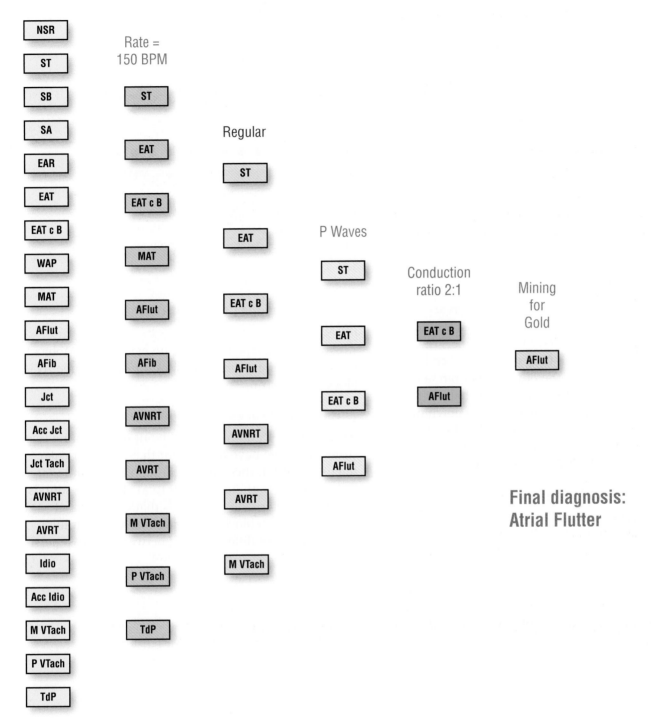

Figure 37-5: The differential diagnosis of the rhythm shown in Figure 37-4 as it is narrowed down by answering some simple questions.

say that those are inverted P waves, then the conduction ratio should be 1:1. If we say that these are F waves, then the conduction ratio would be 2:1. There is one more possibility to consider from looking at our list of possibilities: EAT with block. If this were EAT with block, what would the ratio be? 2:1, just like in atrial flutter.

Let's take another close look at our strip (see Figure 37-6). Place one pin of your calipers at the bottom of the inverted wave before the QRS complex. Now, place the other pin at the bottom of the next inverted wave right before the next QRS complex. That would make 0.38 seconds the presumed P-P interval if the conduc-

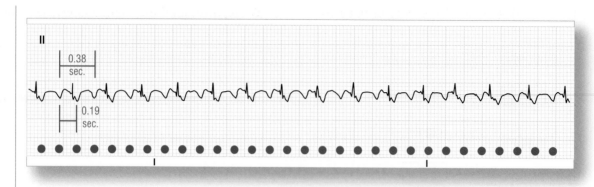

Figure 37-6: The presumed P-P interval is 0.38 seconds. Half of that interval would be 0.19 seconds. Setting your caliper pins to this measurement and walking it through the strip shows a recurrent inverted wave represented by the blue dots. This could be seen in EAT with block or atrial flutter.

tion ratio were 1:1. What would the P-P interval or F-F interval be if the conduction ratio was 2:1? It would be half of the distance that we have in our calipers or 0.19 seconds. Set your calipers to 0.19 seconds and go back to the inverted wave. Does the other caliper pin fall on any other inverted area? Yes! That means that the ratio of conduction is 2:1 and we have narrowed down our list of differentials to two possibilities: either EAT with block or atrial flutter (see blue dots on Figure 37-6). This is a little bit of gold mining. Let's move on.

Question 8: Are the QRS Complexes Narrow or Wide?

Answer: The QRS complexes are narrow. This question really doesn't help us much in this strip.

Question 9: Are the Complexes Grouped or Not Grouped?

Answer: Not grouped. There is no evidence of Mobitz I, Mobitz II second-degree AV block, or third-degree AV block on this strip.

Question 10: Have I Mined for Gold?

Answer: This is another critical point in evaluating this strip. So far, we have figured out that the ventricular rate is 150 BPM, the conduction ratio is 2:1, and that the atrial rate is, therefore, 300 BPM. This sure sounds like atrial flutter. The problem is that ectopic atrial tachycardia with block could also rarely be that high. The key point in differentiating between the two possi-

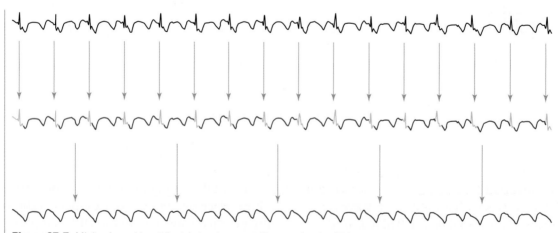

Figure 37-7: Mining for gold on this strip involves mentally removing the QRS complexes from the rhythm strip to see the underlying supraventricular rhythm. As you can clearly see on the blue (bottom) strip, this is atrial flutter because of the constantly undulating baseline formed by the F waves.

bilities is the baseline. If there are isoelectric or flat segments between the P waves, then it is EAT with block. If there is a constant undulating pattern, then it is atrial flutter. So, how do we figure it out? Go mining. . .

We want you to exercise your mind a bit at this point. Look closely at the top strip in Figure 37-7, and mentally remove the QRS complexes. This should be easy to do in this strip because the QRS complexes are so small. When you do that, you see a nice undulating pattern like the one at the bottom of Figure 37-7. The final diagnosis is atrial flutter.

Going through these mental exercises may seem like an exaggeration, but it isn't. An organized approach is the best way to interpret an arrhythmia. Eventually, with time and practice, you will be able to perform this process in seconds. However, you are still learning. Get yourself used to the system, or whatever system you decide to use, and build a strong foundation. We hope that you have enjoyed this chapter and that you will carry the information in it with you forever in your clinical life. Now, let's go practice. . .

CHAPTER **REVIEW**

1. When you are evaluating a strip, you should think about your (mnemonic) _____ _ _ _____!

2. If you see a patient's strip and it shows frequent unifocal PVCs and a rate of 70 BPM, you can assume that the patient is stable and that the rhythm is benign. True or False.

3. You should always let the patient tell you as much information as he or she can, uninterrupted. However, sometimes, you just have to start asking questions. This is especially true when the patient is scared or anxious. Don't be afraid to ask questions! True or False.

4. If the patient is having an arrhythmia that is hemodynamically stable according to his vital signs, but tells you that he is "going to die," you can assume that he is going to be all right. True or False.

5. You should get in the habit of always checking both the heart rate on the monitor and the pulse rate on the patient. True or False.

6. The presence of __ waves is something that is critical in the evaluation of any rhythm abnormality.

7. The PR interval should be between _____ and _____ seconds wide.

8. Rhythms with upright P waves with short PR intervals are very rare and can be found in (pick all that are correct):
   A. Sinus tachycardia
   B. Junctional rhythms
   C. WPW pattern
   D. AVRT
   E. Lown-Ganong-Levine (LGL) syndrome
   F. Accelerated idioventricular

9. When you mine for gold, you should think about two basic principles: (1) Concentrate on the abnormality; and (2) the "_____ __ _____".

10. In general, all of your findings will fit into one arrhythmia. True or False.

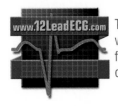

To enhance the knowledge you gain in this book, access this text's website at www.12leadECG.com! This valuable resource provides flashcards, an online glossary, web links, and more. Simply click on the Arrhythmias book cover once at the site.

Final Test

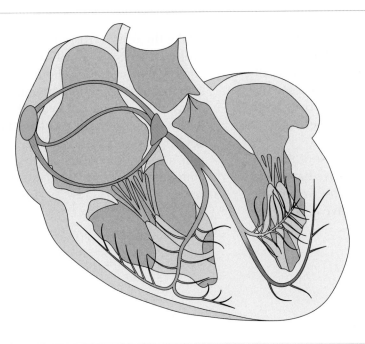

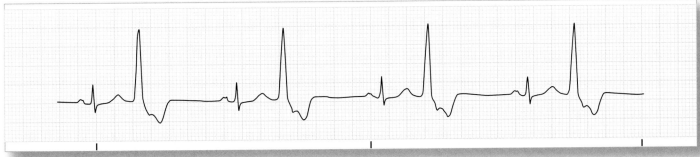

The interpretation of arrhythmias and ECGs is an art form more than it is a science. This final test is intended to bring these concepts out by challenging you and making you use all of your reasoning powers and newfound knowledge. Don't worry if you don't get every strip correct. In order for this test to be challenging, some strips have to push you to the limit. Many times, the strip will only allow you to narrow the differential down to just a few possibilities. This is the way that it should be, because this emulates real situations. Narrowing the possibilities down to a final one usually requires clinical correlation with your patient, evaluating a full 12-lead ECG, or comparison to old strips. Right now, concentrate on the process rather than on scoring 100% correct.

When you are faced with a tough strip, take some time, take a deep breath, and above all don't panic. Begin to analyze the rhythm slowly and methodically, just as we taught you in Chapter 37. You will see that every bit of uncovered information will narrow your list of differentials down a little bit further. Eventually, the answer will become clear.

We are making an effort to cover most of the arrhythmias we have seen in this text. We have, however, weighted the test to reflect the most frequently clinically observed arrhythmias. We have also used some strips to reinforce some of the main take-home messages that we have presented in the individual chapters. When you are done, turn to the answers and analyze the way that we approached the strip. It may not be the same way that you did, but that's OK. There are many paths to the same answer. The object is to examine the thought process involved; you can adjust it to fit your personal pattern as you progress. If you find that you are missing any particular arrhythmia with any frequency, spend a few minutes and go back and review that section again. Practice makes perfect in arrhythmia recognition.

When you have reviewed the material and you feel comfortable with your skills, put the book away for a while. In a couple of months, pick it up again and retake the tests. (Trust me, you won't remember most of the answers.) This will reinforce the knowledge that you have gained and solidify your clinical skills at arrhythmia recognition. In your clinical practice, read as many strips as you can every day. Over time, you will notice how proficient you have become and you will develop the confidence needed to confront any situation. That said, remember the old adage "know your limitations." *When you find a strip you are not sure about, don't ever be afraid to ask for help.*

Final Test ECG 1

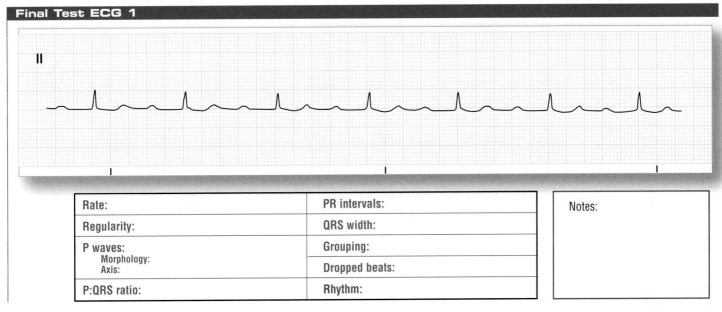

Rate:	PR intervals:	Notes:
Regularity:	QRS width:	

P waves:
  Morphology:
  Axis:
	Grouping:	

	Dropped beats:	
P:QRS ratio:	Rhythm:	

Final Test ECG 2

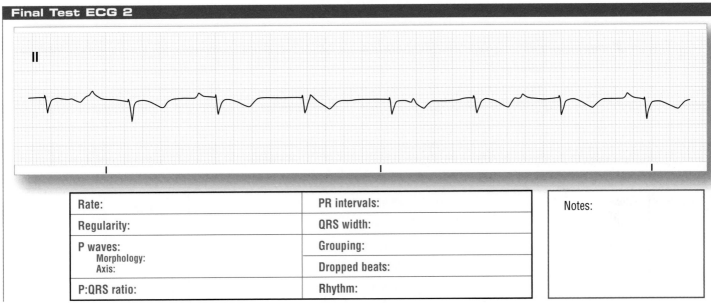

Rate:	PR intervals:	Notes:
Regularity:	QRS width:	

P waves:
  Morphology:
  Axis:
	Grouping:	

	Dropped beats:	
P:QRS ratio:	Rhythm:	

Final Test ECG 3

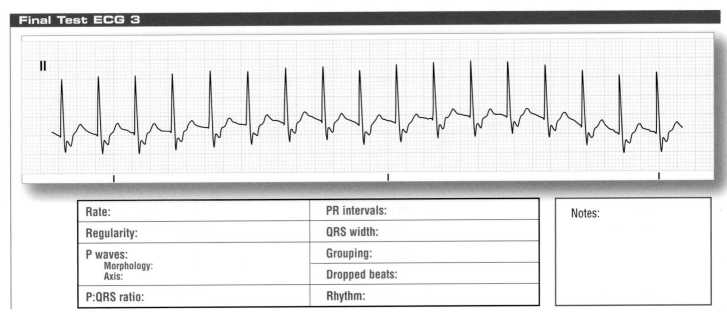

Rate:	PR intervals:	Notes:
Regularity:	QRS width:	

P waves:
  Morphology:
  Axis:
	Grouping:	

	Dropped beats:	
P:QRS ratio:	Rhythm:	

Final Test ECG 4

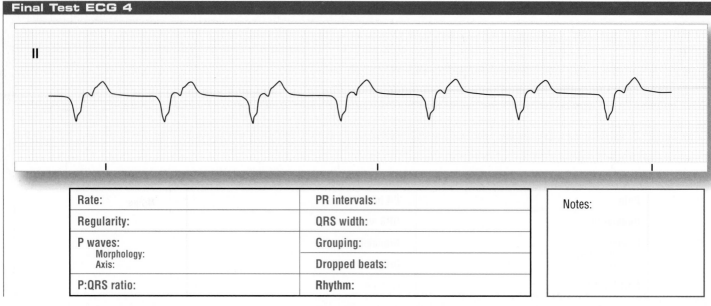

Rate:	PR intervals:
Regularity:	QRS width:
P waves:	Grouping:
Morphology:	
Axis:	Dropped beats:
P:QRS ratio:	Rhythm:

Notes:

Final Test ECG 5

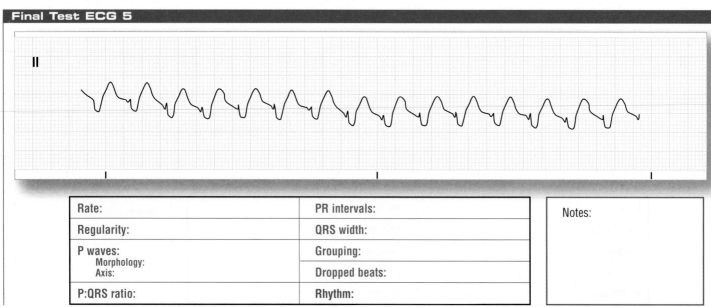

Rate:	PR intervals:
Regularity:	QRS width:
P waves:	Grouping:
Morphology:	
Axis:	Dropped beats:
P:QRS ratio:	Rhythm:

Notes:

Final Test ECG 6

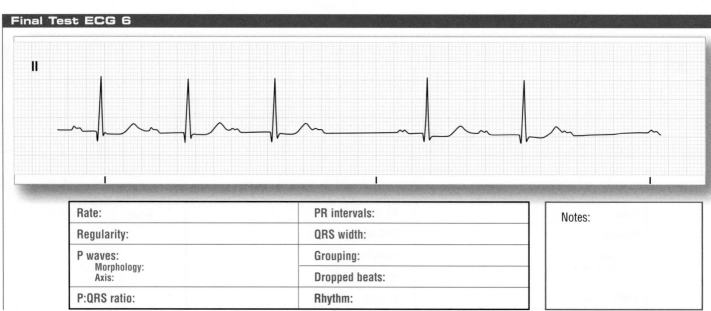

Rate:	PR intervals:
Regularity:	QRS width:
P waves:	Grouping:
Morphology:	
Axis:	Dropped beats:
P:QRS ratio:	Rhythm:

Notes:

Final Test ECG 7

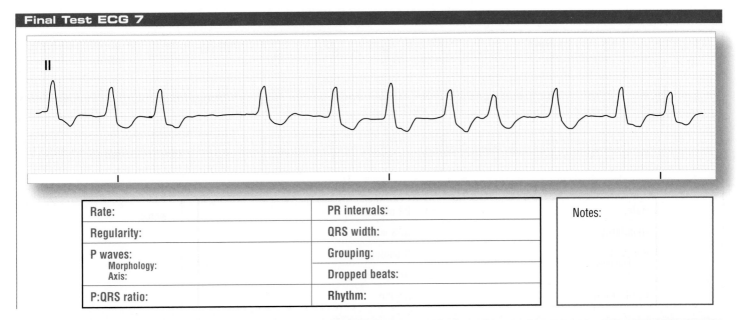

Rate:		PR intervals:		Notes:
Regularity:		QRS width:		
P waves:		Grouping:		
Morphology:				
Axis:		Dropped beats:		
P:QRS ratio:		Rhythm:		

Final Test ECG 8

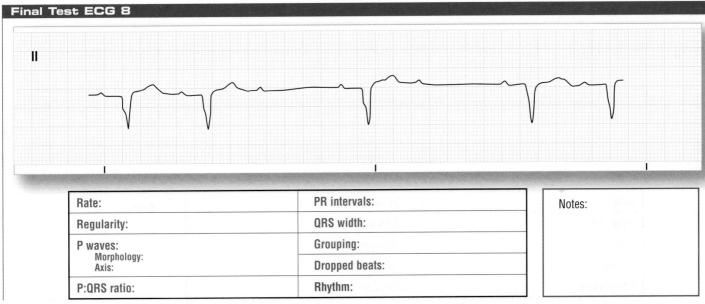

Rate:		PR intervals:		Notes:
Regularity:		QRS width:		
P waves:		Grouping:		
Morphology:				
Axis:		Dropped beats:		
P:QRS ratio:		Rhythm:		

Final Test ECG 9

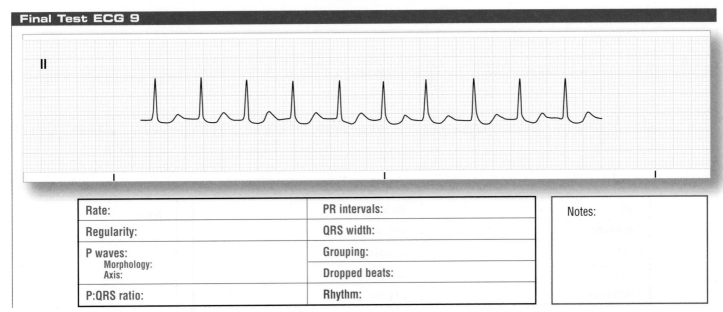

Rate:		PR intervals:		Notes:
Regularity:		QRS width:		
P waves:		Grouping:		
Morphology:				
Axis:		Dropped beats:		
P:QRS ratio:		Rhythm:		

Final Test ECG 10

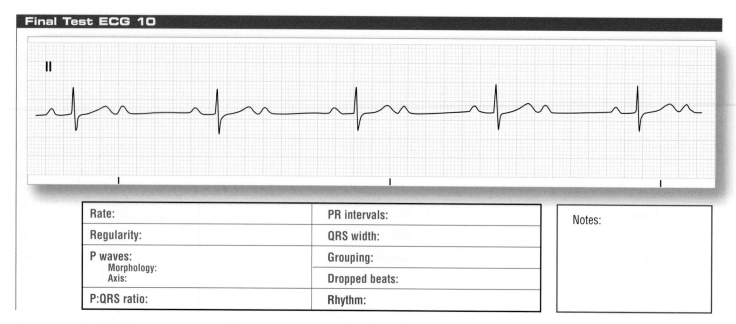

Rate:	PR intervals:	Notes:
Regularity:	QRS width:	
P waves:	Grouping:	
Morphology:		
Axis:	Dropped beats:	
P:QRS ratio:	Rhythm:	

Final Test ECG 11

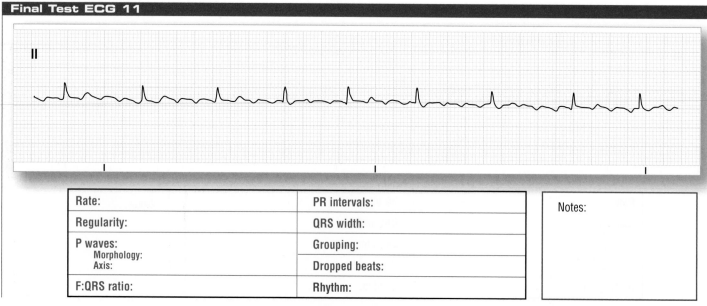

Rate:	PR intervals:	Notes:
Regularity:	QRS width:	
P waves:	Grouping:	
Morphology:		
Axis:	Dropped beats:	
F:QRS ratio:	Rhythm:	

Final Test ECG 12

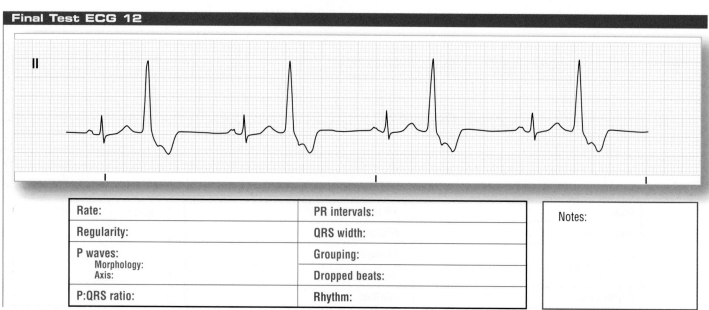

Rate:	PR intervals:	Notes:
Regularity:	QRS width:	
P waves:	Grouping:	
Morphology:		
Axis:	Dropped beats:	
P:QRS ratio:	Rhythm:	

Final Test ECG 13

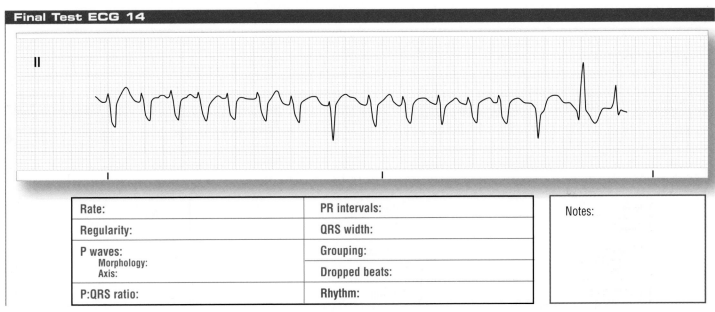

V₁

Rate:	PR intervals:	Notes:	
Regularity:	QRS width:		

P waves:
    Morphology:
    Axis:
	Grouping:		

	Dropped beats:		
P:QRS ratio:	Rhythm:		

Final Test ECG 14

II

Rate:	PR intervals:	Notes:	
Regularity:	QRS width:		

P waves:
    Morphology:
    Axis:
	Grouping:		

	Dropped beats:		
P:QRS ratio:	Rhythm:		

Final Test ECG 15

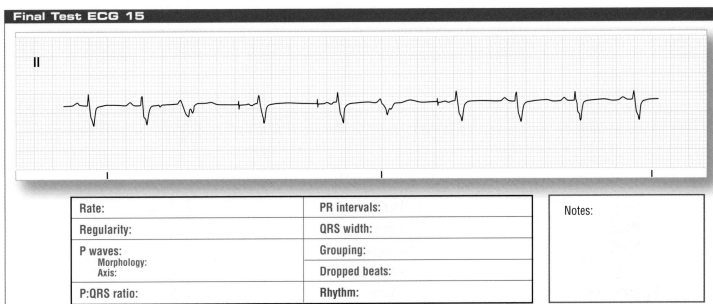

II

Rate:	PR intervals:	Notes:	
Regularity:	QRS width:		

P waves:
    Morphology:
    Axis:
	Grouping:		

	Dropped beats:		
P:QRS ratio:	Rhythm:		

Final Test ECG 16

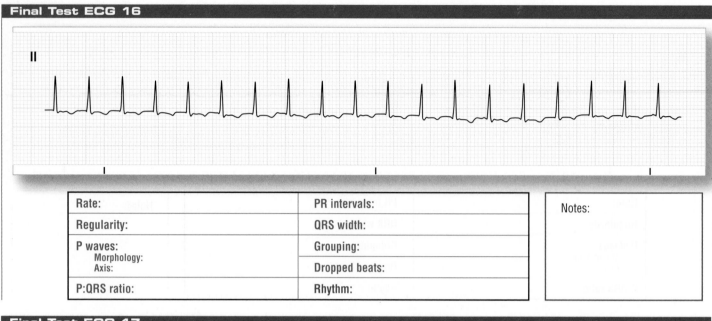

Rate:	PR intervals:	Notes:
Regularity:	QRS width:	

P waves:
    Morphology:
    Axis:
	Grouping:	

	Dropped beats:	
P:QRS ratio:	Rhythm:	

Final Test ECG 17

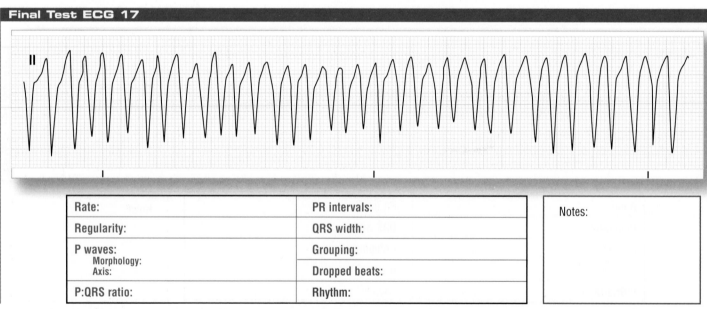

Rate:	PR intervals:	Notes:
Regularity:	QRS width:	

P waves:
    Morphology:
    Axis:
	Grouping:	

	Dropped beats:	
P:QRS ratio:	Rhythm:	

Final Test ECG 18

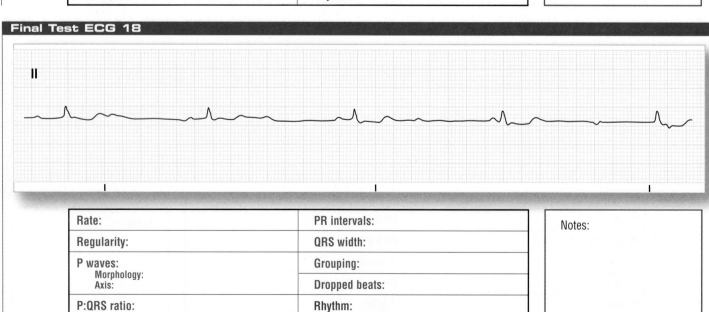

Rate:	PR intervals:	Notes:
Regularity:	QRS width:	

P waves:
    Morphology:
    Axis:
	Grouping:	

	Dropped beats:	
P:QRS ratio:	Rhythm:	

Final Test ECG 19

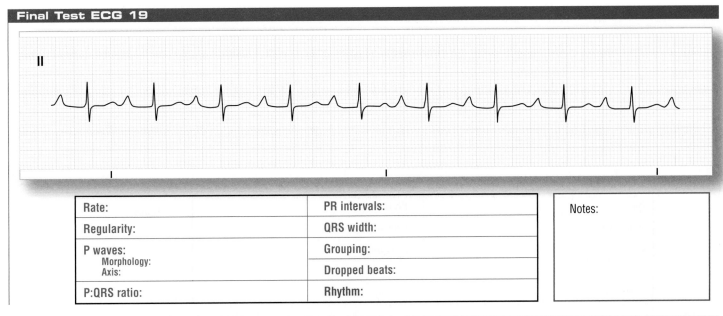

Rate:	PR intervals:	Notes:
Regularity:	QRS width:	

P waves:
   Morphology:
   Axis:
	Grouping:
	
	 Dropped beats:	

P:QRS ratio:	Rhythm:	

Final Test ECG 20

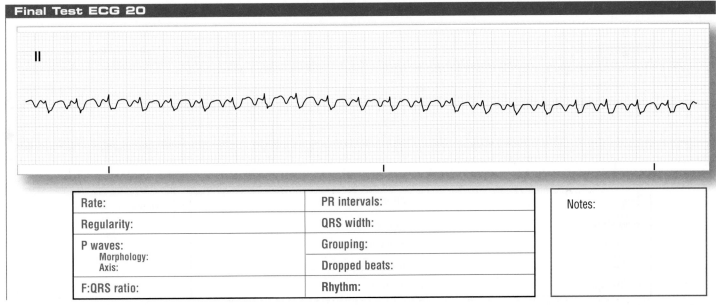

Rate:	PR intervals:	Notes:
Regularity:	QRS width:	

P waves:
   Morphology:
   Axis:
	Grouping:
	
	 Dropped beats:	

F:QRS ratio:	Rhythm:	

Final Test ECG 21

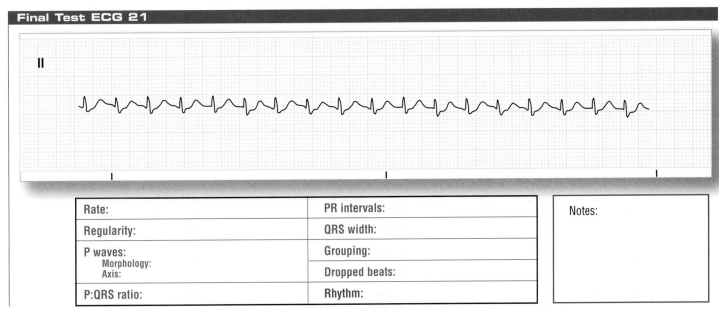

Rate:	PR intervals:	Notes:
Regularity:	QRS width:	

P waves:
   Morphology:
   Axis:
	Grouping:
	
	 Dropped beats:	

P:QRS ratio:	Rhythm:	

Final Test ECG 22

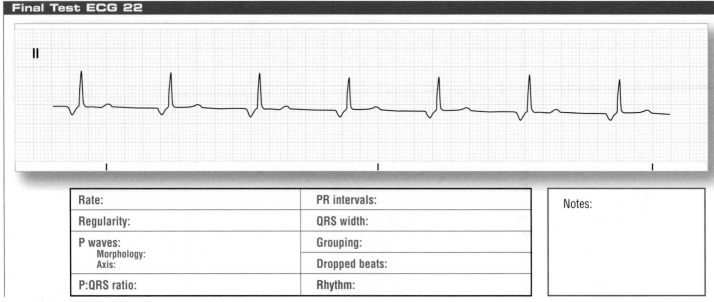

Rate:		PR intervals:	Notes:
Regularity:		QRS width:	
P waves:		Grouping:	
Morphology:			
Axis:		Dropped beats:	
P:QRS ratio:		Rhythm:	

Final Test ECG 23

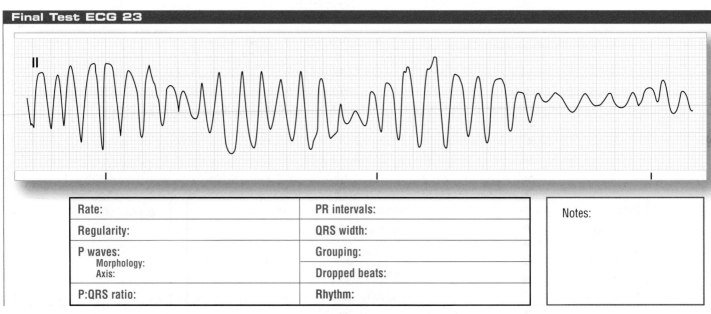

Rate:		PR intervals:	Notes:
Regularity:		QRS width:	
P waves:		Grouping:	
Morphology:			
Axis:		Dropped beats:	
P:QRS ratio:		Rhythm:	

Final Test ECG 24

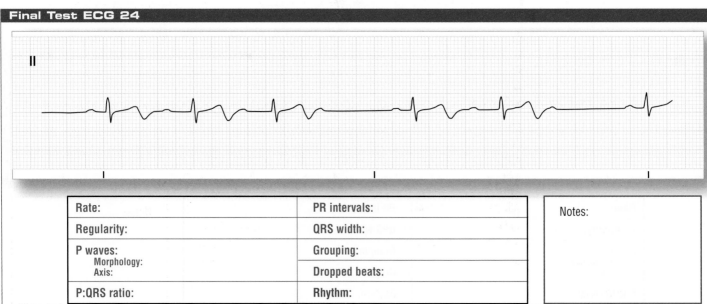

Rate:		PR intervals:	Notes:
Regularity:		QRS width:	
P waves:		Grouping:	
Morphology:			
Axis:		Dropped beats:	
P:QRS ratio:		Rhythm:	

Final Test ECG 25

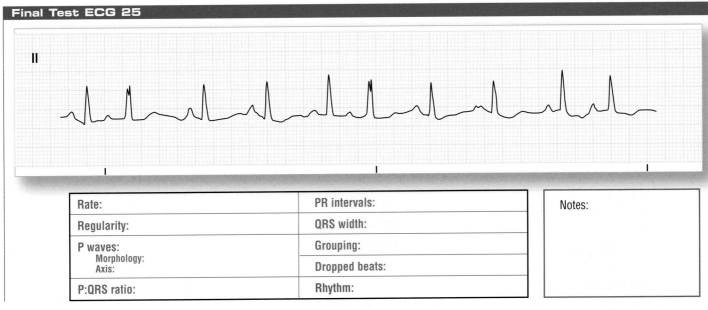

Rate:	PR intervals:
Regularity:	QRS width:
P waves:	Grouping:
Morphology:	
Axis:	Dropped beats:
P:QRS ratio:	Rhythm:

Notes:

Final Test ECG 26

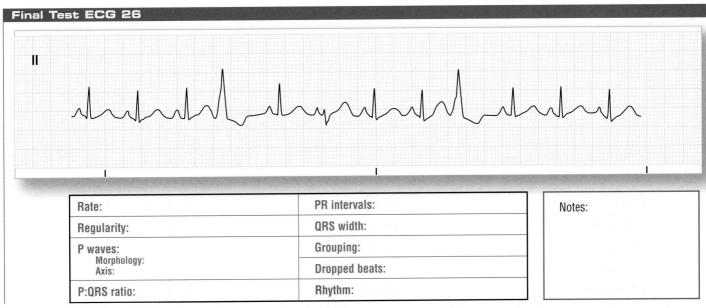

Rate:	PR intervals:
Regularity:	QRS width:
P waves:	Grouping:
Morphology:	
Axis:	Dropped beats:
P:QRS ratio:	Rhythm:

Notes:

Final Test ECG 27

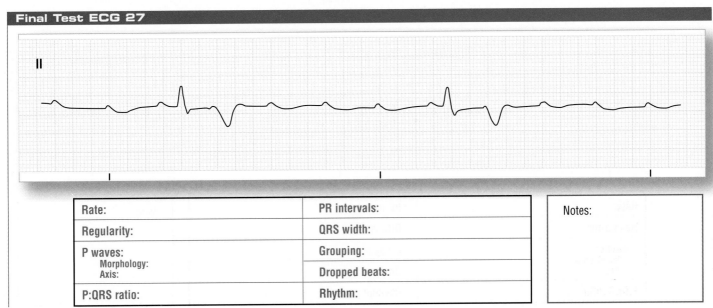

Rate:	PR intervals:
Regularity:	QRS width:
P waves:	Grouping:
Morphology:	
Axis:	Dropped beats:
P:QRS ratio:	Rhythm:

Notes:

Final Test ECG 28

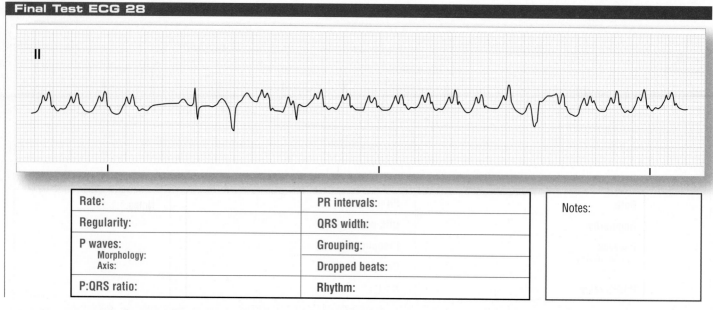

Rate:	PR intervals:	Notes:
Regularity:	QRS width:	
P waves:	Grouping:	
Morphology:		
Axis:	Dropped beats:	
P:QRS ratio:	Rhythm:	

Final Test ECG 29

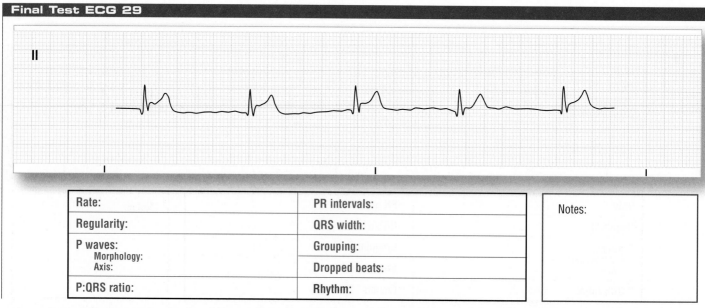

Rate:	PR intervals:	Notes:
Regularity:	QRS width:	
P waves:	Grouping:	
Morphology:		
Axis:	Dropped beats:	
P:QRS ratio:	Rhythm:	

Final Test ECG 30

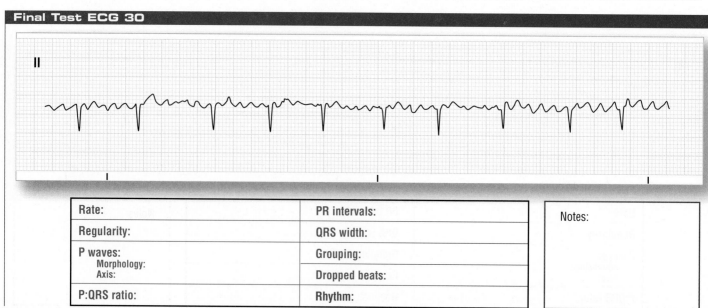

Rate:	PR intervals:	Notes:
Regularity:	QRS width:	
P waves:	Grouping:	
Morphology:		
Axis:	Dropped beats:	
P:QRS ratio:	Rhythm:	

Final Test ECG 31

II

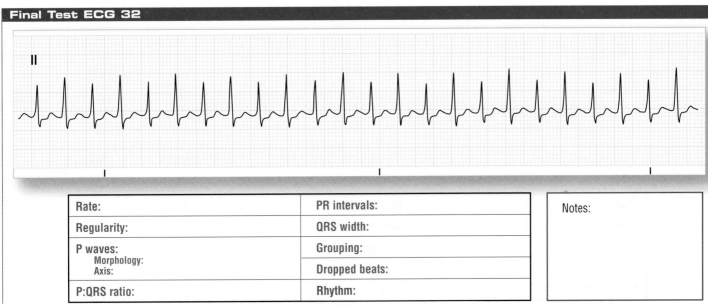

Rate:		PR intervals:	Notes:
Regularity:		QRS width:	
P waves:		Grouping:	
Morphology:			
Axis:		Dropped beats:	
F:QRS ratio:		Rhythm:	

Final Test ECG 32

II

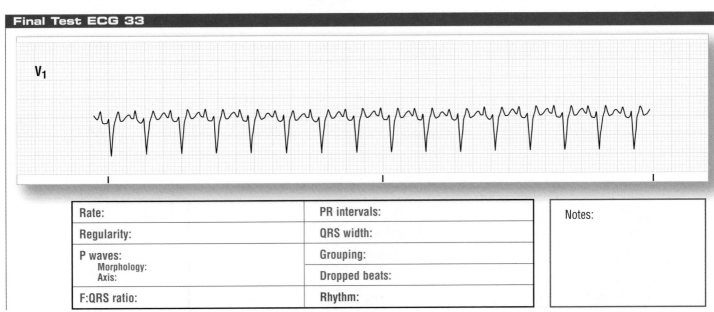

Rate:		PR intervals:	Notes:
Regularity:		QRS width:	
P waves:		Grouping:	
Morphology:			
Axis:		Dropped beats:	
P:QRS ratio:		Rhythm:	

Final Test ECG 33

V₁

Rate:		PR intervals:	Notes:
Regularity:		QRS width:	
P waves:		Grouping:	
Morphology:			
Axis:		Dropped beats:	
F:QRS ratio:		Rhythm:	

Final Test ECG 34

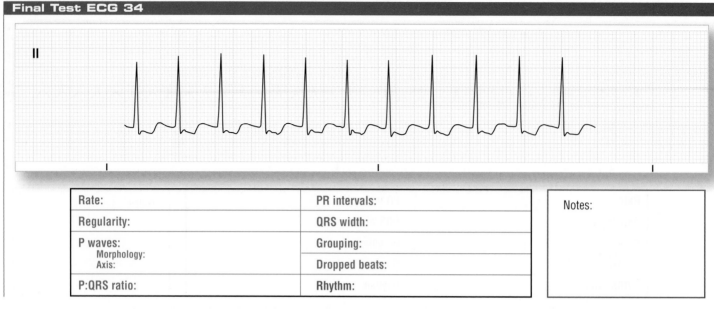

Rate:	PR intervals:
Regularity:	QRS width:
P waves:	Grouping:
Morphology:	
Axis:	Dropped beats:
P:QRS ratio:	Rhythm:

Notes:

Final Test ECG 35

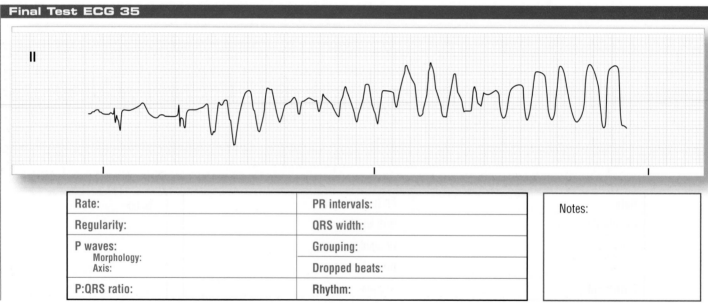

Rate:	PR intervals:
Regularity:	QRS width:
P waves:	Grouping:
Morphology:	
Axis:	Dropped beats:
P:QRS ratio:	Rhythm:

Notes:

Final Test ECG 36

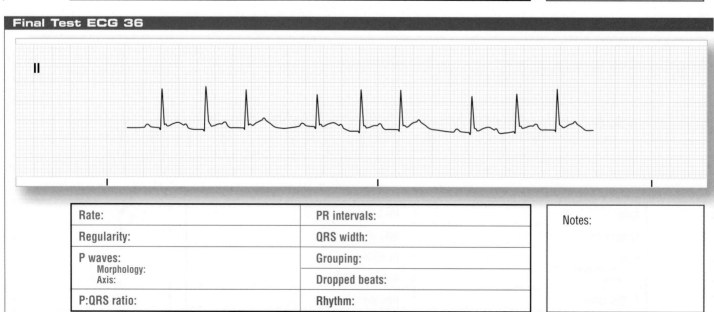

Rate:	PR intervals:
Regularity:	QRS width:
P waves:	Grouping:
Morphology:	
Axis:	Dropped beats:
P:QRS ratio:	Rhythm:

Notes:

Final Test ECG 37

II

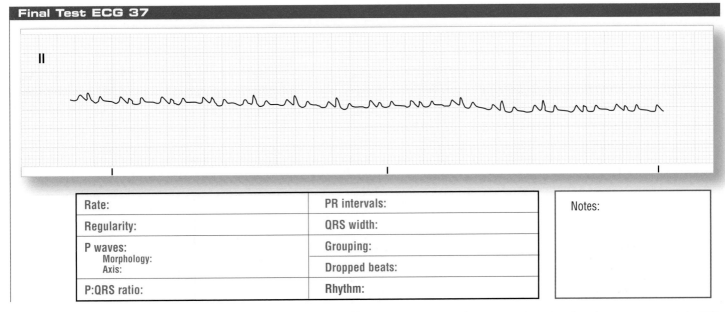

Rate:		PR intervals:	Notes:
Regularity:		QRS width:	
P waves:		Grouping:	
	Morphology:	Dropped beats:	
	Axis:		
P:QRS ratio:		Rhythm:	

Final Test ECG 38

II

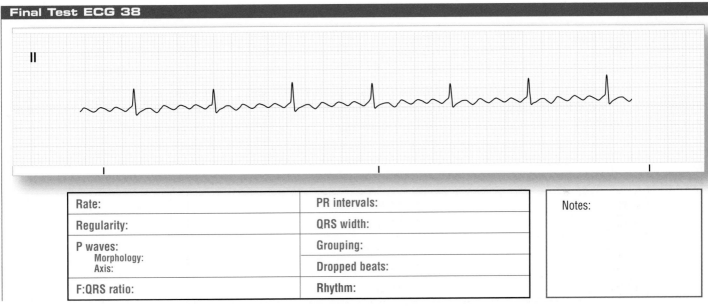

Rate:		PR intervals:	Notes:
Regularity:		QRS width:	
P waves:		Grouping:	
	Morphology:	Dropped beats:	
	Axis:		
F:QRS ratio:		Rhythm:	

Final Test ECG 39

II

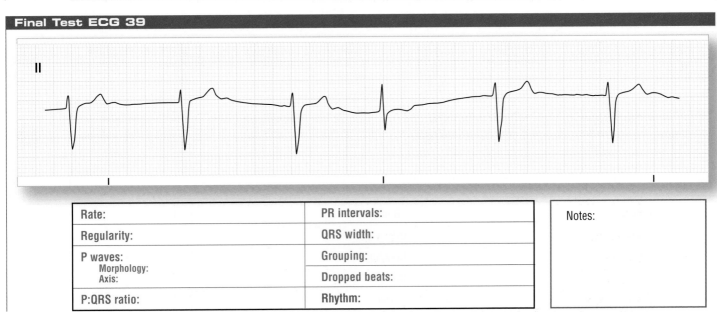

Rate:		PR intervals:	Notes:
Regularity:		QRS width:	
P waves:		Grouping:	
	Morphology:	Dropped beats:	
	Axis:		
P:QRS ratio:		Rhythm:	

Final Test ECG 40

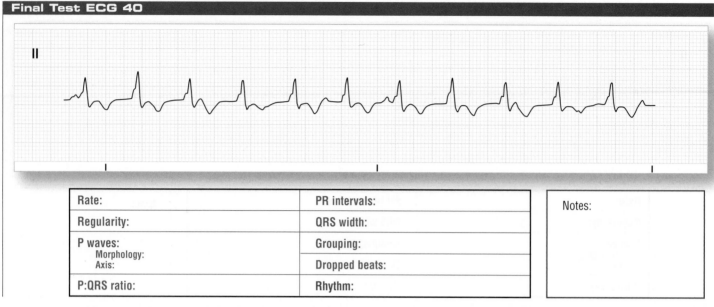

Rate:	PR intervals:	Notes:
Regularity:	QRS width:	
P waves:	Grouping:	
Morphology:		
Axis:	Dropped beats:	
P:QRS ratio:	Rhythm:	

Final Test ECG 41

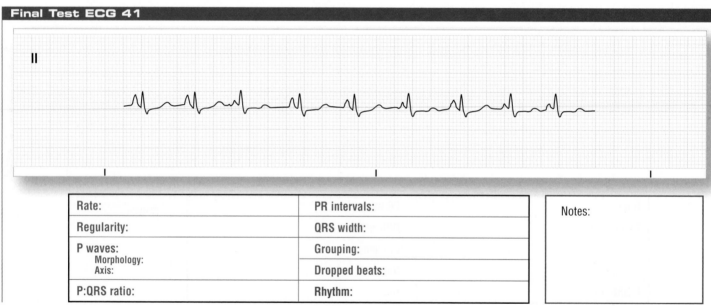

Rate:	PR intervals:	Notes:
Regularity:	QRS width:	
P waves:	Grouping:	
Morphology:		
Axis:	Dropped beats:	
P:QRS ratio:	Rhythm:	

Final Test ECG 42

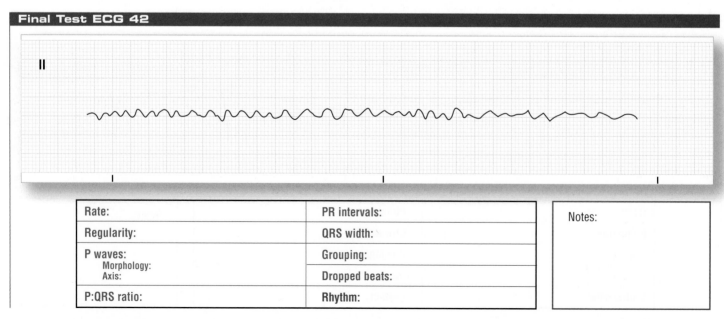

Rate:	PR intervals:	Notes:
Regularity:	QRS width:	
P waves:	Grouping:	
Morphology:		
Axis:	Dropped beats:	
P:QRS ratio:	Rhythm:	

Final Test ECG 43

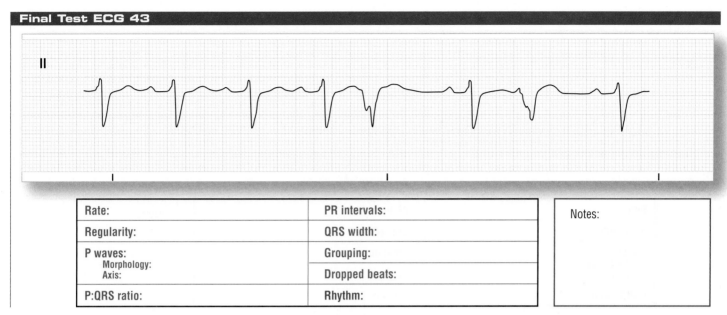

Rate:		PR intervals:		Notes:
Regularity:		QRS width:		
P waves: Morphology: Axis:		Grouping:		
		Dropped beats:		
P:QRS ratio:		Rhythm:		

Final Test ECG 44

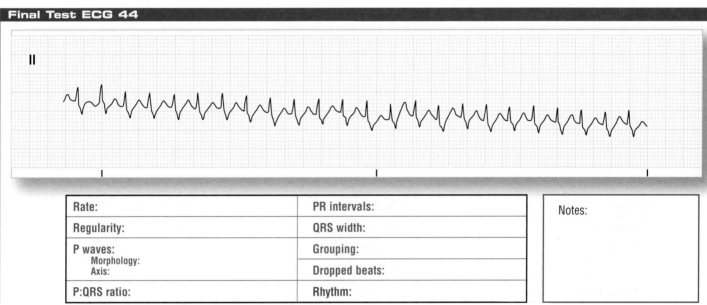

Rate:		PR intervals:		Notes:
Regularity:		QRS width:		
P waves: Morphology: Axis:		Grouping:		
		Dropped beats:		
P:QRS ratio:		Rhythm:		

Final Test ECG 45

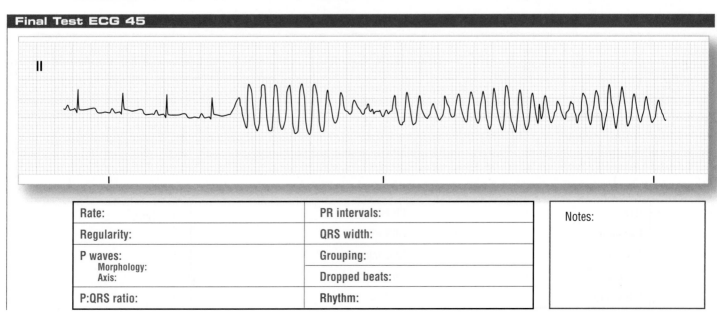

Rate:		PR intervals:		Notes:
Regularity:		QRS width:		
P waves: Morphology: Axis:		Grouping:		
		Dropped beats:		
P:QRS ratio:		Rhythm:		

Final Test ECG 46

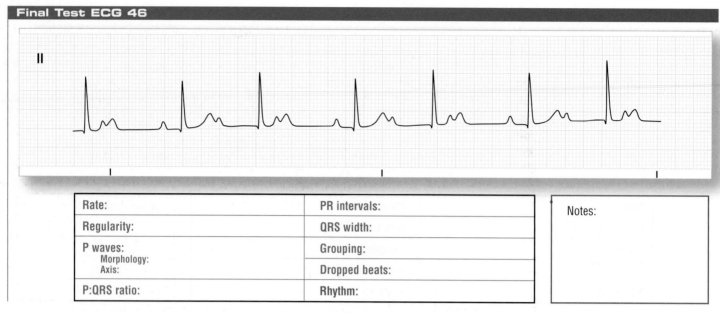

Rate:		PR intervals:	Notes:
Regularity:		QRS width:	
P waves:		Grouping:	
	Morphology:		
	Axis:	Dropped beats:	
P:QRS ratio:		Rhythm:	

Final Test ECG 47

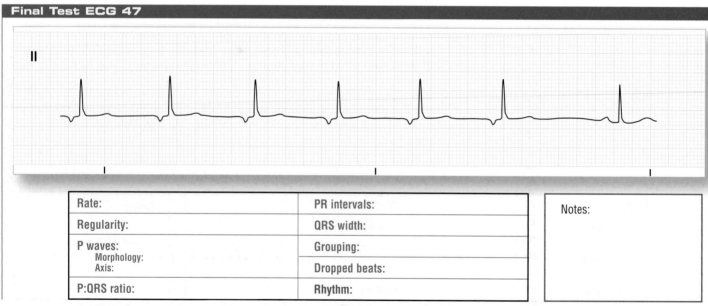

Rate:		PR intervals:	Notes:
Regularity:		QRS width:	
P waves:		Grouping:	
	Morphology:		
	Axis:	Dropped beats:	
P:QRS ratio:		Rhythm:	

Final Test ECG 48

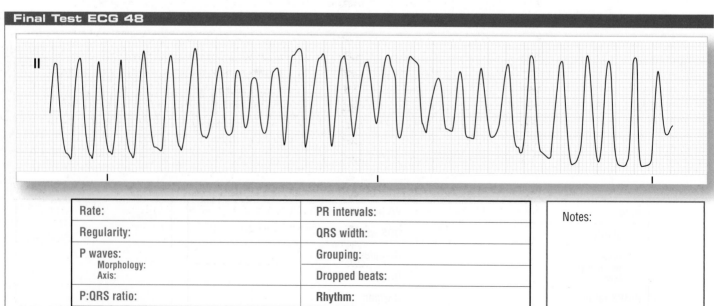

Rate:		PR intervals:	Notes:
Regularity:		QRS width:	
P waves:		Grouping:	
	Morphology:		
	Axis:	Dropped beats:	
P:QRS ratio:		Rhythm:	

Final Test ECG 49

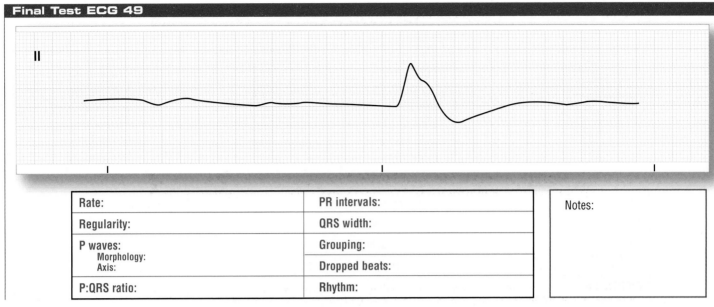

Rate:	PR intervals:	Notes:
Regularity:	QRS width:	

P waves:
  Morphology:
  Axis:
	Grouping:	

	Dropped beats:	
P:QRS ratio:	Rhythm:	

Final Test ECG 50

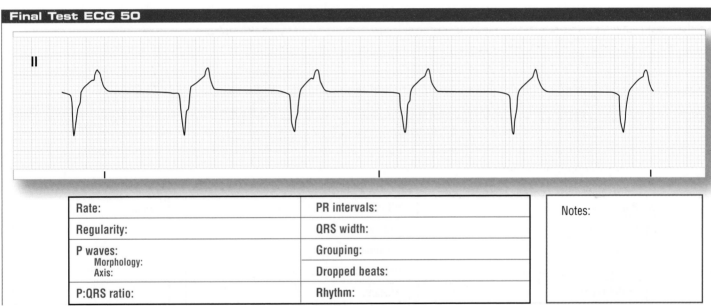

Rate:	PR intervals:	Notes:
Regularity:	QRS width:	

P waves:
  Morphology:
  Axis:
	Grouping:	

	Dropped beats:	
P:QRS ratio:	Rhythm:	

Final Test ECG 51

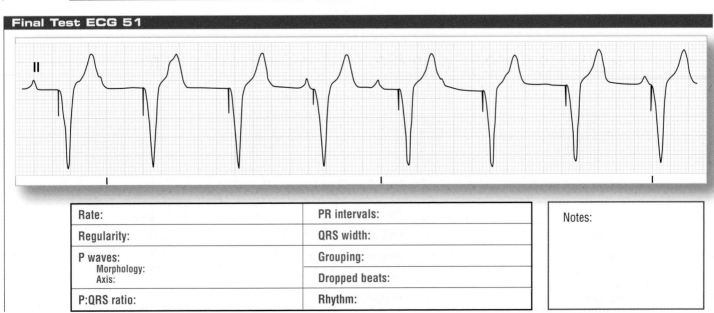

Rate:	PR intervals:	Notes:
Regularity:	QRS width:	

P waves:
  Morphology:
  Axis:
	Grouping:	

	Dropped beats:	
P:QRS ratio:	Rhythm:	

Final Test ECG 52

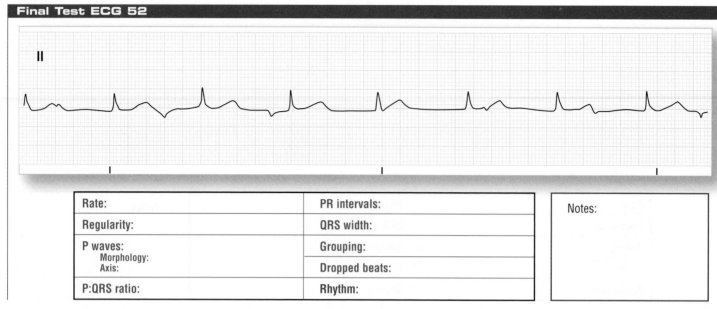

Rate:		PR intervals:	Notes:
Regularity:		QRS width:	
P waves: Morphology: Axis:		Grouping:	
		Dropped beats:	
P:QRS ratio:		Rhythm:	

Final Test ECG 53

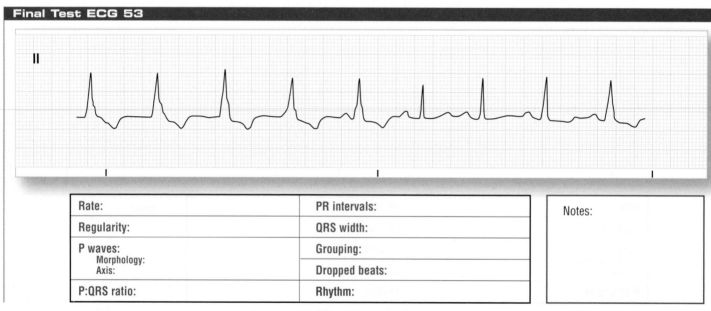

Rate:		PR intervals:	Notes:
Regularity:		QRS width:	
P waves: Morphology: Axis:		Grouping:	
		Dropped beats:	
P:QRS ratio:		Rhythm:	

Final Test ECG 54

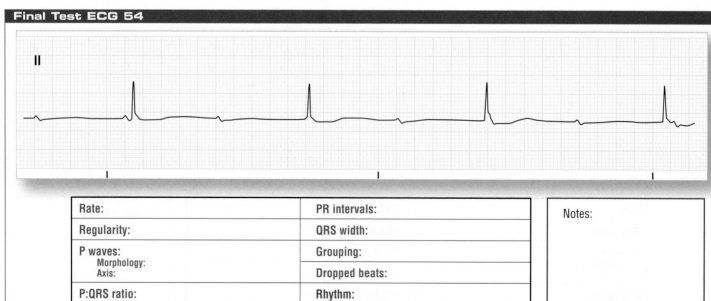

Rate:		PR intervals:	Notes:
Regularity:		QRS width:	
P waves: Morphology: Axis:		Grouping:	
		Dropped beats:	
P:QRS ratio:		Rhythm:	

Final Test ECG 55

II

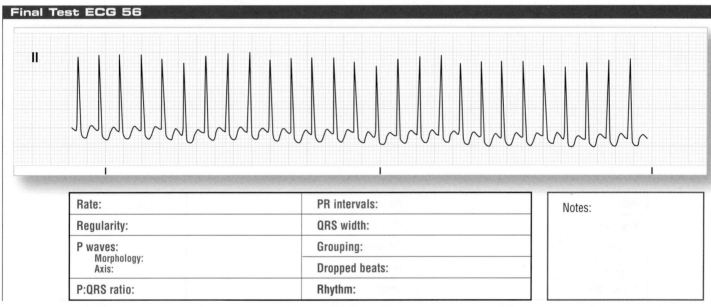

Rate:	PR intervals:	Notes:
Regularity:	QRS width:	
P waves:	Grouping:	
Morphology: Axis:	Dropped beats:	
P:QRS ratio:	Rhythm:	

Final Test ECG 56

II

Rate:	PR intervals:	Notes:
Regularity:	QRS width:	
P waves:	Grouping:	
Morphology: Axis:	Dropped beats:	
P:QRS ratio:	Rhythm:	

Final Test ECG 57

II

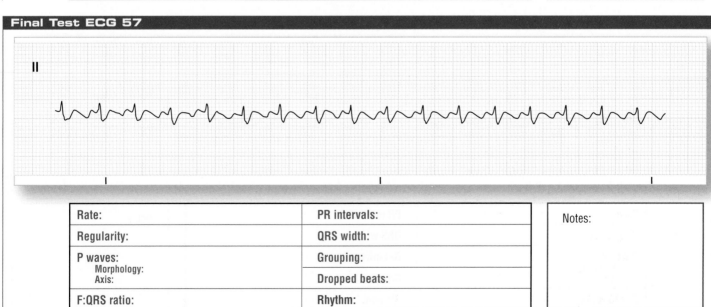

Rate:	PR intervals:	Notes:
Regularity:	QRS width:	
P waves:	Grouping:	
Morphology: Axis:	Dropped beats:	
F:QRS ratio:	Rhythm:	

Final Test ECG 58

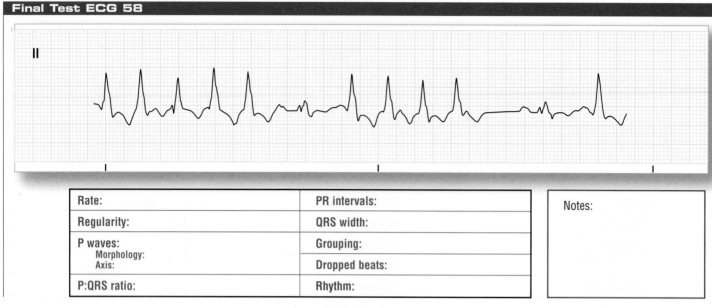

Rate:		PR intervals:		Notes:
Regularity:		QRS width:		
P waves:		Grouping:		
Morphology:				
Axis:		Dropped beats:		
P:QRS ratio:		Rhythm:		

Final Test ECG 59

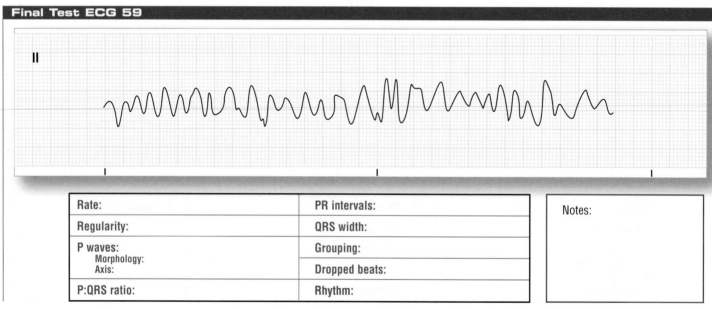

Rate:		PR intervals:		Notes:
Regularity:		QRS width:		
P waves:		Grouping:		
Morphology:				
Axis:		Dropped beats:		
P:QRS ratio:		Rhythm:		

Final Test ECG 60

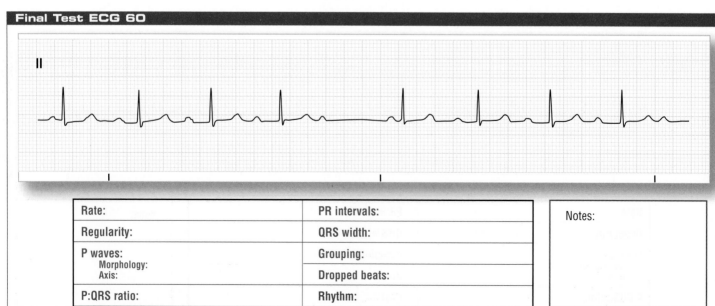

Rate:		PR intervals:		Notes:
Regularity:		QRS width:		
P waves:		Grouping:		
Morphology:				
Axis:		Dropped beats:		
P:QRS ratio:		Rhythm:		

Final Test ECG 61

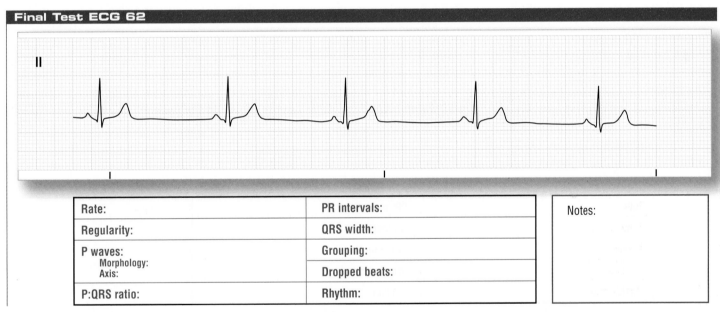

Rate:		PR intervals:		Notes:
Regularity:		QRS width:		
P waves: Morphology: Axis:		Grouping:		
		Dropped beats:		
P:QRS ratio:		Rhythm:		

Final Test ECG 62

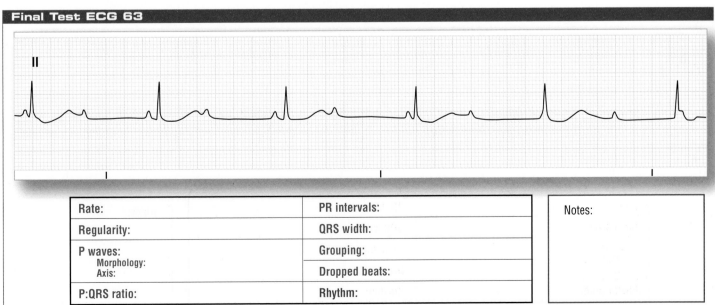

Rate:		PR intervals:		Notes:
Regularity:		QRS width:		
P waves: Morphology: Axis:		Grouping:		
		Dropped beats:		
P:QRS ratio:		Rhythm:		

Final Test ECG 63

Rate:		PR intervals:		Notes:
Regularity:		QRS width:		
P waves: Morphology: Axis:		Grouping:		
		Dropped beats:		
P:QRS ratio:		Rhythm:		

Final Test ECG 64

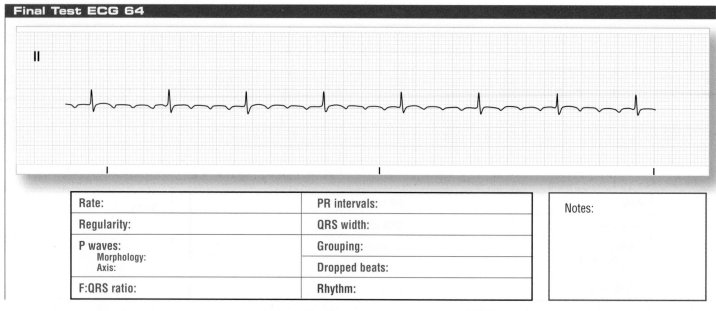

Rate:	PR intervals:	Notes:
Regularity:	QRS width:	

P waves:
    Morphology:
    Axis:
	Grouping:	

	Dropped beats:	
F:QRS ratio:	Rhythm:	

Final Test ECG 65

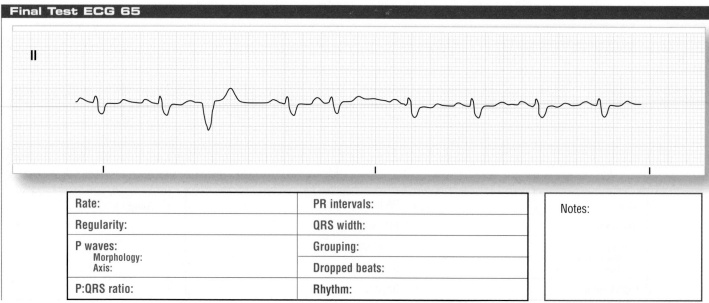

Rate:	PR intervals:	Notes:
Regularity:	QRS width:	

P waves:
    Morphology:
    Axis:
	Grouping:	

	Dropped beats:	
P:QRS ratio:	Rhythm:	

Final Test ECG 66

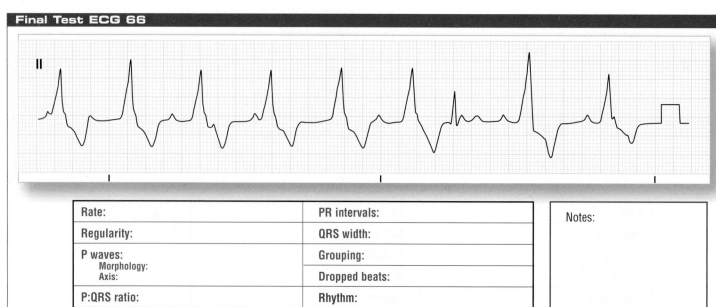

Rate:	PR intervals:	Notes:
Regularity:	QRS width:	

P waves:
    Morphology:
    Axis:
	Grouping:	

	Dropped beats:	
P:QRS ratio:	Rhythm:	

Final Test ECG 67

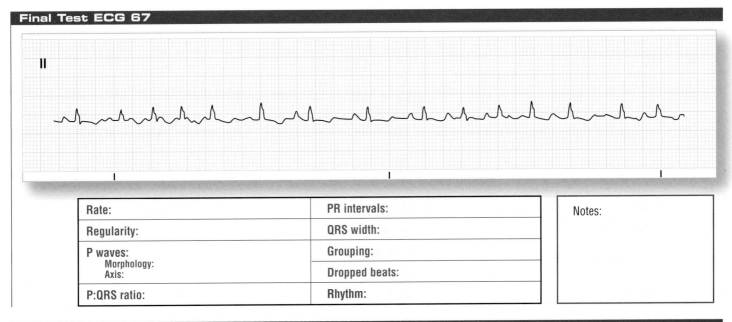

Rate:	PR intervals:	Notes:
Regularity:	QRS width:	
P waves:	Grouping:	
Morphology:	Dropped beats:	
Axis:		
P:QRS ratio:	Rhythm:	

Final Test ECG 68

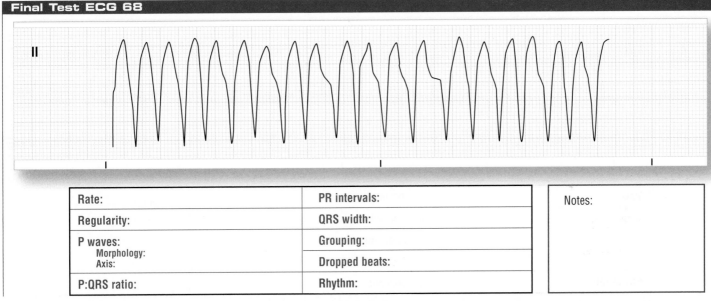

Rate:	PR intervals:	Notes:
Regularity:	QRS width:	
P waves:	Grouping:	
Morphology:	Dropped beats:	
Axis:		
P:QRS ratio:	Rhythm:	

Final Test ECG 69

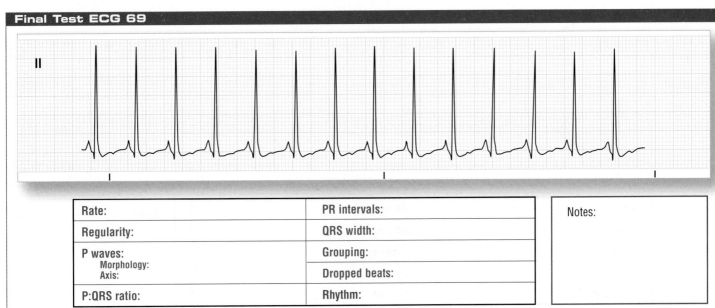

Rate:	PR intervals:	Notes:
Regularity:	QRS width:	
P waves:	Grouping:	
Morphology:	Dropped beats:	
Axis:		
P:QRS ratio:	Rhythm:	

Final Test ECG 70

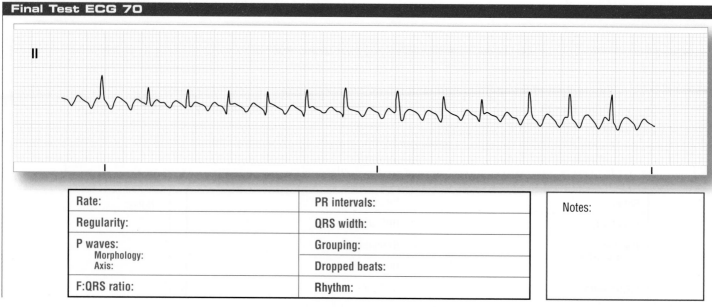

Rate:		PR intervals:	Notes:
Regularity:		QRS width:	
P waves:		Grouping:	
	Morphology:		
	Axis:	Dropped beats:	
F:QRS ratio:		Rhythm:	

Final Test ECG 71

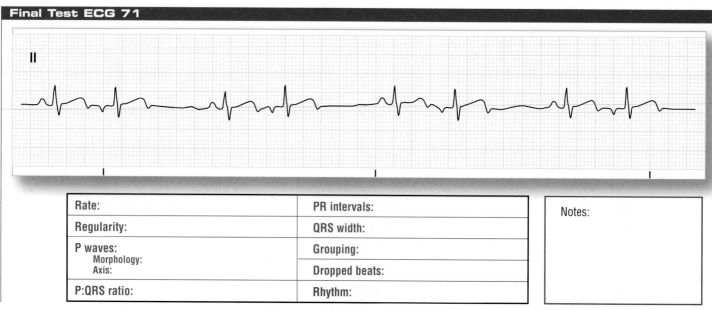

Rate:		PR intervals:	Notes:
Regularity:		QRS width:	
P waves:		Grouping:	
	Morphology:		
	Axis:	Dropped beats:	
P:QRS ratio:		Rhythm:	

Final Test ECG 72

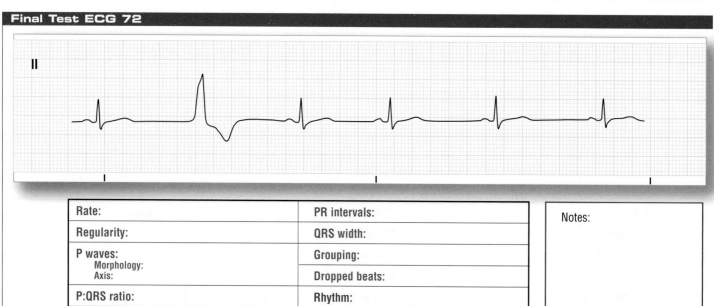

Rate:		PR intervals:	Notes:
Regularity:		QRS width:	
P waves:		Grouping:	
	Morphology:		
	Axis:	Dropped beats:	
P:QRS ratio:		Rhythm:	

Final Test ECG 73

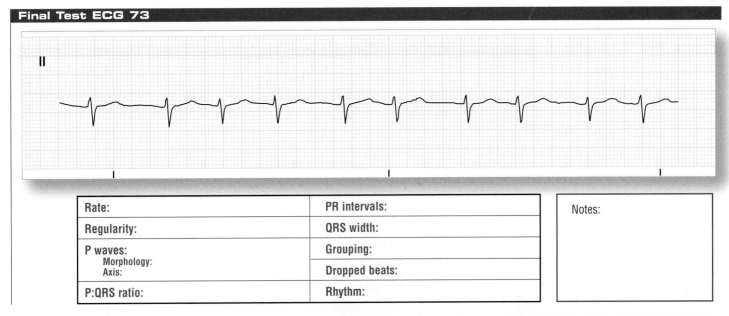

Rate:		PR intervals:	
Regularity:		QRS width:	

P waves:
  Morphology:
  Axis:
		Grouping:	

		Dropped beats:	
P:QRS ratio:		Rhythm:	

Notes:

Final Test ECG 74

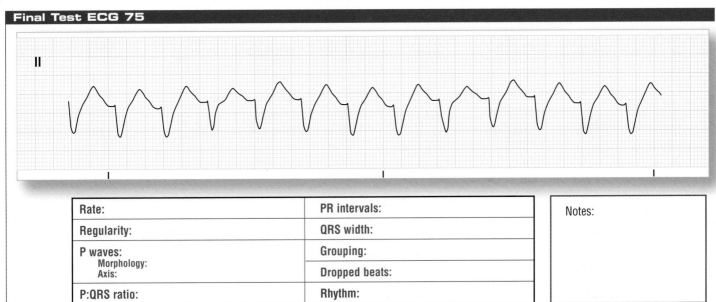

Rate:		PR intervals:	
Regularity:		QRS width:	

P waves:
  Morphology:
  Axis:
		Grouping:	

		Dropped beats:	
P:QRS ratio:		Rhythm:	

Notes:

Final Test ECG 75

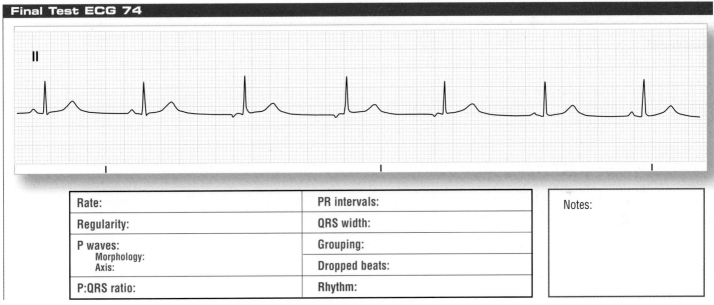

Rate:		PR intervals:	
Regularity:		QRS width:	

P waves:
  Morphology:
  Axis:
		Grouping:	

		Dropped beats:	
P:QRS ratio:		Rhythm:	

Notes:

Final Test Answers

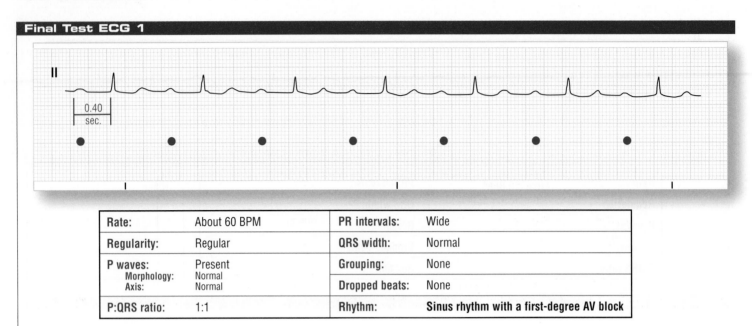

Rate:	About 60 BPM	PR intervals:	Wide
Regularity:	Regular	QRS width:	Normal

P waves:
  Morphology:
  Axis:
	Present
	Normal
	Normal
		Grouping:	None

		Dropped beats:	None
P:QRS ratio:	1:1	Rhythm:	**Sinus rhythm with a first-degree AV block**

Discussion:

The most important thing to do when approaching Final Test ECG 1 is to clearly identify which are the P waves and which are the T waves because of their similar morphologies (P waves are labeled with the blue dots). This is not that difficult to do on this ECG, but if you were to have this problem in another strip, you could examine the morphologies in some different leads. The P waves are associated with very prolonged, consistent PR intervals at 0.40 seconds, making this is a first-degree AV block in a patient with an underlying sinus rhythm.

Since the P wave and T wave morphologies are so similar, mistaking them for each other could confuse some of you into thinking that there was a third P wave buried inside the QRS complex. The rhythm would then be an atrial tachycardia with block. This is a good thought, but it is not the case. If this were the case, the timing of the P wave would be such that you would see the beginning of the buried P wave appear as a slurring or slow upstroke of the R wave. In our strip, the R wave begins with a sharp take-off and there is no evidence of any buried P wave.

Final Test ECG 2

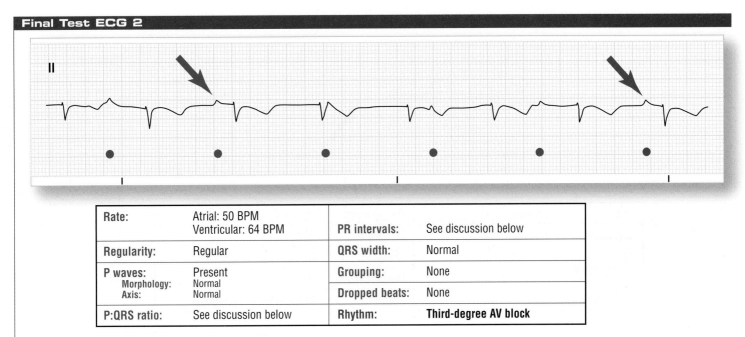

Rate:	Atrial: 50 BPM Ventricular: 64 BPM	PR intervals:	See discussion below
Regularity:	Regular	QRS width:	Normal
P waves: Morphology: Axis:	Present Normal Normal	Grouping:	None
		Dropped beats:	None
P:QRS ratio:	See discussion below	Rhythm:	**Third-degree AV block**

Discussion:

We can only see two P waves before any of the QRS complexes and they each are associated with different PR intervals (see blue arrows). On closer examination, we see that there are some morphological changes in the QRS complexes that recur at regular intervals and are consistent with buried P waves (atrial rate of 50 BPM; see blue dots). The P waves are upright in lead II but they are completely dissociated from the QRS complexes. The lack of associated P waves and the narrow, regular ventricular response at a rate of about 64 BPM are consistent with an accelerated junctional ventricular response. Putting this all together, we have a complete or third-degree AV block with an underlying sinus bradycardia and an accelerated junctional escape rhythm.

Final Test ECG 3

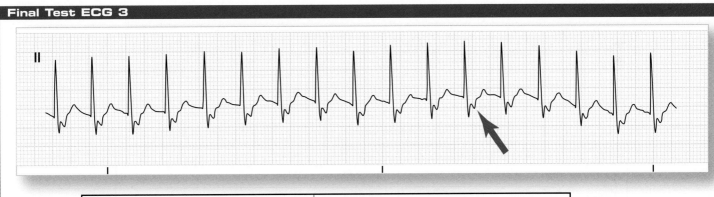

Rate:	About 150 BPM	PR intervals:	Not applicable
Regularity:	Regular	QRS width:	Normal
P waves: Morphology: Axis:	Present Inverted Not applicable	Grouping:	None
		Dropped beats:	None
P:QRS ratio:	1:1	Rhythm:	**AVRT**

Discussion:

The first thing to ask yourself when you see a rate of about 150 BPM is: Could this be atrial flutter? In this case, the answer is no because there are neither flutter waves nor evidence of at least a 2:1 conduction ratio. The QRS complexes are narrow and very regular. There is an inverted area (see blue arrow) which is probably an inverted, retrograde P wave. There is a slightly prolonged R-P interval, suggesting the presence of an orthodromic reentry cycle and, therefore, AVRT. Clinical correlation with the patient, a full 12-lead ECG, and comparison with the morphology of the complexes seen in an old ECG would be needed to completely confirm your suspicions based on this one strip.

Final Test ECG 4

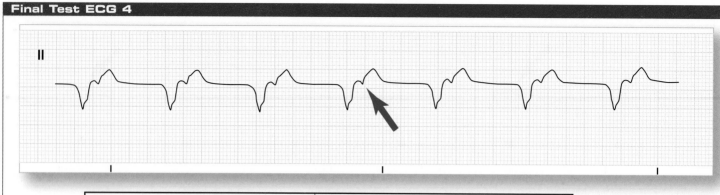

Rate:	About 61 BPM	PR intervals:	Not applicable
Regularity:	Regular	QRS width:	Wide
P waves: Morphology: Axis:	Present Inverted Not applicable	Grouping:	None
		Dropped beats:	None
P:QRS ratio:	1:1	Rhythm:	**Accelerated idioventricular**

Discussion:

Final Test ECG 4 shows a wide-complex rhythm with a morphology consistent with a ventricular origin. The rate is about 61 BPM, which is a little fast for a typical ventricular rhythm but is consistent with an accelerated idioventricular rhythm. The blue arrow is pointing to an inverted, retrogradely conducted P wave on the ST segment. Notice the presence of a long R-P interval, which would be expected because of the long transit times needed by the depolarization wave to travel from the ectopic ventricular site of origin to the atria.

Final Test ECG 5

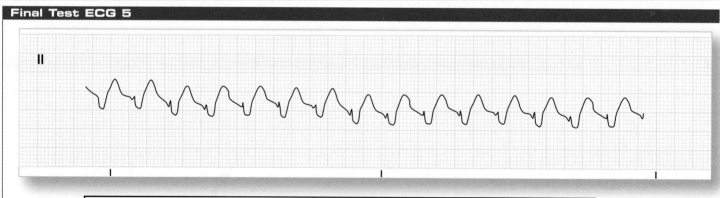

Rate:	About 150 BPM	PR intervals:	None
Regularity:	Regular	QRS width:	Wide
P waves: Morphology: Axis:	None None None	Grouping:	None
		Dropped beats:	None
P:QRS ratio:	None	Rhythm:	**Monomorphic ventricular tachycardia**

Discussion:

Final Test ECG 5 is a tough one. This is a wide-complex tachycardia at a rate of about 150 BPM. This could represent a ventricular tachycardia, an atrial flutter, an AVNRT, or an AVRT. It is almost impossible based on this strip to rule out any of these possibilities. Because of that reason, you should treat the patient as if she were in VTach. If she is unstable, shock her. If not, obtaining a full 12-lead ECG or looking at multiple leads would be extremely helpful. A full 12-lead ECG verified the diagnosis as VTach.

Remember, lead II can be quite deceptive in many patients because the QRS complexes tend to be small in that lead. A monomorphic VTach will, therefore, have small QRS complexes in those patients. As in this case, differentiation between the rhythm possibilities can be made even more difficult when there is no AV dissociation present. You need to always have a high index of suspicion when you approach any wide-complex tachycardia and assume the worst.

Final Test ECG 6

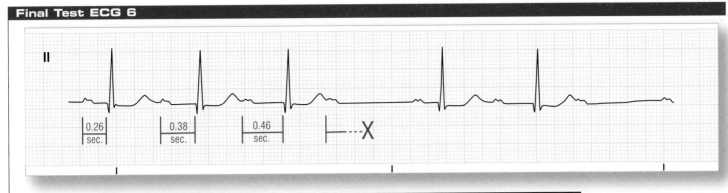

Rate:	About 55 BPM	PR intervals:	See discussion below
Regularity:	Regularly irregular	QRS width:	Normal
P waves: Morphology: Axis:	Present Normal Normal	Grouping:	Yes
		Dropped beats:	Yes
P:QRS ratio:	See discussion below	Rhythm:	**Mobitz I second-degree AV block**

Discussion:

Final Test ECG 6 definitely shows some grouping of the complexes. This should immediately make you think of the AV blocks. It doesn't matter that the first group has a 4:3 conduction ratio and the second group has only a 3:2 conduction ratio. They are still grouped and variability in the conduction ratios is normal in AV blocks. Now, take a look at the P waves. Notice that all of the P waves have the same morphology, but their associated PR intervals are different. The PR intervals appear to lengthen until one of the P waves is eventually blocked from conducting. This is the hallmark of a Mobitz I second-degree AV block. The R-R intervals remain the same, which is atypical for a Wenckebach rhythm.

Final Test ECG 7

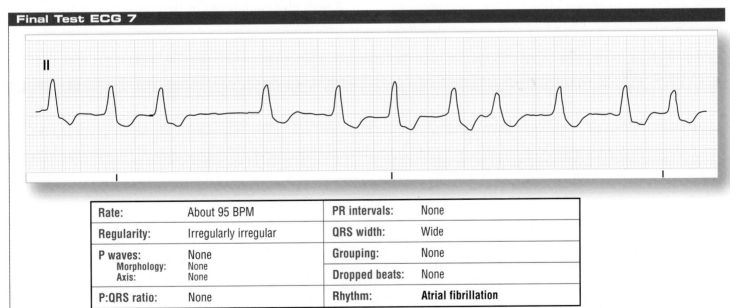

Rate:	About 95 BPM	PR intervals:	None
Regularity:	Irregularly irregular	QRS width:	Wide
P waves: Morphology: Axis:	None None None	Grouping:	None
		Dropped beats:	None
P:QRS ratio:	None	Rhythm:	**Atrial fibrillation**

Discussion:

Final Test ECG 7 shows a wide-complex, irregularly irregular rhythm. The key words in that statement are irregularly irregular. There are three main irregularly irregular rhythms: atrial fibrillation, wandering atrial pacemaker, and multifocal atrial tachycardia. There are no obvious P waves visible on the strip, so WAP and MAT are immediately ruled out from your differential. This leaves you with atrial fibrillation. Could atrial fibrillation have wide complexes? Yes, if there were a pre-existing bundle branch block, if there is aberrancy involved, or if there were significant electrolyte problems. Comparison with an old ECG showed that this patient had a pre-existing left bundle branch block accounting for the wide complexes. Remember, monomorphic VTach is regular except for a few seconds at the onset of the strip or in the presence of fusion and capture beats.

Final Test ECG 8

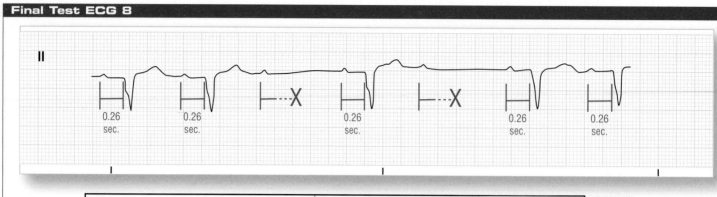

Rate:	About 50 BPM	PR intervals:	Prolonged
Regularity:	Regularly irregular	QRS width:	Normal
P waves: Morphology: Axis:	Present Normal Normal	Grouping:	Yes
		Dropped beats:	Yes
P:QRS ratio:	1:1	Rhythm:	**Mobitz II, second-degree AV block**

Discussion:

Final Test ECG 8 can be quite deceptive. At first glance the QRS complexes appear wide, but close measurement shows that they are within the normal range. Next, there is grouping with two dropped beats. The grouping makes you think of an AV block, and you would be correct. But, which one? On gross examination, the PR intervals appear to be progressively widening, but this is an optical illusion. Close measurement shows that all of the PR intervals are the same at 0.26 seconds. The optical illusion is caused by the slight fluctuations in the morphologies of the P and the QRS waves that are normally seen in almost every patient. This rhythm strip is just one of the reasons why we always suggest that you first form a quick original impression, but then use a set of ECG calipers and closely measure the intervals to verify your impressions. Rough observation can be deceptive, as it was in this case.

Final Test ECG 9

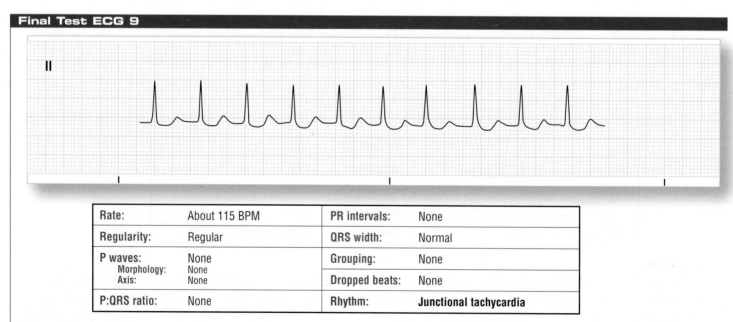

Rate:	About 115 BPM	PR intervals:	None
Regularity:	Regular	QRS width:	Normal
P waves: Morphology: Axis:	None None None	Grouping:	None
		Dropped beats:	None
P:QRS ratio:	None	Rhythm:	**Junctional tachycardia**

Discussion:

This is a regular narrow-complex tachycardia with no visible P waves at a rate of about 115 BPM. The only possible rhythm that fits these parameters is a junctional tachycardia.

Final Test ECG 10

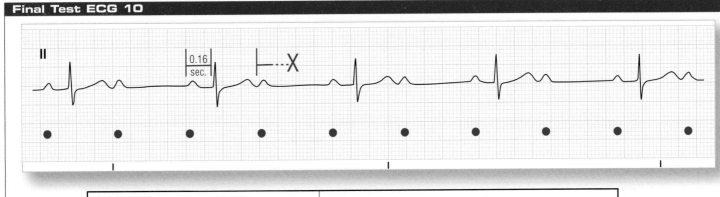

Rate:	Atrial: 76 BPM Ventricular: 38 BPM	PR intervals:	See discussion below
Regularity:	Regular	QRS width:	Normal

P waves:
  Morphology:
  Axis:
	Present
	Normal
	Normal
		Grouping:	Yes

		Dropped beats:	Yes
P:QRS ratio:	2:1	Rhythm:	**2:1 or untypable second-degree AV block**

Discussion:

This strip shows a patient who has a normally conducted P wave with a PR interval of 0.16 seconds. Then, there is another P wave that is blocked and nonconducted. Since the ratio of AV conduction is 2:1, you cannot tell which of the two kinds of type II block is involved, Mobitz I or Mobitz II. This, by definition, is an untypable or 2:1 second-degree AV block. Sometimes, longer strips in these patients will show some groupings that meet either Mobitz I or Mobitz II, allowing you to make a call as to the type involved.

Final Test ECG 11

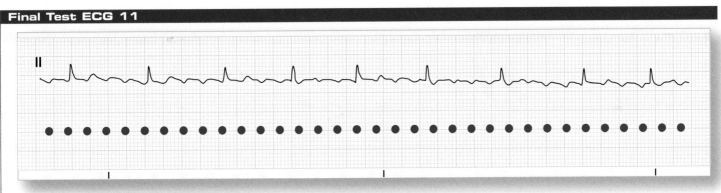

Rate:	Atrial: 300 BPM Ventricular: 70 BPM	PR intervals:	Not applicable
Regularity:	Regularly irregular	QRS width:	Normal

P waves:
  Morphology:
  Axis:
	F waves are present
	Not applicable
	Not applicable
		Grouping:	None

		Dropped beats:	None
F:QRS ratio:	Variable	Rhythm:	**Atrial flutter with variable block**

Discussion:

Final Test ECG 11 shows a rapid atrial flutter at a rate of 300 BPM. Notice the lack of any isoelectric segment between the negative deflection, which is classic for atrial flutter. The ventricular rate in atrial flutter typically occurs at some multiple of the F-F interval, for example two, three, four, and so on times the F-F interval. However, in these uncommon cases, the R-R interval is not a direct multiple but comes at variable conduction rates. This creates a regularly irregular, or even an irregularly irregular ventricular response. Atrial flutter with variable block is one of those rare exceptions to the irregularly irregular rule we are constantly bringing up. (There are three *main* irregularly irregular rhythms: Afib, WAP and MAT.)

Final Test ECG 12

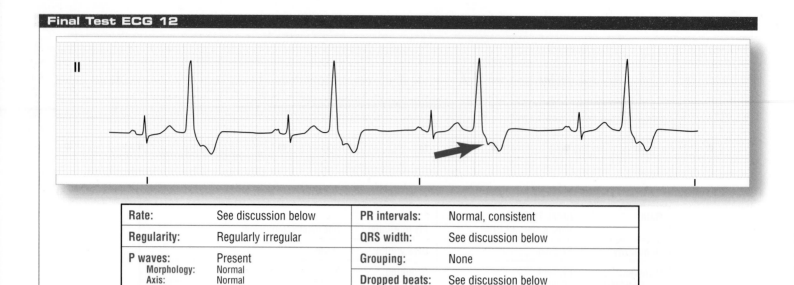

Rate:	See discussion below	PR intervals:	Normal, consistent
Regularity:	Regularly irregular	QRS width:	See discussion below

P waves:
  Morphology:
  Axis:
	Present
	Normal
	Normal
		Grouping:	None

		Dropped beats:	See discussion below
P:QRS ratio:	See discussion below	Rhythm:	**Sinus rhythm with ventricular bigeminy**

Discussion:

Final Test ECG 12 is a great example of ventricular bigeminy. There is one normally conducted beat and one PVC in a recurring pattern. The blue arrow points to an inverted, retrogradely conducted P wave, which is associated with a very prolonged R-P interval. Remember to always check the pulse on these patients. If the PVC is causing a mechanical contraction, then the overall ventricular rate is about 80 BPM (8 beats in a 6-second strip multiplied by 10 = 80 BPM). If only the normally conducted complexes cause a mechanical contraction, then the effective ventricular rate is only 40 BPM, which could be a cause of significant hemodynamic compromise.

Final Test ECG 13

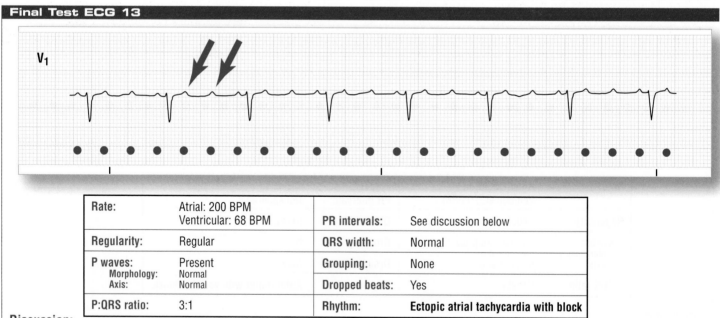

Rate:	Atrial: 200 BPM Ventricular: 68 BPM	PR intervals:	See discussion below
Regularity:	Regular	QRS width:	Normal

P waves:
  Morphology:
  Axis:
	Present
	Normal
	Normal
		Grouping:	None

		Dropped beats:	Yes
P:QRS ratio:	3:1	Rhythm:	**Ectopic atrial tachycardia with block**

Discussion:

The atrial complexes in Final Test ECG 13 are fairly normal in appearance. There is a normal isoelectric segment between the P waves, so atrial flutter is not in the differential. This is an ectopic atrial tachycardia. The P waves conduct at a 3:1 ratio and the PR interval before the conducted beat is normal. The ventricular rate is about 68 BPM and the QRS complexes are narrow, which is consistent with a supraventricular origin to the complexes. The conduction ratio and the presence of the nonconducted P waves make the final diagnosis ectopic atrial tachycardia with block.

Final Test ECG 14

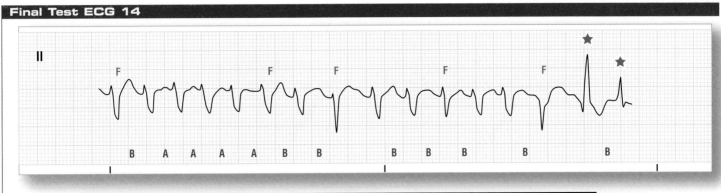

Rate:	About 160 BPM	PR intervals:	Not applicable
Regularity:	Regularly irregular	QRS width:	Wide
P waves:	None	Grouping:	None
Morphology:	None		
Axis:	None	Dropped beats:	None
P:QRS ratio:	Not applicable	Rhythm:	**Monomorphic ventricular tachycardia**

Discussion:

Final Test ECG 14 is one of the toughest in this book. To begin with, you have a wide-complex tachycardia at about 160 BPM. The rhythm is regularly irregular rather than irregularly irregular because there are recurrent R-R intervals. The presence of this many recurrent R-R intervals essentially rules out atrial fibrillation as a possible cause. Ventricular tachycardia, however, is a big possibility. There are some morphological changes in the appearance of the complexes due to fusion. (Fusion beats typically appear different from each other depending on the level of fusion between the normally conducted complex and the ventricular ectopic complex.)

Could the fusion complexes account for the slight variations in regularity noted in the strip? Yes.

The two complexes at the end, labeled with the red stars, represent the last conundrum that we will need to address. The axis of the ventricular complexes seemed to have shifted. Morphologic shifts in appearance from LBBBs to RBBBs and axis shifts can be seen in ventricular tachycardia, although they are uncommon occurrences. This is an example of a monomorphic ventricular tachycardia. A full 12-lead ECG verified the diagnosis in this patient.

Final Test ECG 15

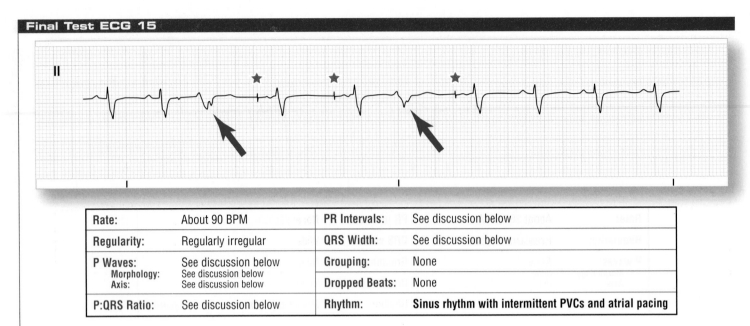

Rate:	About 90 BPM	PR Intervals:	See discussion below
Regularity:	Regularly irregular	QRS Width:	See discussion below
P Waves:	See discussion below	Grouping:	None
Morphology:	See discussion below		
Axis:	See discussion below	Dropped Beats:	None
P:QRS Ratio:	See discussion below	Rhythm:	**Sinus rhythm with intermittent PVCs and atrial pacing**

Discussion:

Final Test ECG 15 is an example of a sinus rhythm that is complicated by some events. Two of those events (labeled with the blue arrows) are either PVCs or aberrantly conducted PJCs. It is impossible to determine if the pauses involved are compensatory or noncompensatory because the pauses are cut short by an atrial pacer spike (see red stars). That thin line under the red stars represents a pacemaker spike that is triggering an atrial depolarization. The atrial depolarization is then normally conducted to the ventricles, causing normal-looking, narrow QRS complexes. The type of pacemaker involved is not evident from this short strip but we do know that it senses the ventricles and paces the atria. The pacer does appears to be functioning normally.

Final Test ECG 16

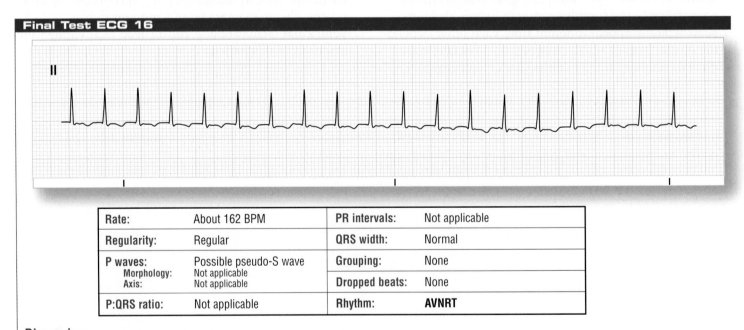

Rate:	About 162 BPM	PR intervals:	Not applicable
Regularity:	Regular	QRS width:	Normal
P waves:	Possible pseudo-S wave	Grouping:	None
Morphology:	Not applicable		
Axis:	Not applicable	Dropped beats:	None
P:QRS ratio:	Not applicable	Rhythm:	**AVNRT**

Discussion:

Final Test 16 shows a rapid narrow-complex tachycardia at about 162 BPM. There is a small deflection at the end of the QRS complex, which could be a part of the patient's normally occurring QRS morphology or could represent a pseudo-S wave. Comparison with old strips or a reevaluation of the area after the tachycardia is broken will answer the question. This patient was having an episode of AVNRT at the time this strip was taken and the pseudo-S wave disappeared when the tachycardia was broken.

Final Test ECG 17

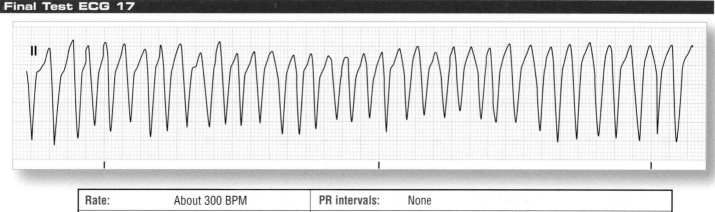

Rate:	About 300 BPM	PR intervals:	None
Regularity:	Irregularly irregular	QRS width:	Wide
P waves: Morphology: Axis:	None None None	Grouping:	None
		Dropped beats:	None
P:QRS ratio:	None	Rhythm:	**Atrial fibrillation in a patient with Wolff-Parkinson-White**

Discussion:

Final Test ECG 17 brings up a commonly misdiagnosed rhythm. The initial impression of most clinicians when they look at this strip is that it is ventricular tachycardia or ventricular flutter. However, the rhythm is too irregular and too rapid to be either of these two possibilities. This rhythm is irregularly irregular even though the amount of variability between the complexes is very small. Normally, these small changes could be written off as being trivial but when the rate is this rapid, these very small distances represent a great overall change in these small R-R intervals. In other words, the smaller the R-R interval, the greater the chance that even a small variability in the interval is significant. A difference of even 0.04 seconds or less can be very significant at rates of 300 BPM.

Now, let's discuss some issues about the rate itself. As the rate increases over 250 BPM for *any* rhythm, the chances that the complexes are being conducted through an accessory pathway increase. (Any rates over 200 BPM in atrial fibrillation should raise the same suspicion.) Normally, the AV node would never allow these rapid rates to be conducted but would interject some sort of AV block to slow the ventricles down. The rapid rates have to be going through some other pathway that does not have an intrinsic physiologic block. That other pathway is typically an accessory pathway. Rates over 250 BPM have been associated with the presence of an accessory pathway in about 85% of the cases. At rates of about 300 BPM, the chances of conduction through an accessory pathway are around 97%. To put this all together, Final Test ECG 17 is an example of a very rapid atrial fibrillation being conducted through an accessory pathway at a rate of 300 BPM.

Final Test ECG 18

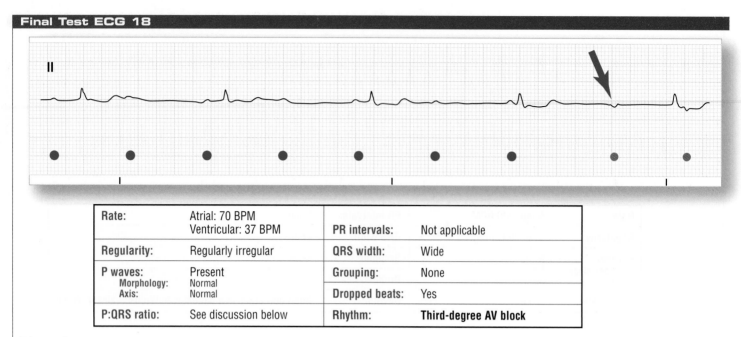

Rate:	Atrial: 70 BPM Ventricular: 37 BPM	PR intervals:	Not applicable
Regularity:	Regularly irregular	QRS width:	Wide
P waves: Morphology: Axis:	Present Normal Normal	Grouping:	None
		Dropped beats:	Yes
P:QRS ratio:	See discussion below	Rhythm:	**Third-degree AV block**

Discussion:

This strip shows a PR interval that is progressively getting shorter in front of each QRS complex. Wenckebach has progressively *widening* PR intervals, so that is not the answer. If you notice, there is another small positive deflection between the QRS complexes. Using your calipers, you see that these small deflections map out to be P waves. In addition, the P waves have no correlation or influence whatsoever over the QRS complexes. The QRS complexes are wider than 0.12 seconds and very slow, at about 37 BPM. This is an example of a third-degree AV block with both an underlying sinus rhythm controlling the atria and a ventricular escape rhythm controlling the ventricles.

The blue arrow represents a change in the morphology, and timing, of the P waves after this point. This morphological and timing shift is due to another ectopic atrial pacemaker picking up the pacemaking function of the atria due to its faster intrinsic rate. This new and faster rate is represented by the red dots at the bottom of the strip.

Final Test ECG 19

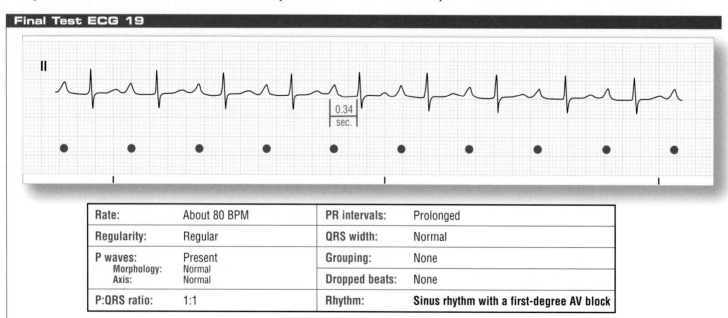

Rate:	About 80 BPM	PR intervals:	Prolonged
Regularity:	Regular	QRS width:	Normal
P waves: Morphology: Axis:	Present Normal Normal	Grouping:	None
		Dropped beats:	None
P:QRS ratio:	1:1	Rhythm:	**Sinus rhythm with a first-degree AV block**

Discussion:

Final Test ECG 19 shows a sinus rhythm with an obvious P wave occurring before each QRS complex. The P waves are tall, but otherwise normal, and the waves are positive in lead II. The PR intervals are constant but very prolonged at 0.34 seconds. Final diagnosis: Sinus rhythm with a first-degree AV block.

Final Test ECG 20

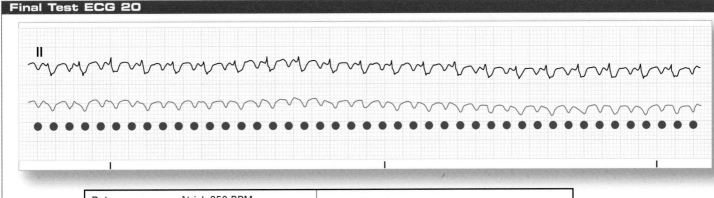

Rate:	Atrial: 350 BPM Ventricular: 135 BPM	PR intervals:	None
Regularity:	Regular	QRS width:	See discussion below

P waves:
    Morphology:
    Axis:
	None, F waves are present
	None
	None
		Grouping:	None

		Dropped beats:	None
F:QRS ratio:	2:1	Rhythm:	**Atrial flutter**

Discussion:

Final Test ECG 20 above shows a rapid tachycardia with a ventricular response of 135 BPM. We have taken the liberty of graphically removing the QRS complexes from the strip, so that you can clearly see the underlying the saw-tooth pattern of the F or flutter waves (see pink strip). You should get into the habit of mentally "cleaning up" the strip whenever atrial flutter is suspected. It is a mental exercise that is easy to do, and you will be able to continuously do it during your clinical career.

Are the QRS complexes wide or narrow? It is really difficult to tell on this strip. Because the F:QRS ratio is 2:1, there is a fusion between the F waves from the atrial flutter and the small voltage QRS complexes, giving the appearance of deep and wide slurred S waves. Additional leads or a full 12-lead ECG will help you answer the question about the width of the ventricular complexes. These QRS complexes were indeed narrow in the other leads.

Final Test ECG 21

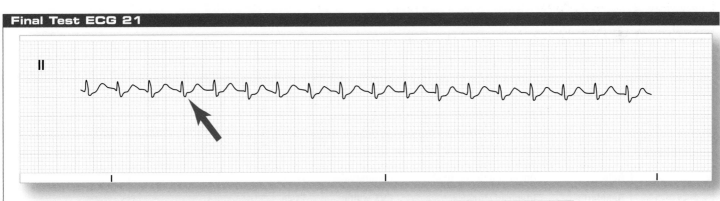

Rate:	About 175 BPM	PR intervals:	Small R-P interval
Regularity:	Regular	QRS width:	Normal

P waves:
    Morphology:
    Axis:
	Pseudo-S wave present
	Not applicable
	Not applicable
		Grouping:	None

		Dropped beats:	None
P:QRS ratio:	1:1	Rhythm:	**AVNRT**

Discussion:

The presence of a rapid narrow-complex tachycardia with obvious pseudo-S waves in lead II should make you immediately think of AVNRT. Remember, both the pseudo-S and the pseudo-R' waves are caused by the retrograde P wave occurring almost immediately after the QRS complex. (Pseudo-R' waves would be visible in lead V_1.)

Final Test ECG 22

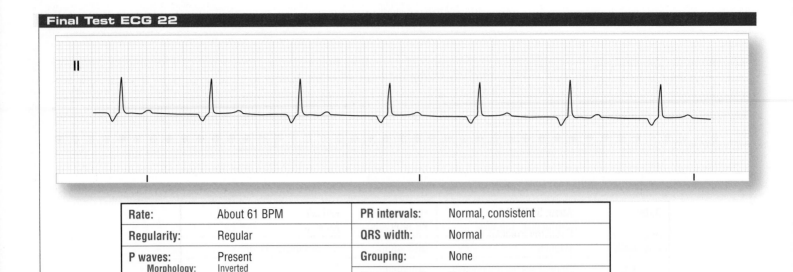

Rate:	About 61 BPM	PR intervals:	Normal, consistent
Regularity:	Regular	QRS width:	Normal

P waves:
   Morphology:
   Axis:
	Present
	Inverted
	Abnormal
		Grouping:	None

		Dropped beats:	None
P:QRS ratio:	1:1	Rhythm:	**Ectopic atrial rhythm**

Discussion:

Final Test ECG 22 shows inverted P waves with normal PR intervals right before each QRS complex. In general, inverted P waves can be due to either ectopic atrial pacemakers from the lower part of the right atria or junctional pacemakers. Recall that the deciding factor between choosing from these two possibilities was the width of the PR interval. Normal or prolonged PR inter-vals are associated with ectopic atrial pacemakers. Short PR intervals are associated with junctional pacemakers. Since our patient has normal PR intervals, the rhythm is consistent with an ectopic atrial rhythm. The overall rate of the rhythm is 61 BPM, which makes the final diagnosis an ectopic atrial rhythm.

Final Test ECG 23

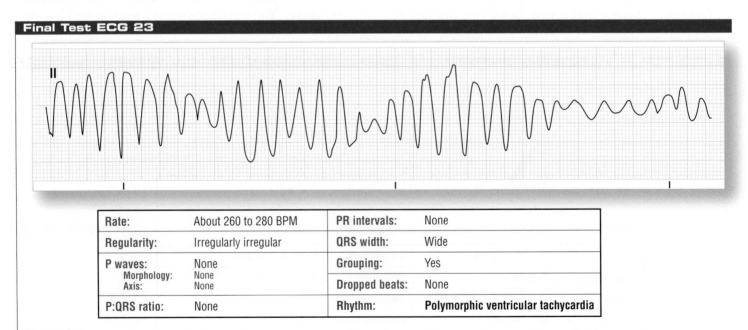

Rate:	About 260 to 280 BPM	PR intervals:	None
Regularity:	Irregularly irregular	QRS width:	Wide

P waves:
   Morphology:
   Axis:
	None
	None
	None
		Grouping:	Yes

		Dropped beats:	None
P:QRS ratio:	None	Rhythm:	**Polymorphic ventricular tachycardia**

Discussion:

This is a wide-complex tachycardia with constantly changing morphology. The rhythm is irregularly irregu-lar and has an undulating pattern with both amplitude and polarity changes. These are the classic attributes for polymorphic VTach and torsade de pointes. The final diagnosis depends on the presence of the QT interval when the patient is in sinus rhythm and/or the clinical correlation. Polymorphic VT is associated with normal QT intervals and is strongly associated with myocardial infarctions. Torsade de pointes is associated with pro-longed QT intervals and is caused by various clinical conditions (see page 416).

Final Test ECG 24

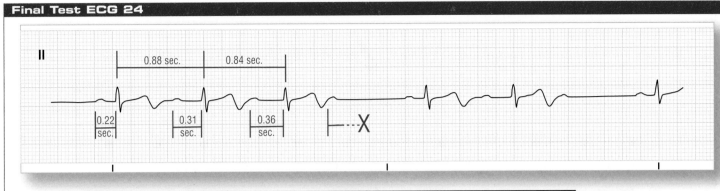

Rate:	About 50 BPM	PR intervals:	Variable
Regularity:	Regularly irregular	QRS width:	Normal
P waves:	Present	Grouping:	Yes
Morphology:	Normal		
Axis:	Normal	Dropped beats:	Yes
P:QRS ratio:	4:3 then 3:2	Rhythm:	**Mobitz I second-degree AV block**

Discussion:

Final Test ECG 24 has all of the earmarks of a Mobitz I second-degree AV block. There is a progressive lengthening of the PR interval from 0.22 seconds to 0.31 seconds to 0.36 seconds, leading up to a dropped beat. The R-R interval decreases, as would be typically expected, from 0.88 seconds to 0.84 seconds. The conduction ratio of the two visible groups varies from 4:3 for the first group, to 3:2 for the second group. Note that the shortest PR interval is borderline prolonged at 0.20 seconds. (Yes, you can have both first-degree and either second-degree AV block occurring simultaneously in the same patient.)

Final Test ECG 25

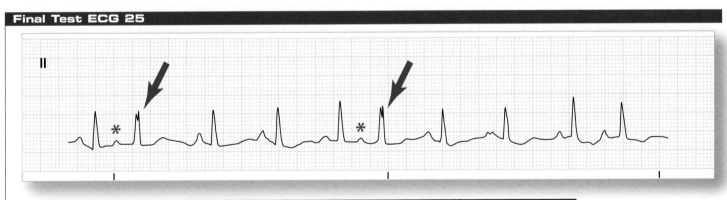

Rate:	About 100 BPM	PR intervals:	Multiple
Regularity:	Irregularly irregular	QRS width:	Normal
P waves:	Present	Grouping:	None
Morphology:	Multiple		
Axis:	Normal	Dropped beats:	None
P:QRS ratio:	1:1	Rhythm:	**Multifocal atrial tachycardia**

Discussion:

There are 10 complexes in a six-second strip. This makes the overall rate of the rhythm exactly 100 BPM. The rhythm is irregularly irregular with at least three P-wave morphologies each with a different PR interval. This is a multifocal atrial tachycardia. There are two buried P waves scattered throughout the strip (see blue asterisks). The blue arrow points to two QRS complexes that are aberrantly conducted. These two complexes are aberrantly conducted because the early occurring, buried P waves of these two complexes arrived at the right bundle branch before it was ready to receive it. This is an example of Ashman's phenomenon (a long R-R interval followed by a short R-R interval; the QRS complex at the end of the short R-R interval tends to be aberrantly conducted). Ashman's phenomenon is typically found in atrial fibrillation and MAT.

Final Test ECG 26

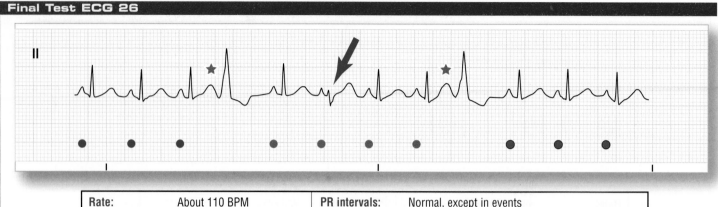

Rate:	About 110 BPM	PR intervals:	Normal, except in events
Regularity:	Regularly irregular	QRS width:	Normal, except in events
P waves: Morphology: Axis:	Present Normal Normal	Grouping:	None
		Dropped beats:	None
P:QRS ratio:	1:1	Rhythm:	**Sinus tachycardia with multiple PACs and a PJC**

Discussion:

This strip is full of small pathological events that require a keen eye and a good set of calipers. There are two obviously different complexes in the strip: the fourth and ninth complexes. Are they PVCs? The answer is no—they are aberrantly conducted PACs. Notice the morphology of the T wave immediately before those two wide QRS complexes. They are taller and wider than the others on the strip because of prematurely occurring, buried P waves. The QRS complexes of these PACs are being aberrantly conducted because the early arrival of the PAC reached a right bundle that was not ready to normally conduct them. The pauses of these two PACs are noncompensatory pauses that reset the underlying sinus rate (see red dots and green dots).

If you were really observant, you would have noticed the complex to which the blue arrow is pointing. What is that complex? It is narrow, starts off in the same direction as the normally conducted QRS complexes, and is a bit premature. This is a PJC. Notice that the PJC arrives just a tiny bit before expected and gives the illusion that it is associated with a short PR interval. Why isn't this a PAC with its own PR interval? Well, the P wave is not premature and has the same morphology as the surrounding normal P waves. Remember to always look at every part of the strip. Sometimes it is the most obscure change that provides a wealth of information.

Final Test ECG 27

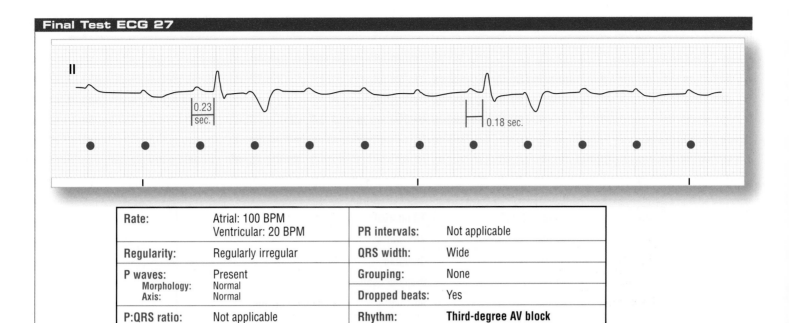

Rate:	Atrial: 100 BPM Ventricular: 20 BPM	PR intervals:	Not applicable
Regularity:	Regularly irregular	QRS width:	Wide
P waves: Morphology: Axis:	Present Normal Normal	Grouping:	None
		Dropped beats:	Yes
P:QRS ratio:	Not applicable	Rhythm:	**Third-degree AV block**

Discussion:

This strip shows an obvious AV block. The atrial rate is 100 BPM, making the atrial rhythm either a sinus tachycardia or an atrial tachycardia. The ventricular rate of 20 BPM makes the ventricular response a ventricular escape rhythm. On first glance, the PR intervals right before the ventricular complexes appear to be the same. That, however, is not the case. The first PR interval measures 0.23 seconds, while the second one measures 0.18. This is not an advanced second-degree AV block, but a complete or third-degree AV block.

Final Test ECG 28

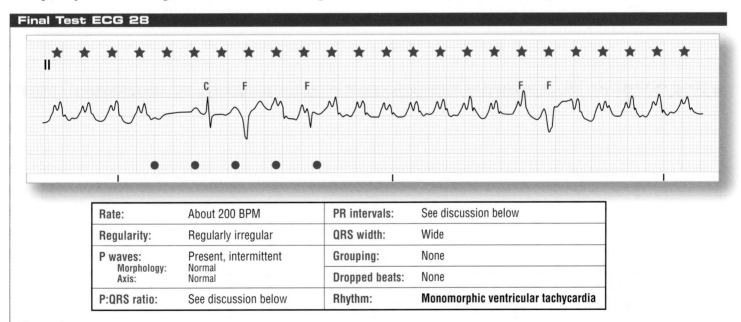

Rate:	About 200 BPM	PR intervals:	See discussion below
Regularity:	Regularly irregular	QRS width:	Wide
P waves: Morphology: Axis:	Present, intermittent Normal Normal	Grouping:	None
		Dropped beats:	None
P:QRS ratio:	See discussion below	Rhythm:	**Monomorphic ventricular tachycardia**

Discussion:

Final Test ECG 28 is a classic example of monomorphic ventricular tachycardia. First of all, it is a wide-complex tachycardia clipping along at about 200 BPM. There is one normally conducted capture beat (labeled "C") and many fusion beats (labeled "F"), which are indirect evidence of AV dissociation. The P waves map out for a short time (see blue dots), but it is impossible to map them out any further.

You have read many times during this book that monomorphic VT is a regular rhythm. At first glance, this strip appears to have its cadence or timing disrupted by the capture and fusion beats, but take a look at the blue stars above the strip. The timing of the blue stars shows that the underlying ventricular reentry loop causing the tachycardia is not interrupted by the capture or fusion beats. In other words, the cadence of the rhythm is never reset. It remains as regular as clockwork.

Final Test ECG 29

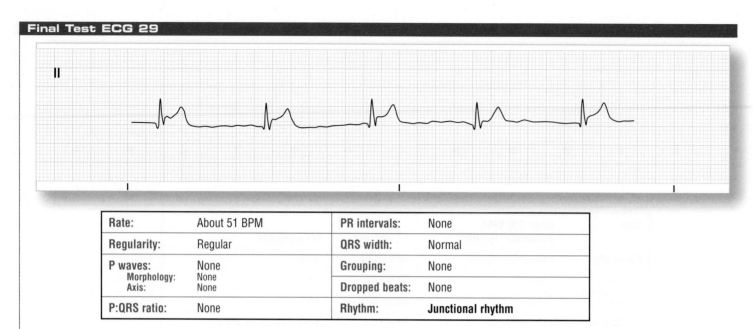

Rate:	About 51 BPM	PR intervals:	None
Regularity:	Regular	QRS width:	Normal
P waves:	None	Grouping:	None
Morphology:	None		
Axis:	None	Dropped beats:	None
P:QRS ratio:	None	Rhythm:	**Junctional rhythm**

Discussion:

This patient has a narrow-complex rhythm at a rate of 51 BPM. There are no visible P waves and the rhythm is regular. This is a junctional rhythm. Two things to mention: First of all, don't let a wavy baseline fool you into thinking that the rhythm is an atrial fibrillation. Look at the regularity of the rhythm. The only time that atrial fibrillation can be regular is if there is complete AV block with a junctional or ventricular escape. The second thing to mention is that this person appears to have some serious ST segment elevation. You should not use a rhythm strip to make any ST segment evaluations, so get a full 12-lead ECG. This person is probably having a big MI.

Final Test ECG 30

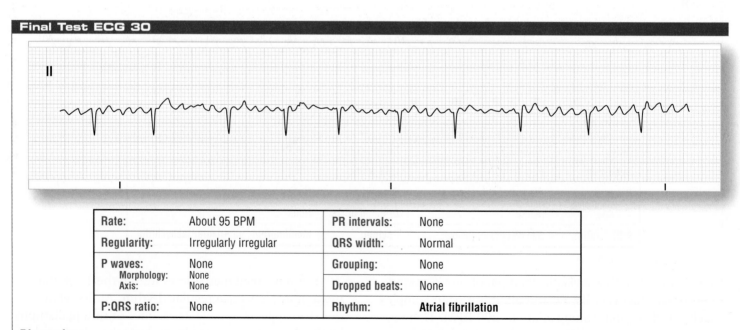

Rate:	About 95 BPM	PR intervals:	None
Regularity:	Irregularly irregular	QRS width:	Normal
P waves:	None	Grouping:	None
Morphology:	None		
Axis:	None	Dropped beats:	None
P:QRS ratio:	None	Rhythm:	**Atrial fibrillation**

Discussion:

This ECG strip shows an irregularly irregular rhythm with a very coarse baseline. This is an atrial fibrillation. It is important in these patients, however, to obtain multiple leads to make sure that P waves are not hidden by the coarseness of the baseline.

Final Test ECG 31

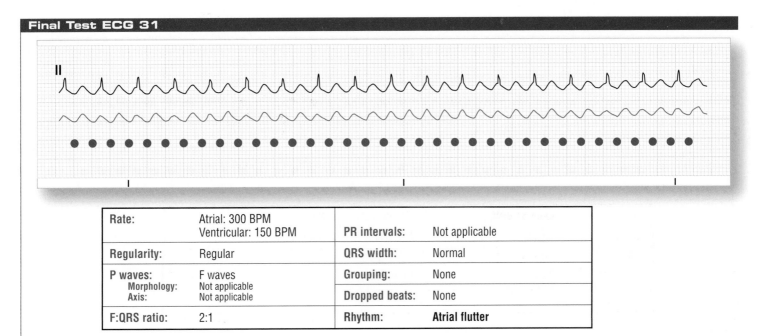

Rate:	Atrial: 300 BPM Ventricular: 150 BPM	PR intervals:	Not applicable
Regularity:	Regular	QRS width:	Normal

P waves:
  Morphology:
  Axis:
	F waves
	Not applicable
	Not applicable
		Grouping:	None

		Dropped beats:	None
F:QRS ratio:	2:1	Rhythm:	**Atrial flutter**

Discussion:

This patient has a ventricular rate of 150 BPM. This figure should trigger in your mind an instant search for the flutter waves of atrial flutter. If you remove the QRS complexes from the strip, you end up with an obvious saw-tooth pattern at a rate of 300 BPM consistent with atrial flutter (see pink strip).

Final Test ECG 32

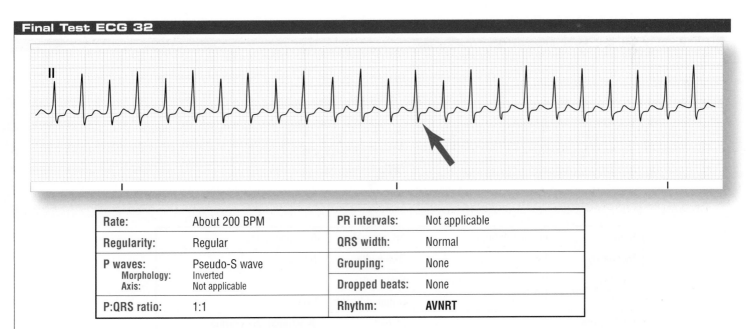

Rate:	About 200 BPM	PR intervals:	Not applicable
Regularity:	Regular	QRS width:	Normal

P waves:
  Morphology:
  Axis:
	Pseudo-S wave
	Inverted
	Not applicable
		Grouping:	None

		Dropped beats:	None
P:QRS ratio:	1:1	Rhythm:	**AVNRT**

Discussion:

This strip shows a narrow-complex tachycardia at a rate of about 200 BPM. There is a small negative deflection at the end of the QRS complexes which could represent a pseudo-S wave. The presumptive diagnosis is AVNRT.

Clinical correlation and a full 12-lead ECG during and after the tachycardia will help confirm AVNRT as the final diagnosis.

Final Test ECG 33

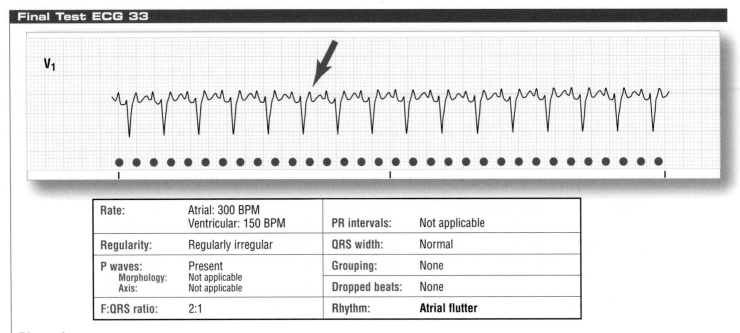

Rate:	Atrial: 300 BPM Ventricular: 150 BPM	PR intervals:	Not applicable
Regularity:	Regularly irregular	QRS width:	Normal
P waves: Morphology: Axis:	Present Not applicable Not applicable	Grouping:	None
		Dropped beats:	None
F:QRS ratio:	2:1	Rhythm:	**Atrial flutter**

Discussion:

First of all, notice that this strip was obtained from lead V_1. There is an obvious P wave before each QRS complex, but there is another one right after the QRS complex that is not so obvious (see blue arrow). The atrial rate is 300 BPM and the conduction ratio is 2:1, making the ventricular rate 150 BPM. There's that number again. . . Once again, when you see a rate of around 150 BPM, think atrial flutter. To confirm your diagnosis, you should obtain a full 12-lead ECG or multiple leads. Many times, however, you will not see anything in lead II, and the only lead where you can see any atrial activity is lead V_1. As a reminder, typically, the best lead to see atrial activity is lead V_1.

Final Test ECG 34

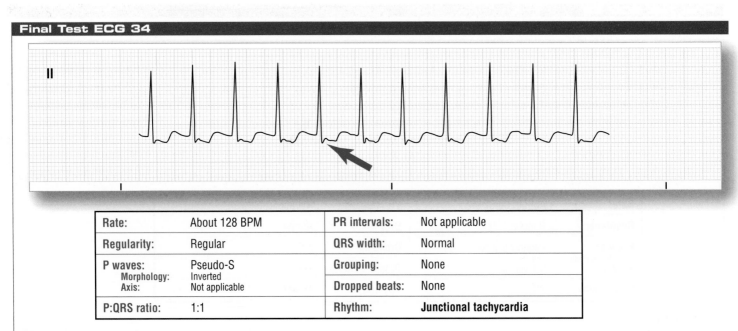

Rate:	About 128 BPM	PR intervals:	Not applicable
Regularity:	Regular	QRS width:	Normal
P waves: Morphology: Axis:	Pseudo-S Inverted Not applicable	Grouping:	None
		Dropped beats:	None
P:QRS ratio:	1:1	Rhythm:	**Junctional tachycardia**

Discussion:

This strip shows a rapid narrow-complex tachycardia with a pseudo-S wave (see blue arrow). The rate of 128 BPM is still within the range for a junctional tachycar- dia. Remember, by tradition, rates above 130 BPM are labeled AVNRT.

Final Test ECG 35

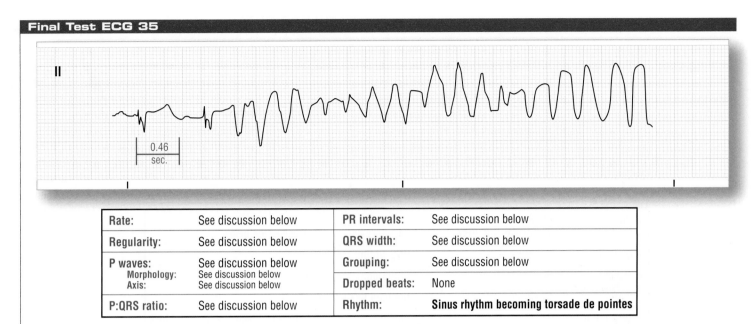

Rate:	See discussion below	PR intervals:	See discussion below
Regularity:	See discussion below	QRS width:	See discussion below
P waves:	See discussion below	Grouping:	See discussion below
Morphology:	See discussion below		
Axis:	See discussion below	Dropped beats:	None
P:QRS ratio:	See discussion below	Rhythm:	**Sinus rhythm becoming torsade de pointes**

Discussion:

The start of this strip shows a sinus rhythm with a QT interval at 0.46 seconds. The rate of the sinus rhythm is about 84 BPM, making the QT interval prolonged. The patient then has some event, most likely a PVC, which triggers off a run of torsade de pointes at a rate of between 240 and 280 BPM. The initial PVC is not clearly different morphologically from the subsequent ventricular complexes in this lead, but it did arrive during the relative refractory period of the ST-T wave area. The undulations and polarity shifts of the torsade de pointes are evident in the middle and latter parts of the strip.

Final Test ECG 36

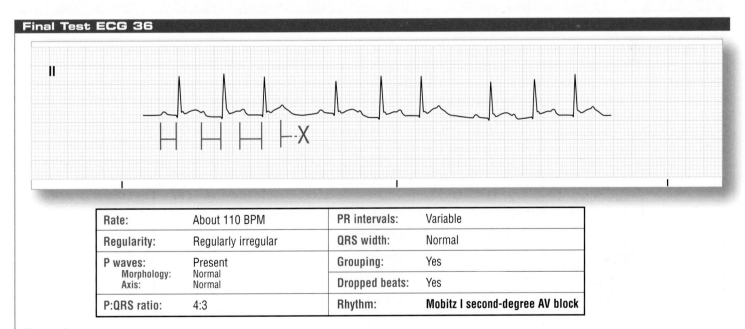

Rate:	About 110 BPM	PR intervals:	Variable
Regularity:	Regularly irregular	QRS width:	Normal
P waves:	Present	Grouping:	Yes
Morphology:	Normal		
Axis:	Normal	Dropped beats:	Yes
P:QRS ratio:	4:3	Rhythm:	**Mobitz I second-degree AV block**

Discussion:

Final Test ECG 36 shows a series of groupings that are conducted at a 4:3 ratio. The PR intervals are progressing between each complex in a group as the R-R intervals are decreasing. The final P wave in each group is not conducted. The longest PR interval in each group is the one before the dropped beat and the shortest is the one immediately after the pause. These are the hallmarks for a Wenckebach or Mobitz I second-degree AV block.

Final Test ECG 37

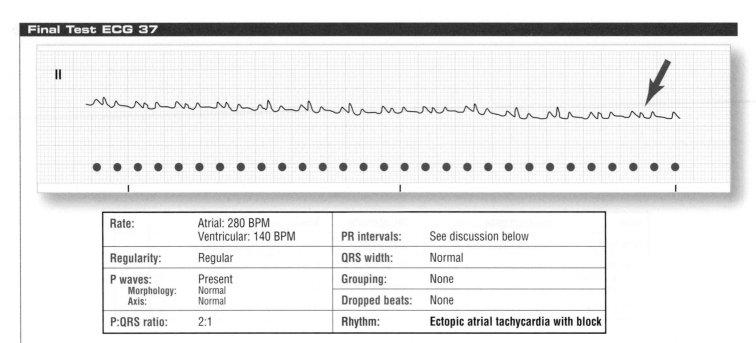

Rate:	Atrial: 280 BPM Ventricular: 140 BPM	PR intervals:	See discussion below
Regularity:	Regular	QRS width:	Normal

P waves:
   Morphology:
   Axis:
	Present
	Normal
	Normal
		Grouping:	None

		Dropped beats:	None
P:QRS ratio:	2:1	Rhythm:	**Ectopic atrial tachycardia with block**

Discussion:

This rhythm strip can be quite deceptive at first glance. The reason for this is that the height of the R waves is very short and they are almost the same size as the P waves that surround it (the blue arrow points to a low-amplitude QRS complex). There are two P waves surrounding each QRS complex, forming a nice recurring pattern of 2:1 conduction with the QRS complexes in the middle. Once again, if you can mentally remove the QRS complexes from the strip, you will notice an atrial tachycardia. But, in comparison to an atrial flutter, there is an isoelectric segment between the P waves. The presence of this isoelectric segment makes this rhythm an ectopic atrial tachycardia with block.

Final Test ECG 38

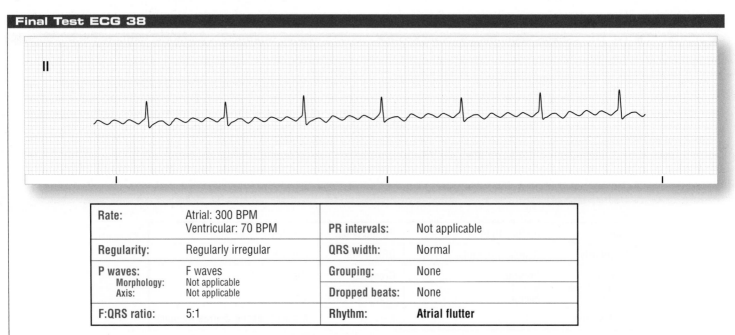

Rate:	Atrial: 300 BPM Ventricular: 70 BPM	PR intervals:	Not applicable
Regularity:	Regularly irregular	QRS width:	Normal

P waves:
   Morphology:
   Axis:
	F waves
	Not applicable
	Not applicable
		Grouping:	None

		Dropped beats:	None
F:QRS ratio:	5:1	Rhythm:	**Atrial flutter**

Discussion:

The underlying saw-tooth pattern of the F waves is evident on this strip. The conduction ratio of this rhythm is 5:1. An easy way to figure out the ratio is to count the number of negative F waves clearly visible between the QRS complexes and then add one to that figure. You add one because there is always one F wave buried within the previous QRS complex. In this example, we have four easily identifiable F waves, so there has to be one more F wave buried in the previous QRS complex, giving you a 5:1 conduction ratio.

Final Test ECG 39

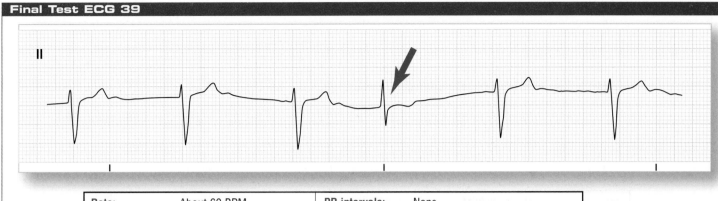

Rate:	About 60 BPM	PR intervals:	None
Regularity:	Regular with event	QRS width:	Wide
P waves: Morphology: Axis:	None None None	Grouping:	None
		Dropped beats:	None
P:QRS ratio:	None	Rhythm:	**Accelerated idioventricular rhythm**

Discussion:

Final Test ECG 39 shows a wide-complex rhythm at about 60 BPM. There are no visible P waves anywhere on the strip. The small positive deflections at the end of the T waves are U waves, not P waves. At this point, our list of possibilities includes an accelerated idioventricular rhythm or a junctional rhythm in a patient with a pre-existing bundle branch block.

The blue arrow is pointing to a QRS complex that is narrow and arrives prematurely. Could this be a PJC? Yes, it could be. But what are the chances of having a wide junctional rhythm with a pre-existing bundle branch block and then having a normally conducted, narrow PJC? Pretty slim. Which brings us to our second possibility. . . Remember when we were talking about

accelerated idioventricular rhythms back in Chapter 30? We mentioned that AV dissociation is a common finding in accelerated idioventricular. Could this narrow complex represent a capture beat? Yes, it could. This diagnosis would fit with the wide complexes, the lack of visible P waves, and the narrow QRS complex right in the middle of the strip. Not bad. . .now, how do we prove it?

Obtaining a full 12-lead ECG, and then comparing that one to an old one, would provide the proof we would need to verify our presumptive diagnosis. This information was easily obtained and the diagnosis of accelerated idioventricular rhythm was confirmed in this patient.

Final Test ECG 40

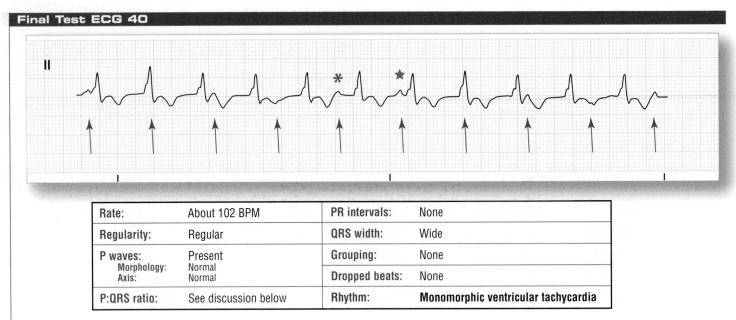

Rate:	About 102 BPM	PR intervals:	None
Regularity:	Regular	QRS width:	Wide

P waves:
  Morphology:
  Axis:
	Present
	Normal
	Normal
		Grouping:	None

		Dropped beats:	None
P:QRS ratio:	See discussion below	Rhythm:	**Monomorphic ventricular tachycardia**

Discussion:

This is a wide-complex rhythm. In addition, it has a rate of 102 BPM, making it a tachycardia. With just those two bits of information, you should be thinking VTach initially. Now, let's prove or disprove it. The first thing to look for is evidence of AV dissociation. Do you see anything that looks like a P wave? Take a look at the wave under the red star. This is an obvious P wave. Can you see any other deflections near that area that resembles another P wave? If you look at the area under the

asterisk, there appears to be another P wave peeking out after the T wave of the previous complex. Now, take your calipers and measure out that distance. Map that distance back and forth across the strip and you will notice irregularities in the strip at those exact sites (see thin blue arrows). These are buried P waves and this is direct proof of AV dissociation. This rhythm, therefore, is ventricular tachycardia.

Final Test ECG 41

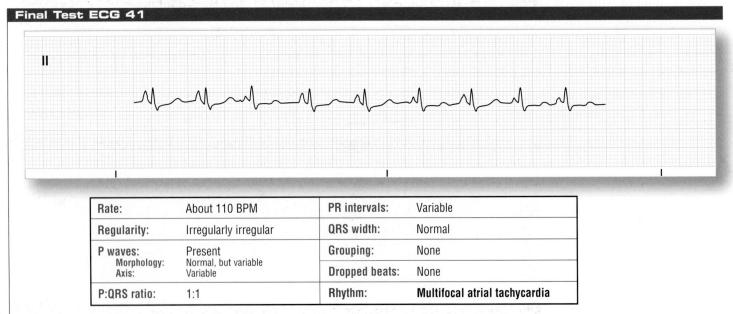

Rate:	About 110 BPM	PR intervals:	Variable
Regularity:	Irregularly irregular	QRS width:	Normal

P waves:
  Morphology:
  Axis:
	Present
	Normal, but variable
	Variable
		Grouping:	None

		Dropped beats:	None
P:QRS ratio:	1:1	Rhythm:	**Multifocal atrial tachycardia**

Discussion:

This is an irregularly irregular rhythm with P waves. There are two main possibilities for this: Multifocal atrial tachycardia and wandering atrial pacemaker. The rate on this strip is about 110 BPM, making multifocal atrial

tachycardia the most probable diagnosis. Now, to confirm our diagnosis. Are there at least three different P wave morphologies, each with their own distinctive PR interval? Yes. We have confirmed MAT as the final diagnosis.

Final Test ECG 42

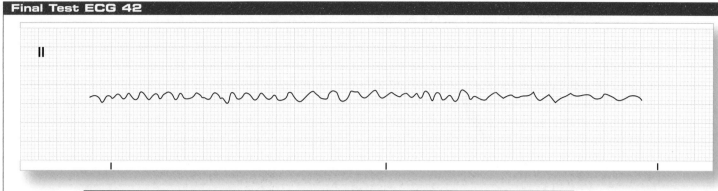

Rate:	Not applicable	PR intervals:	None
Regularity:	None	QRS width:	None

P waves:
    Morphology:
    Axis:
	None
	None
	None
		Grouping:	None

		Dropped beats:	None
P:QRS ratio:	None	Rhythm:	**Ventricular fibrillation**

Discussion:

This rhythm strip shows a completely chaotic ventricular response. This is typical of only two possibilities: Ventricular fibrillation and artifact. Take a look at the patient. If he is unconscious or unresponsive, it is Vfib. If he is talking and having a good time, it is artifact. One more important clinical point. . .make sure that you quickly change leads on the monitor anyway to make sure that artifact is not hiding some other potentially lethal arrhythmia.

Final Test ECG 43

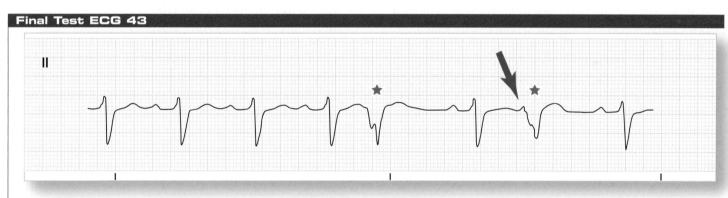

Rate:	About 74 BPM	PR intervals:	Prolonged
Regularity:	Regular with frequent events	QRS width:	Normal

P waves:
    Morphology:
    Axis:
	Present
	Normal
	Normal
		Grouping:	None

		Dropped beats:	None
P:QRS ratio:	1:1	Rhythm:	**Sinus rhythm with a first-degree AV block with frequent PVCs**

Discussion:

This strip shows a patient with an underlying sinus rhythm with a first-degree AV block due to the prolonged PR interval. The patient has two PVCs (see complexes with the red stars) that are associated with fully compensatory pauses. The blue arrow is pointing to the normally occurring P wave that was starting when the second PVC fired. The result is that the P wave was buried at the start of the PVC, thereby altering its morphology slightly. The two PVCs are probably unifocal despite the different coupling intervals (the distance from the previous complex to the start of the PVC).

Final Test ECG 44

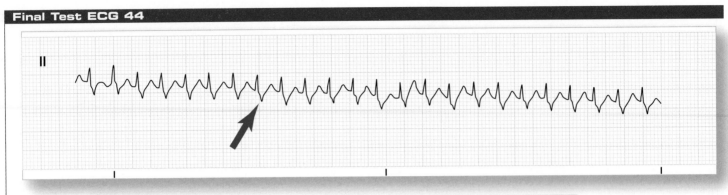

Rate:	About 215 BPM	PR intervals:	See discussion below
Regularity:	Regular	QRS width:	Wide
P waves:	See discussion below	Grouping:	None
Morphology:	See discussion below		
Axis:	See discussion below	Dropped beats:	None
P:QRS ratio:	See discussion below	Rhythm:	**AVRT**

Discussion:

Final Test ECG 44 is a diagnostic dilemma. It is a wide-complex tachycardia at about 215 BPM. The QRS complexes are a little narrower than you would expect to see for a ventricular origin, but VTach is still in the differential. There is a deflection at the bottom of the S wave, which either could be a morphological feature of the aberrancy or could represent an inverted P wave with a long R-P interval. Based on this one strip, you can't narrow it down any further between VTach, AVNRT with aberrancy, or antidromic AVRT with any great degree of certainty. Remember to never gamble with a patient's life...in other words, **_NEVER GUESS!_**

A full 12-lead ECG was able to move VTach down our list from #1 to #3. The possible inverted P wave was visible as a separate structure in almost every lead,

making you lean toward an antidromic AVRT because of the longer R-P interval. The clinical history, if available, could also be a major decision point.

The moral of this strip is that sometimes you can't narrow down a rhythm completely. In those cases, you need to use all available means to arrive at a feasible conclusion. In this case, the patient needed to be treated as if he had VTach, with a strong suspicion that there may be an accessory tract involved and that it could actually be an AVRT. If the patient is unstable, direct cardioversion or defibrillation is indicated in either case. If the patient is stable, obtain a history and use drugs that work on both possibilities, like IV amiodarone (if there are no contraindications).

Final Test ECG 45

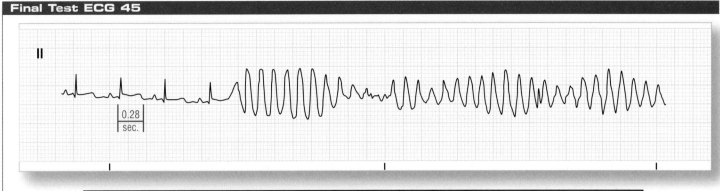

Rate:	About 110 BPM at onset	PR intervals:	Normal, at onset
Regularity:	See discussion below	QRS width:	Normal, at onset
P waves: Morphology: Axis:	Present. at onset Normal. at onset Normal. at onset	Grouping:	Yes, at the end of the strip
		Dropped beats:	None
P:QRS ratio:	1:1. at onset	Rhythm:	**Sinus tachycardia becoming torsade de pointes**

Discussion:

This strip shows a sinus tachycardia that changes into a run of torsade de pointes. The torsade de pointes is triggered by an R-on-T PVC. The rhythm cannot be called polymorphic VTach because the sinus tachycardia has a QT interval of 0.28 seconds, which is prolonged for a rate of 110 BPM. Notice the grouping quality of the torsade de pointes and the constant fluctuation of the morphology and the polarity of the QRS complexes, giving the rhythm an undulating or wavelike quality.

Final Test ECG 46

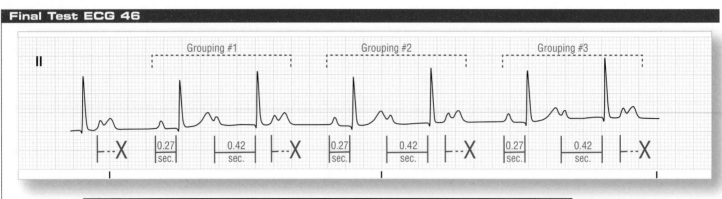

Rate:	About 70 BPM	PR intervals:	Variable
Regularity:	Regularly irregular	QRS width:	Normal
P waves:	Present	Grouping:	Yes
Morphology:	Normal		
Axis:	Normal	Dropped beats:	Yes
P:QRS ratio:	3:2	Rhythm:	**Mobitz I second-degree AV block**

Discussion:

Final Test ECG 46 is a very deceptive strip. At first glance, the rhythm appears to be a simple third-degree AV block. However, close observation and some measurements quickly change this initial evaluation. To start off, is the rhythm regular? No, it is regularly irregular. That fact just about completely rules out third-degree AV block because all of the possible escape rhythms depolarizing the ventricles, either junctional or ventricular, are always regular. Is there any grouping? Yes, but it is difficult to spot. There are two different R-R intervals throughout the strip. One R-R interval is 0.84 seconds and the other is 1.08 seconds and they both alternate throughout the strip.

At this point, let's turn our attention to the PR intervals. There are two measurable PR intervals; one is 0.27 seconds and the other is 0.42 seconds. Now, let's go back and take a look at the groups we isolated in the paragraph above. First there is a P wave with a PR interval of 0.27. Then, there is a PR interval of 0.42 sec-

onds. Then, then there is a nonconducted P wave. This is a recurring pattern in each group, clinching the diagnosis of Wenckebach or Mobitz I second-degree AV block.

What makes this rhythm strip difficult to interpret is the small difference between the two R-R intervals. Usually, there is a larger difference between the groupings, reflecting the dropped beat. However, just because the groups are closer together than expected, it is still a Wenckebach. As mentioned above, a third-degree AV block would give you an escape rhythm of some sort that would have to be regular. When you are approaching a rhythm strip, it is essential to form an initial impression of the rhythm. However, you now have to go and confirm your diagnosis. Checking the regularity and the intervals is a critical step in this confirmation process. Initial impressions are right in most cases, but as this strip exemplifies, they can also be wrong.

Final Test ECG 47

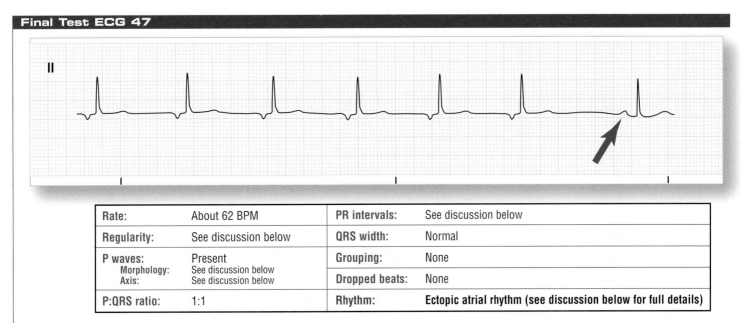

Rate:	About 62 BPM	PR intervals:	See discussion below
Regularity:	See discussion below	QRS width:	Normal
P waves:	Present	Grouping:	None
Morphology:	See discussion below		
Axis:	See discussion below	Dropped beats:	None
P:QRS ratio:	1:1	Rhythm:	**Ectopic atrial rhythm (see discussion below for full details)**

Discussion:

Final Test ECG 47 possibly shows a transition between two different regular rhythms. The first is an ectopic atrial rhythm at about 62 BPM. Note the inverted P waves with normal PR intervals, which are consistent with an ectopic atrial pacemaker, which occur at the front end of the strip. The P wave highlighted by the blue arrow, however, comes after a longer pause than the previous R-R intervals. In addition, the P wave changes to upright and it has a different PR interval. This P wave either can be an atrial escape complex or it can signify a change to a sinus rhythm, or even a different ectopic atrial rhythm (caused by a different atrial pacemaker). Statistically, a new rhythm is more likely than an atrial escape complex, but a longer strip is needed to verify the change.

Final Test ECG 48

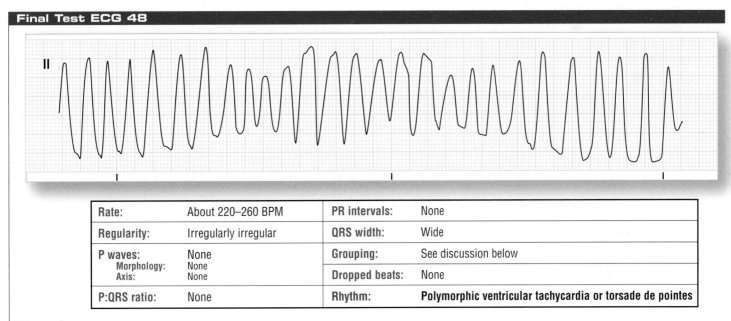

Rate:	About 220–260 BPM	PR intervals:	None
Regularity:	Irregularly irregular	QRS width:	Wide
P waves:	None	Grouping:	See discussion below
Morphology:	None		
Axis:	None	Dropped beats:	None
P:QRS ratio:	None	Rhythm:	**Polymorphic ventricular tachycardia or torsade de pointes**

Discussion:

Final Test ECG 48 shows the typical undulating pattern either of polymorphic VTach or of torsade de pointes. Which one of these is the final diagnosis depends on the underlying QT interval of the patient when in a sinus rhythm. Note the continuous change in the size, morphology, and polarity of the QRS complexes in this strip. The undulating pattern caused by the changes gives the strip an appearance of having grouping.

Final Test ECG 49

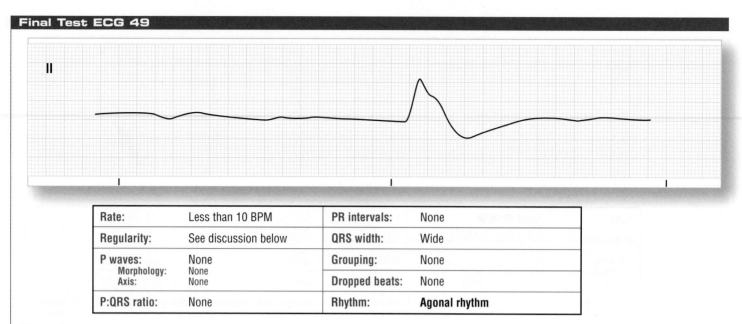

Rate:	Less than 10 BPM	PR intervals:	None
Regularity:	See discussion below	QRS width:	Wide
P waves:	None	Grouping:	None
Morphology:	None		
Axis:	None	Dropped beats:	None
P:QRS ratio:	None	Rhythm:	**Agonal rhythm**

Discussion:

Final Test ECG 49 shows an agonal rhythm. Notice the width of the QRS complexes and the totally abnormal and bizarre appearance of the one complex. Agonal rhythms are terminal events and are a close precursor to complete asystole. Most of the time, the ventricular depolarizations are strictly an electrical event and there is no resultant mechanical contraction.

Final Test ECG 50

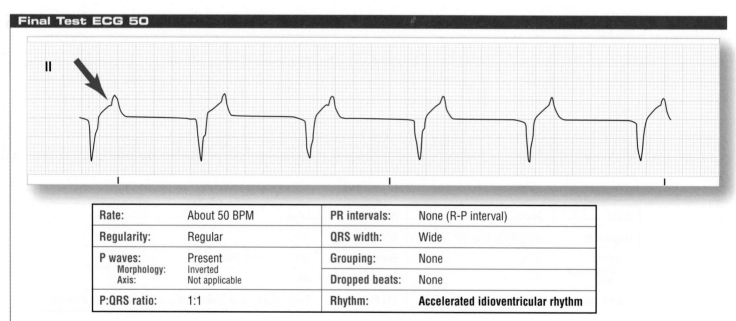

Rate:	About 50 BPM	PR intervals:	None (R-P interval)
Regularity:	Regular	QRS width:	Wide
P waves:	Present	Grouping:	None
Morphology:	Inverted		
Axis:	Not applicable	Dropped beats:	None
P:QRS ratio:	1:1	Rhythm:	**Accelerated idioventricular rhythm**

Discussion:

Final Test ECG 50 shows a wide, bizarre-looking rhythm, which is obviously ventricular in origin. There are no visible P waves before the QRS complexes, but there is an inverted P wave near the top of the T wave (see blue arrow). Note the very prolonged R-P interval, which is commonly seen in ventricular rhythms for these retrogradely conducted P waves.

Final Test ECG 51

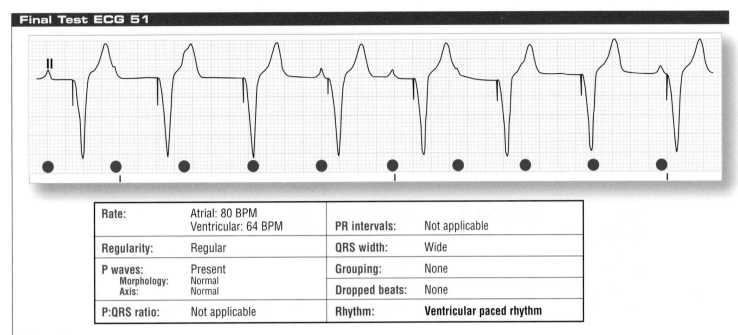

Rate:	Atrial: 80 BPM Ventricular: 64 BPM	PR intervals:	Not applicable
Regularity:	Regular	QRS width:	Wide

P waves:
  Morphology:
  Axis:
	Present
	Normal
	Normal
		Grouping:	None

		Dropped beats:	None
P:QRS ratio:	Not applicable	Rhythm:	**Ventricular paced rhythm**

Discussion:

Final Test ECG 51 shows a sharp deflection immediately before each ventricular complex that is caused by an artificial pacer. The pacer appears to be completely ignoring the underlying atrial rhythm below (see blue dots). As there is no atrial sensing or pacing evident on this strip, the paced rhythm is consistent with a VVI pacer.

Final Test ECG 52

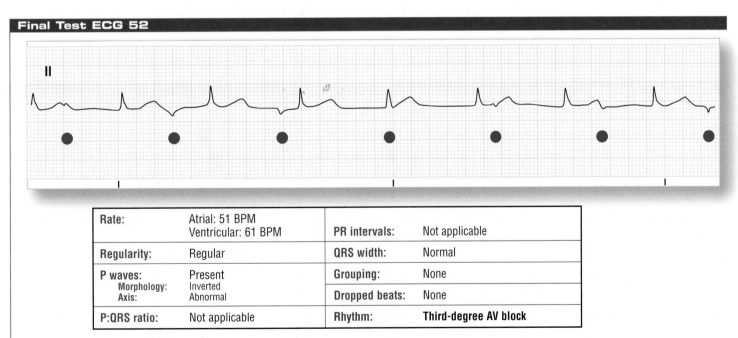

Rate:	Atrial: 51 BPM Ventricular: 61 BPM	PR intervals:	Not applicable
Regularity:	Regular	QRS width:	Normal

P waves:
  Morphology:
  Axis:
	Present
	Inverted
	Abnormal
		Grouping:	None

		Dropped beats:	None
P:QRS ratio:	Not applicable	Rhythm:	**Third-degree AV block**

Discussion:

The ventricular response is regular and about 61 BPM. The atrial rhythm is actually slower at 51 BPM. There are some inverted P waves, but there is no association at all between the P waves and the QRS complexes. Notice the morphological changes that develop when the inverted P waves fuse with the QRS complexes, ST segments, and T waves. This is a third-degree AV block with a sinus bradycardic atrial rhythm and an accelerated junctional escape rhythm.

Final Test ECG 53

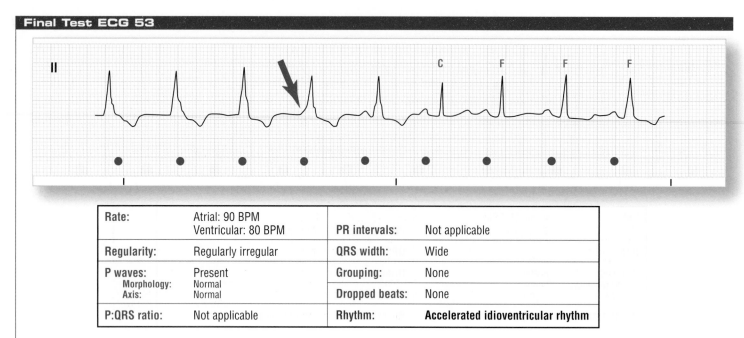

Rate:	Atrial: 90 BPM Ventricular: 80 BPM	PR intervals:	Not applicable
Regularity:	Regularly irregular	QRS width:	Wide

P waves:
  Morphology:
  Axis:
	Present
	Normal
	Normal
		Grouping:	None

		Dropped beats:	None
P:QRS ratio:	Not applicable	Rhythm:	**Accelerated idioventricular rhythm**

Discussion:

Final Test ECG 53 shows a wide-complex rhythm with a ventricular rate of about 90 BPM. The start of the strip shows some wide, bizarre complexes that are obviously of ventricular origin. Then there is a narrow capture beat with a P wave before it (see complex labeled "C"). Followed by several fusion complexes (see complex labeled "F"). These are indirect evidence for the presence of AV dissociation. The P waves map through throughout the entire strip and cause some fusion with the ventricular complexes. For example, take a look at the area highlighted by the blue arrow. This area is slurred upward because of a fusion between the P wave and the ventricular complex. This is indirect evidence of AV dissociation.

Because the rate is less than 100 BPM, this is not a ventricular tachycardia. Instead, the slower rate makes this rhythm an accelerated idioventricular rhythm. Remember, idioventricular, accelerated idioventricular, and VTach can all have AV dissociation.

Final Test ECG 54

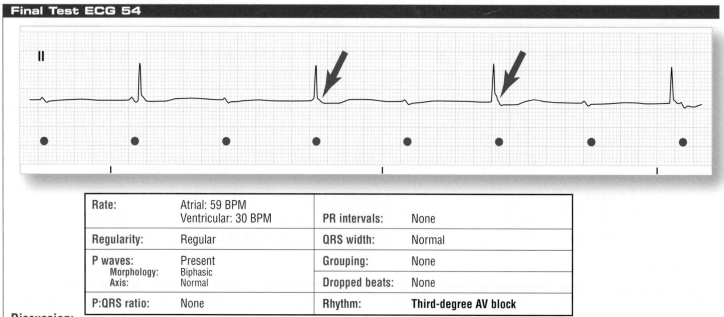

Rate:	Atrial: 59 BPM Ventricular: 30 BPM	PR intervals:	None
Regularity:	Regular	QRS width:	Normal

P waves:
  Morphology:
  Axis:
	Present
	Biphasic
	Normal
		Grouping:	None

		Dropped beats:	None
P:QRS ratio:	None	Rhythm:	**Third-degree AV block**

Discussion:

Final Test ECG 54 shows a complete or third-degree AV block with a sinus bradycardia and a very slow junc-tional escape rhythm. The blue arrows point to buried P waves inside of the QRS complex.

Final Test ECG 55

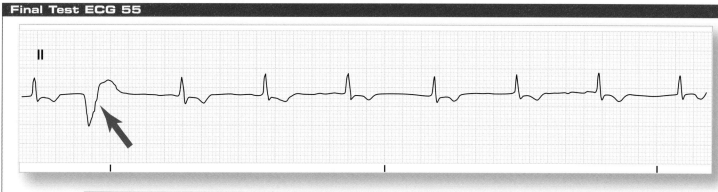

Rate:	About 66 BPM	PR intervals:	None
Regularity:	Regular with an event	QRS width:	Normal
P waves: Morphology: Axis:	None None None	Grouping:	None
		Dropped beats:	None
P:QRS ratio:	None	Rhythm:	**Accelerated junctional rhythm with a PVC**

Discussion:

Final Test ECG 55 shows a narrow-complex rhythm at about 66 BPM. There are no visible P waves on the strip. There could be a pseudo-S wave pattern at the end of the QRS complex, but it could also represent part of the normal morphology for the QRS complex in that lead. There is one PVC (see blue arrow) near the start of the strip. A full 12-lead ECG will help you decide whether or not there is a pseudo-S wave. In either case, verification of the pseudo-S wave is not necessary for you to make the diagnosis of an accelerated junctional rhythm with a PVC.

Final Test ECG 56

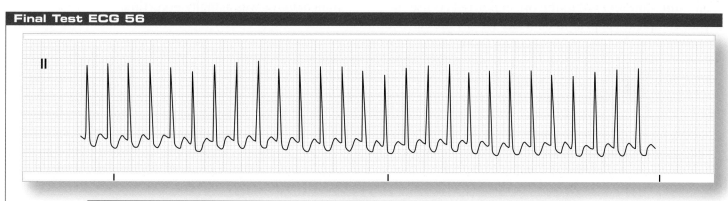

Rate:	About 270 BPM	PR intervals:	None
Regularity:	Regular	QRS width:	Normal
P waves: Morphology: Axis:	None None None	Grouping:	None
		Dropped beats:	None
P:QRS ratio:	None	Rhythm:	**AVRT**

Discussion:

Final Test ECG 56 shows a very, very rapid narrow-complex tachycardia with no visible P waves. The rhythm is very regular. There is some electrical alternans noted, which would be expected in many tachycardias, especially at this rate. The rhythm is too fast for an AVNRT. The only other logical possibility is an ortho-dromic AVRT. Clinical correlation and a full 12-lead ECG once the patient is stable would be highly recommended. Be careful treating this patient and keep in mind that there is a tremendously high probability that you are dealing with a patient who has an accessory pathway.

Final Test ECG 57

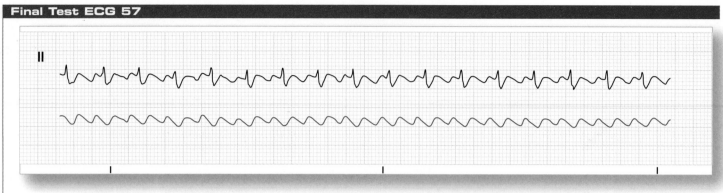

Rate:	Atrial: 300 BPM Ventricular: 150 BPM	PR intervals:	Not applicable
Regularity:	Regular	QRS width:	See discussion below
P waves: 　Morphology: 　Axis:	F waves None None	Grouping:	None
		Dropped beats:	None
F:QRS ratio:	2:1	Rhythm:	**Atrial flutter**

Discussion:

The ventricular rate of 150 BPM should immediately make you think of an atrial flutter. Can we rule this possibility in? Yes. Take a look at the strip and mentally remove the QRS complexes...the result is the strip in blue above. There is an obvious saw-tooth pattern on this modified strip. The saw-tooth pattern, however, is a bit more camouflaged in the original strip because the QRS complexes appear to be wide. We say appear to be wide, because we cannot be sure if this is an illusion caused by a fusion of the F wave with the overlying QRS in this lead. A full 12-lead ECG or looking at some other leads will help to clarify this issue. In this case, the 12-lead ECG showed very clear evidence that the QRS complexes were narrow, and the illusion we mentioned above was actually occurring.

Final Test ECG 58

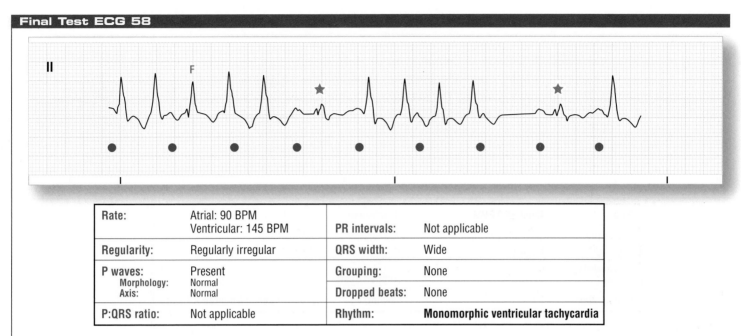

Rate:	Atrial: 90 BPM Ventricular: 145 BPM	PR intervals:	Not applicable
Regularity:	Regularly irregular	QRS width:	Wide

P waves:
  Morphology:
  Axis:
	Present
	Normal
	Normal
		Grouping:	None

		Dropped beats:	None
P:QRS ratio:	Not applicable	Rhythm:	**Monomorphic ventricular tachycardia**

Discussion:

This strip is another tough one. The important thing is your initial logic. It is a wide-complex tachycardia; therefore VTach should be #1 on your differential diagnosis list. The last two complexes hold the initial key to proving your original impression because they have obvious P waves right before the QRS complexes. Mapping this distance with your calipers, and then walking that distance over the rest of the strip, brings up irregularities in the strip, which are caused by buried P waves. This is direct evidence of AV dissociation. A wide-complex tachycardia with AV dissociation is VTach for all intents and purposes.

It is unclear whether the complexes marked by the red star are capture complexes in a patient with an underlying bundle branch block or whether they are fusion complexes. Statistically, they should be fusion complexes because that is the most common possibility. However, you will need to obtain some old strips to be absolutely sure of this before making that call. The complex labeled with the "F" represents an obvious fusion complex.

Final Test ECG 59

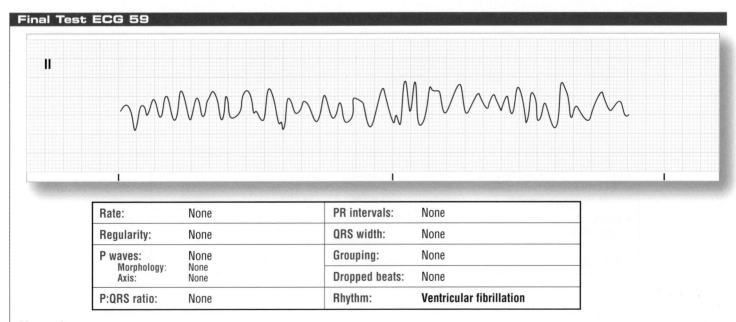

Rate:	None	PR intervals:	None
Regularity:	None	QRS width:	None

P waves:
  Morphology:
  Axis:
	None
	None
	None
		Grouping:	None

		Dropped beats:	None
P:QRS ratio:	None	Rhythm:	**Ventricular fibrillation**

Discussion:

This ECG shows a completely chaotic ventricular response. The only possibility is ventricular fibrillation. Once again, clinical correlation is required to rule out artifact.

Final Test ECG 60

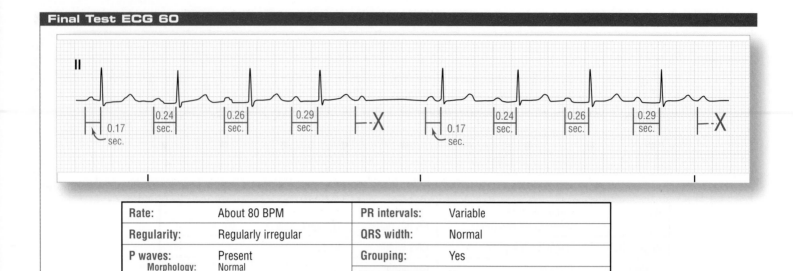

Rate:	About 80 BPM	PR intervals:	Variable
Regularity:	Regularly irregular	QRS width:	Normal
P waves:	Present	Grouping:	Yes
Morphology:	Normal		
Axis:	Normal	Dropped beats:	Yes
P:QRS ratio:	5:4	Rhythm:	**Mobitz I second-degree AV block**

Discussion:

Final Test ECG 60 shows some obvious grouping of four ventricular complexes and then a pause. The P waves are all morphologically similar, but the PR intervals are different in each complex in the group. The PR intervals show the typical lengthening pattern seen in Wenckebach or Mobitz I second-degree AV block. Note that the widest incremental change in the PR intervals occurs between the first and second complexes. In addition, the PR interval immediately following the pause is the shortest, and the one before the pause is the longest. Finally, the R-R intervals shorten along the grouping, as would be expected. Final diagnosis is Mobitz I second-degree AV block.

Final Test ECG 61

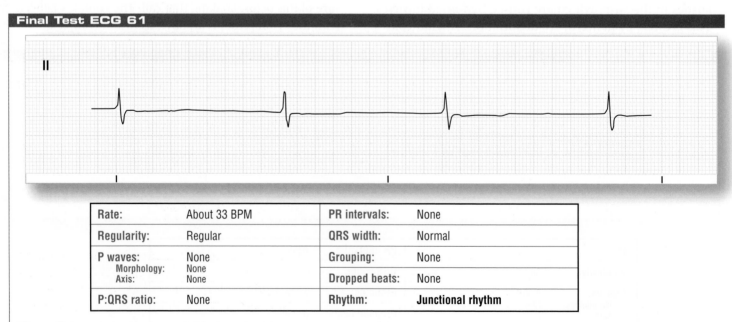

Rate:	About 33 BPM	PR intervals:	None
Regularity:	Regular	QRS width:	Normal
P waves:	None	Grouping:	None
Morphology:	None		
Axis:	None	Dropped beats:	None
P:QRS ratio:	None	Rhythm:	**Junctional rhythm**

Discussion:

This is a very slow junctional rhythm. Junctional rhythm usually has rates between 40 and 60 BPM, but can be slower at times. This is one of those times. It is important to try to figure out why this patient's rate is so slow. Clinical correlation is needed to see if there is drug use or toxicity, a CNS event, ischemia, or an electrolyte problem, among other things, as the cause of the slower rate.

Final Test ECG 62

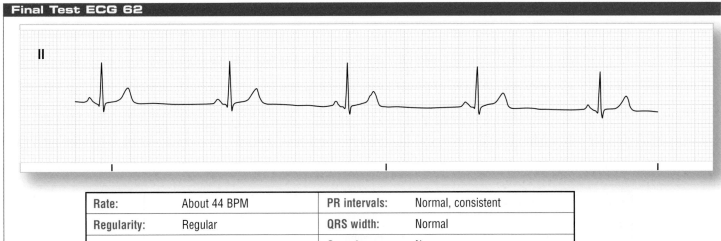

Rate:	About 44 BPM	PR intervals:	Normal, consistent
Regularity:	Regular	QRS width:	Normal
P waves:	Present	Grouping:	None
Morphology:	Normal		
Axis:	Normal	Dropped beats:	None
P:QRS ratio:	1:1	Rhythm:	**Sinus bradycardia**

Discussion:

This strip shows your typical sinus bradycardia. Notice the P wave in front of each QRS. The P waves are the same morphology and have the same PR intervals. The QRS complexes are narrow, and there are no major abnormalities or irregularities noted anywhere else along the strip.

Final Test ECG 63

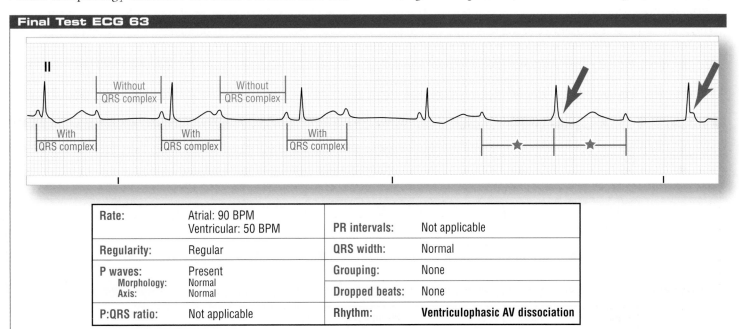

Rate:	Atrial: 90 BPM Ventricular: 50 BPM	PR intervals:	Not applicable
Regularity:	Regular	QRS width:	Normal
P waves:	Present	Grouping:	None
Morphology:	Normal		
Axis:	Normal	Dropped beats:	None
P:QRS ratio:	Not applicable	Rhythm:	**Ventriculophasic AV dissociation**

Discussion:

It is easy to spot the AV block in this strip, but note that this is not a typical third-degree AV block. The ventricular rate is regular, narrow, and consistent with a junctional escape rhythm. The atrial rhythm is another matter. At the start of the strip there appear to be two different P-P intervals: One P-P interval occurs when there is a QRS complex falling between the two P waves. The other P-P interval occurs when there is no QRS complex falling between the two P waves. This part of the strip is a classic example of what is known as a *ventriculophasic* AV dissociation (see page 500 for further details).

The exact P-P intervals start to fall apart in the middle of the strip for some reason. The two P-P intervals labeled with the red stars are exactly even because the P wave falls right in the middle of the QRS complex (see first blue arrow). The green arrow also points to a buried P wave, but this time, the QRS complex does exert some influence on the underlying P-P interval, causing it to narrow slightly. Notice that the ventriculophasic influence remains throughout the strip, but is less classic toward the latter half of the strip.

Final Test ECG 64

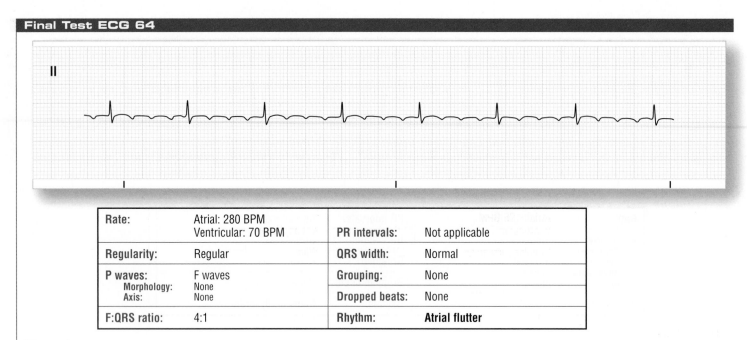

Rate:	Atrial: 280 BPM Ventricular: 70 BPM	PR intervals:	Not applicable
Regularity:	Regular	QRS width:	Normal
P waves: Morphology: Axis:	F waves None None	Grouping:	None
		Dropped beats:	None
F:QRS ratio:	4:1	Rhythm:	**Atrial flutter**

Discussion:

This rhythm strip shows the very obvious saw-tooth pattern of atrial flutter along the baseline. The ratio of conduction is 4:1 with an atrial rate of 280 BPM and a ventricular response of 70 BPM.

Final Test ECG 65

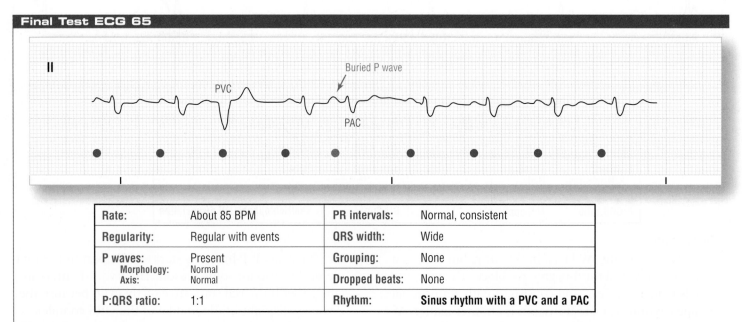

Rate:	About 85 BPM	PR intervals:	Normal, consistent
Regularity:	Regular with events	QRS width:	Wide
P waves: Morphology: Axis:	Present Normal Normal	Grouping:	None
		Dropped beats:	None
P:QRS ratio:	1:1	Rhythm:	**Sinus rhythm with a PVC and a PAC**

Discussion:

Final Test ECG 65 shows an underlying sinus rhythm that is broken up by a PVC and a PAC. The PVC and the PAC are both associated with compensatory pauses, which means that the underlying atrial cadence is not broken by the two events. In other words, the sinus node is not reset by either the PVC or the PAC. The PAC is associated with a buried P wave.

Final Test ECG 66

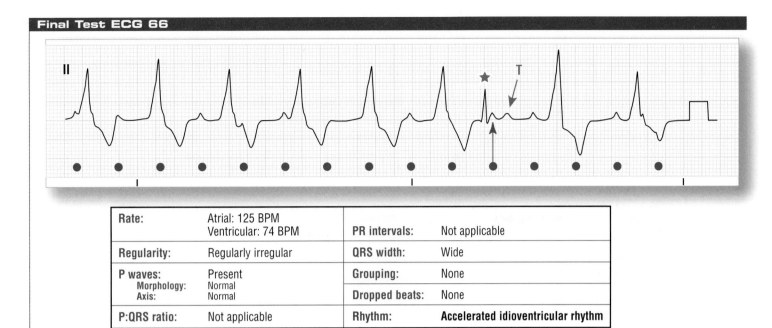

Rate:	Atrial: 125 BPM Ventricular: 74 BPM	PR intervals:	Not applicable
Regularity:	Regularly irregular	QRS width:	Wide

P waves:
  Morphology:
  Axis:
	Present
	Normal
	Normal
		Grouping:	None

		Dropped beats:	None
P:QRS ratio:	Not applicable	Rhythm:	**Accelerated idioventricular rhythm**

Discussion:

Final Test ECG 66 shows a wide-complex rhythm that is broken up by one narrow complex (see red starred complex). This is a capture beat and indirect evidence of AV dissociation. When we look at the rest of the strip, we notice some P waves scattered throughout. These P waves map out at a tachycardic rate of 125 BPM (see blue dots). One of the P waves falls right after the QRS complex of the capture beat (see small blue arrow). Due to the ventricular rate of 74 BPM, this rhythm is an accelerated idioventricular rhythm.

Notice anything else unusual about the strip? The strip was recorded at half-standard (see calibration mark at the end of the strip). This means that all of the waves are actually twice as tall as they appear on this strip. These are some really big waves!

Final Test ECG 67

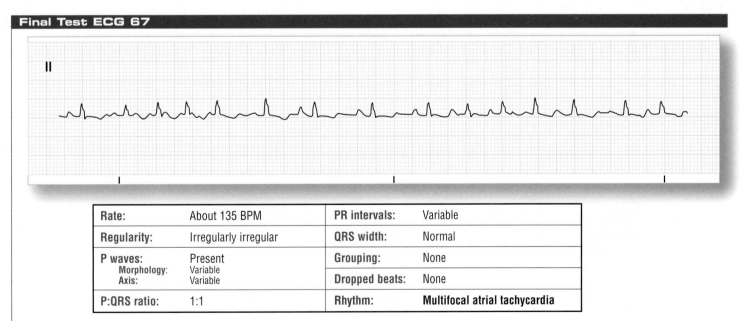

Rate:	About 135 BPM	PR intervals:	Variable
Regularity:	Irregularly irregular	QRS width:	Normal

P waves:
  Morphology:
  Axis:
	Present
	Variable
	Variable
		Grouping:	None

		Dropped beats:	None
P:QRS ratio:	1:1	Rhythm:	**Multifocal atrial tachycardia**

Discussion:

Final Test ECG 67 shows a rapid narrow-complex tachycardia that is irregularly irregular. Are there P waves? Yes. Then it is probably MAT. Are there at least three different P wave morphologies each with their own PR interval? Yes. Then it is definitely MAT.

Final Test ECG 68

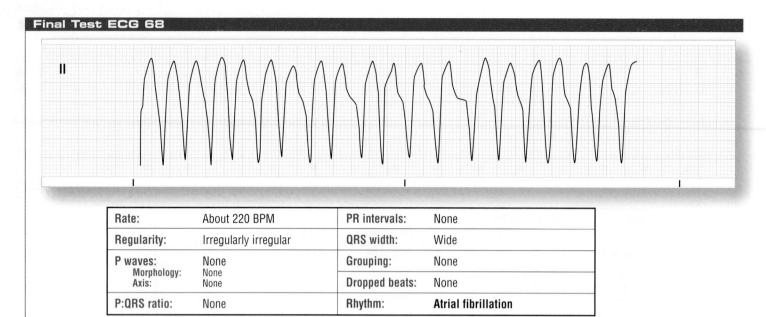

Rate:	About 220 BPM	PR intervals:	None
Regularity:	Irregularly irregular	QRS width:	Wide
P waves:	None	Grouping:	None
Morphology:	None		
Axis:	None	Dropped beats:	None
P:QRS ratio:	None	Rhythm:	**Atrial fibrillation**

Discussion:

This is a wide-complex tachycardia. But, it is an *irregularly irregular* wide-complex tachycardia. This is atrial fibrillation. Because of the very fast rates, you need to think about the fact that you may also be dealing with an accessory pathway. (As a rule, you need to think about accessory pathways in atrial fibrillation when the rate is greater than 200 BPM.) Don't be fooled into thinking that this is VTach or VFlutter! Those two rhythms are regular (except at the very start of the rhythm).

Final Test ECG 69

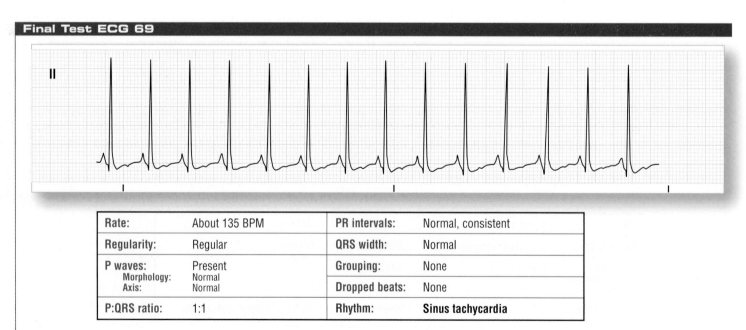

Rate:	About 135 BPM	PR intervals:	Normal, consistent
Regularity:	Regular	QRS width:	Normal
P waves:	Present	Grouping:	None
Morphology:	Normal		
Axis:	Normal	Dropped beats:	None
P:QRS ratio:	1:1	Rhythm:	**Sinus tachycardia**

Discussion:

Don't let the size of the QRS complexes fool you. This is a rapid, regular narrow-complex tachycardia with P waves before each of the QRS complexes. The P waves are all identical and so are the PR intervals. This is a sinus tachycardia.

Final Test ECG 70

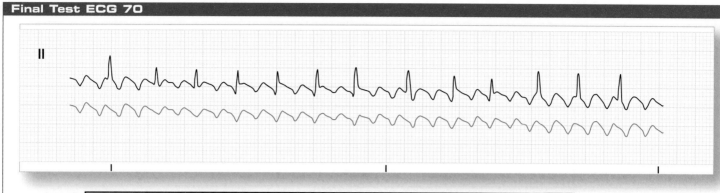

Rate:	Atrial: 280 BPM Ventricular: 125 BPM	PR intervals:	Not applicable
Regularity:	Regularly irregular	QRS width:	Normal
P waves: 　Morphology: 　Axis:	F waves Not applicable Not applicable	Grouping:	None
		Dropped beats:	None
F:QRS ratio:	Variable	Rhythm:	**Atrial flutter with variable block**

Discussion:

Final Test ECG 70 shows a narrow-complex tachycardia with a ventricular response of about 125 BPM. The rhythm is regularly irregular with one particular R-R interval recurring frequently throughout most of the strip. Once again, imagine mentally removing the QRS complexes from the rhythm strip. What you would be left with is the pink strip. The saw-tooth pattern of atrial flutter is evident on this strip. This is an atrial flutter with variable block.

Final Test ECG 71

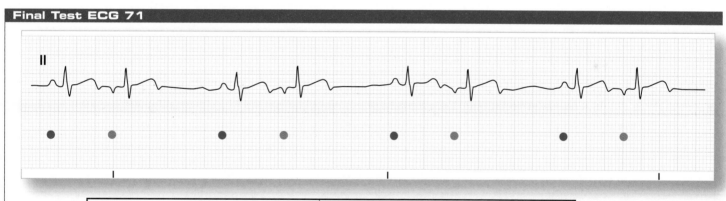

Rate:	About 70 BPM	PR intervals:	Variable
Regularity:	Regularly irregular	QRS width:	Normal
P waves: 　Morphology: 　Axis:	Present Variable Variable	Grouping:	Yes
		Dropped beats:	None
P:QRS ratio:	1:1	Rhythm:	**Supraventricular bigeminy**

Discussion:

Final Test ECG 71 shows a rhythm that has one complex with a normal upright P wave followed by a complex with an inverted P wave. This causes a grouping pattern to develop, but this time, it is not due to an AV block. This is a rhythm known as a supraventricular bigeminy. It is a bigeminy because every other beat is premature; it is supraventricular because the premature beat is a PAC. If you cannot remember the term supraventricular bigeminy, it is OK to call it sinus rhythm with frequent PACs.

This is usually a stable rhythm as long as the PACs are causing a mechanical contraction. Checking the patient's pulse for the same pattern as seen on the strip will answer that question. To treat it, find the underlying cause and treat that. It may be too much caffeine, drugs (legal and illegal), anxiety, hypoxemia, and many other causes. A good history, physical exam, and a full 12-lead ECG will usually help you spot the culprit.

Final Test ECG 72

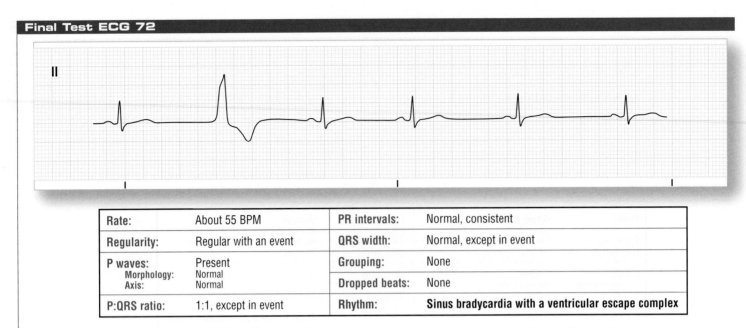

Rate:	About 55 BPM	PR intervals:	Normal, consistent
Regularity:	Regular with an event	QRS width:	Normal, except in event

P waves:
   Morphology:
   Axis:
	Present
	Normal
	Normal
		Grouping:	None

		Dropped beats:	None
P:QRS ratio:	1:1, except in event	Rhythm:	**Sinus bradycardia with a ventricular escape complex**

Discussion:

The event in question on Final Test ECG 72 is obviously a ventricular complex. But, is it a PVC? No. It doesn't arrive earlier than expected; it arrives later than expected. The ventricular fired as a failsafe mechanism because the sinus node took too long to fire. This is a ventricular escape complex. The underlying rhythm is a sinus bradycardia since the rate is 55 BPM.

Final Test ECG 73

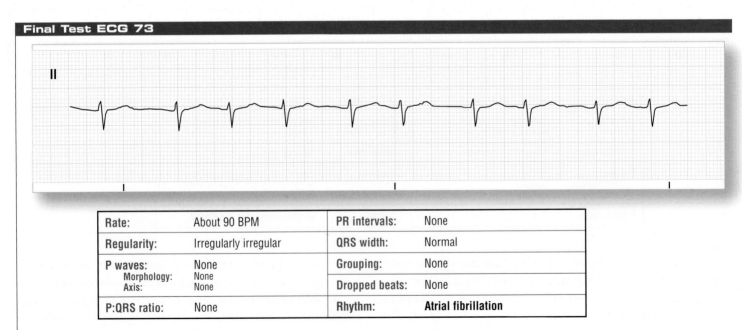

Rate:	About 90 BPM	PR intervals:	None
Regularity:	Irregularly irregular	QRS width:	Normal

P waves:
   Morphology:
   Axis:
	None
	None
	None
		Grouping:	None

		Dropped beats:	None
P:QRS ratio:	None	Rhythm:	**Atrial fibrillation**

Discussion:

Final Test ECG 73 shows an irregularly irregular rhythm with no obvious P waves. The rhythm is an atrial fibrillation. The QRS complexes are narrow and the rate is about 90 BPM.

Final Test ECG 74

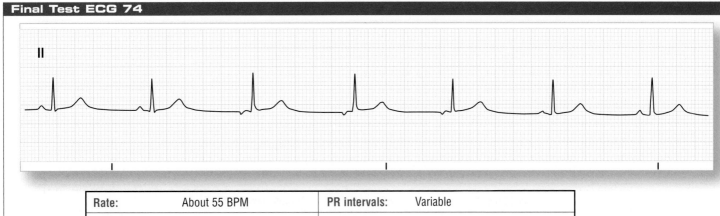

Rate:	About 55 BPM	PR intervals:	Variable
Regularity:	Regularly irregular	QRS width:	Normal
P waves:	Variable	Grouping:	None
Morphology:	Variable		
Axis:	Variable	Dropped beats:	None
P:QRS ratio:	1:1	Rhythm:	**Wandering atrial pacemaker**

Discussion:

This strip shows a rhythm where the P waves are slowly transitioning from upright to inverted and then back again in a continuous pattern. This is the hallmark of a wandering atrial pacemaker.

Final Test ECG 75

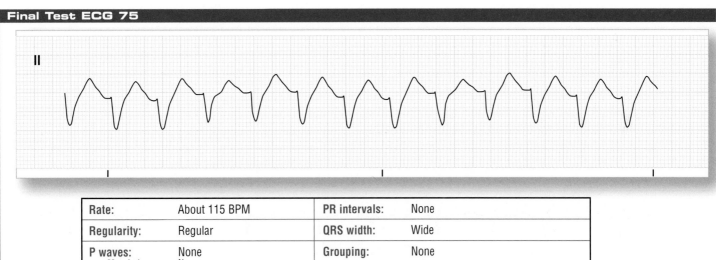

Rate:	About 115 BPM	PR intervals:	None
Regularity:	Regular	QRS width:	Wide
P waves:	None	Grouping:	None
Morphology:	None		
Axis:	None	Dropped beats:	None
P:QRS ratio:	None	Rhythm:	**Monomorphic ventricular tachycardia**

Discussion:

This strip shows a wide-complex tachycardia at a rate of 115 BPM. The complexes are regular and have the same morphological presentation. There is no direct or indirect evidence of AV dissociation present. The differential diagnosis is short for this rhythm. It could either be a monomorphic ventricular tachycardia or a junctional tachycardia in a patient with a pre-existing condition that widens the QRS complex. Statistically, the second possibility is very rare. So, for all intents and purposes, you can make the call of a monomorphic ventricular tachycardia.

A full 12-lead ECG could possibly help you confirm the diagnosis, if you have the time to get one. You could look for Josephson's sign, Brugada's sign, or concordance in the precordial leads. You may also be able to see some evidence of AV dissociation in another lead. All in all, it is worthwhile to get one if the patient is clinically stable.

Section 1: Introduction to Arrhythmia Recognition

Chapter 1: Anatomy

1. True
2. False
3. C
4. C
5. E
6. F
7. A
8. D
9. B
10. C

Chapter 2: Electrophysiology

1. B
2. False
3. False
4. D
5. True
6. C
7. True
8. False
9. A
10. True
11. autonomic nervous system
12. sympathetic; parasympathetic
13. increases; increases; decreases; decreases
14. epinephrine
15. acetylcholine
16. Epinephrine
17. Acetylcholine

Chapter 3: Vectors and the Basic Beat

1. C
2. True
3. D
4. True
5. C
6. False
7. False
8. C
9. B
10. C
11. True
12. True
13. False
14. True

Chapter 4: The Rhythm Strip, Tools, and Calculating Rates

1. D
2. A
3. D
4. A
5. B
6. C
7. B
8. True

9. B
10. C
11. C

Chapter 5: Basic Concepts in Arrhythmia Recognition

1. False
2. B, D, and E
3. True
4. C
5. True
6. E
7. True
8. True
9. E
10. True
11. C
12. True
13. False
14. True

Chapter 6: Relevant Topics in Basic Electrocardiography

1. D
2. True
3. C
4. D
5. A
6. C
7. False
8. D
9. False
10. A

Chapter 7: Arrhythmias: A Quick Review

1. True
2. E
3. D
4. B
5. True
6. True
7. A
8. False
9. True
10. C
11. True
12. False
13. C
14. D
15. E

Section 2: Sinus Rhythms

Chapter 8: Normal Sinus Rhythm

1. Sinoatrial (SA)
2. A, C
3. Less than 60 BPM
4. 60 and 100 BPM
5. Greater than 100 BPM
6. True
7. C
8. II, III, and aVF

9. C
10. True
11. True
12. B
13. False
14. True
15. True
16. A
17. A, B, C, D
18. 1, 5
19. True
20. D

Chapter 9: Sinus Bradycardia

1. A
2. less than
3. True
4. False
5. D
6. True
7. D
8. II, III, and aVF
9. True
10. False! Always treat any hemo-dynamically significant arrhythmia as a cardiac emergency.

Chapter 10: Sinus Tachycardia

1. 100 BPM
2. 100 and 160/200/220
3. 220
4. False
5. True
6. PR
7. amplitude or height
8. False
9. E
10. E
11. TP
12. True
13. treat the underlying cause
14. decrease; decrease; decrease
15. F
16. True
17. True
18. False
19. False!
20. False. You use cardioversion to shock someone into a sinus rhythm. Sinus tachycardia is a sinus rhythm, it is just fast.

Chapter 11: Sinus Arrhythmia

1. True
2. True
3. E
4. B
5. True
6. A
7. F
8. False

Chapter 12: Sinus Blocks, Pauses, and Arrests

1. P
2. atrial
3. False
4. P-P interval
5. False
6. D
7. Pause
8. arrest
9. True
10. True

Section 3: Atrial Rhythms

Chapter 13: Premature Atrial Contraction

1. atria
2. False
3. D
4. True
5. P wave axis
6. upright or positive
7. inverted or negative
8. False
9. True
10. C
11. True
12. True
13. reset
14. A
15. C
16. True
17. B
18. False
19. True
20. True

Chapter 14: Ectopic Atrial Rhythm

1. False
2. False
3. D
4. D
5. True
6. True
7. False
8. E
9. A
10. B

Chapter 15: Ectopic Atrial Tachycardia

1. E
2. True
3. True
4. C
5. False
6. True
7. True
8. False
9. False
10. E

Chapter 16: Ectopic Atrial Tachycardia with Block

1. D
2. False
3. E

4. True
5. False
6. A
7. True
8. True
9. False
10. False!

Chapter 17: Wandering Atrial Pacemaker

1. irregularly irregular
2. A, C, D
3. True
4. Three
5. C
6. True
7. False
8. E
9. chaotic
10. less than

Chapter 18: Multifocal Atrial Tachycardia

1. atrial fibrillation, wandering atrial pacemaker, and multifocal atrial tachycardia
2. True
3. False
4. True
5. False
6. C
7. right
8. True
9. False
10. True

Chapter 19: Atrial Flutter

1. True
2. C
3. D
4. Flutter or F waves
5. False
6. macroreentry, right
7. True
8. E
9. False
10. MAD RAT PPP

Chapter 20: Atrial Fibrillation

1. Irregularly irregular/P waves
2. B, D
3. D
4. True
5. False
6. True
7. 100/200
8. False
9. True
10. long/short

Section 4: Junctional Rhythms

Chapter 21: Introduction to Junctional Rhythms

1. False
2. junctional
3. True
4. D
5. shorter

6. RP
7. ectopic atrial, junctional
8. 60
9. 60 and 100
10. 100

Chapter 22: Junctional Rhythm

1. True
2. B and D
3. E
4. Escape
5. False
6. False
7. True
8. False
9. Digitalis
10. E

Chapter 23: Premature Junctional Contraction

1. narrow, 0.12 seconds
2. inverted
3. True
4. False
5. B
6. E
7. T
8. A
9. False
10. True

Chapter 24: Rapid Junctional Rhythms

1. True
2. True
3. 60 and 100
4. 100 and 130
5. True

Chapter 25: AV Nodal Reentry Tachycardia

1. D
2. fast, slow
3. fast
4. True
5. PR intervals
6. True
7. C
8. before, immediately behind, buried in
9. False
10. True

Chapter 26: AV Reentry Tachycardia

1. AV node/accessory pathway
2. True
3. E
4. True
5. A
6. B
7. E
8. False
9. Concealed conduction
10. Orthodromic
11. Antidromic
12. True
13. True

14. False
15. True

Chapter 27: How to Approach a Narrow-Complex Tachycardia

1. B
2. focused
3. False
4. A. Atrial fibrillation
   B. Multifocal atrial tachycardia
   C. Atrial flutter with variable block
5. False
6. atrial fibrillation
7. True
8. AVNRT
9. False
10. The correct answer is E. Electrical cardioversion is never indicated for a sinus tachycardia. Find the underlying cause of the sinus tachycardia and treat that problem, not the rhythm itself. If the patient is hypoxemic, give oxygen. If the patient is hypotensive or dehydrated, give fluids. If the patient has a fever, give acetaminophen. If the patient is in pain, give morphine or an agent to control pain.

Section 5: Ventricular Rhythms

Chapter 28: Introduction to Ventricular Rhythms

1. True
2. 0.12
3. E
4. False
5. E
6. False
7. True, the interval is always the same no matter what the lead. The measurement of the interval, however, does vary due to iso-electric segments.
8. inverted
9. True
10. third-degree

Chapter 29: Premature Ventricular Contraction

1. D
2. E
3. False
4. True
5. P wave
6. compensatory
7. False
8. bigeminy
9. couplet
10. E

Chapter 30: Ventricular Escape and Idioventricular Rhythms

1. three
2. False

3. ventricles
4. C
5. E
6. D
7. AMI
8. True
9. False
10. accelerated idioventricular or ventricular tachycardia

Chapter 31: Ventricular Tachycardia

1. three, 100
2. 100, 200
3. ventricular flutter
4. monomorphic
5. nonsustained
6. sustained
7. D
8. D
9. E
10. False
11. True
12. D
13. 50%
14. B
15. acute myocardial infarction

Chapter 32: Polymorphic Ventricular Tachycardia and Torsade de Pointes

1. True
2. True
3. normal
4. prolonged
5. E (notice this trick question asks about polymorphic VTach and not torsade de pointes)
6. True
7. 150–300 BPM
8. False
9. True
10. D

Chapter 33: How to Approach a Wide-Complex Tachycardia

1. 80%
2. 90%
3. atrioventricular dissociation
4. True
5. ventricular tachycardia
6. B and D
7. False (Think of atrial fibrillation in a patient with an accessory pathway.)
8. True
9. 0.14
10. B
11. D
12. PVCs
13. A
14. D
15. concordance

Chapter 34: Ventricular Fibrillation and Asystole

1. True
2. True

3. Fine
4. acute myocardial infarction
5. defibrillation
6. True
7. True
8. agonal

Section 6: Additional Rhythms and Information

Chapter 35: Atrioventricular Block

1. Incompletely or completely
2. first
3. second
4. complete or third
5. E
6. 0.20
7. True
8. False
9. D
10. A
11. C
12. F
13. B
14. E
15. False
16. True
17. False
18. B
19. narrow
20. E
21. True
22. narrow or wide
23. True
24. False. Capture and fusion beats are indicative of AV dissociation, not a complete block.
25. True

Chapter 36: Artificially Paced Rhythms

1. True!
2. D
3. D
4. B
5. C
6. True

Chapter 37: Putting It All Together

1. patient's IQ points!
2. False
3. True
4. False! (**Clinical pearl:** If a patient ever tells you that he or she is going to die…believe it! It may just be nerves but the patient can also be sensing something that you are not able to pick up yet.)
5. True
6. P
7. 0.12/0.20
8. C and E
9. company it keeps
10. True

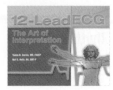

12-Lead ECG: The Art of Interpretation
by Tomas B. Garcia and Neil E. Holtz
1ˢᵗ Edition, 2001, Jones and Bartlett Publishers

This is the companion text to this arrhythmia book. It is a graphics-intensive programmed learning text that covers the entire spectrum of electrocardiography from beginner to expert. There are hundreds of actual full-sized ECGs to guide your training.

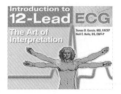

Introduction to 12-Lead ECG:
The Art of Interpretation
by Tomas B. Garcia and Neil E. Holtz
1ˢᵗ Edition, 2003, Jones and Bartlett Publishers

This is an introductory companion to this arrhythmia book. It is also a graphics-intensive teaching text that introduces the student to the basics of clinical electrocardiography.

Chou's Electrocardiography in Clinical
Practice: Adult and Pediatric
by Borys Surawicz and Timothy K Knilans
5ᵗʰ Edition, 2001, W.B. Saunders Company

Arrhythmias
by John A. Kastor
2ⁿᵈ Edition, 2000, W.B. Saunders Company

Cardiac Arrhythmias: Mechanism, Diagnosis, and Management
by Phillip J. Podrid and Peter Kowey
2ⁿᵈ Edition, 2001, Lippincott, Williams, and Wilkins

Advanced Concepts in Arrhythmias
by Henry J.L. Marriott and Mary B. Conover
3ʳᵈ Edition, 1998, Mosby

Advanced ECG: Boards and Beyond
by Brendon P. Phibbs
1st Edition, 1997, Little, Brown and Co.

A

A	atrial response pacemaker
AAI	atrial demand pacemaker
ACLS	advanced cardiac life support
AEI	atrial escape interval
Afib	atrial fibrillation
AMI	acute myocardial infarction
ANS	autonomic nervous system
AV	atrioventricular
AVB	AV block
AVNRT	AV nodal reentry tachycardia
AVRT	AV reentry tachycardia

B

BP	blood pressure
BPM	beats per minute

C

CAD	coronary artery disease
CHF	congestive heart failure
CNS	central nervous system
COPD	chronic obstructive pulmonary disease

D

D	dual response pacemaker
DDD	automatic pacemaker
DVI	AV sequential pacemaker

E

EAT	ectopic atrial tachycardia
ECG	electrocardiogram
EPS	electrophysiology

I

I	inhibited response pacemaker

ICHD	Intersociety Commission for Heart Disease
IWMI	inferior wall myocardial infarction

J

JVD	jugular vein distention

L

LA	left arm (lead)
LAF	left anterior fascicle
LBB	left bundle branch
LBBB	left bundle branch block
LGL	Lown-Ganong-Levine syndrome
LL	left leg (lead)
LPF	left posterior fascicle
LV	left ventricle

M

MAT	multifocal atrial tachycardia
MI	myocardial infarction

N

NSR	normal sinus rhythm
NSVT	nonsustained ventricular tachycardia

O

O	no response pacemaker

P

PAC	premature atrial contraction
PAT	paroxysmal atrial tachycardia
PJC	premature junctional contraction

PNS	peripheral nervous system
PSVT	paroxysmal supraventricular tachycardia
PVC	premature ventricular contraction

R

RA	right arm (lead)
RBB	right bundle branch
RBBB	right bundle branch block
RL	right leg (lead)
RV	right ventricle

S

SA	sinoatrial
SSS	sick sinus syndrome
SVT	supraventricular tachycardia

T

T	triggered response pacemaker

V

V	ventricular response pacemaker
VEI	ventricular escape interval
Vfib	ventricular fibrillation
VTach	ventricular tachycardia
VVI	ventricular demand pacemaker

W

WAP	wandering atrial pacemaker
WPW	Wolff-Parkinson-White pattern

A

aberrancy – The abnormal conduction of the electrical impulse through the heart. This aberrant conduction gives rise to wide complexes that are morphologically different from those that have gone through the normal pathways.

absolute refractory period – That period in the cell firing cycle at which it is impossible to restimulate a cell to fire off another impulse.

accessory pathway – A pathway, other than the AV node, for the transmission of the impulse from the atria to the ventricles.

acetylcholine – A chemical neurotransmitter used by the parasympathetic system.

acidosis – The acid state on the pH balance scale.

actin – A muscle protein that is part of the contractile element.

action potential – The electrical firing of the myocyte, which leads to contraction. Consists of four phases.

afferent nerves – Nerves that bring information into the CNS.

amplitude – The total height of a wave or complex.

antegrade conduction – Normal conduction of the electrical impulse through the AV node from the atria to the ventricles.

anterior – Before or towards the front.

anterior wall – The vertical wall that lies along the anatomical front of the heart, that is, closest to the anterior chest wall.

antidromic conduction – A circus movement of the electrical impulse found in patients with Wolff-Parkinson-White syndrome in which the impulse travels down the Kent bundle and then reenters the atria via the AV node. Leads to a wide-complex morphology of the QRS complexes.

approach – When related to the AV node, the approaches or tracts are the path-ways that lead to the AV node. (also known as *tract*)

arrhythmia – An abnormal rhythm of the heart. Also can be called a dysrhythmia.

arrhythmogenic – Can potentiate arrhythmias.

arteries – Vessels of the circulatory system that carry blood away from the heart.

Ashman's phenomenon – The propensity of a complex to be transmitted aberrantly if it arrives prematurely after a long pause. In other words, if there is a long pause and then a short pause (the premature complex), the QRS complex of the short pause is usually transmitted aberrantly.

asynchronous – The events do not occur at the same time.

atria – Small, thin-walled, chambers of the heart. They act as priming pumps for the ventricles. There are two: the left atrium and the right atrium. (singular = *atrium*)

atrioventricular (AV) node – Part of the electrical conduction system. It is responsible for slowing down conduction from the atria to the ventricles just long enough for atrial contraction to occur. This slowing allows the atria to "overfill" the ventricles and helps maintain the output of the heart at a maximum level.

atrium – Small, thin-walled, chamber of the heart. Each atrium acts as a priming pump for the ventricles. There are two: the left atrium and the right atrium. (plural = *atria*)

augmented limb leads – The limb leads aVR, aVL, and aVF.

automaticity – The ability of a pacemaker to repolarize and automatically trigger another interval by itself.

autonomic nervous system – The part of the nervous system that is responsible for unconscious or involuntary body functions (such as heart rate).

AV dissociation – An incomplete block of the AV node leading to the independent firing of the atria and the ventricles. The atrial impulse exerts some minimal control over the ventricular rate. In AV dissociation, the atrial rate is the same as or close to the ventricular rate.

AV junction – The area immediately surrounding and encompassing the AV node.

B

Bachman bundle – Part of the electrical conduction system that transmits the impulses through the inter-atrial septum.

bigeminy – A premature complex that occurs at every second beat. The complexes can be either supraventricular or ventricular.

biphasic – A term used to describe a wave with both negative and positive components. Usually used in conjunction with P and T waves.

block – Obstruction to flow of the impulse or depolarization wave.

bradycardia – A slow rhythm (< 60 BPM).

Brugada's sign – Brugada's sign, by definition, is the presence of an abnormally long interval from the R wave to the bottom of the S wave ≥ 0.10 seconds long. This is an abnormality that, if present, will help identify a wide-complex tachycardia as VTach in comparison to an aberrantly conducted supraventricular tachycardia.

bundle branch block (BBB) – A physiologic block of either the left or right bundle branch of the electrical conduction system.

bundle of His – Part of the electrical conduction system. It originates in the AV node and ends in the bundle branches.

C

calibration box – A box or step-like displacement of the ECG baseline at the end of the ECG that is used to ensure that the ECG conforms to a standard format. The standard calibration box is 10 mm high and 0.20

seconds wide. The calibration box can also be set at half-standard or double-standard when evaluating height, or 25-mm or 50-mm standard in regard to width.

calipers – A tool with two identical legs whose terminal points (pins) are used to evaluate distance. A measuring tool used in electrocardiography, architecture, and navigation.

cannon A waves – A very large and obvious distention of the jugular vein caused by the extra blood volume regurgitating back up the jugular system when the atria contract against closed AV valves (mitral and tricuspid).

capillary refill – The capillary refill is obtained by pushing down on the nail until the nail bed turns white. The pressure is then released and the number of seconds it takes for the normal pink color to return is measured. Capillary refill should be less than 2 seconds in the normal patient. It is a sign of a hypoperfused cardiovascular state.

capture beat – Sometimes in AV dissociation a P wave falls during a period that enables it to innervate the ventricles. These complexes are narrower (identical to or close to the appearance of the normal complexes) than the ectopic ventricular beats due to the transmission of the electrical impulse down the normal conduction pathway.

cardiac output – The amount of blood that the heart pumps per minute from either the left or right ventricles. Cardiac output = stroke volume *x* heart rate.

central nervous system (CNS) – The brain and spinal cord.

circus movement – A self-propagating, recurrent looping pattern of impulse transmission in which the depolarization wave continuously restimulates itself.

coarse atrial fibrillation – A morphological type of atrial fibrillation in which the baseline shows grossly large fibrillatory (f) waves. The coarse f waves may sometimes be mistaken for atrial flutter.

collateral circulation – Shared arterial perfusion areas that occur between the arteries of the heart. In other words, one area is perfused by multiple different arteries or arterioles.

compact zone – The center or core of the AV node. This area is composed of cells very similar in histologic appearance and function to those cells found in the sinoatrial node.

compensatory pause –A pause immediately following a premature complex that is longer than the interval between two normally conducted beats, allowing the rhythm to proceed, without any alteration of cycle length, around the premature complex. In essence, the pause compensates for the short interval preceding the premature complex and allows the rate to proceed on schedule.

complete block – Complete blockage of all transmission through the AV node. The result is that the atria and the ventricles are functioning completely isolated from each other electrically.

concealed conduction pathway – Conduction through an accessory pathway which does not create a delta wave. This type of conduction is electrocardiographically silent and there is no way (short of electrophysiologic testing) to identify the presence of these silent conduction pathways. Note that the potential for tachyarrhythmias and abnormal transmission exists in these cases. This type of conduction is the most common presentation for patients with accessory pathways.

concordance – All going in the same direction, either positive or negative.

conduction – The process by which bioelectricity is transferred through the myocardial tissue. It refers to a successive stimulation of cells which, in essence, create an electrical current.

controlled atrial fibrillation – Atrial fibrillation at normal rates.

couplet – Two PVCs occurring sequentially.

D

decompensated atrial fibrillation – Atrial fibrillation with rates between 100

and 200 BPM. (also known as *uncontrolled atrial fibrillation*)

delta wave – A slurring of the upstroke of the first part of the QRS complex that occurs in Wolff-Parkinson-White syndrome.

depolarization – A state in which the cell becomes more positive, moving toward equilibrium with the extracellular fluid. Depolarization takes place during the latter part of resting state and is completed during activation by the action potential.

diastole – The normal "resting" phase of the heart when the heart is not actively contracting.

digitalis effect – A scooped-out appearance of the ST segment and the T waves in patients taking digoxin or digitalis-like substances.

distal – Anatomically, describes the direction and relative distance away from midline. An object that is distal is further away from the midline than one that is proximal; the hand is distal to the elbow.

dual response – A type of response from a pulse generator or pacemaker in which the device responds in a triggered manner for some pre-programmed cases and in an inhibitory manner for other pre-programmed events.

E

electrical alternans – A finding associated with a fluctuation of the electrical axis of the ventricles over two or more beats. It is usually associated with large pericardial effusions.

electrical axis – The summation of the individualized vectors for all of the ventricular myocytes during activation.

electrical conduction system – A specialized collection of cells that coordinate the bioelectrical activity of the heart. They are involved in initiating (pacemaking) and conducting the electrical impulse. They also coordinate the sequencing of the atrial and ventricular contractions to allow efficient pumping of blood.

electrical potential – The difference between the charges on the outside and the inside of the cell wall. The electric potential of the resting myocyte is usually about –70 to –90 mV.

electrocardiogram (ECG) – A 12-lead electrocardiographic recording used to evaluate the heart and its rhythm.

electrode – The electrical sensors placed on the chest to record the bioelectrical activity of the heart.

electrolyte – A chemical agent or molecule that can conduct an electrical current.

end-diastolic PVCs – When a PVC falls after the next normally occurring sinus P wave. These PVCs are known as end-diastolic PVCs because they occur during the late diastolic phase of the previous complex.

endocardial ischemia – Relative or absolute hypoxemia of the endocardial surface of the heart.

endocardium – The internal lining of the atrial and ventricular walls.

epinephrine – Chemical neurotransmitter used by the sympathetic system.

escape complex – A beat that occurs after a normal pacemaker fails to fire. The R-R interval is longer in these cases.

escape rhythm – A rhythm that occurs after a normal pacemaker fails to fire.

extreme right quadrant – The quadrant of the hexaxial system represented by the area from –90° to –180°.

F

fibrillatory (f) waves – The fine or coarse waves caused by the wavelet depolarizations in atrial fibrillation.

fine atrial fibrillation – A morphological type of atrial fibrillation in which the baseline shows very small fibrillatory (f) waves. The coarse f waves may sometimes be mistaken for a complete absence of atrial activity.

flutter (F) waves – The sawtooth waves formed by the circus movements found in atrial flutter. They can be either in a positive or negative direction.

flutter-fibrillation pattern – A rhythm which switches between atrial flutter and atrial fibrillation often.

fusion beat – Occurs when two complexes with different inciting pacemakers fuse to form a complex unlike either the normal or the ectopic complex. Commonly seen in VTach.

fusion complex – Occurs when two complexes with different inciting pacemakers fuse to form a complex unlike either the normal or the ectopic complex. Commonly seen in premature complexes, VTach, idioventricular rhythms, and multifocal atrial tachycardias.

G

gap junction – The small area where a nerve ending and the muscle tissue come together. Communication occurs between the cells via neurotransmitters which are released into the extracellular space at the junction.

H

heart rate – The rate at which the heart contracts per minute.

hexaxial system – The system developed to describe the coronal plane that is created by the limb leads (I, II, III, aVR, aVL, and aVF).

hyperkalemia – Elevated potassium level.

hypocalcemia – Low level of calcium.

hypomagnesemia – Low level of magnesium.

hypovolemia – Low fluid or volume of the blood or circulatory system.

hypoxemia – Low oxygen level in the blood.

I

incessant ventricular tachycardia – Ventricular tachycardia that is present most of the time.

inferior wall – Anatomically, the inferior wall of the heart, which lies on the diaphragm.

inhibited response – The pacemaker responds to a sensed event by not firing a response for a certain interval of time (the VEI).

innervation – Activation of the myocardial cells by an electrical impulse.

internodal pathways – Three pathways of the electrical conduction system found in the atria that transmit the impulse from the SA node to the AV node.

interpolated PVC – A PVC that falls exactly between two sinus complexes and does not alter the cadence of the rhythm in any way.

intrinsicoid deflection – The amount of time it takes the electrical impulse to travel from the Purkinje system in the endocardium to the surface of the epicardium. It is measured from the beginning of the QRS complex to the beginning of the downslope of the R wave, and is usually measured in leads with no Q wave.

ion – An atom or molecule that carries an electrical charge.

isoelectric – When referring to a wave, the wave is neither positive nor negative. When referring to a lead, the lead in question is exactly 90° from the electrical axis. It is usually the lead with the smallest amplitude and the one that is the closest to being neither positive nor negative.

J

Josephson's sign – A small notching near the low point of the S wave in ectopic ventricular complexes.

K

Kent bundle – An accessory pathway found in patients with Wolff-Parkinson-White syndrome.

L

lateral wall – The lateral wall of the heart, along its left side.

lead – 1. Any of the electrodes or conductors used to measure the biochemical activity of the heart. 2. The actual representation of the electrical activity of the heart based on the placement of the electrodes, analogous to camera angles.

lead placement – The exact position on the body of the ECG electrodes.

left anterior fascicle (LAF) – Part of the electrical conduction system.

Responsible for innervating the anterior and superior areas of the left ventricle. It is a single-stranded cord terminating in the Purkinje cells.

left bundle branch (LBB) – The bundle branch that branches towards the left side. The LBB is responsible for depolarizing the right side of the interventricular septum and the right ventricle.

left bundle branch block (LBBB) – A physiologic block of the left bundle branch causing the characteristic ECG pattern of a QRS complex > 0.12 seconds, monomorphic S wave in V_1 and monomorphic R wave in leads I and V_6.

left posterior fascicle (LPF) – Part of the electrical conduction system. Responsible for innervating the posterior and inferior areas of the left ventricle. It is a widely distributed, fan-like structure terminating in the Purkinje cells.

limb leads – The leads that form the hexaxial system, dividing the heart along a coronal plane into anterior and posterior segments. These leads include I, II, III, aVR, aVL, and aVF.

Lown-Ganong-Levine (LGL) syndrome – A syndrome characterized by a short PR interval and a normal QRS complex.

M

microcollateral circulation – A shared arterial perfusion area that occurs between the arteries of the heart. In other words, one area is perfused by multiple different arterioles.

monomorphic – One morphological appearance.

morphology – The physical appearance of a wave or complex.

multifocal PVCs – PVCs that are morphologically different because they either originate in separate ventricular ectopic foci or are transmitted through different depolarization routes.

myocardial infarction (MI) – A process, acute or chronic, that is characterized by the formation or presence of dead myocardial tissue.

myocardium – A specialized term to describe the muscle tissue of the heart.

myocyte – An individual heart muscle cell.

myofibrils – Another term for the individual muscle cells or myocytes.

myosin – A muscle protein that is part of the contractile element.

N

noncompensatory pause – A pause, immediately following a premature complex, that alters the rhythm, causing a resetting of the pacemaker and an alteration of cycle length, after the premature complex. In essence, this pause does not compensate for the short interval preceding the premature complex, and the rate is completely reset after the event.

nonsustained ventricular tachycardia – Ventricular tachycardia that lasts less than 30 seconds.

norepinephrine – A chemical neurotransmitter used by the sympathetic system.

normal quadrant – The quadrant of the hexaxial system represented by 0° to 90°.

O

orthodromic conduction – A circus movement of the electrical impulse found in patients with Wolff-Parkinson-White syndrome, in which the impulse travels normally down the AV node and then reenters the atria via the Kent bundle.

P

P wave – The deflection used to identify atrial depolarization. It is the first wave of a complex or beat.

P wave axis – The calculated electrical axis for the P waves.

pacemaker – The location that initiates cardiac depolarization and dictates the rate at which the heart will cycle. Pacemaking function is usually performed by the cells of the electrical conduction system, although any myocardial cell can perform this function. The pacemaker can be an intrinsic part of the heart or an external unit.

pacemaker syndrome – The clinical syndrome that occurs because of a lack of atrial contribution to ventricular filling and the inability of the heart rate to compensate for any form of exertion or exercise, giving rise to various clinical symptoms related to decreased cardiac output and hypotension. These include fatigue, light headedness, syncope, dyspnea, exercise intolerance, congestive heart failure, and anginal symptoms due to myocardial ischemia.

parasympathetic nervous system – The part of the nervous system that causes a slowing down or calming effect. Its main chemical messenger is acetylcholine.

pericardium – The external lining or surface of the heart.

peripheral nerves – The nerves that are outside of the central nervous system and are responsible for bringing information to and from the brain and spinal cord.

physiologic block – The normal delay period in the conduction of the electrical impulse caused by the AV node in order to allow the atria and the ventricles to contract synchronously.

posterior wall – Anatomically in the heart, the vertical wall that lies closest to the posterior wall of the chest or thorax.

P-P interval – The interval represented by the space between the P waves of two consecutive complexes.

PR interval – That interval of time that occupies the space between the beginning of the P wave and the beginning of the QRS complex.

PR segment – The segment of the complex that occupies the space between the end of the P wave and the beginning of the QRS complex.

precordial leads – Another term used to describe the chest leads. They are labeled from V_1 through V_6. They divide the heart along a sagittal plane.

precordial system – Another term used to describe the chest leads. They are labeled from V_1 through V_6. They divide the heart along a sagittal plane.

premature complex – A complex that arrives earlier than expected for the cadence of the rhythm.

proximal – Anatomically, describes the direction and relative distance away from midline. An object that is proximal is closer to the midline than one that is distal; the elbow is proximal to the hand.

pseudo-R wave – See *pseudo-R' wave*.

pseudo-R' wave – The fusion of the P wave with the QRS complex of another complex to give the appearance of the presence of an R wave.

Purkinje system – Specialized cells that act as the final pathway of the electrical conduction system of the heart. They directly innervate the ventricular myocytes.

Q

Q wave – The first negative wave of the QRS complex.

QRS complex – The wave complex represented by ventricular depolarization. It may consist of individual or multiple waves in succession, which may appear in any combination: the Q wave, R wave, and S wave.

QRS interval – The interval of time occupied by the QRS complex.

QT interval – The interval of time represented by the space from the beginning of the QRS complex to the end of the T wave; may vary with heart rate.

QTc interval – The QT interval, corrected mathematically for the heart rate.

quadrants – The hexaxial system can be broken down into four quadrants: the normal, left, right, and extreme right quadrants. Each represents 90° of the hexaxial system.

quadrigeminy – A premature complex every fourth beat. The complexes can be either supraventricular or ventricular.

R

R wave – The first positive wave of the QRS complex.

R' wave – A second positive wave inside a QRS complex.

rabbit ears – A slang term for the RSR' pattern traditionally found in V_1 in an RBBB.

rapid filling phase – Part of the cardiac filling cycle that occurs during early diastole. It starts when the AV valves open and blood rushes in to fill the ventricles. The phase ends when the atria begin to contract. Most of the blood enters the ventricles during this period.

rate – The number of beats per minute.

reentry – A self-propagating, recurrent looping pattern of impulse transmission in which the depolarization wave continuously restimulates itself. (see *circus movement*)

refractory state – A short period of time, immediately after depolarization, in which the myocytes are not yet repolarized and are unable to fire or conduct an impulse

relative hypotension – A hypoperfusion state that occurs in hypertensive patients due to their need for higher perfusion pressures. The term "relative" refers to the fact that the actual pressures would be considered normal in most patients.

relative refractory period – That period in the cell firing cycle at which it is possible but difficult to restimulate the cell to fire another impulse. The pattern taken by the depolarization wave is usually abnormal in these cases.

reperfusion arrhythmia – An arrhythmia that develops in a patient after a thrombolytic or an external device has reopened a clotted artery in a patient undergoing an acute myocardial infarction.

repolarization – A state in which the cell becomes more negative, moving away from equilibrium with the extracellular fluid. This is an active process.

retrograde conduction – The conduction of the electrical impulse backward through the AV node, from the ventricles or AV node to the atria.

rhythm strip – A single lead electrocardiographic recording used to evaluate the patient's rhythm.

right bundle branch (RBB) – The bundle branch that branches towards the right side. The RBB is responsible for depolarizing the right side of the interventricular septum and the right ventricle.

right bundle branch block (RBBB) – A physiologic block of the right bundle branch causing the characteristic ECG pattern of a QRS complex > 0.12 seconds, slurred S wave in leads I and V_6 and an RSR' pattern in V_1.

R-on-T phenomenon – When a premature ventricular contraction falls on the T wave of the previous complex.

R-R interval – The interval represented by the space between the R waves of two consecutive complexes.

S

S wave – The second negative wave of the QRS complex. (The first one would be the Q wave, and next would be the S wave.)

S' wave – The third negative wave inside a QRS complex. (The first one would be the Q wave, next would be the S wave, then the third would be an S'.)

salvo – When three or more PVCs occur sequentially. Commonly used when the presence of ventricular tachycardia is suspected.

second marks – Small marks at the bottom of the ECG to represent an interval of time. They are usually found every three or six seconds depending on the system. At a 25-mm standard, five large boxes represent one second.

septum – The muscular or fibrous wall that separates the atria or the ventricles in the heart. When the word is used by itself it usually refers to the ventricular septum.

sick sinus syndrome – A diseased state of the sinoatrial node that leads to multiple abnormal rhythm states. In this diseased state, the rhythms can quickly alternate between tachycardia and bradycardia, and atrial flutter and fibrillation are common.

sinoatrial (SA) node – The main pacemaker of the heart. Located anatomically in the right atrium.

slurred S wave – A slow upstroke of the S wave noted in RBBB in leads I and V_6. Slurred S waves can have various morphologies.

somatic nervous system – The part of the nervous system that is responsible for conscious and controllable muscle movement and functions.

ST segment – The section of the complex from the end of the QRS complex to the beginning of the T wave. Electrically, it represents the period of inactivity between ventricular depolarization and repolarization. Mechanically, it represents the time that the myocardium is maintaining contraction.

stroke volume – The amount of blood ejected from the ventricle during a single ventricular contraction.

supraventricular – Refers to an impulse or rhythm that originated above the ventricles.

sustained ventricular tachycardia – Ventricular tachycardia that lasts greater than 30 seconds or is shorter than 30 seconds but required either electrical or pharmaceutical intervention to terminate.

sympathetic nervous system – The part of the nervous system that is responsible for the fight-or-flight response. Uses epinephrine and norepinephrine as the chemical messengers.

sympatholytic – Interfering with or inhibiting the effect of the impulses from the sympathetic nervous system.

sympathomimetic – Effects resembling those caused by stimulation of the sympathetic nervous system, such as the effects seen following the injection of epinephrine into a patient.

synchronized – All events occur at the same time.

T

T wave – The wave that represents ventricular repolarization.

tachycardia – A rapid rhythm (≥100 BPM).

threshold potential – The electrical value at which an action potential is triggered.

TP segment – The area of baseline between the end of the T wave and the beginning of the next P wave. A line drawn from one TP segment to the TP segment of a consecutive complex is the true baseline of the ECG.

Tp wave – A wave representing the repolarization of the atria. It usually presents as PR depression or the ST segment depression seen in very fast tachycardias.

tract – When related to the AV node, the approaches or tracts are the pathways that lead to the AV node. (also known as *approach*)

transitional cell zone – a small area of tissue that surrounds the tip of the AV node. This zone is full of autonomic fibers and is very arrhythmogenic.

trigeminy – A premature complex every third beat. The complexes can be either supraventricular or ventricular.

triggered response – The pacemaker activates a depolarization wave or "fires" to a sensed event.

triplet – Three PVCs occurring sequentially.

T-wave alternans – Alternating polarity of the T wave between positive and negative that occurs on an ECG or rhythm strip.

U

U wave – A small, flat wave sometimes seen after the T wave and before the next P wave. It could represent ventricular afterdepolarization and endocardial repolarization.

uncontrolled atrial fibrillation – Atrial fibrillation with rates between 100 and 200 BPM. (also known as *decompensated atrial fibrillation*)

unifocal PVCs – Singly occurring PVCs or PVCs that share the same common morphological appearance because they originate in the same ectopic focus.

V

vagus nerve – Main nerve or pathway of the parasympathetic nervous system.

vector – A diagrammatic term used to show the strength and direction of an electrical impulse.

ventricle – Large, thick-muscled chambers of the heart, the primary pumping chambers. There are two: the left and right ventricles.

ventricular escape interval (VEI) – The interval of time during which a pacemaker is dormant before triggering the next response.

W

wave – A deflection from the baseline in either a positive or negative direction, representing an electrical event of the cardiac cycle.

wavelet – A small depolarization wave that is found in cases of atrial fibrillation.

wide-complex tachycardia – A tachycardia in which the QRS complexes are morphologically wider than 0.12 seconds.

Wolf-Parkinson-White pattern – An electrocardiographic pattern characterized by short PR intervals, delta waves, and nonspecific ST-T wave changes caused by the presence of an accessory pathway.

Wolf-Parkinson-White syndrome (WPW) – A syndrome characterized by short PR intervals, delta waves, nonspecific ST-T wave changes, and paroxysmal episodes of tachycardia caused by the presence of an accessory pathway.

Q

R

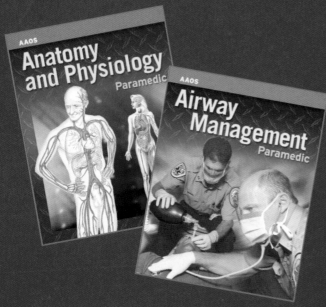
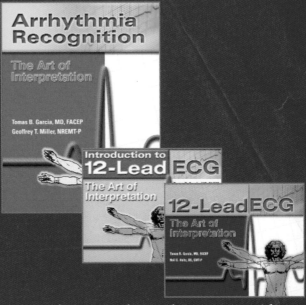
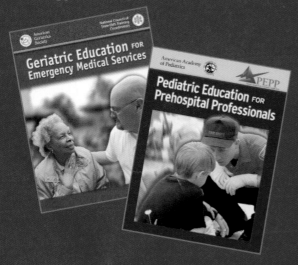
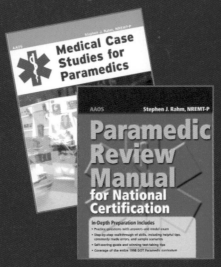
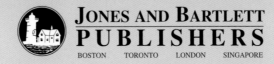